Metabolic Diseases: A Clinical Approach

Metabolic Diseases: A Clinical Approach

Editor: Wade Chambers

FOSTER
ACADEMICS
www.fosteracademics.com

www.fosteracademics.com

FOSTER ACADEMICS

Cataloging-in-Publication Data

Metabolic diseases : a clinical approach / edited by Wade Chambers.
p. cm.
Includes bibliographical references and index.
ISBN 978-1-63242-646-8
1. Metabolism--Disorders. 2. Diseases. 3. Clinical medicine. I. Chambers, Wade.
RC627.54 .M48 2019
616.3--dc23

Foster Academics,
118-35 Queens Blvd., Suite 400,
Forest Hills, NY 11375, USA

ISBN 978-1-63242-646-8 (Hardback)

Printed and bound in China.

Contents

Preface

I am honored to present to you this unique book which encompasses the most up-to-date data in the field. I was extremely pleased to get this opportunity of editing the work of experts from across the globe. I have also written papers in this field and researched the various aspects revolving around the progress of the discipline. I have tried to unify my knowledge along with that of stalwarts from every corner of the world, to produce a text which not only benefits the readers but also facilitates the growth of the field.

Metabolic diseases arise when there is an alteration in the normal metabolic process caused due to abnormal chemical reactions in the body. The symptoms of metabolic diseases can be classified into four categories, namely, acute symptoms, permanent symptoms, late-onset acute symptoms and progressive general symptoms. However, some of the most common symptoms include jaundice, weight loss, seizures and lethargy. Enzyme deficiency caused due to a defective gene, and problems in the functioning of the liver or pancreas are some common causes of metabolic diseases. Diagnostic methods include routine screening, specific blood tests and DNA tests. Nutrition management is a common and effective strategy to treat metabolic diseases. This book attempts to understand various metabolic diseases and their causes along with the ways to diagnose and treat them. It brings forth some of the most innovative concepts and elucidates the unexplored aspects of metabolic diseases. The book is appropriate for students seeking detailed information in this area as well as for doctors and researchers.

Finally, I would like to thank all the contributing authors for their valuable time and contributions. This book would not have been possible without their efforts. I would also like to thank my friends and family for their constant support.

Editor

1

HELP LDL Apheresis Reduces Plasma Pentraxin 3 in Familial Hypercholesterolemia

Michela Zanetti[1]*, Mariagrazia Zenti[2], Rocco Barazzoni[1], Federica Zardi[2], Annamaria Semolic[1], Michele Giuseppe Messa[3], Filippo Mearelli[1], Gianpaolo Russi[5], Maurizio Fonda[4], Luca Scarano[5], Enzo Bonora[2], Luigi Cattin[4]

1 Clinica Medica, Department of Medical, Surgical and Health Sciences, University of Trieste, Trieste, Italy, **2** Endocrinology, Diabetes and Metabolism, University and Azienda Ospedaliera Universitaria Integrata of Verona, Verona, Italy, **3** Nephrology, University and Azienda Ospedaliera Universitaria Integrata of Verona, Verona, Italy, **4** Diabetes and Metabolic Diseases Unit, Department of Medical, Surgical and Health Sciences, University of Trieste, Trieste, Italy, **5** Immunohematology and Transfusion Unit, Ospedale Santa Maria Nuova, Reggio Emilia, Italy

Abstract

Background: Pentraxin 3 (PTX3), a key component of the humoral arm of innate immunity, is secreted by vascular cells in response to injury, possibly aiming at tuning arterial activation associated with vascular damage. Severe hypercholesterolemia as in familial hypercholesterolemia (FH) promotes vascular inflammation and atherosclerosis; low-density lipoprotein (LDL) apheresis is currently the treatment of choice to reduce plasma lipids in FH. HELP LDL apheresis affects pro- and antiinflammatory biomarkers, however its effects on PTX3 levels are unknown. We assessed the impact of FH and of LDL removal by HELP apheresis on PTX3.

Methods: Plasma lipids, PTX3, and CRP were measured in 19 patients with FH undergoing chronic HELP LDL apheresis before and after treatment and in 20 control subjects. In the patients assessment of inflammation and oxidative stress markers included also plasma TNFα, fibrinogen and TBARS.

Results: At baseline, FH patients had higher ($p = 0.0002$) plasma PTX3 than matched control subjects. In FH PTX3 correlated positively ($p \leq 0.05$) with age, gender and CRP and negatively ($p = 0.01$) with HELP LDL apheresis vintage. The latter association was confirmed after correction for age, gender and CRP. HELP LDL apheresis acutely reduced ($p \leq 0.04$) plasma PTX3, CRP, fibrinogen, TBARS and lipids, but not TNFα. No association was observed between mean decrease in PTX3 and in LDL cholesterol. PTX3 paralleled lipids, oxidative stress and inflammation markers in time-course study.

Conclusion: FH is associated with increased plasma PTX3, which is acutely reduced by HELP LDL apheresis independently of LDL cholesterol, as reflected by the lack of association between change in PTX3 and in LDL levels. These results, together with the finding of a negative relationship between PTX3 and duration of treatment suggest that HELP LDL apheresis may influence both acutely and chronically cardiovascular outcomes in FH by modulating PTX3.

Editor: Harald HHW Schmidt, Maastricht University, Netherlands

Funding: Funding provided by Grant LR26/2005, Regione FVG to L. Cattin. The funders had no role in study design, data collection and analysis, decision to publish, or preparation of the manuscript.

Competing Interests: The authors have declared that no competing interests exist.

* Email: zanetti@units.it

Introduction

A body of clinical and experimental evidence supports a link between LDL cholesterol, inflammation and atherosclerosis [1–3]. Cholesterol accumulation in the artery triggers a local and systemic inflammatory reaction by activating multiple pathways, including native and adaptive immune responses [4–5]. Pentraxin 3 (PTX3), a component of the humoral arm of native immunity, is a TNFα-inducible molecule selectively produced following activation of the vessel wall by several cell types at the site of injury [6–8]. PTX3 is strictly associated with vascular disease, as high levels have been detected in atherosclerotic plaques and in plasma from patients with elevated LDL cholesterol and extensive atherosclerosis [9–11]. In hypercholesterolemia PTX3 correlates with the severity of vascular disease and statin therapy reduces plasma PTX3 [11], suggesting its involvement in the mechanisms by which LDL cholesterol triggers vascular inflammation. So far, the precise role of PTX3 in atherosclerosis is unclear. The finding that PTX3 deficiency amplifies tissue damage and inflammation after vascular injury [12] suggests a protective activity, which however needs to be proven in human studies.

LDL apheresis is the treatment of choice for severe hypercholesterolemia not adequatelly controlled by maximal statin treatment, as in familial hypercholesterolemia (FH) [13–14]. Patients affected by FH undergoing LDL apheresis are a paradigmatic model since LDL cholesterol rapidly drops from elevated to normal levels and then slowly rebounds to pre-apheresis concentrations [15]. In addition to LDL cholesterol, LDL apheresis acutely reduces inflammation and oxidative stress markers, including pro-inflammatory cytokines, adhesion molecules, oxidative products as well as coronary endothelial dysfunction [16–19]; therefore positive effects overwhelm possible detrimental consequences of endothelial activation following blood-biomaterial interaction during the procedure. For these reasons LDL apheresis has been proposed in the acute treatment of acute coronary syndromes (ACS) [20]. Chronic LDL apheresis delays the progression of atherosclerosis, stabilizes atherosclerotic plaques and reduces clinical events in FH [21–22]. These beneficial effects are paralleled by long-term reduction in several inflammatory biomarkers including CRP, which is notably associated with clinical endpoints [23–24].

Whether FH and LDL apheresis impact PTX3 levels is currently unknown. Therefore we assessed the effects of HELP LDL apheresis on plasma PTX3, selected pro-inflammatory cytokines and markers of oxidative stress in FH patients and their mutual associations.

Materials and Methods

Ethics Statement

The study was approved by the Ethical Committee of Verona University Hospital, and all participants gave written informed consent to it.

Patients

19 heterozygous FH patients (M/F:11/8) undergoing regular HELP LDL apheresis every two weeks because of severe hypercholestereolemia inadequatelly controlled by maximal statin treatment for at least 6 months and previous cardiovascular events were recruited. 20 age- and sex- matched subjects were studied as control. Inclusion criteria were outpatients who were 18 years old or older. LDL elimination from plasma was achieved through HELP apheresis (LDL precipitation by acetic acid and heparin, Braun, Melsungen, Germany). Anticoagulation was performed with heparin (1000–5000 IU as a bolus and up to 3000 IU/h continuously). Exclusion criteria were the diagnosis of malignancies, chronic autoimmune, liver, thyroid and concomitant acute inflammatory diseases. Patient characteristics are shown in Table 1.

Clinical data

On a baseline visit from each patient a detailed medical history and a physical examination were obtained. Then, in the morning of the scheduled day, FH patients were admitted to the Clinic for their regular HELP LDL apheresis. A blood sample was withdrawn immediately before and at the end of apheresis. In a subgroup of patients a time-course study was performed and additional blood samples were collected after 5, 10 and 14 days.

Laboratory data

Plasma glucose, triglycerides, total, HDL and LDL cholesterol were assessed with standard techniques. Plasma fibrinogen was determined by the Clauss method.

Plasma TBARS were measured using a commercially available kit (Oxitek, Zeptometrix Co, Buffalo, NY) following the manufacturer's recommendations. Plasma high-sensitivity C-reactive protein and PTX3 were measured using ELISA kits (Diagnostics Biochem, London, Ontario, Canada; Perseus Proteomics, Tokyo, Japan intra-assay coefficient of variation: <4.1%, inter-assay coefficient of variation: <4.3%). TNFα was measured by using MILLIPLEX MAP Kit Human High Sensitivity Cytokine (EMD, Millipore, Billerica MA, USA); intra-assay coefficient of variation was <10.6%, inter-assay coefficient of variation: <9.8%. The minimum detectable concentration for TNFα was 0.07 pg/mL.

Statistical analysis

Data are expressed as mean±SEM. ANOVA followed by Student's t test for paired or unpaired data were used as appropriate to compare variables between the experimental groups. Post-hoc analysis was performed, when appropriate, using Bonferroni's adjustment. Multivariate regression analysis was performed to adjust the relationship between PTX3 and apheresis vintage for age, gender and CRP. StatView software was used for statistical analysis. P values of 0.05 or less were considered statistically significant.

Results

At baseline, FH patients had threefold higher ($p = 0.0002$) plasma PTX3 than matched control subjects (Fig.1). In the patients higher PTX3 was positively associated with increasing age ($p = 0.001$), female gender ($p = 0.047$) and higher CRP ($p = 0.05$)

Table 1. Anthropometric and clinical characteristics of study subjects.

	FH	Control
n	**19**	**20**
Gender (M/F)	11/8	11/9
Age (years)	60±2	56±5
Body mass index (kg/m^2)	27±1	27±3
SBP (mm Hg)	131±2	139±4
DBP (mm Hg)	80±2	83±6
Smoking status	3 current/16 never	2 current/18 never
Diabetes	1	-
Family history CAD	All	-
Previous cardiovascular events	All	-
LDL apheresis vintage (years)	7.8±1.6	-

FH: familial hypercholesterolemia. Data are means±SEM. SBP: systolic blood pressure; DBP: diastolic arterial pressure; CAD: coronary artery disease.

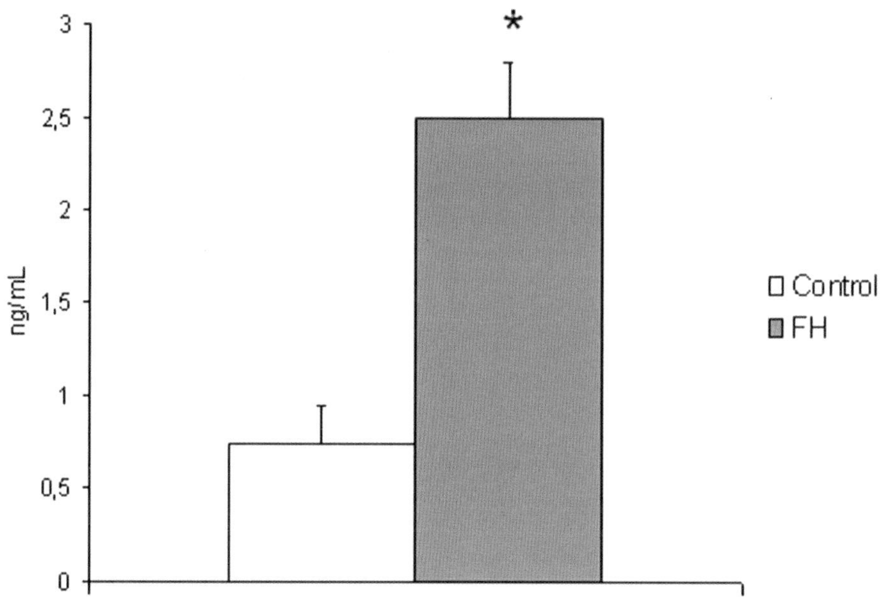

Figure 1. Plasma levels of PTX3 in control (n = 20) and FH patients (n = 19). P = 0.0002.

and negatively with HELP LDL apheresis vintage (p = 0.01) (Table 2). The latter association held true (p = 0.05) in multivariate modeling including CRP as well as age and gender (Table 3). In contrast, no correlation was detected with plasma lipids, TNFα and TBARS.

A single HELP LDL apheresis treatment acutely decreased ($p \leq 0.0001$) plasma total (from 268±11 to 125±7 mg/dL, −52±2%), LDL (from 176±10 to 65±6 mg/dL, −63±3%) and HDL cholesterol (from 52±4 to 45±4 mg/dL, −17±2%) as well as triglycerides (from 195±26 to 104±22 mg/dL, −50±4%), as expected. Substantial reductions in acute phase proteins CRP, fibrinogen and PTX3 were also observed by respectively 55, 65, and 20% ($p \leq 0.04$) (Fig. 2) as well as in the oxidative stress marker TBARS (by 19%, from 1.7±0.1 to 1.4±0.1 mmol/mL, p = 0.02). In contrast, TNFα did not decrease following HELP LDL apheresis (Fig. 2).

A time-course experiment in a subgroup of 9 patients demonstrated that within 14 days all parameters rebounded to pre-treatment values: plasma LDL, fibrinogen, CRP, TBARS and PTX3 (Fig. 3). In univariate analysis, no association was detected between HELP LDL apheresis-induced mean decrease in PTX3 and CRP and mean reduction in LDL cholesterol (PTX3: r = 0.38, p = 0.16; CRP: r = 0.48, p = 0.06).

Table 2. Univariate analysis of plasma baseline PTX3 with anthropometric and laboratory parameters in FH patients.

	r	p
Gender (F/M)	0.46	0.047
Age (years)	0.69	0.001
Body mass index (kg/m^2)	−0.41	0.08
SBP (mm Hg)	−0.39	0.3
DBP (mm Hg)	−0.49	0.17
Blood glucose (mg/dL)	−0.12	0.63
Duration of apheresis (years)	−0.63	0.01
Total cholesterol (mg/dL)	0.11	0.66
LDL cholesterol (mg/dL)	0.09	0.82
HDL cholesterol (mg/dL)	0.05	0.7
Triglycerides (mg/dL)	−0.05	0.8
Fibrinogen (mg/dL)	0.40	0.14
CRP (mg/L)	0.50	0.05
TNFα (pg/mL)	0.27	0.4
TBARS (nmol/mL)	0.11	0.8

FH: familial hypercholesterolemia. SBP: systolic blood pressure; DBP: diastolic arterial pressure; CRP: C reactive protein.

Discussion

This study provides the first evidence of the effects of FH and of HELP LDL apheresis on PTX3 plasma levels. FH patients on chronic statin and HELP LDL apheresis treatment show higher PTX3 levels than healthy subjects. HELP LDL apheresis acutely determines a rapid decrease of PTX3, which rebounds to pretreatment levels within 5 days after treatment. In addition, a negative association between PTX3 and apheresis vintage was observed.

Higher plasma PTX3 represent a consistent finding in this group of FH patients. Mean concentrations of PTX3 were over threefold higher in FH than those measured in control subjects, in spite of concomitant maximal statin treatment, which significantly reduces PTX3 concentrations [11,25]. Indeed, measured PTX3 values in both groups are in line with those documented in subjects with cardiovascular risk factors including hypercholesterolemia [11,26]. Statins are routinely administered to reduce LDL cholesterol and vascular inflammation in FH. When they fail to achieve LDL cholesterol target levels, LDL apheresis is considered [13,14]. Extracorporeal treatment as in HELP is hampered by blood-biomaterial interaction, which may trigger inflammation; however acute adverse events during the procedure are rare [15]. In this study PTX3, a specific and sensitive marker of vascular activation decreased by about 20% following HELP LDL apheresis. The underlying mechanisms are unclear; either low

Table 3. Multiple regression model predicting LDL apheresis vintage in FH patients.

	Coefficient	P value
FH patients (n = 19, r = 0.69)		
Age (years)	0.18	0.35
Gender (female)	0.84	0.8
PTX3 (ng/mL)	−3.55	0.05

PTX3: pentraxin 3, CRP: C reactive protein.

buffer pH or heparin used in HELP may precipitate PTX3 along with several other molecules which are non-selectively removed during the procedure [27]. Since percent reduction of LDL cholesterol, triglycerides and fibrinogen was similar to previous data [18,23,28] and since plasma albumin did not differ before and after each session (data not shown), as expected [28], it is unlikely that dilution is responsible for PTX3 reduction in HELP apheresis. Based on these observations it is currently unknown whether acute PTX3 decrease is HELP-specific or other apheresis systems share the same effect.

LDL apheresis is the most efficient approach to achieve a rapid drop not only in plasma LDL but also in several procoagulatory, prooxidative and proinflammatory mediators, including fibrinogen, plasminogen, oxidative stress markers, adhesion molecules and CRP [17]. In addition, a single session has been demonstrated to increase coronary artery blood flow and luminal diameter [16]. For all these reasons LDL apheresis has been proposed as a potential therapeutic strategy in acute coronary syndromes [20]. In this setting however acute elevations of PTX3 may represent a protective, counteractive response to vascular injury and lowering PTX3 may be detrimental to clinical outcome [12]. Therefore the overall effect of HELP LDL apheresis in the acute setting is currently unclear.

TNFα is a known stimulator of PTX3 expression [6,7] and variable effects on its plasma levels have been described during LDL apheresis [17,29]. In this study however no correlation was found between baseline and post-apheresis PTX3 and TNFα, and unlike PTX3, TNFα did not decrease following HELP LDL apheresis. Likewise, no correlation was found between PTX3 and plasma HDL, which have been reported to induce PTX3 expression in endothelial cells [30]. In contrast with previous studies [8,26], we did detect an association between baseline PTX3 and CRP. The reason for the discrepancy is not fully understood. One hypothesis is that the peculiar clinical characteristics of our patients (FH) can account for the finding. As such, a previous study confirmed an association between PTX3, CRP, LDL cholesterol and coronary artery disease severity in patients with intermediate-high atherosclerosis severity [31].

Chronic LDL apheresis is extremely effective in reducing the burden of atherosclerosis in FH [32,21] as a result of modified lipid, proinflammatory and procoagulant profile despite rebounding to pretreatment levels after each session. Serum PTX3 is

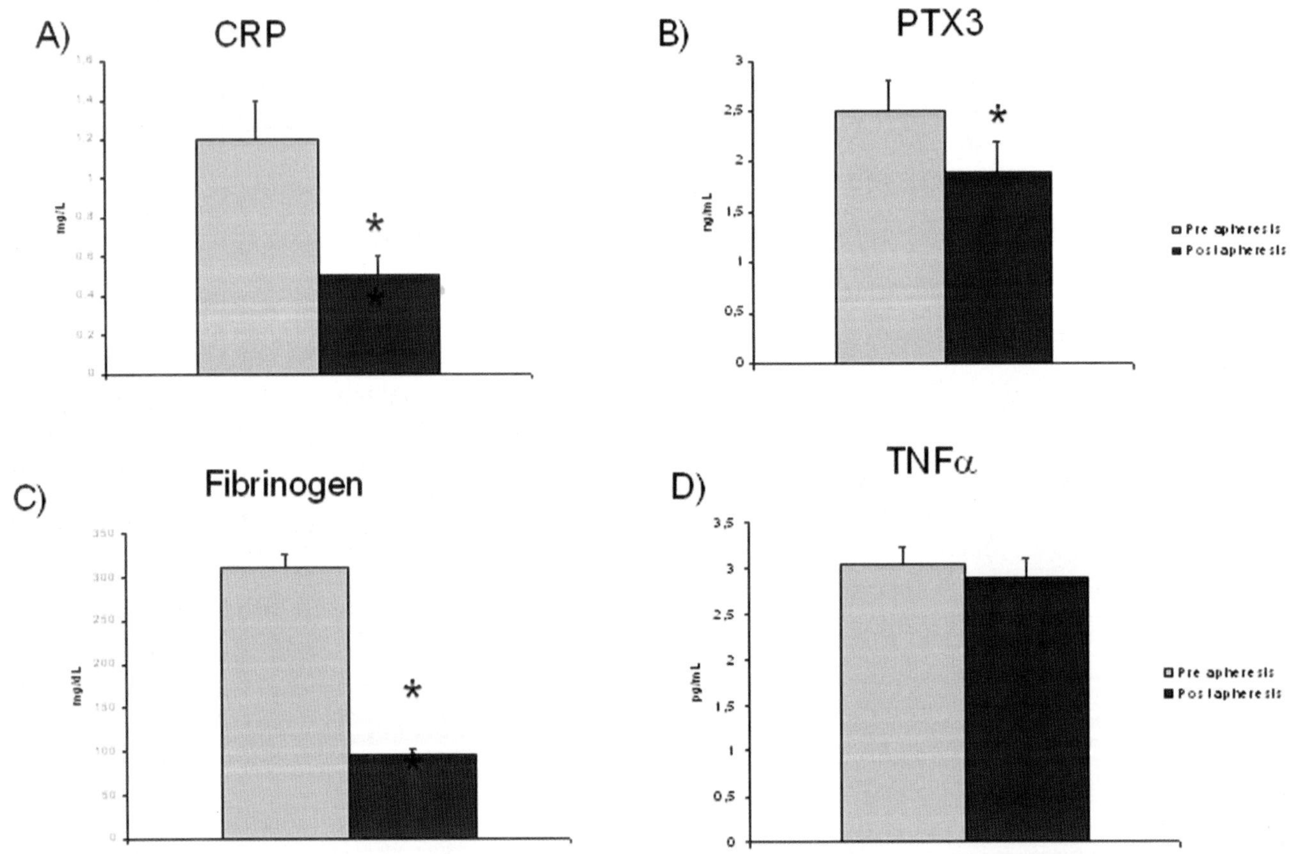

Figure 2. Plasma concentrations of inflammatory proteins A) CRP, B) PTX3, C) fibrinogen, D) TNFα in study patients. n = 19 both before and after HELP LDL-apheresis. *P≤0.04; **P≤0.003.

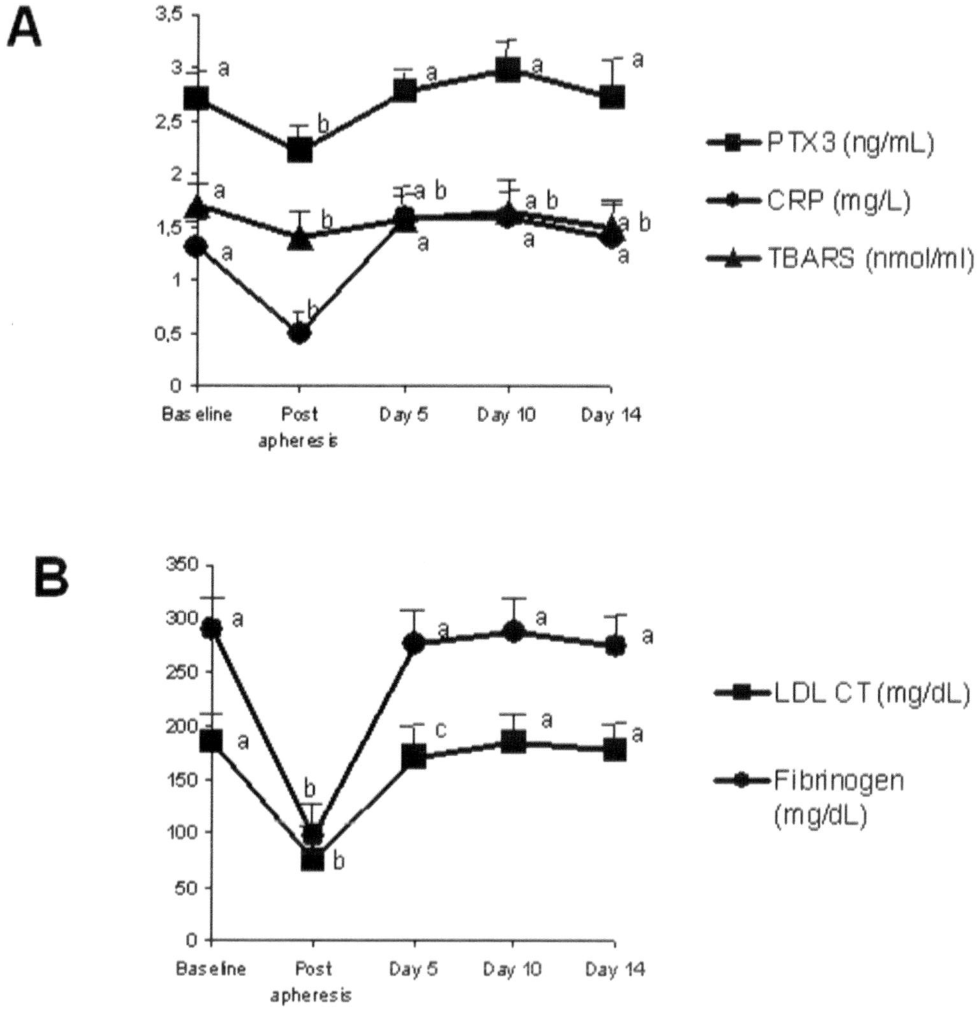

Figure 3. Fourteen-days trend analysis of pre- and post-treatment A) PTX3, CRP and TBARS plasma levels and B) LDL-cholesterol (LDL-CT) and fibrinogen in nine patients on chronic HELP LDL-apheresis. Within each curve, values sharing the same superscript letter do not differ significantly ($P<0.05$).

acutely elevated in critically ill and chronic cardiovascular patients [10,33] correlating with clinical scores that reflect disease extension and complexity [31,33]. The current data confirm these observations, as higher PTX3 was observed in subjects with shorter duration of treatment; this inverse relationship was independent from other clinical factors known to influence PTX3 levels, namely age and gender [34]. Lowering PTX3 level in high risk patients is associated with disease regression and reduced incidence of cardiovascular events [11,35]; whether reduced PTX3 in patients with longer duration of treatment is a direct or indirect effect of HELP LDL apheresis remains to be elucidated.

In this study overall reduction rates of LDL cholesterol, triglycerides, fibrinogen and CRP were similar to results from previous studies [18,22,23]. However, mean reductions in plasma total and LDL cholesterol induced by HELP LDL apheresis were not related with the decrease in plasma PTX3 and CRP, indicating that plasma lipid pattern is not a major drive in the LDL-apheresis related changes of the inflammatory proteins PTX3 and CRP.

Our study has some limitations. First, direct assessment of atherosclerosis severity was not available at the time of the study, although a positive relationship between the extension of vascular disease and PTX3 levels in subjects with cardiovascular risk factors is well established [31,33]. Second, due to small variations in PTX3 concentrations over time, a further sample collection for trend analysis of PTX3 levels was not acquirable within the study period. Despite these observations, the negative association between PTX3 and HELP LDL apheresis vintage suggests that chronic intensive lipid-lowering with HELP LDL apheresis has beneficial effects in patients with extensive cardiovascular disease.

Acknowledgments

The authors are grateful to Mrs. Anna De Santis and Cristina Bernetti for skillful technical and patient assistance.

Author Contributions

Conceived and designed the experiments: M. Zanetti LC M. Zenti RB EB. Performed the experiments: FZ LS MGM GR MF. Analyzed the data: M. Zanetti RB M. Zenti FM. Contributed reagents/materials/analysis tools: AS FM. Wrote the paper: M. Zanetti RB FM M. Zenti EB LC.

References

1. Narverud I, Ueland T, Nenseter MS, Retterstøl K, Telle-Hansen VH, et al. (2011) Children with familial hypercholesterolemia are characterized by an inflammatory imbalance between the tumor necrosis factor α system and interleukin-10. Atherosclerosis 214: 163–168.
2. Charakida M, Tousoulis D, Skoumas I, Pitsavos C, Vasiliadou C, et al. (2009) Inflammatory and thrombotic processes are associated with vascular dysfunction in children with familial hypercholesterolemia. Atherosclerosis 204: 532–7.
3. El Messal M, Beaudeux JL, Drissi A, Giral P, Chater R, et al. (2006) Elevated serum levels of proinflammatory cytokines and biomarkers of matrix remodeling in never-treated patients with familial hypercholesterolemia. Clin Chim Acta 366: 185–9.
4. Libby P, Lichtman AH, Hansson GK (2013) Immune effector mechanisms implicated in atherosclerosis: from mice to humans. Immunity 38: 1092–1104.
5. Bondarenko S, Catapano AL, Norata GD (2014) The CD1d-Natural Killer T Cell Axis in Atherosclerosis. J Innate Immun 6: 3–12.
6. Abderrahim-Ferkoune A, Bezy O, Chiellini C, Maffei M, Grimaldi P, et al. (2003) Characterization of the long pentraxin PTX3 as a TNF alpha-induced secreted protein of adipose cells. J Lipid Res 44: 994–1000.
7. Basile A, Sica A, d'Aniello E, Breviario F, Garrido G, et al. (1997) Characterization of the promoter for the human long pentraxin PTX3. Role of NF-kappaB in tumor necrosis factor-alpha and interleukin-1beta regulation. Biol Chem 272: 8172–8178.
8. Mantovani A, Valentino S, Gentile S, Inforzato A, Bottazzi B, et al. (2011) Pentraxins and atherosclerosis: the role of PTX3. The long pentraxin PTX3: a paradigm for humoral pattern recognition molecules. Curr Pharm Des 17: 38–46.
9. Savchenko A, Imamura M, Ohashi R, Jiang S, Kawasaki T, et al. (2008) Expression of pentraxin 3 (PTX3) in human atherosclerotic lesions. J Pathol 215: 48–55.
10. Bosutti A, Grassi G, Zanetti M, Aleksova A, Zecchin M, et al. (2007) Relation between the plasma levels of LDL-cholesterol and the expression of the early marker of inflammation long pentraxin PTX3 and the stress response gene p66ShcA in pacemaker-implanted patients. Clin Exp Med 7: 16–23.
11. Ohbayashi H, Miyazawa C, Miyamoto K, Sagara M, Yamashita T, et al. (2009) Pitavastatin improves plasma pentraxin 3 and arterial stiffness in atherosclerotic patients with hypercholesterolemia. J Atheroscler Thromb 16: 490–500.
12. Norata GD, Marchesi P, Pulakazhi Venu VK, Pasqualini F, Anselmo A, et al. (2009) Deficiency of the long pentraxin PTX3 promotes vascular inflammation and atherosclerosis. Circulation 120: 699–708.
13. Leren TP, Berge KE (2011) Subjects with molecularly defined familial hypercholesterolemia or familial-defective apoB-100 are not being adequately treated. PLoS One Feb 18; 6: 616721, doi: 10.1371/journal.pone.0016721.
14. Hemphill LC (2010) Familial hypercholesterolemia: Current treatment options and patient selection for low-density lipoprotein apheresis. J Clin Lipidol 4: 346–349.
15. McGowan MP (2013) Emerging low-density lipoprotein (LDL) therapies: Management of severely elevated LDL cholesterol—the role of LDL-apheresis. J Clin Lipidol 7: S21–S26.
16. Mellwig KP, Pulawski E, Horstkotte D, van Buuren F (2012) Lipid apheresis: oxidative stress, rheology, and vasodilatation. Clin Res Cardiol Suppl 7: S45–S49.
17. Hovland A, Lappegård KT, Mollnes TE (2012) LDL apheresis and inflammation-implications for atherosclerosis. Scand J Immunol 76: 229–236.
18. Cattin L, Petrucco A, Cazzolato G, Bon GB, Borelli V, et al. (1997) Low density lipoprotein-apheresis decreases oxidized low density lipoproteins and monocyte adhesion to endothelial cells. ASAIO J 43: 209–213.
19. Wang Y, Blessing F, Walli AK, Uberfuhr P, Fraunberger P, et al. (2004) Effects of heparin-mediated extracorporeal low-density lipoprotein precipitation beyond lowering proatherogenic lipoproteins-reduction of circulating proinflammatory and procoagulatory markers. Atherosclerosis 175: 145–150
20. Banerjee S, Abu Fadel M, Sarode R, Terada L, Moritz T, et al. (2013) Plaque regression and progenitor cell mobilization with intensive lipid elimination regimen (PREMIER) trial design. J Clin Apher Oct 4. doi: 10.1002/jca.21298.
21. van Buuren F, Kreickmann S, Horstkotte D, Kottmann T, Mellwig KP (2012) HELP apheresis in hypercholesterolemia and cardiovascular disease: efficacy and adverse events after 8,500 procedures. Clin Res Cardiol 7: 24–30.
22. Koga N (1999) The retardation of progression, stabilization, and regression of coronary and carotid atherosclerosis by low-density lipoprotein apheresis in patients with familial hypercholesterolemia. J Intern Med 246: 35–43.
23. Moriarty PM, Gibson CA, Shih J, Matias MS (2001) C-reactive protein and other markers of inflammation among patients undergoing HELP LDL apheresis. Atherosclerosis 158: 495–498.
24. Emerging Risk Factors Collaboration, Kaptoge S, Di Angelantonio E, Pennells L, Wood AM, et al. (2012) C-reactive protein, fibrinogen, and cardiovascular disease prediction. N Engl J Med 367: 1310–1320.
25. Iwata A, Miura S, Tanaka T, Ike A, Sugihara M, et al. (2012) Plasma pentraxin-3 levels are associated with coronary plaque vulnerability and are decreased by statin. Coron Artery Dis 23: 315–321.
26. Jylhävä J, Haarala A, Kähönen M, Lehtimäki T, Jula A, et al. (2011) Pentraxin 3 (PTX3) is associated with cardiovascular risk factors: the Health 2000 Survey. Clin Exp Immunol 164: 211–217.
27. Bambauer R, Bambauer C, Lehmann B, Latza R, Schiel R (2012) LDL-apheresis: technical and clinical aspects. Scientific World Journal 2012: 314283 doi: 10.1100/2012/314283.
28. Schaumann D, Welch-Wichary M, Voss A, Schmidt H, Olbricht CJ (1996) Prospective cross-over comparisons of three low-density lipoprotein (LDL)-apheresis methods in patients with familial hypercholesterolaemia.Eur J Clin Invest 26: 1033–1038.
29. Suzuki M, Yamane S, Matsugane T, Nobuto T, Azuma N, et al. (1996) Evaluation of double filtration plasmapheresis, thermofiltration, and low density lipoprotein adsorptive methods by crossover test in the treatment of familial hypercholesterolemia patients. Artif Organs 20: 296–302.
30. Norata GD, Marchesi P, Pirillo A, Uboldi P, Chiesa G, et al. (2008) Long pentraxin 3, a key component of innate immunity, is modulated by high-density lipoproteins in endothelial cells. Arterioscler Thromb Vasc Biol 28: 925–933.
31. Karakas MF, Buyukkaya E, Kurt M, Motor S, Akcay AB, et al. (2013) Serum pentraxin 3 levels are associated with the complexity and severity of coronary artery disease in patients with stable angina pectoris. J Investig Med 61: 278–285.
32. Matsuzaki M, Hiramori K, Imaizumi T, Kitabatake A, Hishida H, et al. (2002) Intravascular ultrasound evaluation of coronary plaque regression by low density lipoprotein-apheresis in familial hypercholesterolemia: the Low Density Lipoprotein-Apheresis Coronary Morphology and Reserve Trial (LACMART). J Am Coll Cardiol 40: 220–227.
33. Knoflach M, Kiechl S, Mantovani A, Cuccovillo I, Bottazzi B, et al. (2012) Pentraxin-3 as a marker of advanced atherosclerosis results from the Bruneck, ARMY and ARFY Studies. PLoS One;7:e31474. doi: 10.1371/journal.-pone.0031474.
34. Yamasaki K, Kurimura M, Kasai T, Sagara M, Kodama T, et al. (2009) Determination of physiological plasma pentraxin 3 (PTX3) levels in healthy populations. Clin Chem Lab Med 47: 471–477.
35. Latini R, Maggioni AP, Peri G, Gonzini L, Lucci D, et al. (2004) prognostic significance oft he long pentraxin 3 PTX3 in acute myocardial infarction. Circulation 110: 2349–2354.

2

Cardiomyopathy and Response to Enzyme Replacement Therapy in a Male Mouse Model for Fabry Disease

Aurelie Nguyen Dinh Cat[1,2], Brigitte Escoubet[1,3,4], Vincent Agrapart[1,2], Violaine Griol-Charhbili[1,2], Trenton Schoeb[5], Wenguang Feng[5], Edgar Jaimes[5], David G. Warnock[5], Frederic Jaisser[1,2]*

1 Inserm U872 Team 1, Paris, France, **2** University Pierre et Marie Curie, Paris, France, **3** AP-HP Hôpital Bichat, Paris, France, **4** *Centre d'Explorations Fonctionnelles-Imagerie*, Bichat Federative Research Institute 02, University Denis Diderot, Paris, France, **5** University of Alabama at Birmingham, Birmingham, Alabama, United States of America

Abstract

Fabry disease is an X-linked disorder of glycosphingolipid metabolism that results in progressive accumulation of neutral glycosphingolipids, (predominately globotriaosylceramide; GL-3) in lysosomes, as well as other cellular compartments and the extracellular space. Our aim was to characterize the cardiac phenotype of male knock-out mice that are deficient in alpha-galactosidase A activity, as a model for Fabry disease and test the efficacy of Enzyme Replacement Therapy with agalsidase-beta. Male mice (3–4 months of age) were characterized with awake blood pressure and heart rate measurements, cardiac echocardiography and electrocardiography measurements under light anesthesia, histological studies and molecular studies with real-time polymerase chain reaction. The Fabry knock-out mouse has bradycardia and lower blood pressure than control wild type (CB7BL/6J) mice. In Fabry knock-out mice, the cardiomyopathy associated mild hypertrophy at echography with normal systolic LV function and mild diastolic dysfunction. Premature atrial contractions were more frequent in without conduction defect. Heart weight normalized to tibial length was increased in Fabry knock-out mice. Ascending aorta dilatation was observed. Molecular studies were consistent with early stages of cardiac remodeling. A single dose of agalsidase-beta (3 mg/kg) did not affect the LV hypertrophy, function or heart rate, but did improve the mRNA signals of early cardiac remodeling. In conclusion, the alpha-galactosidase A deficient mice at 3 to 4 months of age have cardiac and vascular alterations similar to that described in early clinical stage of Fabry disease in children and adolescents. Enzyme replacement therapy affects cardiac molecular remodeling after a single dose.

Editor: Raphael Schiffmann, Baylor Research Institute, United States of America

Funding: This work was supported by grants to FJ from Institut National de la Santé et de la Recherche Médicale, the GENZYME Investigator Sponsored Research Program and the Centre de Recherche Industrielle et Technique. ANDC held a PhD grant from INSERM/Conseil Regional Ile de France; VG-C held a Lefoulon-Delalande postdoctoral fellowship. DGW received support from the Division of Nephrology and Department of Medicine at the University of Alabama at Birmingham, Birmingham Alabama, United States of America, and Genzyme Corporation, Cambridge, Massachusetts, United States of America. The funders had no role in study design, data collection and analysis, decision to publish, or preparation of the manuscript.

Competing Interests: Part of the work was financed by GENZYME Corporation through the GENZYME Investigator Sponsored Research Program. This does not alter the authors' adherence to all the PLoS ONE policies on sharing data and materials.

* E-mail: frederic.jaisser@crc.jussieu.fr

Introduction

After initial clinical descriptions, mutations in the alpha-galactosidase A (AGAL) gene were found to be responsible for Fabry disease, which is an X-linked disorder of glycosphingolipid metabolism that results in progressive accumulation of neutral glycosphingolipids, (predominately globotriaosylceramide; GL-3) in lysosomes, as well as other cellular compartments and the extracellular space [1]. The prevalence of Fabry mutation ranges from 1 in 40,000 to 1:117,000 in United States and Australia to 1:833,000 in Northern Portugal, the majority of them Caucasians [2]. These figures may underestimate the real prevalence of the disease as many patients go undiagnosed due to rarity of this disorder and phenotypic variation of the clinical features, especially in females. Much higher estimates of prevalence (e.g., 1 in 4,000) have been obtained from a newborn screening project, most of which were so-called "late-onset" variants with some residual enzyme activity [3]. Most affected males have little, if any, alpha-galactosidase A activity, and the deposition of GL-3 occurs primarily in vascular endothelial cells as well as epithelial and smooth muscle cells throughout the body. Early clinical manifestations of the disease include angiokeratoma, acroparesthesias, episodic pain "crises", hypohydrosis, and gastrointestinal complaints [1].

Progressive GL-3 accumulation in the microvasculature and parenchyma leads to microvascular dysfunction, occlusion, and ischemia. Recent reports have described increased inflammation, oxidative stress, and circulating myeloperoxidase [4] which appears to be associated with vasculopathic events [5]. In adult males with Fabry disease, the renal, cardiovascular and cerebrovascular manifestations such as proteinuria, chronic kidney disease and kidney failure, cardiac arrhythmias, hypertrophic cardiomyopathy and strokes lead to early death during the fourth and fifth decade of life [1,6,7]. A late onset cardiac variant has been described in male patients which is associated with progressive cardiac fibrosis and ultimate death in the 6th decade of life from the cardiac disease with preserved renal function [8,9].

Recent studies have emphasized the importance of controlling proteinuria with inhibitors of the renin-angiotensin-aldosterone system in patients receiving enzyme replacement therapy (ERT)

[10] but even with stabilization of kidney function, some of these patients still experience cardiac events, including bradyarrhythmias, ventricular premature contractions and sustained ventricular arrhythmias and conduction delays [11,12] as have been described in untreated patients [8,13]. The cardiac manifestations in adults with Fabry disease, with emphasis on the non-obstructive, concentric hypertrophic cardiomyopathy are well described [8,14,15,16]. Kampmann *et al.* have studied a large number of adolescents with Fabry disease; some present with early symptoms and signs of cardiac involvement [17], findings that have been confirmed by reports from Fabry registries [18,19].

Mouse knock-out (KO) models for Fabry disease have been described [20,21]. Shayman *et al.* have studied large vessel reactivity and pathology in this model [4,22,23,24,25]. Recent work by Rozenfeld et al has described myocardial alterations in this model, and the response to ERT given at biweekly intervals for 2 months [26]. In the present study, we found that Fabry KO male mice have bradycardia, low systemic blood pressure and mild hypertrophic cardiomyopathy when compared to the control wild-type (WT) C57BL/6J mice. Molecular studies are consistent with early cardiac remodelling, and these changes were reversed rapidly in response to a single dose of ERT.

Methods

Ethics Statement

This study conforms to European Union Council Directives (86/609/EEC) regarding the care and use of laboratory animals, and the Guide for the Care and Use of Laboratory Animals published by the US National Institutes of Health (NIH Publication No. 85–23, revised 1996. The Institutional Animal Care and Use Committee approved live animal procedures conducted at the University of Alabama at Birmingham (Animal Project Number 10XX08339).

Animal Model

Breeding pairs of the Fabry KO mouse were obtained from the National Institutes of Health (Bethesda, MD). This model as been previously used by Eitzman et al. to analyze vascular function [22]. Control WT animals were gender- and age-matched C57BL/6J mice obtained from the Charles River Laboratories. Male animals were used, and mice were provided standard chow (A04, Scientific Animal Food Engineering, Epinay sur Orge, France) and drank tap water *ad libitum.*

Blood Pressure, Electrocardiography and Echocardiography Measurements

Systolic blood pressure (SBP) on trained conscious mice was measured by tail cuff plethysmography using a BP2000 Visitech model as published previously [27]. Conscious heart rate (HR) was extracted from the pulse signal. Electrocardiograms (ECGs) were recorded over a 10 min period in 3–4-month-old mice under light anesthesia with isoflurane. Arrhythmia was detected by analysis of the tachogram of the recording (10 min tracings). Tachograms were constructed from automatic R wave detection (ECG-Auto EMKA, France) and RR plotted against time. All abnormal RR intervals were checked for validation and labeling. ECG intervals were measured from short recordings on average beats, constructed from 200 consecutive QRST complexes. Intervals were determined semi-automatically from a library of QRST waveforms sampled from the tracing. Average beats were checked and intervals set using the first derivative of the tracing. PQ was measured from the onset of P wave to the onset of the QRS wave. QRS duration was measured from the onset of the Q wave to the end of high-amplitude electrical events, as detected on the first derivative. The QT interval was measured from the onset of the Q wave to the last detectable electrical event on the first derivative. QT interval was corrected for heart rate by drawing the linear regression line from individual beats for each mouse, and was expressed as the value at a RR of 150 msec [28].

Echocardiography was performed on lightly anesthetized mice (isoflurane, Abbott, in oxygen), as described previously [29]. A small number of animals appeared to have more severe bradycardia in response anesthesia, and these animals were not included in the analysis of the echocardiograhy results to avoid non-specific rate-related changes. Briefly, the heart was visualized in the long axis parasternal view for M-mode left ventricle (LV) dimension measurement and posterior wall pulse wave tissue Doppler measurement. An apical 4- to 5-chamber view was obtained from the subcostal view for diastolic function assessment with pulse wave spectral LV inflow and outflow and for pulse wave tissue Doppler measurement of the mitral annulus velocities [29]. Relative wall thickness was calculated as (IVST+LVPWT)/LV EDD (IVST, interventricular wall thickness; LVPWT, LV posterior wall thickness).

Histochemistry and Quantification of Non-Vascular Collagen

Following intra-aortic perfusion with phosphate-buffered saline, hearts were excised from mice anesthetized with pentobarbital (50 mg/kg, i.p.) and fixed in 10% neutral buffered formalin. Fixed hearts were transected perpendicular to the long axis through the ventricles at their widest point and processed routinely for paraffin sectioning. Both portions were embedded so that sections contained 2 cross sections. Sections were cut 5 μm thick and stained with hematoxylin and eosin or Pirosirius Red [30]. Fields of the anterior, posterior and lateral left ventricle and the intraventricular septum were digitally photographed at 10x objective magnification with routine transmitted light and with polarization. For each field, myocardial area was determined by extraction of the green color channel, thresholding, and measurement with Image Pro Plus 6.2 software (MediaCybernetics, Inc. Bethesda MD). Myocardial collagen was determined by inverting polarized images, thresholding, deleting normal perivascular collagenous tissue and measurement of remaining areas. Collagen area was expressed as a percentage of the total myocardial area for each field. Myocyte diameters were measured perpendicular to the long axis of the sarcomeres from unbranched areas of the myocytes near an intercalated disk.

RNA Purification, cDNA Synthesis and Reverse Transcriptase-Polymerase Chain Reaction (RT-PCR)

Total RNA was extracted from the hearts of control and Fabry KO mice after being homogenized in Trizol (Trisol Reagent, Invitrogen), following the instructions of the manufacturer. Total RNA samples were treated with DNase I (Ambion®, Applied Biosystems, Courtaboeuf, France) and reverse-transcribed using random hexamers (Invitrogen, Cergy Pontoise, France) and the DNA polymerase SuperScriptII (Invitrogen). Real-time PCR was carried out on the iCycler (Biorad) using gene-specific primers to quantify the relative abundance of each gene with SYBR Green I as the fluorescent molecule as described [31]. The primers used are listed in Table S1. The GAPDH gene was used as reference gene for normalization. Relative copy number of the target genes was calculated with the $2^{(-\Delta\Delta Ct)}$ method, as described [31].

Enzyme Replacement Therapy (ERT)

Mice were inject via tail vein with a single injection of agalsidase-beta (Fabrazyme®, Genzyme Corporation, Cambridge MA, USA) at a dose of 3 mg/kg, as previously described [20]; GL-3 levels in the heart reached a nadir at 3 weeks following a single intravenous injection of agalsidase-beta at 3 mg/kg, which is the timing and dose of agalsidase-beta used in the present study. Control animals received similar volumes of normal saline. Mice underwent physiologic and echocardiographic assessment prior to injection, and then at 3 weeks following injection, at which point the cardiac GL-3 content was stably reduced by 80% [20].

Statistics

Data are expressed as mean ± SE. Student's two-tailed t tests were used to compare unpaired data between two groups. If the global test was significant, pair-wise comparisons were performed with a Tuckey-Kramer test. P * 0.05 was considered significant.

Results

Systolic Blood Pressure, Heart Rate, ECG and Cardiac Weight Measurements

Systolic blood pressure was lower for male Fabry KO mice than for male wild-type mice (WT) (Figure *1A*). In addition, heart rate was significantly slower in the Fabry KO mice than the WT controls (*Figure 1B*).

The measurements of RR intervals with surface ECG recordings showed prolonged RR intervals for Fabry KO mice compared to WT controls (Table 1). and the standard deviations of the RR intervals (SDNN) were significantly increased in the Fabry KO mice compared to the WT controls after normalization for heart rate (Fabry KO: 12% vs WT: 5%). There were no differences in PQ, QRS, or corrected QT intervals (Table 1). Premature atrial contractions were more frequently observed in Fabry KO mice than WT mice (Table 1).

Heart weight was increased for Fabry KO mice, compared to WT mice when normalized to body weight (Figure *2A*) or tibial length (*Figure 2B*).

Left Ventricle and Aortic Structural Alterations

The echocardiography results for 4 month-old mice are summarized in Table 2. There were significant increases in LV mass normalized to body weight (LV mass/BW) for Fabry KO mice compared to the WT age-matched controls (4.8±0.32 versus 4.2±0.14 mg/g; p<0.05). Despite the lower systolic blood pressure measurements, there was also a significant increase in the aortic diameter during diastole for Fabry KO mice compared to the WT controls (1.6±0.07 versus 1.4±0.03 mm; p<0.01). Aortic dilation was not associated with aortic valvular regurgitation (data not shown).

Left Ventricular Functional Alteration

Global LV systolic function was similar in Fabry KO mice as compared to age-matched WT mice, as assessed with echographic analysis of ejection fraction and systolic velocity of the mitral annulus by tissue Doppler (Table 2). Fabry KO mice had mild diastolic LV dysfunction as depicted with the decrease in Ea velocity, without change in the isovolumic relaxation time.

Left Ventricular Histologic Alteration

Routine histological stains (*Figure 3A*) did not reveal any structural difference between 4 month-old Fabry KO and wild type mice. Morphometric analysis showed identical myocyte diameters (Table 3), and electron micrographs showed occasional electron dense lamelated inclusion bodies, similar to previous descriptions (data not shown) [20].

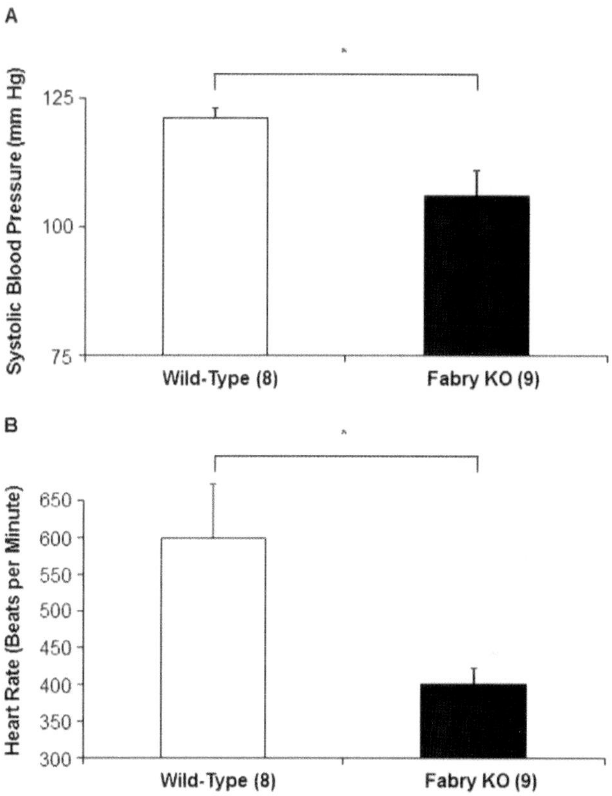

Figure 1. Comparison of Fabry Knock-out (KO) mice to wild type C57BL/6NJ mice: Tail Cuff Measurements. (A) Systolic blood pressures (mm Hg) and (B) Heart rates (beats per minute) were determined with tail-cuff measurements in awake animals. Data represent the means ± SE for 9 Fabry KO and 8 wild type male mice. Statistical significance was determined by unpaired, two-tailed t-test: *P<0.05.

Table 1. ECG results in 3–4 month old WT and Fabry KO mice.

	WT Controls	Fabry KO
Number	12	16
RR interval (msec)	117±4.5	135±5.6*
SDNN (msec)	6.4±0.7	16.2±1.4*
PR interval (msec)	36±0.4	37±0.8
QRS interval (msec)	16±0.5	16±0. 6
QT_{c150} interval (msec)	49±1.2	47±2.0
APC (%)	33	93**

Surface ECGs were obtained in lightly anesthesized mice. Data represent the means ± SE. Statistical significance was determined by pair-wise comparisons with a Tuckey-Kramer test, or χ^2 analysis.
WT, wild-type; KO, knockout; SDNN, standard deviation of normal RR intervals; APC, %of animals with atrial premature contractions during 10 min recording.
*P<0.05,
**P<0.05 by for χ^2 analysis.

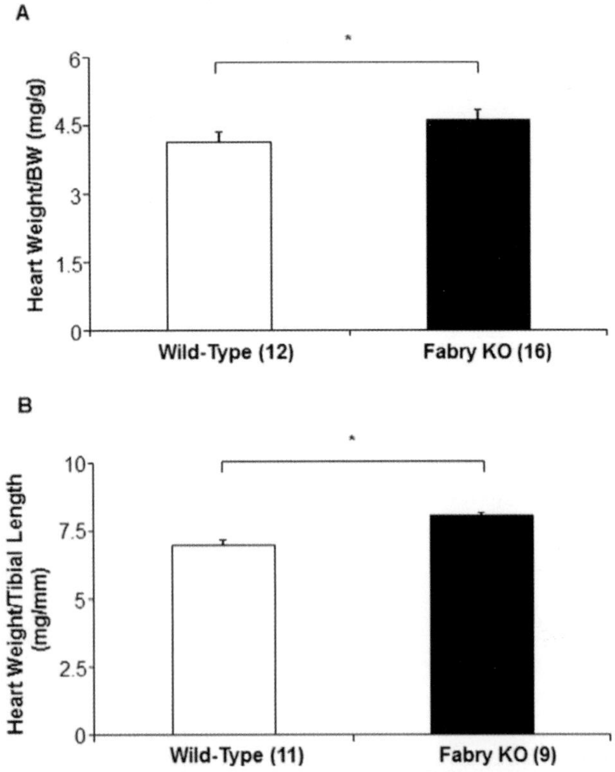

Figure 2. Comparison of Fabry Knock-out (KO) mice to wild type C57BL/6NJ mice: Heart Weights. Body weights (g), heart weights (mg) and tibial lengths (mm) were measured at sacrifice. Data represent the means ± SE for 9 Fabry KO and 11 wild type male mice. Statistical significance was determined by unpaired, two-tailed *t*-test: *P<0.05.

Staining with Picrosirius Red showed no significant differences in non-vascular collagen staining in the myocardium of male Fabry KO mice compared to WT mice (*Figure 3C–B*) and no predominant area of fibrosis in Fabry KO mice.

LV Molecular Alterations in Fabry KO Mice

We examined myocardial alterations that could be associated with cardiac remodeling and dysfunction by analyzing mRNA expression for atrial natriuretic factor (ANF) brain natriuretic peptide (BNP), plasminogen activator inhibitor-1 (PAI-1); connective tissue growth factor (CTGF), thrombospondin 1 (TSP1), and thrombospondin 2 (TSP2). As shown in Figure 4A, ANF and BNP mRNA levels normalized to GAPDH levels were significantly increased in male Fabry KO mice compared to wild type controls. PAI-1 and CTGF mRNA levels were increased in male Fabry KO mice, as compared to wild type. Also shown in Figure 4 are the normalized values for TSP1 and TSP2, members of the matricellular protein family, which are up-regulated during cardiac stress, injury and remodeling [32]. TSP2 but not TSP1 mRNA levels were increased in male Fabry KO mice compared to wild type controls. The mRNA levels for collagen 1a and collagen 3a, the matrix metallo-proteinases 2 and 9 were not altered in Fabry KO mice (data not shown).

Table 2. Echocardiographic evaluation of 3 to 4 month-old Wild type and Fabry Knock Out (KO) mice.

	Wild Type	Fabry KO
Number	12	11
Body Weight (g)	27.6±0.4	31.1±0.5
Age (weeks)	18.8±0.1	18.2±0.3
Heart Rate (beats per min)	518±7	521±9.4
Cardiac and vascular remodeling		
LA Diameter (mm)	2.2±0.08	2.7±0.10
LA Diameter/BW (mm/g)	0.1±0.01	0.1±0.03
LV EDD/BW (mm/g)	0.15±0.01	0.15±0.01
LV mass/BW (mg/g)	4.2±0.14	4.8±0.32*
Relative Wall Thickness	0.4±0.02	0.4±0.02
Diastolic Ao (mm)	1.4±0.03	1.6±0.07**
Left Ventricular Systolic Function		
LV Ejection Fraction (%)	82±2	79±3
Vcfc, circumference/sec	3.25±0.12	3.15±0.31
Sa (cm/s)	2.7±0.20	2.9±0.12
Spw (cm/s)	3.1±0.20	3.2±0.16
Left Ventricular Diastolic Function		
IVRT (ms)	17.0±0.60	17.0±1.1
Ea (cm/s)	5.5±0.24	4.5±0.40**
Epw (cm/s)	4.4±0.19	4.0±0.40
E/Ea	19.1±0.8	21.7±1.7

Data represent the means ± SE. Statistical significance was determined by unpaired, two-tailed *t*-test: *P<0.05: **P<0.01.
Abbreviations: LA, left atrium; LV, left ventricle; LV EDD, left ventricular end diastolic diameter; Vcfc, velocity of shortening of circumferential fibers; Sa, Spw: maximal systolic velocity of the mitral annulus and posterior wall; IVRT: isovolumic relaxation time; Ea and Epw: maximal diastolic velocity of the mitral annulus and posterior wall; E, maximal velocity of LV inflow.

Systolic Blood Pressure, Heart Rate, ECG and Cardiac Weight Measurements: Effects of ERT

The measurements of RR intervals with surface ECG recordings showed identical RR intervals and the standard deviation of the RR intervals, and the frequency of premature atrial contractions for Fabry KO mice compared to Fabry KO mice treated with 3 mg/kg intravenous ERT 3 weeks before (Table 4). There were no significant differences in PQ, QRS, or corrected QT intervals (data not shown).

ERT had no effect 3 weeks after injection on heart weight for Fabry KO mice, when normalized to body weight (Figure *5A*) or tibial length (*Figure* 5C). There was no effect 3 weeks after injection on heart weight for WT mice, when normalized to body weight (Figure *5B*) or tibial length (*Figure 5D*).

Left Ventricle and Aortic Structural Alterations with ERT

The echocardiography results for 6–7 month-old Fabry KO mice are summarized in Table 5 for untreated mice and those who received a single injection of ERT 3 weeks before evaluation. While there was no significant effect on the LV mass estimates, there was a significant increase in relative wall thickness for Fabry KO mice treated with ERT compared to the untreated KO

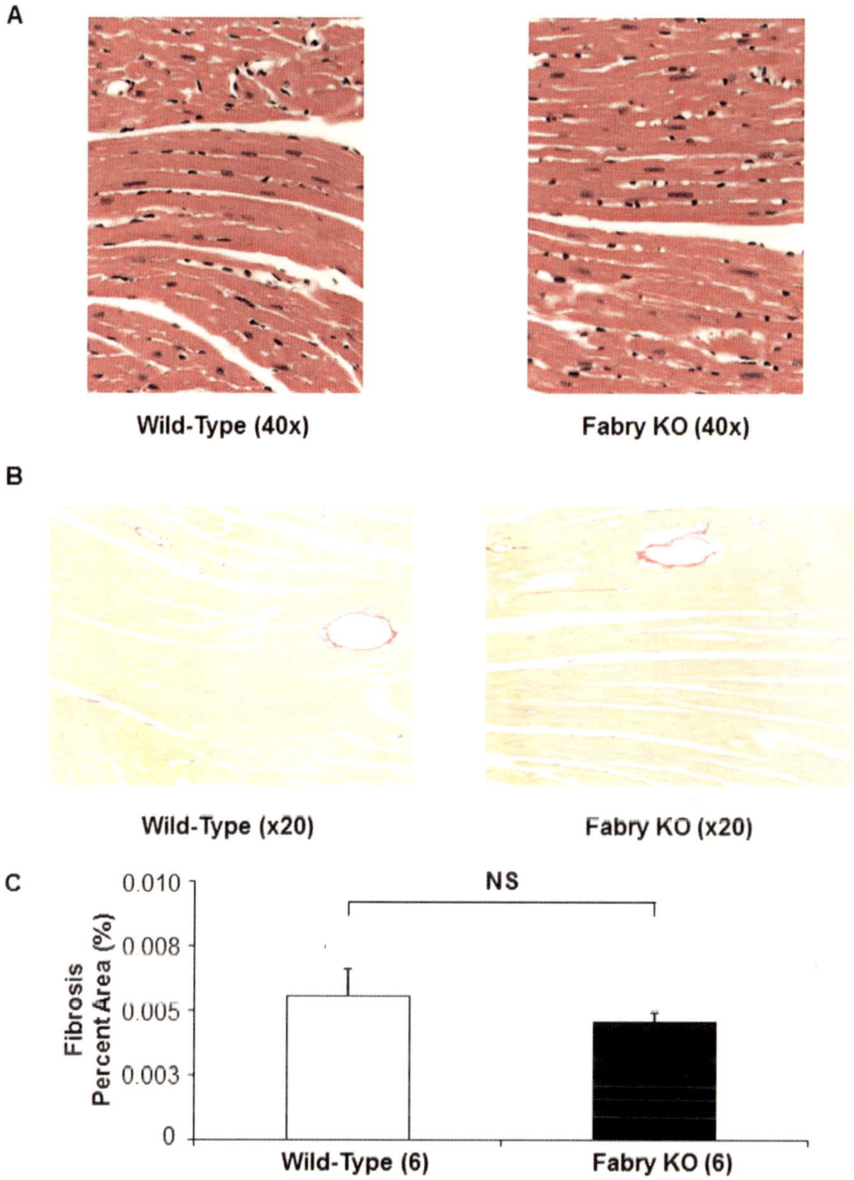

Figure 3. Left Ventricular Histology of wild type C57BL/6NJ mice to Fabry Knock-out (KO) mice. (A) Wild type mouse, left panel; Fabry KO mouse, right panel; 40×magnification. Hearts were perfusion fixed and sections obtained for staining for hematoxylin and eosin. (B) Pirosirius Red staining for non-vascular collagen (Wild type mouse, left panel; Fabry KO mouse, right panel; 20×magnification). (C) Pirosirius Red staining for non-vascular collagen, expressed as the percentage of the total myocardial area for each field.

age-matched controls according to a trend toward decrease in LV diameter after treatment (3.9±0.6 vs 4.2±0.15, ns) without change in wall thickness (septum: Fabry mice ERT 1.0±0.03, Fabry mice: 0.9±0.02; posterior wall Fabry mice ERT 0.8±0.04, Fabry mice: 0.7±0.03). There was a significant decrease in the aortic diameter during diastole for Fabry KO mice treated with ERT compared to the age-matched KO controls (1.7±0.05 versus 1.6±0.04 mm; $p<0.01$).

Table 3. Myocyte Diameter and Picrosirius Red Staining of 4-month old Fabry KO and WT mice.

	WT Controls	Fabry KOs
Myocyte diameter (μm)	82.6±9.9	79.1±4.9
Collagen content (%)	0.0056±0.0025	0.0046±0.0008

Left Ventricular Functional Alterations in Fabry KO Mice with ERT

The heart rates obtained in 6–7 week old mice undergoing echocardiography with isoflurane anesthesia were the same for untreated Fabry KO mice compared to age-matched Fabry KO mice that had received ERT (3 mg/kg) as a single IV injection 3 weeks before evaluation (Table 5).

LV systolic function, as assessed by echocardiography was similar in ERT-treated Fabry KO mice as compared to age-matched untreated KO mice (Table 4). ERT-treated Fabry KO

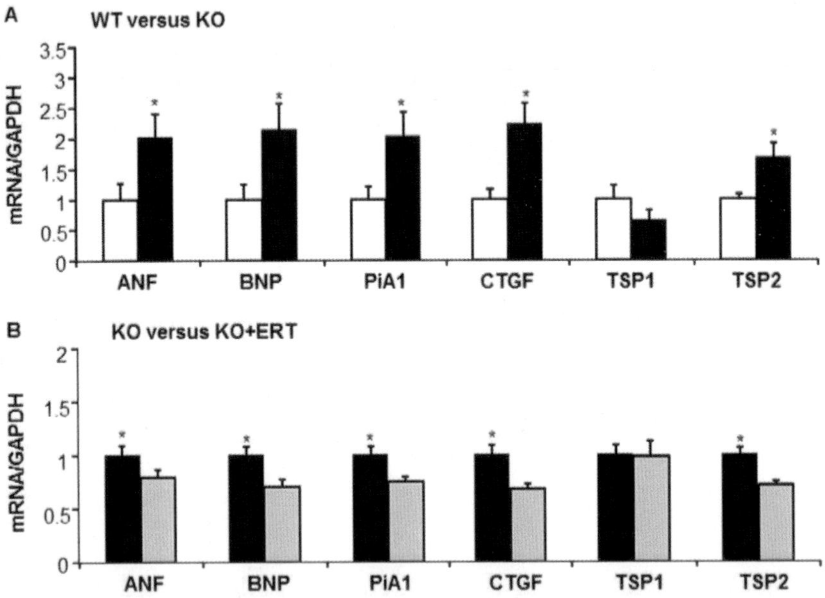

Figure 4. Comparison of wild type C57BL/6NJ mice (open bars) to Fabry Knock-out (KO) mice (black bars): mRNA levels. Real-time PCR amplification of indicated mRNA targets, normalized to GAPDH mRNA level. ANF, atrial natriuretic factor; BNP, brain natriuretic peptide; PAI-1, plasminogen activator inhibitor -1; CTGF, connective tissue growth factor; TSP1, thrombospondin 1; TSP2, thrombospondin 2; Statistical significance was determined by unpaired, two-tailed *t*-test: *$P<0.05$. (A). Comparison of wild type C57BL/6NJ mice (open bars) to Fabry Knock-out (KO) mice (black bars): mRNA levels. (B). Comparison of Fabry Knock-out (KO) mice (black bars) to Fabry Knock-out (KO) mice (gray bars) 3 weeks after a single intravenous treatment with agalsidase-beta at 3 mg/kg: mRNA levels.

mice had similar diastolic LV function as the untreated KO controls.

LV Molecular Alterations in Fabry KO and WT Mice Treated with ERT

As shown in Figure 4B, ANF and BNP mRNA levels normalized to GAPDH levels were significantly decreased in male Fabry KO mice 3 weeks after ERT treatment compared to untreated KO controls. PAI-1 and CTGF mRNA levels were decreased in ERT-treated male Fabry KO mice, as compared to untreated KO controls. TSP2 but not TSP1 mRNA levels were decreased in ERT-treated male Fabry KO mice compared to untreated KO controls.

The effects of ERT were also examined in WT controls 3 weeks after a single IV injection (3 mg/kg), compared to untreated age-matched WT controls. There was a significant decrease in BNP mRNA normalized to GAPDH levels in ERT-treated WT mice, but there were not any effects of ERT on any of the mRNA levels examined in this series compared to WT concurrent control male mice (Figure S1).

Table 4. ECG results in 6–7 month old Fabry KO mice: effects of ERT.

	KO Controls	KO ± ERT
Number	11	11
RR (msec)	135±5.6	143±4
SDNN (ms)	16.7±2	19.7±2.2
APC (%)	45.6	54

Surface ECGs were obtained in lightly anesthesized mice. Data represent the means ± SE. Statistical significance was determined by pair-wise comparisons with a Tuckey-Kramer test, or χ^2 analysis.
WT, wild-type; KO, knockout; SDNN, standard deviation of normal RR intervals;APC, % of animals with atrial premature contractions during 10 min recording.

Discussion

In the present study, we define the cardiac phenotype in male Fabry KO mice. We found that these mice have bradycardia and low systemic blood pressures compared to the control WT strain, as well as mild hypertrophic cardiomyopathy on echocardiography and gravimetry. The heart rates and systolic blood pressures reported herein for the WT mice are very similar to previous reports [33,34].

Thus KO Fabry mice displayed a mild hypertrophic cardiomyopathy with structural and functional alteration similar to that described for the early stages of human myocardiopathies. Our results are similar to and extend the findings of Rozenfeld et al., who have described changes in passive pressure volume curves and contractility measurements in the male mouse KO model of Fabry disease, but did not document hypertrophy as assessed by cardiac weight normalized to tibial length or echo cardiographic assessment of left ventricular mass [26].

The initial descriptions of the KO model of Fabry disease were used for pharmacokinetic studies of ERT, and did not evaluate the phenotype of these animals (".no clinical disease phenotype and survived a normal laboratory lifespan"[20]). Shayman et al. have studied large vessel reactivity and pathology in this model [4,22,23,24,25,35] but did not evaluated the cardiac findings.

The most striking aspect of the cardiac phenotype in the KO mice was hypotension and bradycardia, compared to the WT controls. Autonomic nervous system alteration, as assessed on heart rate variability, was described in children and adolescents with decreased heart rate variability in boys [17] and could

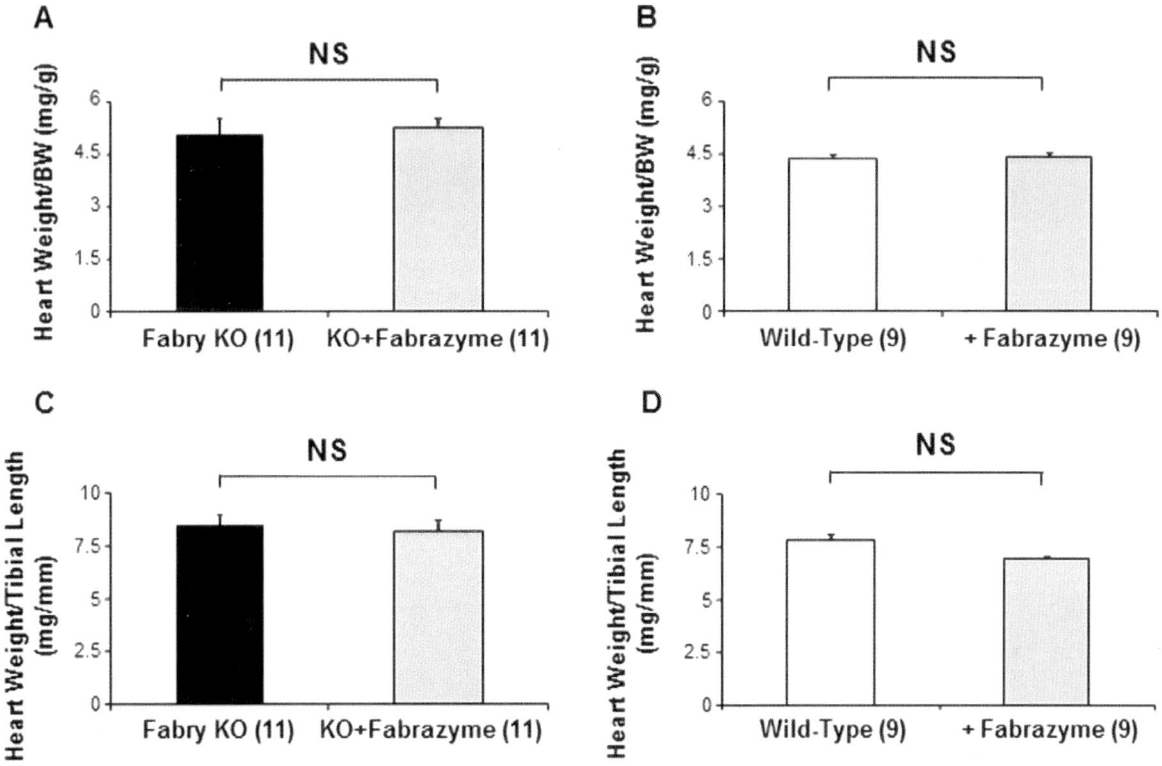

Figure 5. Comparison of untreated Fabry Knock-out (KO) and WT mice to ERT-treated KO mice and ERT-treated WT mice: Heart Weights. Body weights (g), heart weights (mg) and tibial lengths (mm) were measured at sacrifice. Data represent the means ± SE for 11 Fabry KO and 9 wild type male mice. Statistical significance was determined by unpaired, two-tailed *t*-test: $*P<0.05$.

represent early findings of the cardiac involvement in Fabry disease. Our results suggest that the mouse model have also alteration of the autonomic nervous system, as depicted by bradycardia and time domain parameters of heart rate variability suggesting increase in variability. The change in time domain parameter (SDNN) could be partly accounted for by bradycardia itself with increasing dispersion of the RR but also by a greater influence of parasympathetic activity which could also be responsible for the lower blood pressure. Comparison with the human findings would need a complete autononic nervous system evaluation in mice.

Endothelial dysfunction was described in human Fabry disease with inflammation and increased oxidative stress within the vessel wall [4]. GL-3 accumulation occurs primarily in endothelial cells with impairment of vessel reactivity [4,25]. Alteration in endothelial function, with the consequent change in smooth muscle cells, could be related to our findings of ascending aorta dilatation in the KO model that does not appear to be explained by hemodynamic changes. This has also been recently described in the human disease [36].

Cardiac abnormalities in Fabry disease are characterized mainly by LV wall thickening without significant dilatation, and LV hypertrophy [14]. Systolic function is largely preserved in most affected individuals, but diastolic dysfunction is a relatively common finding even at early stage of the disease [14,17]. In the mouse model, we found LV functional alterations with mild alteration of diastolic function, as depicted with Tissue Doppler interrogation, and no systolic alteration. This is very similar to the findings in human at early stages of the cardiac disease [37,38,39]. Moreover, a good relationship was shown between tissue Doppler echocardiographic data and mechanical properties of human cardiac myofilaments obtained from myocardial biopsies [38]. The findings that the mouse model has mild cardiac involvement detectable with tissue Doppler suggest that this specific interrogation in human has to be performed for early detection of cardiac involvement, inasmuch as the efficiency of the replacement therapy is dependent on early onset of treatment [15]. We also found evidence of cardiac remodeling at the molecular level, with increased mRNA levels, for atrial natriuretic factor (ANF) brain natriuretic peptide (BNP), plasminogen activator inhibitor-1 (PAI-1); connective tissue growth factor (CTGF), and thrombospondin 2 (TSP2).

Our results suggest that atrial arrhythmias could be associated with early cardiac involvement in Fabry disease. Although more than 60% of patients with Fabry disease have evidence of cardiac involvement, the prevalence and clinical significance of arrhythmia in Fabry disease are unknown. Shah and colleagues studied 78 consecutive patients (mean age 43.5±15.0 years, 43 males) with Fabry disease [40]. Three patients (3.9%) had persistent atrial fibrillation, and 8 (13.3%) had paroxysmal atrial fibrillation. Five males (8.3%) had nonsustained ventricular tachycardia with a maximal left ventricular wall thickness >20 mm. Age, left atrial diameter, maximal left ventricular wall thickness, left ventricular mass index, and angina were univariate predictors of atrial fibrillation. During follow-up, there was 1 sudden cardiac death, 4 patients received pacemakers for bradyarrhythmias, and 1 patient received a biventricular pacemaker and an internal cardiac defibrillator. The high incidence of arrhythmias and pacemaker implantation and sudden cardiac death suggests that arrhythmia has a significant impact on the natural history of Fabry disease. The mouse model did not, however, displayed ventricular arrhythmias possibly because the mice were relatively young.

Table 5. Echocardiographic evaluation of 6–7 month-old Fabry Knock Out (KO) mice: response to enzyme replacement therapy (ERT).

	Fabry KO	Fabry KO + ERT
Number	11	11
Body Weight (g)	31.1±0.5	29.6±0.6
Age (weeks)	28	27
Heart Rate (beats per min)	521±9.4	530±12
Cardiac and vascular remodeling		
LA Diameter (mm)	2.7±0.19	2.4±0.13
LA Diameter/BW (mm/g)	0.1±0.03	0.1±0.03
LV EDD/BW (mm/g)	0.1±0.01	0.1±0.01
LV mass/BW (mg/g)	4.4±0.22	4.6±0.16
Relative Wall Thickness	0.4±0.02	0.5±0.02*
Diastolic Ao (mm)	1.7±0.05	1.6±0.04*
Left Ventricular Systolic Function		
LV Ejection Fraction (%)	84±2	81±2
Vcfc, circumference/sec	3.41±0.20	3.33±0.18
Sa (cm/s)	2.90±0.12	3.13±0.10
Spw (cm/s)	3.4±0.23	3.3±0.17
Left Ventricular Diastolic Function		
IVRT (ms)	17.0±0.54	17.8±0.83
Ea (cm/s)	5.0±0.15	5.0±0.19
Epw (cm/s)	4.1±0.18	4.8±0.27
E/Ea	19.5±0.78	19.0±0.71

Data represent the means ± SE. Statistical significance was determined by unpaired, two-tailed *t*-test: *P<0.05.
Abbreviations: LA, left atrium; LV, left ventricle; LV EDD, left ventricular end diastolic diameter; Vcfc, velocity of shortening of circumferential fibers; Sa, Spw: maximal systolic velocity of the mitral annulus and posterior wall; IVRT: isovolumic relaxation time; Ea and Epw: maximal diastolic velocity of the mitral annulus and posterior wall; E, maximal velocity of LV inflow.

Despite the describe phenotype, the mouse model did not recapitulate all cardiac feature of human Fabry disease: 1) Ventricular arrhythmias or conduction (atrioventricular or intraventricular) defect were not found; 2) LV hypertrophy and GL-3 accumulation was mild or absent; and 3) Accelerated arteriosclerosis and vascular thrombosis was not evident in the mouse model, at least at the ages we examined in this series.

Over the last decade, the natural history of Fabry disease appears to have changed. With the use of ERT and antiproteinuric therapy, renal outcomes have improved and currently the most common cause of death is cardiac involvement and sudden cardiac death [41,42] Electrocardiographic changes that have been described in Fabry disease include atrial fibrillation, atrioventricular conduction abnormalities, left ventricular hypertrophy, and repolarization abnormalities [17,43]; [44]. Cardiac symptoms in patients with Fabry disease include bradycardia, shortness of breath with exertion, vasospastic and/or exertional angina pectoris, and syncope [45,46]. Long term treatment with ERT has been shown to reduce LV hypertrophy, and suggested that early treatment may yield better long-term cardiac outcomes and exercise capacity [15].

Whether or not these abnormalities in heart rhythm or rate, as well as the cardiac remodeling will respond to ERT, and/or other forms of adjunctive therapy [47] are questions that can be addressed in the Fabry KO mouse despite the limitations of the model [1]. We have found changes in the cellular phenotype in this model, 3 weeks following a single intravenous injection of 3 mg/kg agalsidase-beta, a dose and interval chosen to maximize the reduction in cardiac GL3 content [20]. Rozenfeld et al. observed improvement in left ventricular contractility following longer treatment periods (4 injections over 2 months) of a much lower dose of ERT (0.5 mg/kg) [26]. Alternate dosing schedules as well as consideration of alternative forms of therapy [48] for this condition are important avenues for future research.

Supporting Information

Figure S1 Comparison of WT mice treated with ERT to WT mice 3 weeks after a single intravenous injection with agalsidase-beta at 3 mg/kg: mRNA levels. Wild type C57BL/6NJ mice (open bars) compared to ERT-treated WT mice (gray bars). Real-time PCR amplification of indicated mRNA targets, normalized to GAPDH mRNA level. ANF, atrial natriuretic factor; BNP, brain natriuretic peptide; PAI-1, plasminogen activator inhibitor -1; CTGF, connective tissue growth factor; TSP1, thrombospondin 1; TSP2, thrombospondin 2; Statistical significance was determined by unpaired, two-tailed *t*-test: *P<0.05.

Table S1 Primers sequences.

Acknowledgments

We acknowledge the assistance of Gary Murray, PhD of the National Institute of Neurologic Dieseases and Stroke with establishing the Fabry KO breeding colony at the University of Alabama at Birmingham, under a Materials Transfer Agreement between the NIH and UAB. Histology services were provided by the UAB Animal Resources Program Comparative Pathology Laboratory. We thank James Oliver of the Gnotobiotic and Genetically-Engineered Mouse Core Facility (Director: C. Weaver, MD PhD) at UAB for maintaining the breeding colony, and Darren Duvall, ARP Transfer Coordinator for assistance in shipping mice from UAB to Paris.

Author Contributions

Conceived and designed the experiments: FJ DGW EJ. Performed the experiments: ANDC VG-C VA BE TS WF EJ. Analyzed the data: ANDC VA BE DGW FJ EJ. Wrote the paper: FJ DGW EJ BE.

References

1. Desnick RJ, Ioannou YA, Eng CM (2001) Alpha-Galactosidase A deficiency: Fabry disease. In: Scriver C, Beaudet A, Sly W, Valle D, eds. The Metabolic Bases of Inherited Disease. 8th ed. New York: McGraw-Hill. pp 3733–3774.
2. Meikle PJ, Hopwood JJ, Clague AE, Carey WF (1999) Prevalence of lysosomal storage disorders. J Am Med Assoc 281: 249–254.
3. Spada M, Pagliardini S, Yasuda M, Tukel T, Thiagarajan G, et al. (2006) High incidence of later-onset fabry disease revealed by newborn screening. Am J Hum Genet 79: 31–40.
4. Shen JS, Meng XL, Moore DF, Quirk JM, Shayman JA, et al. (2008) Globotriaosylceramide induces oxidative stress and up-regulates cell adhesion molecule expression in Fabry disease endothelial cells. Mol Genet Metab 95: 163–168.
5. Kaneski CR, Moore DF, Ries M, Zirzow GC, Schiffmann R (2006) Myeloperoxidase predicts risk of vasculopathic events in hemizgygous males with Fabry disease. Neurology 67: 2045–2047.
6. Schiffmann R, Warnock DG, Banikazemi M, Bultas J, Linthorst GE, et al. (2009) Fabry disease: progression of nephropathy, and prevalence of cardiac and cerebrovascular events before enzyme replacement therapy. Nephrol Dial Transplant 24: 2102–2111.

7. Wanner C, Oliveira JP, Ortiz A, Mauer M, Germain DP, et al. (2010) Prognostic indicators of renal disease progression in adults with fabry disease: natural history data from the fabry registry. Clin J Amer Soc Nephrol 5: 2220–2228.
8. Takenaka T, Teraguchi H, Yoshida A, Taguchi S, Ninomiya K, et al. (2008) Terminal stage cardiac findings in patients with cardiac Fabry disease: An electrocardiographic, echocardiographic, and autopsy study. J Cardiol 51: 50–59.
9. Fervenza FC, Torra R, Warnock DG (2008) Safety and efficacy of enzyme replacement therapy in the nephropathy of Fabry disease. Biologics: Targets and Therapy 2: 1–22.
10. Tahir H, Jackson LL, Warnock DG (2007) Antiproteinuric therapy and Fabry nephropathy: Sustained reduction in proteinuria in patients receiving enzyme replacement therapy with agalsidase-beta. J Am Soc Nephrol 18: 2609–2617.
11. Fervenza FC, Torra R, Lager DJ (2008) Fabry disease: an underrecognized cause of proteinuria. Kidney intern 73: 1193–1199.
12. Warnock DG, Ortiz A, Mauer M, Linthorst GE, Oliveira JP, et al. (2011) Renal outcomes of agalsidase beta treatment for Fabry disease: role of proteinuria and timing of treatment initiation. Nephrology, dialysis, transplantation: official publication of the European Dialysis and Transplant Association - European Renal Association.
13. Shah JS, Elliott PM (2005) Fabry disease and the heart: an overview of the natural history and the effect of enzyme replacement therapy. Acta Paediatr Suppl 94: 11–14; discussion 19–10.
14. Linhart A, Kampmann C, Zamorano JL, Sunder-Plassmann G, Beck M, et al. (2007) Cardiac manifestations of Anderson-Fabry disease: results from the international Fabry outcome survey. European Heart J 28: 1228–1235.
15. Weidemann F, Niemann M, Breunig F, Herrmann S, Beer M, et al. (2009) Long-Term Effects of Enzyme Replacement Therapy on Fabry Cardiomyopathy: Evidence for a Better Outcome With Early Treatment. Circulation 119: 524–529.
16. Weidemann F, Niemann M, Warnock DG, Ertl G, Wanner C (2011) The fabry cardiomyopathy: models for the cardiologist. Ann Rev Med 62: 59–67.
17. Kampmann C, Wiethoff CM, Whybra C, Baehner FA, Mengel E, et al. (2008) Cardiac manifestations of Anderson-Fabry disease in children and adolescents. Acta Paediatr 97: 463–469.
18. Hopkin RJ, Bissler J, Banikazemi M, Clarke L, Eng CM, et al. (2008) Characterization of Fabry disease in 352 pediatric patients in the Fabry Registry. Pediatr Res 64: 550–555.
19. Ries M, Gupta S, Moore DF, Sachdev V, Quirk JM, et al. (2005) Pediatric Fabry disease. Pediatrics 115: e344–355.
20. Ioannou YA, Zeidner KM, Gordon RE, Desnick RJ (2001) Fabry disease: preclinical studies demonstrate the effectiveness of alpha-galactosidase A replacement in enzyme-deficient mice. Am J Hum Genet 68: 14–25.
21. Ohshima T, Murray GJ, Swaim WD, Longenecker G, Quirk JM, et al. (1997) alpha-Galactosidase A deficient mice: a model of Fabry disease. Proc Natl Acad Sci U S A 94: 2540–2544.
22. Eitzman DT, Bodary PF, Shen Y, Khairallah CG, Wild SR, et al. (2003) Fabry disease in mice is associated with age-dependent susceptibility to vascular thrombosis. J Am Soc Nephrol 14: 298–302.
23. Bodary PF, Shen Y, Vargas FB, Bi X, Ostenso KA, et al. (2005) Alpha-galactosidase A deficiency accelerates atherosclerosis in mice with apolipoprotein E deficiency. Circulation 111: 629–632.
24. Park JL, Whitesall SE, D'Alecy LG, Shu L, Shayman JA (2008) Vascular dysfunction in the alpha-galactosidase A-knockout mouse is an endothelial cell-, plasma membrane-based defect. Clin Exp Pharmacol Physiol 35: 1156–1163.
25. Shu L, Park JL, Byun J, Pennathur S, Kollmeyer J, et al. (2009) Decreased Nitric Oxide Bioavailability in a Mouse Model of Fabry Disease. J Am Soc Nephrol.
26. Rozenfeld PA, Fritz M, Blanco P, Gonzalez P, Rinaldi GJ (2011) Myocardial alterations in the murine model of fabry disease can be reversed by enzyme replacement therapy. Canadian J Cardiol 27: 339–345.
27. Bichara M, Attmane-Elakeb A, Brown D, Essig M, Karim Z, et al. (2006) Exploring the role of galectin 3 in kidney function: a genetic approach. Glycobiology 16: 36–45.
28. Sainte-Marie Y, Nguyen Dinh Cat A, Perrier R, Mangin L, Soukaseum C, et al. (2007) Conditional glucocorticoid receptor expression in the heart induces atrio-ventricular block. FASEB J 21: 3133–3141.
29. Parlakian A, Charvet C, Escoubet B, Mericskay M, Molkentin JD, et al. (2005) Temporally controlled onset of dilated cardiomyopathy through disruption of the SRF gene in adult heart. Circulation 112: 2930–2939.
30. Whittaker P, Kloner RA, Boughner DR, Pickering JG (1994) Quantitative assessment of myocardial collagen with picrosirius red staining and circularly polarized light. Basic Res Cardiol 89: 397–410.
31. Ouvrard-Pascaud A, Sainte-Marie Y, Benitah JP, Perrier R, Soukaseum C, et al. (2005) Conditional mineralocorticoid receptor expression in the heart leads to life-threatening arrhythmias. Circulation 111: 3025–3033.
32. Schellings MW, Pinto YM, Heymans S (2004) Matricellular proteins in the heart: possible role during stress and remodeling. Cardiovas Res 64: 24–31.
33. Mallon AM, Blake A, Hancock JM (2008) EuroPhenome and EMPReSS: online mouse phenotyping resource. Nucleic Acids Res 36: D715–718.
34. Guo X, Kono Y, Mattrey R, Kassab GS (2002) Morphometry and strain distribution of the C57BL/6 mouse aorta. Am J Physiol Heart Circ Physiol 283: H1829–1837.
35. Shu L, Murphy HS, Cooling L, Shayman JA (2005) An in vitro model of Fabry disease. J Am Soc Nephrol 16: 2636–2645.
36. Barbey F, Qanadli SD, Juli C, Brakch N, Palacek T, et al. (2010) Aortic remodelling in Fabry disease. Eur Heart J 31: 347–353.
37. Sadick N, Thomas L (2007) Cardiovascular manifestations in Fabry disease: a clinical and echocardiographic study. Heart Lung Circ 16: 200–206.
38. Chimenti C, Hamdani N, Boontje NM, DeCobelli F, Esposito A, et al. (2008) Myofilament degradation and dysfunction of human cardiomyocytes in Fabry disease. Am J Pathol 172: 1482–1490.
39. Toro R, Perez-Isla L, Doxastaquis G, Barba MA, Gallego AR, et al. (2009) Clinical usefulness of tissue Doppler imaging in predicting preclinical Fabry cardiomyopathy. Int J Cardiol 132: 38–44.
40. Shah JS, Hughes DA, Sachdev B, Tome M, Ward D, et al. (2005) Prevalence and clinical significance of cardiac arrhythmia in Anderson-Fabry disease. Am J Cardiol 96: 842–846.
41. Mehta A, Clarke JT, Giugliani R, Elliott P, Linhart A, et al. (2009) Natural course of Fabry disease: changing pattern of causes of death in FOS - Fabry Outcome Survey. J Med Genet 46: 548–552.
42. Waldek S, Patel MR, Banikazemi M, Lemay R, Lee P (2009) Life expectancy and cause of death in males and females with Fabry disease: findings from the Fabry Registry. Genet Med 11: 790–796.
43. Kouris NT, Kontogianni DD, Pavlou MT, Babalis DK (2005) Atrioventricular conduction disturbances in a young patient with Fabry's disease without other signs of cardiac involvement. Int J Cardiol 99: 327–328.
44. Olivotto I, Gistri R, Petrone P, Pedemonte E, Vargiu D, et al. (2003) Maximum left ventricular thickness and risk of sudden death in patients with hypertrophic cardiomyopathy. J Am Coll Cardiol 41: 315–321.
45. Bierer G, Kamangar N, Balfe D, Wilcox WR, Mosenifar Z (2005) Cardiopulmonary exercise testing in Fabry disease. Respiration 72: 504–511.
46. Lobo T, Morgan J, Bjorksten A, Nicholls K, Grigg L, et al. (2008) Cardiovascular testing in Fabry disease: exercise capacity reduction, chronotropic incompetence and improved anaerobic threshold after enzyme replacement. Intern Med J 38: 407–414.
47. Tsai CT, Chiang FT, Tseng CD, Hwang JJ, Kuo KT, et al. (2010) Increased expression of mineralocorticoid receptor in human atrial fibrillation and a cellular model of atrial fibrillation. J Am Coll Cardiol 55: 758–770.
48. Marshall J, Ashe KM, Bangari D, McEachern K, Chuang WL, et al. (2010) Substrate reduction augments the efficacy of enzyme therapy in a mouse model of Fabry disease. PLoS One 5: e15033.

A Novel Role for Niemann-Pick Disease Type 2C Protein in Papillae Formation

Masahiro Sugawara[1,2]*, Hidemi Ohye[1], Chisato Tomoda[1], Takahiko Kogai[1], Yoshimasa Kamata[3], Gholam H. Pezeshkpour[4], Farhad Moatamed[4]

1 Endocrinology and Diabetes Division, Department of Medicine, Veterans Affairs Greater Los Angeles Health Care System, David Geffen School of Medicine at University of California Los Angeles, Los Angeles, California, United States of America, **2** Primary Care Service, Department of Medicine, Veterans Affairs Greater Los Angeles Health Care System, David Geffen School of Medicine, University of California Los Angeles, Los Angeles, California, United States of America, **3** Department of Pathology, Hirosaki University School of Medicine, Hirosaki, Japan, **4** Department of Pathology, Veterans Affairs Greater Los Angeles Health Care System, David Geffen School of Medicine, University of California Los Angeles, Los Angeles, California, United States of America

Abstract

Background: Despite the presence of papillary structures and papillary tumors in humans, the mechanism of papillae formation is unknown. We describe herein a novel role for Niemann-Pick disease type 2C (NPC2) protein, a cholesterol binding protein in the lysosome, in papillae formation.

Methodology/Principal Finding: We examined NPC2 protein expression in surgical samples of papillary tissues by immunohistochemical stain, and all papillary tissues expressed NPC2 protein in the epithelium. To examine our hypothesis of NPC2 protein-mediated papillae formation, we carried out xenograft experiments using wild H460 cells (large cell lung carcinoma cell line) that constitutively expressed abundant NPC2 protein and NPC2 protein-depleted H460 cells by *NPC2 shRNA*. The xenografts of wild H460 cells and empty *shRNA* vector cells showed distinct papillae formation, whereas NPC2 protein-depleted H460 cells displayed markedly reduced or no papillae. Since all papillary tissues have open spaces we examined whether NPC2 protein might also contribute to the creation of open spaces. The TUNEL assay in the xenografts of wild and empty *shRNA* vector H460 cells showed massive cell death, and NPC2 protein-depleted cells displayed minimal cell death. Measurement of caspase 3/7 activities in cultured H460 cells supported NPC2 protein-mediated apoptotic cell death. The presence of excess NPC2 protein, however, did not always produce papillae as seen in the xenografts of CHO cells that were stably transfected with *NPC2*.

Conclusions/Significance: The NPC2 protein of certain cells forms papillae coupled with apoptosis that creates open space. This protein may have future applications to modulate papillae formation and papillary growth in tumor tissues.

Editor: Vladimir N. Uversky, University of South Florida College of Medicine, United States of America

Funding: This work was supported by a Veterans Affairs Merit Review grant. The funders had no role in study design, data collection and analysis, decision to publish or preparation of the manuscript.

Competing Interests: The authors have declared that no competing interests exist.

* E-mail: msugawar@ucla.edu

Introduction

In humans, ovarian fimbria, choroid plexus of the brain, villi of the intestine, papillary cancer and papilloma are examples of papillary structure. Papillary structure consists of a fibrovascular core covered by epithelium creating nipple-like projections, called fronds. One unique feature of all papillary tissues is the presence of open spaces. There has been no report describing the mechanism of how papillae and open spaces are formed. We previously reported unique upregulation of *human epididymal protein-1* (*HE-1*) in papillary thyroid carcinoma by two-dimensional cDNA electrophoresis, an unbiased gene screening [1]. This gene was later named as *Niemann-Pick disease type C2* (*NPC2*) because mutation of this gene causes Niemann-Pick disease type 2C, a fatal cholesterol storage disorder of the lysosome [2,3]. Our previous study suggested that the NPC2 could be a specific protein for human papillary structures [1]. In this study, all papillary tissues uniformly expressed NPC2 protein in the epithelium. Then, we hypothesized that the NPC2 protein could be involved in papillae formation. To examine this hypothesis, we carried out xenograft experiments using NPC2 protein-rich and-depleted H460 cells. Our present study revealed the requirement of NPC2 protein for papillary structure formation in certain cells. We describe here new functions of the NPC2 protein—papillae formation and creation of open spaces by apoptosis.

Results

Expression of NPC2 protein in papillary tissues

All papillary tissues examined so far showed cytoplasmic NPC2 protein in the epithelium as representative samples of normal papillae, papilloma and papillary cancer are shown in Figure 1. In addition, choroid plexus of the brain, colon polyps, and papillary carcinomas of breast expressed NPC2 protein (not shown here). Thus, NPC2 protein is associated with all papillary structures; this raised the possibility that NPC2 protein might contribute to

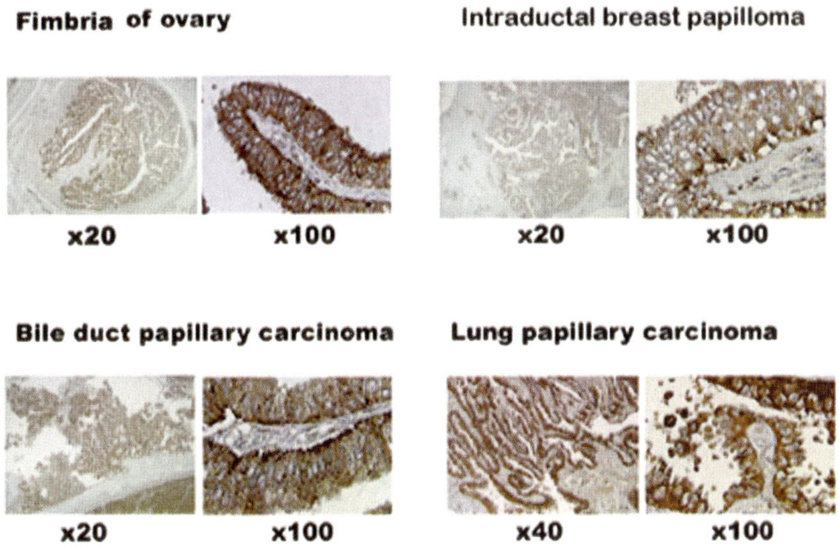

Figure 1. NPC2 protein expression in human papillary tissues. Immunohistochemical stain showed the presence of cytoplasmic NPC2 protein (brown color) in surgical samples of human papillary tissues. All papillary tissues have open spaces outside of papillary projections. The numbers indicate the degree of the magnification.

papillae formation. To examine this hypothesis, we used NPC2 protein-rich and-depleted H460 cells.

Characterization of wild H460 cells, empty vector and *NPC2-shRNA* containing H460 cells

Wild H460 cells and empty *shRNA* vector H460 cells showed the same cell morphology; cells grew attaching each other. H460 cells containing *NPC2-shRNA* grew as separate and individual cells (Figure 2A). Cell proliferation activity in *NPC2-shRNA* containing cells was less than 50% of that of empty vector cells after the 3rd day of culture (Figure 2B). Immunohistochemical stain showed abundant NPC2 protein in wild H460 cells and empty vector cells, whereas *NPC2-shRNA*-containing H460 cells had markedly reduced NPC2 protein expression (Figure 3).

Papillae formation in xenografts

We injected the three types of H460 cells (wild cells, empty vector cells, and *NPC2-shRNA*-containing cells) into nude mice and examined xenografts for papillae formation. The xenografts of wild H460 and empty vector cells showed distinct papillae formation, whereas NPC2-depleted H460 cells failed to show papilla (Figure 4A). The fibrovascular core covered by epithelium was clearly seen in the enlarged papilla. Immunohistochemistry showed localization of NPC2 protein in the entire epithelium of papillae, and little NPC2 protein was seen in NPC2-depleted cells as expected (Figure 4B).

Requirement of apoptosis to form papillary shape

Papillary structures require open spaces between papillary fronds (Figure 1). We speculated that apoptosis might be responsible for creating these open spaces. The TUNEL assay from the xenograft of wild H460 cells showed massive cell death due to DNA fragmentation, whereas the xenograft of NPC2 protein-depleted H4607 cells had minimal cell death (Figure 5). Interestingly, the transition from epithelial cells to apoptotic cells was clearly seen in the outer border of epithelium (middle panel of Figure 5). To validate NPC2 protein-mediated apoptotic cell death, we measured caspase 3/7 activities from cultured H460 cells (empty vector cells and *NPC2-shRNA* containing cells); both cells were cultured under the identical conditions in the presence of hygromycin B. As shown in Table 1, caspase 3/7 activity in NPC2 protein-depleted cells was 13% of that of empty vector cells.

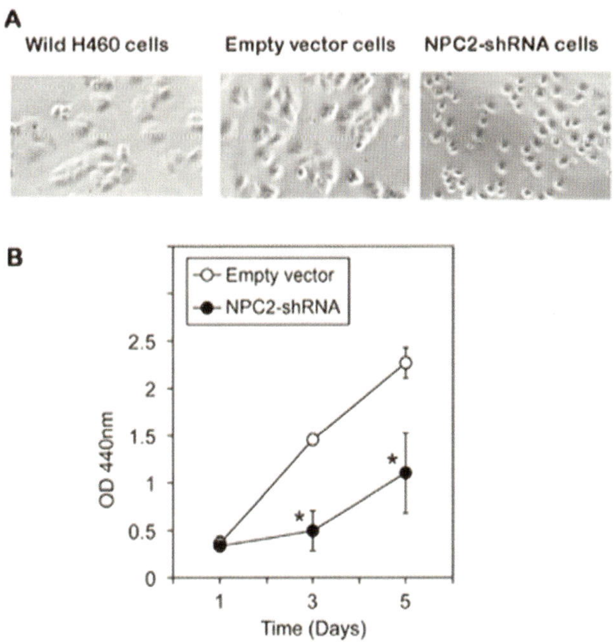

Figure 2. Characterization of three types of cultured H460 cells. Cell morphology: Wild and empty vector cells showed the same cell morphology, whereas cells containing *NPC2-shRNA* displayed clearly separated individual cells. Cell proliferation activity in NPC2-rich and-depleted H460 cells: Cells (1000 cells/well) were plated into a 96-well plate. Cell proliferation activity on each day was measured by incubating cells with the reagents for 2 hours in a CO2 incubator. The results are mean ± SD of quadruplicate samples of one of the three experiments. *$p<0.01$ when compared with the empty vector cells.

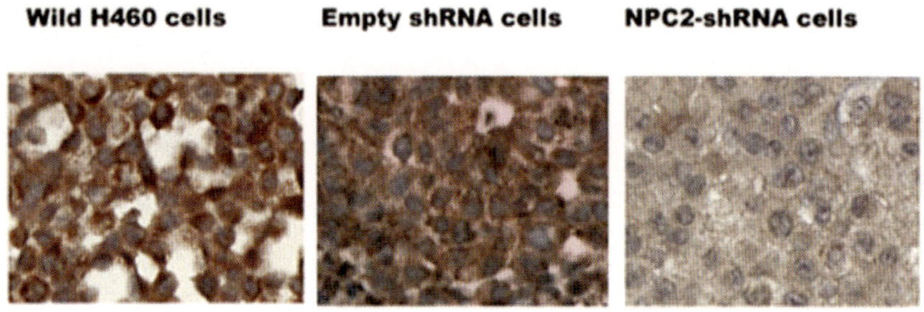

Figure 3. NPC2 protein expression in cultured H460 cells. Immunohistochemical staining showed abundant NPC2 protein in wild and empty vector cells and markedly reduced NPC2 protein in *NPC2-shRNA*-containing cells.

Also, CHO cells stably transfected with *NPC2* showed a distinct caspase 3/7 activity expressed as relative luminescent unit (RLU) of $78\times10^4 \pm 15\times10^4$ (mean ± SD of 3 determinations), whereas wild CHO cells had almost no caspase activity (RLU of 0 to 66). The presence of apoptotic cells was confirmed in surgical samples of human papillary tissues by the TUNEL assay (Figure 6).

Papillae formation by NPC2 protein-enriched CHO cells

We examined whether NPC2 protein-mediated papillae formation takes place regardless of cell types. Wild CHO cells showed very little NPC2 protein, and transfected cells displayed abundant NPC2 protein (Figure 7a, b). The xenograft of CHO cells stably transfected with *NPC2* failed to show visible papilla, despite abundant NPC2 protein expression (Figure 7c). Thus, excessive amount of NPC2 protein does not universally lead to papillae formation in some cells.

Discussion

This study is focused on the mechanism of papillae formation, an unexplored area. Surgical specimens of all papillary tissues examined so far expressed NPC2 protein in the epithelium of papillae without exception (Figure 1). In fact, any form of papillary projections, such as intrafollicular papillary projection in goiter tissues [1] and colon polyps expressed NPC2 protein. Why is NPC2 protein present in all papillary tissues? We speculated that NC2 protein might be involved for formation of papillae. To demonstrate NPC2-mediated papillae formation in xenografts, cells expressing abundant NPC2 protein and depleted NPC2 protein are required. After screening several cancer cell lines, we found wild H460 cell line that constitutively expressed abundant NPC2 protein (Figure 3). To deplete *NPC2* in H460 cells, we constructed *shRNA* for *NPC2*, and our selected clone showed persistent and profound depletion of NPC2 protein (Figure 3). The xenografts of wild H460 cells and empty *shRNA* vector cells showed many papillae, whereas NPC2-depleted cells showed markedly reduced or no papillae formation depending on the microscopic fields examined (Figure 4). We attempted to create different levels of NPC2 protein expression by mixing wild H460 cells and *NPC2-shRNA* containing H460 cells with 1:1 or 1:5 ratios (wild cells: *NPC2-shRNA* treated cells). The xenografts of the mixed cells always showed many papillae as seen in the xenograft of wild H460 cells probably due to overwhelming growth of wild H460 cells over *NPC2-shRNA* containing cells. Decreased cell proliferation activity by *NPC2-shRNA* containing cells (Figure 2B) supports this phenomenon. Restricted localization of NPC2 protein to the

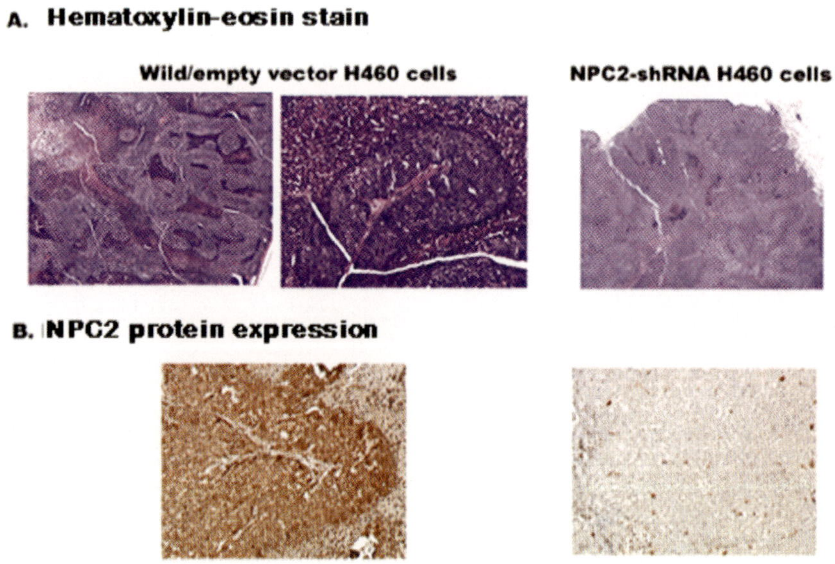

Figure 4. Papillae formation in xenografts of three types of H460 cells. A: Hematoxylin-eosin stain. B: Immunohistochemical stain for NPC2 protein. Distinct papillae formation was seen in wild and empty vector cells. No papilla was seen in *NPC2-shRNA* containing cells (A). NPC2 protein was localized in the epithelium of papillae (B).

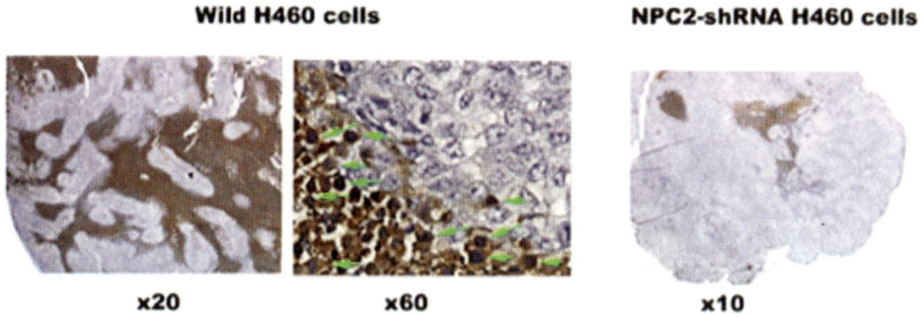

Figure 5. TUNEL assay in xenografts NPC2 protein-rich and-depleted cells. Apoptotic ell death was seen between papillary structures (brown colored areas) in wild H460 cells. The transition from epithelial cells (blue colored cells) to apoptotic cells (brown colored cells) was seen in the outer border of epithelium (middle panel). NPC2 protein-depleted H460 cells showed only small areas of apoptotic cell death.

epithelium suggests a specific role for NPC2 protein in papillary fronds formation. One unique feature of all papillary tissues is the presence of open spaces (Figure 1), and this could be crucial for the growth of papillary fronds. The mechanism of creating these open spaces has never been addressed. The TUNEL assay in the xenografts of wild H460 cells showed massive cell death between papillary fronds and a minimal cell death in NPC2 protein-depleted cells (Figure 5). Apoptosis is defined by caspase-mediated cell death [4]. Measurement of caspase 3/7 activities in cultured H460 cells supports NPC2 protein-mediated apoptosis (Table 1). Also, the TUNEL assay from human samples showed apoptotic cells (Figure 6). Apoptosis in papillary tissues can be summarized as follows. 1) Epithelial cells producing NPC2 protein can become apoptotic. 2) Apoptosis starts from the outer border of the epithelium. 3) Apoptosis should contribute to the formation of open spaces in papillary structures. In addition, apoptotic activity was seen in CHO cells transfected with *NPC2* but not in wild CHO cells. The NPC2 protein is localized in the lysosome for cholesterol binding and transport [2,3], and the lysosome can activate intrinsic and extrinsic pathways of apoptosis under certain conditions [5]. Our study suggests that NPC2 protein itself can cause apoptosis. The mechanism of triggering apoptosis by excessive NPC2 protein has yet to be studied.

The question can be raised whether the expression of abundant NPC2 protein alone is sufficient to form papillae regardless of cell types. We examined this question in CHO cells that were stably transfected with *NPC2*. No papilla formation was seen in the xenografts, despite abundant NPC2 protein (Figure 7C). This finding suggests that an increase in cholesterol binding to NPC2 protein and its transport to the membrane, well known function of NPC2, is not solely responsible for papillae formation. Similarly, human liver highly expresses *NPC2* without papillary structure [2]. Therefore, an enrichment of NPC2 protein alone does not always produce papillae in certain cells. It is conceivable that additional factors or proteins are required to form papillae together with the NPC2 protein. We had an opportunity to examine *NPC2*

Table 1. Caspase 3/7 activities in cultured H460 cells.

Cell types	Caspase 3/7 activities
Empty vector cells	100%±12.5%
NPC2-shRNA cells	13.5%±5.8%

Caspase activity of empty vector cell is considered as 100%. The results are mean ± SD of three different experiments performed in duplicates. *$p<0.0004$.

hypomorphous mouse expressing 0–4% of NPC2 protein; this mouse was kindly provided by Dr. Peter Lobel [6]. We found normal papillae in the choroid plexus of the brain and villi of the intestine in this mouse. Therefore, the discrepancy of papillae formation between xenograft experiments (tumor of *NPC2* depleted cells under the skin) and live animal model (born with *NPC2* defect) exists. It is speculated that this mouse model may have NPC2 independent mechanisms or might have developed alternative mechanisms to form papillae. In humans, patients with Niemann-Pick Disease type 2C represent human model of NPC2 protein depletion. However, there is no autopsy report examining papillary tissues in this disorder.

The clinical application of NPC2 protein in papillae forming diseases has yet to be identified. Upregulation of *NPC2* in human papillary thyroid cancer [1] and significant decrease in cell proliferation in *NPC2*-depleted H460 cells (Figure 2B) suggest that NPC2 protein may also control cell proliferation in papillary tumors. Whether blocking NPC2 action has any therapeutic value for papillary cancer has yet to be studied in vivo. Exogenous NPC2 protein is taken into cells via two mannose 6 phosphate receptors that are ubiquitously present in the membrane [7] and corrected the abnormality of cholesterol handling in fibroblasts from a patient with *NPC2* mutation [2]. Therefore, it is interesting to examine whether addition of exogenous NPC2 protein restores disrupted papillary structures, such as epithelial atrophy of choroid plexus in Alzheimer disease [8].

Methods

Ethical statement

Paraffin sections of surgical samples were obtained from Hirosaki University Hospital, Hirosaki, Japan. The ethical committee of Hirosaki University School of Medicine exempted this human study including obtaining the consent from patients because paraffin section samples are 13 year-old with unidentifiable patients and no direct linkage of this study to the health care management. This is in accord with the human study guidelines established by the Ministry of Education and Science and the Ministry of Health and Welfare in Japan.

The animal experiments proposed here were fully approved by the GLA-VA Institutional Animal Care and Use Committee (IACUC) with protocol number of 02004-05. All animal experiments were carried out under the regulation of IACUC.

Cells and surgical samples

H460 cells (large cell lung cancer cell line) and CHO cells (Chinese ovarian cells) were obtained from ATCC, Manassas, VA., and cultured in RPMI1640 medium and F-12 medium,

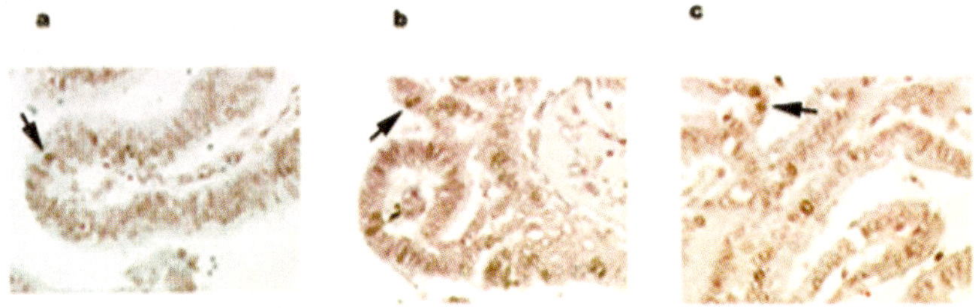

Figure 6. Presence of apoptotic cells in human papillary tissues. TUNEL assay showed the presence of apoptotic cells in representative samples of human papillary tissues; arrows indicate examples of apoptotic cells.

respectively, in the presence of 10% fetal bovine serum and antibiotic cocktail.

Preparation for NPC2 protein-rich and-depleted cells

We used wild H460 cells, since this cell line constitutively expressed abundant NPC2 protein. We also made NPC2 protein-rich CHO cells by stable transfection of CHO cells with *NPC2*. For the *NPC2* transfection experiment, we obtained the entire coding region of human *NPC2 cDNA* (NM_006432) from 3 µg total RNA of BHP 2-7 human papillary thyroid cancer cells by two-step RT-PCR using Superscript III (Invitrogen, CA.), Expand High Fidelity PCR System (Roche Applied Science, Indianapolis, IN), and custom primers (Invitrogen), 5′-GATGCGTTTCCTGGCAGCTA-3′ and 5′-CTGCTAACCAAGTGCTGCAT-3′. We introduced the amplicons into the *pCR 2.1* vector (Invitrogen), confirmed the correct sequences of the insert, and sub-cloned it into a mammalian expression vector *pcDNA3* (Invitrogen) with *Hind*III and *Xba*I (New England Biolabs, Ipswich, MA). We carried out transfection of CHO cells with *NPC2* in *pcDNA3* using Effectene Transfection Reagents (Qiagen, Valencia, CA) and selected clones expressing constant and abundant NPC2 protein in the presence of geneticin. Wild CHO cells contained very little NPC2 protein.

NPC2 knockdown experiments in H460 cells

We designed the target DNA sequences corresponding to *NPC2-shRNA* using the online program (Applied Biosystems/Ambion, Austin, TX) and ligated the target DNA to the *pSilencer3.1-H1 hygro* vector (Applied Biosystems/Ambion). After confirming the correct sequences of the insert from the amplified plasmid, we transfected H460 cells with *NPC2-shRNA* or *shRNA* vector alone (empty vector) using the T-20 program of the Amaxa Nucleofector II (Lonza Group, Ltd., Boston, MA). We selected stably transfected clones by culturing cells in the presence of 500 µg/ml hygromycin B (Invitrogen). The silencing effect of *NPC2-shRNA* on *NPC2* and its protein expression was confirmed by RT-PCR and immunohistochemistry staining, respectively. The most effective *NPC2-shRNA* insert inhibiting NPC2 protein expression contained the following sequences: 5′GATCCGTGGTATCCAGTGATTCGTTCTCAAGAGAAACGAATCACTGGATACCATTTTTTGGAAA-3′, and 5′AGCTTTTCCAAAAAATGGTATCCAGTGATTCGTTTCTCTTGAGAACGAATCACTGGATACCACG-3′.

Animal experiments

We obtained female nude mice (15 g) from Charles-River Laboratories INC, Wilmington, MA, and all animals were kept in sterile cages. We injected 10^6 cells in 0.1 ml phosphate buffered saline (PBS) subcutaneously to the flank region of mice. After tumors grew to 1–1.5 cm in diameter, we sacrificed animals in a CO2 chamber, removed tumors, and kept sliced tumor samples in formalin for immunostaining.

Immunohistochemical staining, TUNEL assay and image analysis

Immunohistochemical studies were performed on formaldehyde-fixed, paraffin-embedded tissues. Deparaffinized sliced sections were incubated for 60 min at room temperature with the rabbit polyclonal anti-human NPC2 antiserum (1:1000). Polyclonal anti-human NPC2 antibody was kindly provided by Dr. Peter Lobel, Rutgers University. Immunostaining was carried out using a Dako autostainer in conjunction with the EnVision™ detection kits (Dako, Carpinteria, CA). Positive controls (human epididymis tissue originally shown to express NPC2) and negative controls (without antibody) were used for NPC2 immunostaining. For TUNEL assay in sliced tissues, we used Apop Tag Peroxidases In Site Apoptosis Detection kit (Millipore Co., Bellireca, MA). For image analysis, we used Metamorph™ image analysis software version 7.5 (Molecular devices, Downingtown, PA).

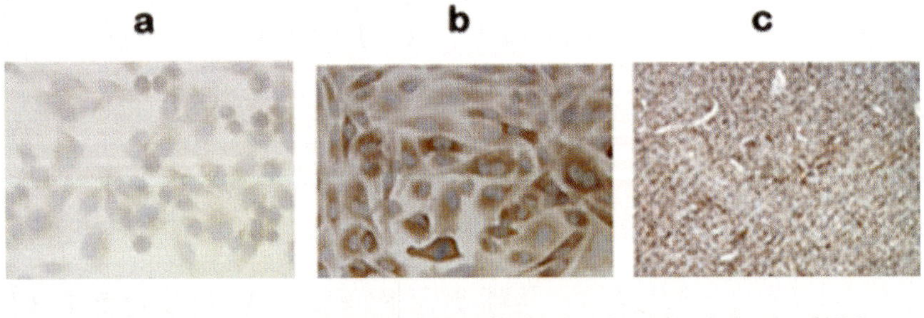

Figure 7. NPC2 protein expression in CHO cells. Immunohistochemical stain of NPC2 protein in wild CHO cell (a), CHO cells stably transfected with *NPC2* (b) and xenograft of CHO cells transfected with *NPC2* (c). No papilla was seen in the xenograft, despite abundant NPC2 protein expression.

Caspase activity assay

Caspase 3/7 activities were measured from cultured cells using Promega caspase-Glo luminescent method (Promega, Madison, WI). We used H460 cells containing empty *shRNA* vector and *NPC2-shRNA*. These cells were thawed on the same day and cultured in 6-well plate in the presence of hygromycin B until 80% confluence was achieved. Cells were washed with PBS twice and sonicated in 1 ml PBS. An aliquot of 50 µl sonicate corresponding to 6×10^4 cells was used immediately for caspase 3/7 assay. Each assay was run with or without 5 units Z-VAD-FMK, caspase inhibitor (Promega), by incubating the reaction mixture for 30 min at 37°C, and relative luminescent unit (RLU) was measured by GloMax 20/20 luminometer (Promega). We defined caspase activity as the RLU that was inhibited in the presence of caspase inhibitor. Similarly, we measured caspase3/7 activities from wild CHO cells and transfected CHO cells with *NPC2*.

Cell proliferation assay

We used empty vector cells and *NPC2-shRNA* cells by plating 1000 cells/well in a 96-well plate; they were cultured under the identical condition in the presence of hygromycin B. Cell proliferation was measured using a quick cell proliferation assay kit (BioVision, Mountain View, CA) on first, third and fifth days of cell culture. The optical density from each well was measured at 440 nm using a microplate reader (Molecular devices, Sunnyvale, CA).

Statistical analysis

The results of caspase activity and cell proliferation assay were analyzed by Student's *t*-test based on difference of variance (F test). The p value less than 0.05 were considered significant.

Acknowledgments

We thank Dr. Peter Lobel for providing us with NPC2 polyclonal antibody and *NPC2* hypomorphous mouse.

Author Contributions

Conceived and designed the experiments: MS HO CT TK YK GHP FM. Performed the experiments: MS HO CT TK YK GHP FM. Analyzed the data: MS TK YK GHP FM. Contributed reagents/materials/analysis tools: MS HO CT TK YK FM. Wrote the paper: MS HO TK GHP. Paraffin preparation of surgical samples: YK. Microscopic examination of xenograft: YK GHP FM.

References

1. Asakawa J, Kodaira M, Ishikawa N, Nagataki S, Motatamed F, et al. (2002) Two-dimensional complementary deoxyribonucleic acid electrophoresis revealing up-regulated human epididymal protein 1 and down-regulated C100 in papillary thyroid carcinoma. Endocrinology 143: 4422–4428.
2. Naureckiene S, Sleat DE, Lackland H, Fensom A, Vanier MT, et al. (2000) Identification of HE1 as the second gene of Niemann-Pick C disease. Science 290: 2298–2301.
3. Storch J, Xu Z (2009) Niemann-Pick C2 (NPC2) and intracellular cholesterol trafficking. Biochim Biophys Acta 1791: 671–678.
4. Samali A, Zhivotovsky B, Jones D, Nagata S, Orrenius S (1999) Apoptosis: cell death defined by caspase activation. Cell Death Differ 6: 495–6.
5. Kurz T, Eaton JW, Brunk UT (2010) Redox activity within the lysosomal compartment: implications for aging and apoptosis. Antioxid Redox Signal 13: 511–523.
6. Sleat DE, Wiseman JA, El-Banna M, Price SM, Verot L, et al. (2004) Genetic evidence for nonredundant functional cooperativity between NPC1 and NPC2 in lipid transport. Proc Natl Acad Sci U S A 101: 5886–5891.
7. Willenborg M, Schmidt CK, Braun P, Landgrebe J, von Figura K, et al. (2005) Mannose 6-phosphate receptors, Niemann-Pick C2 protein, and lysosomal cholesterol accumulation. J Lipid Res 46: 2559–69.
8. Serot JM, Béné MC, Foliguet B, Faure GC (2000) Morphological alterations of the choroid plexus in late-onset Alzheimer's disease. Acta Neuropathol 99: 105–108.

4

Defining Natural History: Assessment of the Ability of College Students to Aid in Characterizing Clinical Progression of Niemann-Pick Disease, Type C

Jenny Shin[1]✉, Katrina Epperson[1]✉, Nicole M. Yanjanin[2], Jennifer Albus[3], Laura Borgenheimer[3], Natalie Bott[3], Erin Brennan[3], Daniel Castellanos[3], Melissa Cheng[3], Michael Clark[3], Margaret Devany[3], Courtney Ensslin[3], Nina Farivari[3], Shanik Fernando[3], Lauren Gabriel[3], Rani Gallardo[3], Moriah Castleman[3], Olimpia Gutierrez[3], Allison Herschel[3], Sarah Hodge[3], Anne Horst[3], Mary Howard[3], Evan James[3], Lindsey Jones[3], Mary Kearns[3], Mary Kelly[3], Christine Kim[3], Kinzie Kiser[3], Gregory Klazura[3], Chris Knoedler[3], Emily Kolbus[3], Lauren Lange[3], Joan Lee[3], Eileena Li[3], Wei Lu[3], Andrew Luttrell[3], Emily Ly[3], Katherine McKeough[3], Brianna McSorley[3], Catherine Miller[3], Sean Mitchell[3], Abbey Moon[3], Kevin Moser[3], Shane O'Brien[3], Paula Olivieri[3], Aaron Patzwahl[3], Marie Pereira[3], Craig Pymento[3], Erin Ramelb[3], Bryce Ramos[3], Teresa Raya[3], Stephen Riney[3], Geoff Roberts[3], Mark Robertshaw[3], Frannie Rudolf[3], Samuel Rund[3], Stephanie Sansone[3], Lindsay Schwartz[3], Ryan Shay[3], Edwin Siu[3], Timothy Spear[3], Catherine Tan[3], Marisa Truong[3], Mairaj Uddin[3], Jennifer VanTrieste[3], Omar Veloz[3], Elizabeth White[3], Forbes D. Porter[2], Kasturi Haldar[1]*

1 Center for Rare and Neglected Diseases, University of Notre Dame, Notre Dame, Indiana, United States of America, **2** Program in Developmental Endocrinology and Genetics, NICHD, National Institutes of Health, DHHS, Bethesda, Maryland, United States of America, **3** NPC Consortium for Community-Based Assessment of Patient Records, Cape Town, South Africa

Abstract

Niemann-Pick Disease, type C (NPC) is a fatal, neurodegenerative, lysosomal storage disorder. It is a rare disease with broad phenotypic spectrum and variable age of onset. These issues make it difficult to develop a universally accepted clinical outcome measure to assess urgently needed therapies. To this end, clinical investigators have defined emerging, disease severity scales. The average time from initial symptom to diagnosis is approximately 4 years. Further, some patients may not travel to specialized clinical centers even after diagnosis. We were therefore interested in investigating whether appropriately trained, community-based assessment of patient records could assist in defining disease progression using clinical severity scores. In this study we evolved a secure, step wise process to show that pre-existing medical records may be correctly assessed by non-clinical practitioners trained to quantify disease progression. Sixty-four undergraduate students at the University of Notre Dame were expertly trained in clinical disease assessment and recognition of major and minor symptoms of NPC. Seven clinical records, randomly selected from a total of thirty seven used to establish a leading clinical severity scale, were correctly assessed to show expected characteristics of linear disease progression. Student assessment of two new records donated by NPC families to our study also revealed linear progression of disease, but both showed accelerated disease progression, relative to the current severity scale, especially at the later stages. Together, these data suggest that college students may be trained in assessment of patient records, and thus provide insight into the natural history of a disease.

Editor: Markus Schuelke, Charité Universitätsmedizin Berlin, NeuroCure Clinical Research Center, Germany

Funding: The work was supported in part by funds to KH (start-up funds from the University of Notre Dame), to FDP (intramural research program of NICHD and via a Bench to Bedside Grant from the Office of Rare Diseases), and to NY (Ara Parseghian Medical Research Foundation, http://www.parseghian.org/, and Dana's Angels Research Trust, www.DanasAngels.org). The funders had no role in study design, data collection and analysis, decision to publish, or preparation of the manuscript.

Competing Interests: The authors have declared that no competing interests exist.

* E-mail: khaldar@nd.edu

✉ These authors contributed equally to this work.

Introduction

Niemann-Pick Disease, type C (NPC) is a lysosomal, cholesterol storage disorder [1]. It is an autosomal, recessive, rare disease with a prevalence in the range of 1:120,000 to 150,000 [2]. Although the earliest manifestations are splenomegaly and hepatomegaly, clinically, it presents as a broad spectrum of neurological problems. This in conjunction with highly variable age of onset (ranging from fetal to adult) makes it difficult to diagnose [3, also reviewed in 2]. Indeed, the average time from initial symptom to diagnosis is approximately 4 years. Even after diagnosis, which comprises of a skin biopsy to obtain fibroblasts to demonstrate accumulation of unesterified cholesterol or genetic testing, there is need for a universally accepted clinical outcome measure for testing urgently needed new therapeutics as well as disease management. Clinical investigators have defined emerging, disease severity scales [4,5], the most comprehensive of which was recently reported by Yanjanin et al., 2010 [6], as part of a natural history study being conducted at the National Institutes of Health (NIH).

However, since the incidence of NPC is low, the number of patients seen in a clinical center is limited. Many patients will not travel to specialized clinical centers (even a national center like the NIH) after diagnosis, because of the paucity of therapies, lack of information about programs, as well as significant logistical issues. In addition to enrolling 18 patients on the current study, Yanjanin et al. [6] were also able to utilize 19 clinical records archived at the NIH, and this led to the suggestion that assessment of patient records donated by families including records of patients who have died from the disease, may be used to rapidly strengthen emerging clinical severity scales.

For a rare disease like NPC, scales derived from a larger set of clinical records would represent a significant advance in capturing a standardized clinical outcome measure. However due to limited resources associated with rare disease research, only a number of physicians specialize in NPC, suggesting that community-based assessment of clinical records by trained volunteers could greatly facilitate generation of disease severity scales and other clinical tools. As a first step towards this goal we undertook to develop a scalable model in which pre-existing medical records may be correctly assessed by non clinical practitioners trained to quantify disease progression and assemble succinct clinical summaries. If successful, this model could be implemented to assist in the collection of natural history data for other rare diseases.

Methods

Ethics statement

The study was an extension of a Natural History study performed at the National Institutes of Health in Bethesda, Maryland. It was approved by the University of Notre Dame Institutional Review Board (09-174), as well as the Eunice Kennedy Shriver National Institute of Child Health and Human Development Institutional Review Board (06-CH-0186, *NCT00344331*). Consent and if appropriate assent, were obtained from guardians and patients. All students received HIPAA training in class, prior to reviewing private patient data.

Participants and procedures

The study was developed to ascertain whether non-clinical practitioners who were trained over a few weeks to recognize NPC clinical disease, could extract clinical severity scores from patient records. The clinical severity scale of Yanjanin et al. 2010 [6] was adopted. This scale has been validated with data from 37 patient records. 18 of these records were from a cross sectional study of current NPC patients. An additional 19 were obtained from longitudinal chart review of a 'historic' cohort at the NIH, and thus the scale is expected to be useful as a long-term outcome measure for biomarkers and therapeutic trials. The scale utilizes nine major and eight minor clinical symptomatic domains, with a Likert-like scale to assign scores of 0-5 and 0-2 in each domain-type respectively. The total scores can range from 0 to 61 and higher scores indicate increased disease burden.

Training of students was done in an in-class room setting because this is an easily scalable format. The class, entitled Developing Health Networks in Rare and Neglected Diseases was developed by the Center for Rare and Neglected Diseases (CRND) at the University of Notre Dame in collaboration with the Eunice Kennedy Shriver National Institute of Child Health and Human Development (NICHD) and consultation with the Center for Social Concerns at the University of Notre Dame, Riley Children's Hospital, the National Niemann Pick Disease Foundation (NNPDF), the Ara Parseghian Medical Research Foundation (APMRF) and the Niemann-Pick Disease Group (UK).

5-30 students were enrolled per class for four classes in Spring 2009, Fall 2009, Spring 2010 and Spring 2011. Registration required the instructor's permission (the class was restricted to upper level undergraduate students). For the initial class in Spring 2009 two graduate students were also allowed to enroll to determine whether the course was better suited to post graduate rather than undergraduate students A total of sixty four undergraduates and two graduate students were enrolled over the indicated semesters. The class met once a week for 3 contact hours.

All students registered for the course indicated no prior experience in clinical research. Thus, for all students, this class represented the first exposure to critical concepts pertinent for developing therapies for rare and neglected diseases in general and specifically Niemann-Pick type C. Students researched multiple NPC family narratives publicly available via the internet, to understand the socioeconomic and cultural impact of NPC disease. Students were then instructed on NPC diagnosis, symptoms and clinical history through a combination of didactic lectures and reading of clinical research papers, as well as discussions with clinical practitioners and researchers in NPC disease (http://nd.edu/crnd/CTSSeriesAnnouncements.html).

In Spring 2009, five students (3 undergraduate and 2 graduate students) were assigned a single clinical history previously assessed by Yanjanin et al., 2010 [6]. In Fall and Spring 2010, the class size was expanded to 16 students and an additional three clinical histories from Yanjanin et al. [6] were also assessed by students working in teams of four. In Spring 2011, each of these four clinical histories as well as three additional histories taken from Yanjanin et al., 2010 [6] were assessed in groups of six students scoring in pairs, creating triplicate values for each case. This was done to directly determine the variability in disease severity assessments ascribed to a medical history, when conducted by a pairs of students in the same class environment. In Spring 2011, we also tested the variability in disease severity assessments across 30 students when each student independently assessed disease severity for a new case directly donated to our study. In all semesters, a single clinical visit was first assessed in class to confirm that the logistics of scoring was uniformly understood by the group. Students then scored the entire clinical history as a take home exercise to generate individual disease severity curves. In Spring 2009, Fall 2009 and Spring 2010, the disease severity curves were subsequently reviewed and finalized in consultation with clinical experts pediatric nurse practitioner Nicole M. Yanjanin and physician-scientist Forbes D. Porter from the intramural research program of Eugene Kennedy Shriver National Institute of Child Health and Human Development (NICHD). The indicated disease severity curves incorporated the concept of the 'carry-over' effect which is based on the principle that increased score for a symptomatic domain in a prior visit is 'carried' through to a subsequent clinical visit in absence of any additional information pertaining to the domain. Thus if a patient is wheel chair dependent on one visit, this is assumed to be true in

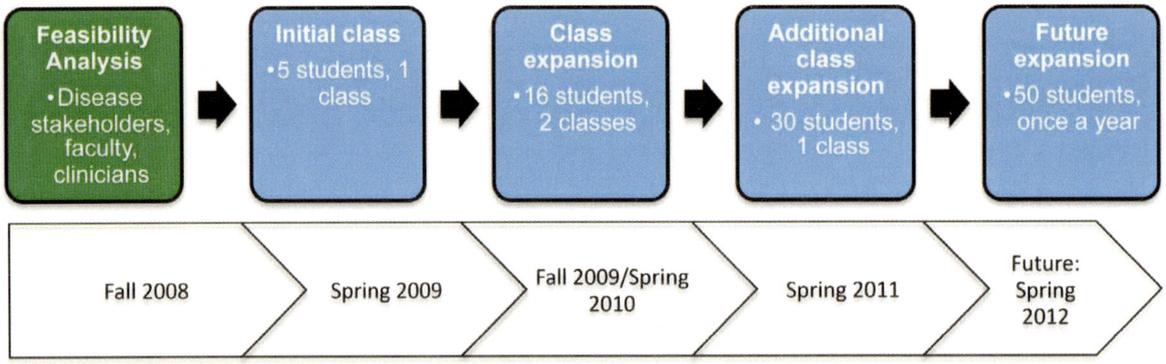

Figure 1. Overall work flow undertaken to assess the ability of college students to assist in characterizing clinical progression of Niemann Pick Type C. The project began in Fall 2008 with discussions with the Center for Social Concerns at the University of Notre Dame, Riley Children's Hospital, Indianapolis, the National Niemann Pick Disease Foundation (NNPDF), the Ara Parseghian Medical Research Foundation (APMRF) and the Niemann-Pick Disease Group (UK), clinical practitioners at Eunice Kennedy Shriver National Institute of Child Health and Human Development (NICHD) and faculty and program staff the Center for Rare and Neglected Diseases (CRND) at the University of Notre Dame.

a subsequent visit, unless specified otherwise. In Spring 2011, the 'carry-over' effect was discussed prior to the visits for Yanjanin and Porter in order to incorporate it as a standard feature of 'in class' training. The overall work flow is summarized in Figure 1.

NPC families were made aware of the study at the 2009 and 2010 NNPDF family meetings in Seattle, Washington and Toronto, Canada, respectively. Consenting families submitted records through NNPDF to the NIHCD team. An amendment was made to the existing protocol, which then allowed for the records to be forwarded from the NIHCD to the CRND at the University of Notre Dame.

Results

Early discussions (in Fall 2008) with major stakeholders in the NPC disease community including, foundations, clinical practitioners and families, led to the concept that direct interactions between students and patient groups may fail to protect vulnerabilities of both groups. However, assessment of disease from clinical records by appropriately trained students and collaboration with clinical practitioners was likely to offer a secure process of engagement, training and research.

Comprehensive training of students in clinical NPC disease manifestation, diagnosis and management and requisite medical terminology required 4 weeks of a 12 week semester, with three hours of in-class time and three to six hours of out-of-class time per week. Followed by one, three hour in-class training session focused on a single clinical visit from one record, all assessments were carried out independently by students as part of 'take-home' exercises. The first specific product generated by the class was a list of medical terminology used to describe major and minor symptomatic domains (Table 1). This assisted understanding and recognition of symptoms by the students. This list was additionally expanded to include clinical terms encountered in patient histories received over four semesters and has evolved as a key, starting reference tool (Table S1) in assessing new clinical records.

Scoring and disease severity curve generated from NPC patient records obtained from Yanjanin et al., 2010 [6]

The first class in Spring of 2009 was limited to five students, three senior undergraduate students who were also Science majors as well as two graduate students in Biological Sciences. The group assessed one medical history. The small group size and close supervision was deemed appropriate since this type of class on clinical research had not previously been offered for undergraduate students. Five independent disease severity curves were extracted from a single clinical history. As shown in Figure 2A, there was close correspondence between student assessments. For any given symptomatic domain the differences in scores assigned were no greater than 1 (not shown). The indicated disease severity curves incorporated of the concept of 'carry-over' (see Methods) The average curve and mean progression score were overlayed on the data of Yanjanin et al. 2010 [6] (Fig. 2B and C). The rate of change for this patient, 1.315 closely corresponds to 1.3 previously reported by Yanjanin et al., 2010 [6].

These data tentatively suggested that upper level undergraduate college students could be trained to recognize disease domains in clinical records and compute disease severity scores. Our impression was that there was no difference in the work product of undergraduate and graduate students. This justified opening subsequent class enrollment to undergraduate juniors and seniors who were declared as Premedical (also referred to as Pre-Professional) and/or majors in Biological Sciences, Chemistry or Biochemistry, and thus an expansion in class size.

With a larger class, we adopted group-wise assessment of clinical records, to minimize operator variability. Thus in Fall 2009 and Spring 2010, when the class sizes were expanded to 14-16, four groups of three to five students were assigned the same clinical record assessed by the initial class as well as three additional medical histories from Yanjanin et al. 2010 [6], for assessment. As shown in Fig. 3A, for a given case, the variation to the mean was comparable across data points in disease progression curves. These data suggested that over two semesters, junior and senior undergraduate students with basic (200 level) background course work in life sciences, could be sufficiently trained in recognition and quantification of disease domains and work in groups of 3–5 to generate consistent disease progression curves from clinical histories.

Since our long term goal is to maximize the capacity of student assessment, in the subsequent semester we increased the class enrollment from 16 to 30. We also investigated the assessment of records by pairs of students. A single case was assigned to three pairs of students within a 'group' to rigorously assess variation between pairs within a single class. Of the seven assigned cases, four had been reviewed by the prior classes. The slopes of the disease severity scales in Spring 2011 (Fig. 3B) were comparable to those seen in prior semesters (Fig. 3A), with an average of ~15%

Table 1. NP-C terms students *must* know.

Ambulation	To walk from place to place; move about.
Auditory Brainstem Response	An electrical output in response to sound, a response to a complex signal.
Biomarkers	A single characteristic that is indicative of a disease.
Cerebellar Ataxia	Gross lack of coordination
Cognition	The mental process of knowing, including aspects such as awareness, perception, reasoning, and judgment.
Cross-sectional	Taken only once
Dysarthria	Motor speech disorder
Dysmetria	Lack of coordination of movement typified by the undershoot and/or overshoot of intended position with the hand, arm, leg, or eye. It is sometimes described as an inability to judge distance or scale.
Dysphagia	Difficulty swallowing
Dystonia	Sustained muscle contractions cause twisting and repetitive movements or abnormal postures.
Fine Motor Skills	Coordination of small muscle movements
Gelastic Cataplexy	Loosening of the muscle, dropping of the jaw during extreme emotion, such as laughter.
Hyperlipidemia, Type IV	A not uncommon inherited metabolic disorder that is characterized by increased blood levels of the triglyceride form of fat that makes up very low-density lipids (VLDL). Abnormally high blood levels of triglycerides or cholesterol may be the result of poor dietary habits, genetic causes, or other metabolic disorders or a side effect of certain drugs. Also known as:
	Carbohydrate-Induced Hyperlipemia
	Hypercholesterolemia, Type IV
	Hyperlipidemia IV
	Hyperprebeta-Lipoproteinemia
	Hypertriglyceridemia, Endogenous
Hyperreflexia	Overactive reflex
Incontinence	The inability of organs to restrain the natural evacuations, so that the discharges are involuntary; as, incontinence of urine. The involuntary discharge of urine or feces.
Likert-like scale	Graded self evaluation
Longitudinal	taken over time, multiple data points from expression
Narcolepsy	Chronic sleep disorder characterized by overwhelming daytime drowsiness and sudden attacks of sleep.
Ophthalmology:	*Distance visual activity (DVA):* Acuteness or clearness of vision, especially form vision, which is dependent on the sharpness of the retinal focus within the eye and the sensitivity of the interpretative faculty of the brain.
	Extra-ocular movement (EOM): Can often identify abnormalities in individual muscles or in particular cranial nerves (oculomotor, trochlear, or abducens) in their course from the brainstem to the orbit, in the brainstem nuclei, or finally, in the higher-order centers and pathways in the cortex and brainstem that control eye movements; an example of EOM is saccades.
	Systemic lupus erythematosus (SLE): A chronic, relapsing autoimmune disease that may affect skin, joints, and internal organs. The most common ocular finding is the presence of cotton wool spots, retinal hemorrhages, and papilledema. Other symptoms such as lid swelling, exophthalmus, and fluctuating weakness of extraocular muscles may occur.
Ophthalmoplegia (horizontal and vertical)	A paralysis or weakness of one or more of the muscles that control eye movement. Eyes don't move togetherà double vision.
Psychotic Episodes	Hallucinating, altered reality
Saccades	Fast movement of an eye, head or other part of an animal's body or device; eye saccades are quick, simultaneous movements of both eyes in the same direction; serve as a mechanism for fixation, rapid eye movement and the fast phase of optokinetic nystagmus (a type of involuntary eye movement).
Seizures	A sudden episode of transient neurologic symptoms such as involuntary muscle movements, sensory disturbances and altered consciousness.
Supranuclear Vertical Gaze Palsy	Cannot look upwards, impaired upward gaze
Xanthoma	A skin condition in which fat builds up under the surface of the skin; common, particularly among older adults and persons with high blood lipids.
Also need to know:	Behavior, eye movement, hearing, memory, psychiatric, speech, swallowing, respiratory problems

variation in progression measured a year apart. In the remainder, the variation along disease severity curve for one case [6] was indeed low (Fig. 3B). This case was not reported in Yanjanin et al. 2010 [6]. However it was partially scored (one visit) before being transferred to the study and is therefore included. In two records (numbered cases 7 and 5) we noticed a significant variation across the triplicates pairs (Fig. 3B; see also Fig. S1). Discussion with the class suggested that for case 7, fine motor (2-4) and cognition (1-4) were the areas of greatest variance. Importantly at one age (29), one group scored consistently higher than the other group in fine

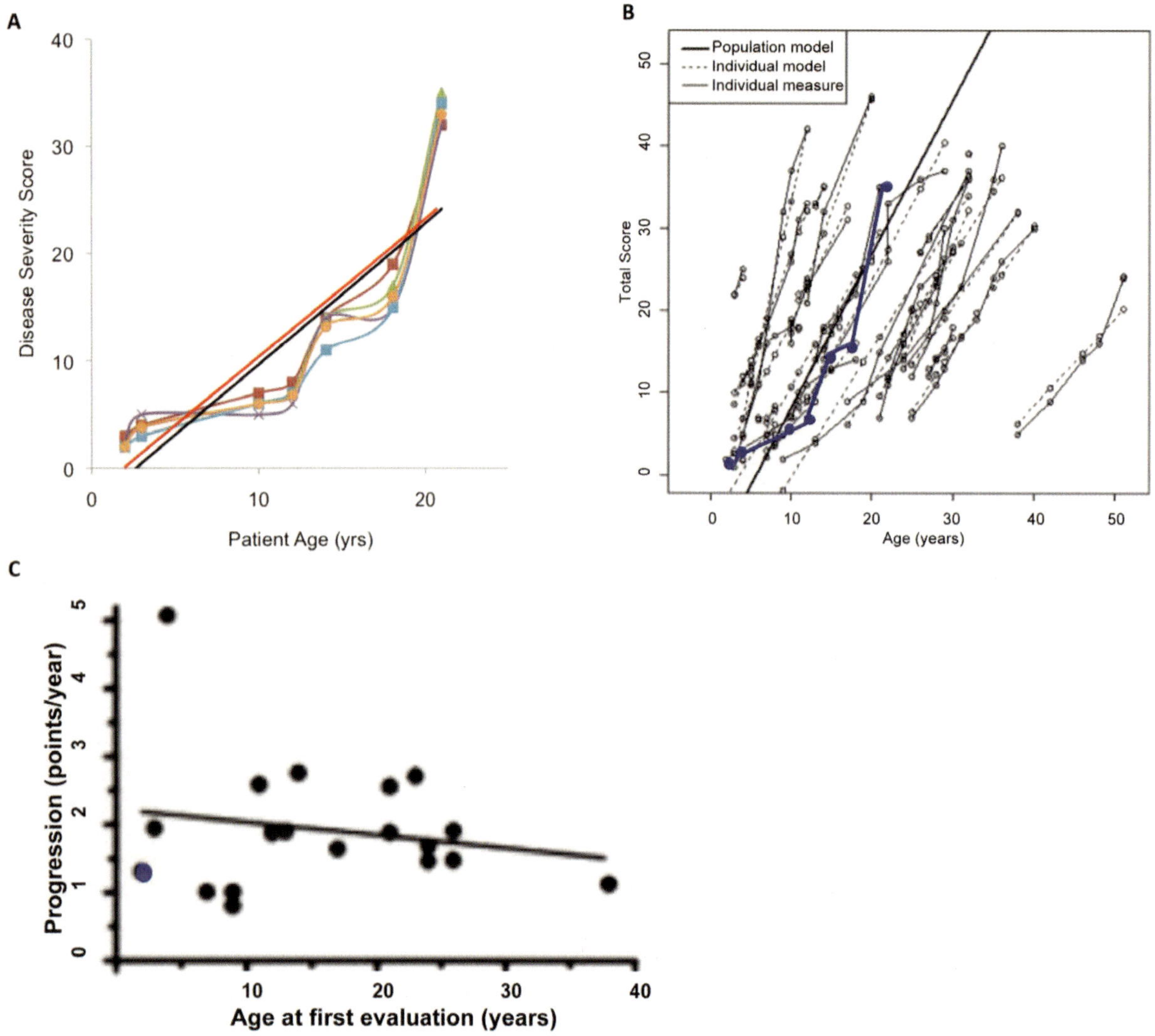

Figure 2. Initial assessment of one NP-C patient medical record by five students in Spring 2009. A. Five students independently scored one NP-C patient's medical record, The disease severity curves were plotted as shown. The correlation among their evaluation is 0.76. The best fit line is shown in black line with a slope of 1.315. In red is the best fit line (with a slope of 1.3 and a correlation of 0.90) obtained by Yanjanin et al. 2010. B. The average of five student scores (show in blue) was overlaid on a summary of disease severity curves obtained by Yanjanin et al 2010 (obtained by combining their historical and current cohorts). C. The progression slope shown in panels A and B was determined by linear regression and overlaid (blue dot) onto the progression slope created by Yanjanin et al. 2010.

motor skills (2–4 variation over the group), cognition (1–4), and speech (the higher scoring group scored speech 1 pt higher than all other individuals (1–2) (Figure S2). In case 5, the discrepancies in scoring occurred in cognition (1-3) and swallow (3–5) (not shown): Even for case 6, where there was little variation in overall scoring (Fig. 3B and Fig. S1), there were scoring discrepancies between cognition and memory. 1 pair consistently scored cognition 1 and memory 3. 2 other pairs scored cognition 3 and memory 0 (not shown). Another problem with case 7 was that it contained data from just four visits and the main source of error appears to be from visit 3, when pair 2 provided an anomalously high score of 21 instead of 14.5 and 15.5 (See Figures S1 and S2). Due to carry over this resulted in continued maintenance of the elevated score by pair 2 in visit 4. In contrast, in case 5, pair 2 appeared to consistently score lower than pairs 1 and 3, through all ten visits and hence the overall slope for pair 2 is closely comparable to pairs 1 and 3 (Figure S1).

In aggregate, the data in Figures 3, suggest that it is probably desirable to have a clinical record assessed by 3-5 (rather than 2) students to flag occasional anomalies in scoring. Moreover we should also flag for greater scrutiny, records with (i) less than 5 visits disease curves and/or (ii) disease where cognition, memory, fine motor skills and speech are the prominent symptoms, since the students sometimes show a range of scores for these phenotypes. Despite these scoring anomalies, all seven disease severity curves mapped back with close correspondence to the progression described by Yanjanin et al. 2010 [6] (Figs. 3 C, D).

In summary the data show that both science-majors and non majors (but who were declared premed), can consistently be trained to assess and quantify NPC major and minor clinical

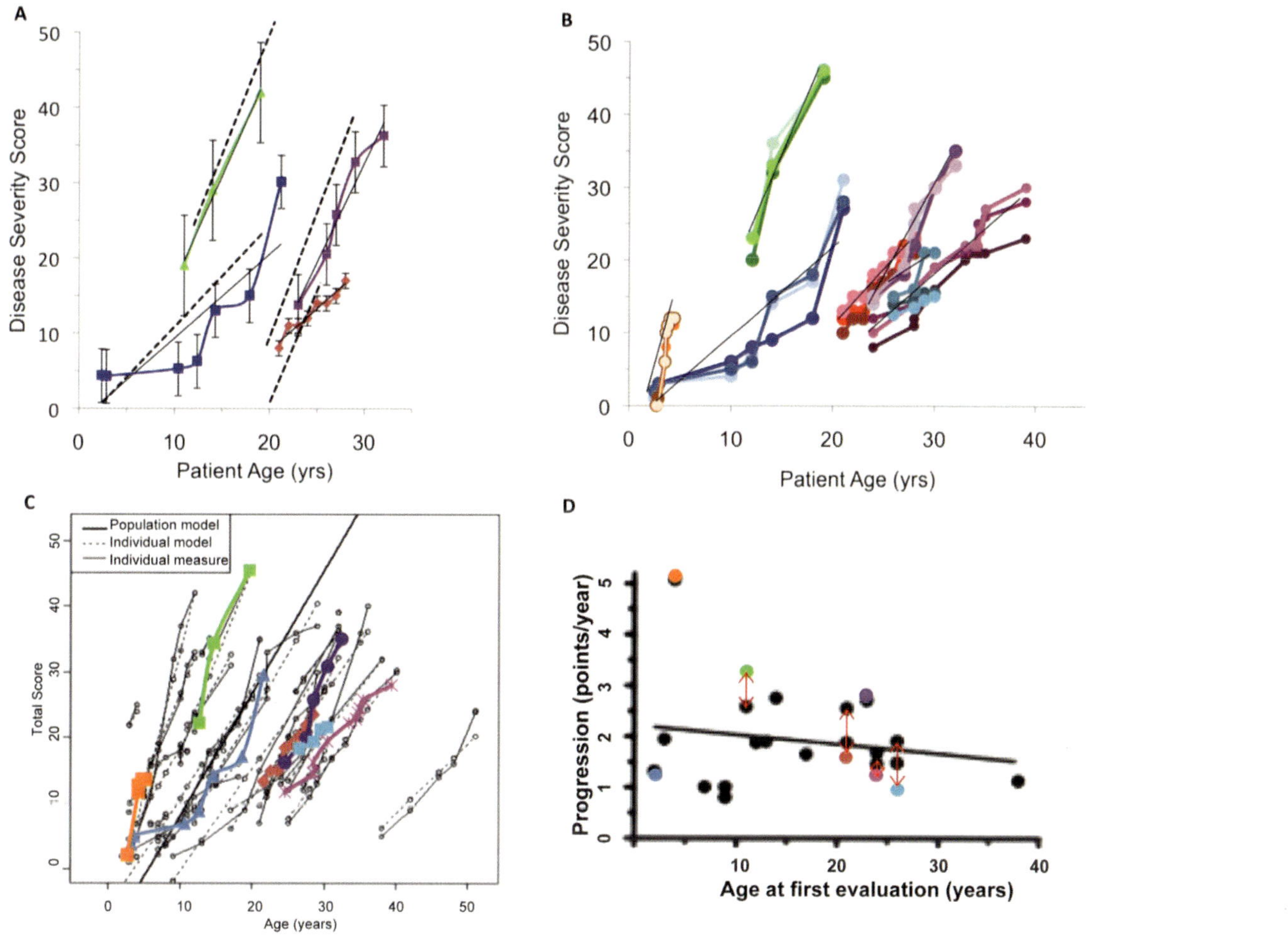

Figure 3. Assessment of four NP-C patient medical records by expanded class sizes. A. Disease severity curves generated by two different classes of sixteen students in Fall 2009 and Spring 2010. From each class groups of three to five students evaluated four NP-C patient's medical records obtained from Yanjanin et al. 2010. Each group evaluated one patient record. Error bars indicate scoring variation between the two classes. Linear best fit shown as solid black line for each record. Hatched line indicates best fit obtained by Yanjanin et al 2010. Color code: case 1, blue; case 2, red; case 3, purple; case 4 green; B. Disease severity curves generated by thirty students in Spring 2011. Five groups of six students scored the four NP-C medical records from panel A as well as three additional records. Scoring was done by pairs of students and triplicate scores were generated for each medical record as shown. Color code as indicated in panel A as well as case 5, magenta; case 6 orange; case 7, teal. Triplicate curves associated with each case, where each curve indicated pair wise scoring. C. The average of curves shown in panel B overlaid a summary of disease severity curves described in Yanjanin et al. 2010. D. The progression slope shown in panel C was determined by linear regression and overlaid onto the progression slope created by Yanjanin et al. 2010. Red arrows indicate extent of displacement of progression obtained from student assessments. Colors as indicated for panel C. When students' progression values were used, the progression slope was found to be 1.907 +/− 0.2374. The original progression slope calculated by Yanjanin et al. 1.923 +/− 0.2200.

disease symptoms and develop disease severity scales from clinical histories in a defined class structure.

Scoring and disease severity curve generated from two new NPC patient records donated directly to our study

Two new clinical histories that were not previously assessed by Yanjanin et al. 2010 [6] were directly donated by families to our study in Spring 2010 and Spring 2011 respectively.

In Spring 2010, a group of four students assessed the record, and progression of severity of disease (Figure S3) was mapped back to the cohort group of Yanjanin et al., 2010 [6] (Fig. 4A–B). Notably the linear regression yielded a slope of 2.676, (Fig. S3), which was greater than three standard deviations from the mean slope originally described by Yanjanin et al., 2010 [6] 1.9±0.2. This appeared to be due to the fact that patient displayed accelerated rapid disease progression in the last two clinical visits recorded. For the remaining data points, the curve and progression slope appeared to be in range (~2.2) with the other patients previously reported by Yanjanin et al. 2010 [6].

The second case directly donated in Spring 2011 was assessed by all 30 students in class because in addition to generating the disease severity curve, we were also interested in investigating the inherent variation across individual students in a larger class. Thus, we had each of the thirty students assess the new record. The average disease severity curve was mapped back to the cohort of Yanjanin et al. 2010 [6] (Fig. 4A–B). The linear regression curve yielded a slope of 2.45, again suggesting accelerated disease progression compared to the cohort.

We therefore examined in detail the individual disease progression curves and scores that were derived from across clinical visits (in Figures S4 and S5). In aggregate these data showed that approximately 3–4 (~10%) of 30 students had

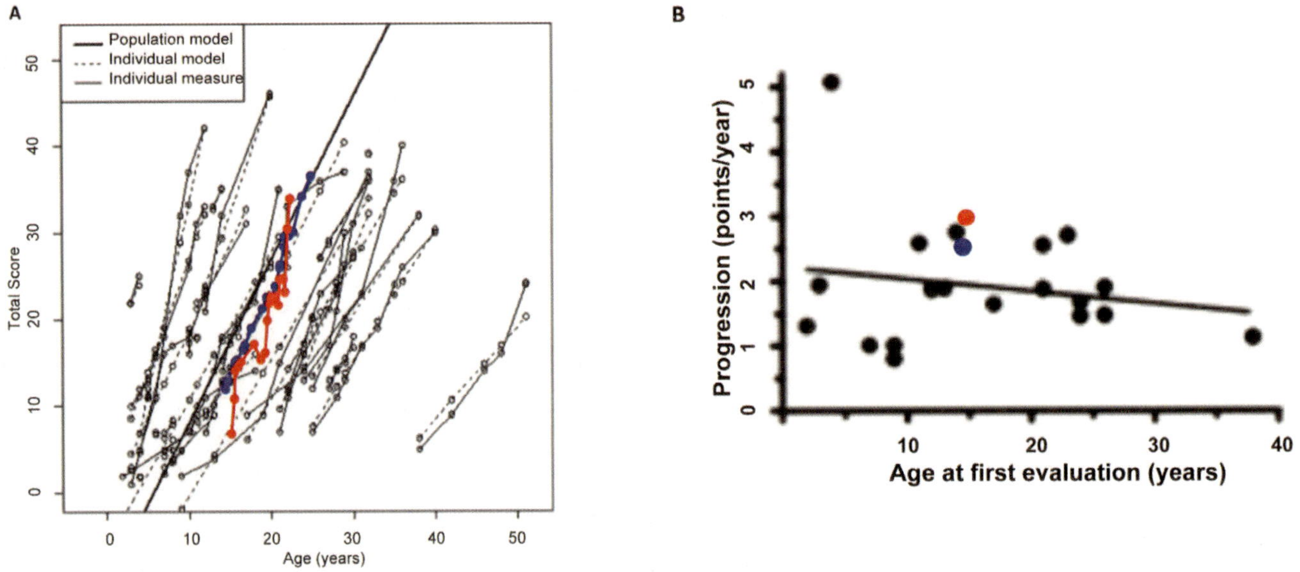

Figure 4. Assessment of two new NP-C patient medical records donated directly to the study. A. Disease severity curves of medical record donated in Spring 2010 (red) and Spring 2011 (blue). The Spring 2010 case was assessed by four students. The Spring 2011 case was assessed by 30 students. The data were overlaid on disease severity curves obtained by Yanjanin et al., 2010. B. The progression slopes of two curves shown in panel A were determined by linear regression and overlaid onto the progression slope created by Yanjanin et al. 2010.

consistently lower scorers, with absolute scores that were as much as 2 standard deviations away from the mode (Fig. S5). However this bias did not change the slope, suggesting that the accelerated disease progression portrayed was consistently observed across operators. This was similar to the accelerated rapid disease progression in the last two clinical visits recorded in the first donated clinical record shown in Fig. 4A

Creation of a clinical summary sheet

For each clinical case, students also created one to two page summary sheet displaying a history of medical visits and lab tests, onset of major and minors systems, utilization of drugs, known contraindication, allergies, hospitalizations, surgical procedures, all physicians and specialists previously visited including reason for visit, and herbal supplements. This summary provides a condensed insight for physicians treating NPC patients and is a service product that could be helpful to families.

Discussion

Our study suggests that college students were able to review and assess clinical records once they achieved understanding of clinical NPC disease manifestation, diagnosis and management and learned the requisite medical terminology indicated and method of scoring. One difficulty was variability and sometimes limited information in individual medical histories. The method is dependent on the quality of existing medical records. The records from the NIH are equivalent to those from a university outpatient clinical setting, with evaluation by neurologists familiar with metabolic disorders. Records from primary care centers were also used, although the charts from standard hospital chart-systems, were relatively well organized since the specialist was integrated into the same system.

In-class discussions also focused on ambiguity of scoring domains and how to score inconsistently recorded data. After students independently graphed the plots, it was apparent that inter-individual variability based on ambiguity of recognizing domains were small and that the scoring process was robust. Discussion with clinical experts Forbes D. Porter M.D., Ph. D. and Nicole Yanjanin N.P. provided guidelines (previously reported in Yanjanin et al. 2010 [6]) on handling inconsistently recorded data. In early phases of the course, direct interaction with clinical practitioners greatly facilitated confidence in utilization and interpretation of scoring methods and data, although the 2011 class was able to complete finals scores prior to their interaction with clinical practitioners.

The take-home assessment of a single patient history was completed within 6 hours of out-of-class time. Assigning a record to three to four students per group would be sufficient to ensure accurate and verifiable assessment. Moreover once the group is trained (in the first four weeks), additional records could be assessed at the rate of one per week per student pair, for the remaining eight weeks. Finally the class size is easily scalable up to 50 students, suggesting significant, future, potential for assessing ~200 patient records in the course of one semester. Thus this approach as the ability to produce a robust database from which the Natural History of a rare disease could be extracted. The limiting factor is obtaining sufficient number of records and thus coordination with a parent support organization (PSO) would be critical. PSOs may also be helpful to prospective studies, by providing attending physicians with a list of questions on clinical history and symptoms that serve as a checklist for the disorder, but mechanisms to ensure that such a list is systematically used, are also needed.

Assessment of the two medical records directly contributed to our study (received in Spring 2010 and 2011) supported the model of Yanjanin et al. (2010; 6) but also revealed, unexpected and accelerated disease progression, especially at later stages, not predicted by the severity scale of Yanjanin et al., 2010 [6]. One possible explanation for this is that the current scale is based on patients who can travel to the NIH, because travel for patients in wheel chairs, needing oxygen and other critical assistance is difficult. Additionally, travel to a tertiary clinical center typically requires travel with family members and a natural history study on late stage disease would need to be sustained over many more years, further complicating logistics and increasing costs to the point that it would be difficult to fund. This is in contrast to relatively low costs of retrospective analysis of a decade or more of existing medical records, by taking advantage of existing university infrastructure and training. The Yanjanin et al study continues to provide a reference point for the linear disease progression model, however additional data is needed to ascertain the relative contribution of quadratic disease progression (Table S2) and accurately model the full disease course.

Additional review of community-based assessment of patient records will reveal whether it can provide specific insight into the natural history at more severe stages of disease, in addition to accelerate the volume of assessments needed to strengthen disease scores to assess urgently needed, emerging therapies for NPC. It will also be of interest to determine whether community based assessment of patient records in other rare diseases can be undertaken to yield insights into disease processes and prognosis.

Supporting Information

Figure S1 Disease severity scores generated by pairs of students for cases 5-7 for curves shown in Figure 3B.

Figure S2 Disease severity scores generated by individual students for case 7. Pair 1 Score, Pair 2 Score, and Pair 3 Score indicate student pairs and individual domain scores for a pair is separated by a comma, as shown.

Figure S3 Disease severity curve for new case donated in Spring 2010.

Figure S4 Individual disease severity curves for new case donated in Spring 2011, as assessed by 30 individual students.

Figure S5 Individual disease severity scores for new case donated in Spring 2011, as assessed by 30 individual students.

Table S1

Table S2 Average linear and quadratic R^2 values for disease severity curves associated with cases 1-7 (numbered as described in Figure 3B). The suffix (Y) indicates that they were obtained from medical records reported in Yanjanin et al (2010). New cases donated directly to our study in 2010 and 2011, not previously reported by Yanjanin et al (2010) and assessed in Figure 4, are also indicated. *Log fit is best fit. (DOCX)

Acknowledgments

We thank Will Hayman at the University of Notre Dame for his participation in this project. Mary Beckman, Center for Social Concerns at the University of Notre Dame, Maureen Clark, Center for Rare and Neglected Disease at the University of Notre Dame, Brian Hainline, Riley Children's Hospital, IUSOM, Indianapolis, the National Niemann Pick Disease Foundation, the Ara Parseghian Medical Research Foundation, and the Niemann-Pick Disease Group (UK) for helpful discussions. We thank the National Niemann Pick Disease Foundation for help in donation of patient records directly to the study. We thank Father James Foster and Dr. Paul Grimstad at the University of Notre Dame, for assistance with advising students about the class and registering them. We thank Dr. Pamela Tamez for help with formatting the manuscript. Finally we would like to express our gratitude to the parents, guardians, and patients who have participated in these studies.

Author Contributions

Conceived and designed the experiments: KH FDP JS KE NY. Performed the experiments: JS KE NY JA LB NB EB DC M. Castleman M. Cheng M. Clark LD CE NF SF LG RG OG WH A. Herschel SH A. Horst MH EJ LJ M. Kearns M. Kelly C. Kim KK GK C. Knoedler EK LL JL E. Li WL AL E. Ly K. McKeough BM CM SM AM K. Moser SO PO AP MP CP ER BR TR GR MR FR S. Riney S. Rund SS LS RS ES TS CDT MT MU JV OV EW FDP KH. Analyzed the data: JS KE NY JA LB NB EB DC M. Castleman M. Cheng M. Clark LD CE NF SF LG RG OG WH A. Herschel SH A. Horst MH EJ LJ M. Kearns M. Kelly C. Kim KK GK C. Knoedler EK LL JL E. Li WL AL E. Ly K. McKeough BM CM SM AM K. Moser SO PO AP MP CP ER BR TR GR MR FR S. Riney S. Rund SS LS RS ES TS CDT MT MU JV OV EW FDP KH. Contributed reagents/materials/analysis tools: KH FDP JS KE NY. Wrote the paper: KH FDP JS KE NY.

References

1. Pentchev PG, Comly ME, Kruth HS, Tokoro T, Butler J, et al. (1987) Group C Niemann-Pick disease: Faulty regulation of low-density lipoprotein uptake and cholesterol storage in cultured fibroblasts. FASEB J 1: 40–45.
2. Vanier MT (2010) Niemann-Pick disease type C. Orphanet J of Rare Diseases 5: 16–18.
3. Imrie J, Dasgupta S, Besley GT, Harris C, Heptinstall I, et al. (2007) The natural history of Niemann Pick disease type C in the UK. J. Inherit Metab Dis 30: 51–59.
4. Iturriaga C, Pineda M, Fernandez-Valero EM, Vanier MT, Coll MJ (2006) Niemann-Pick C disease in Spain: clinical spectrum and development of a disability scale. J. Neurol Sci. 249: 1–6.
5. Pineda M, Wraith JE, Mengel E, Sedel F, Hwu WL, et al. (2009) Miglustat in patients with Niemann-Pick disease Type C (NP-C): a multicenter observational retrospective cohort study. Mol Genet Metab 98: 243–9.
6. Yanjanin NM, Velez JI, Gropman A, King K, Bianconi SE, et al. (2010) Linear Clinical Progression, Independent of Age of Onset, in Niemann-Pick Disease, Type C. Am. J. Med Genet B Neuropsychiatr Genet 153B: 132–40.

5

Receptor-Mediated Endocytosis of α-Galactosidase A in Human Podocytes in Fabry Disease

Thaneas Prabakaran[1], Rikke Nielsen[1], Jakob V. Larsen[2], Søren S. Sørensen[3], Ulla Feldt-Rasmussen[4], Moin A. Saleem[5], Claus M. Petersen[2], Pierre J. Verroust[6], Erik I. Christensen[1]*

1 Section of Cell Biology, Department of Anatomy, Aarhus University, Aarhus, Denmark, **2** Department of Medical Biochemistry, Aarhus University, Aarhus, Denmark, **3** Department P, Rigshospitalet, Copenhagen, Denmark, **4** Department of Medical Endocrinology, Rigshospitalet, Copenhagen, Denmark, **5** Children's Renal Unit and Academic Renal Unit, University of Bristol, Southmead Hospital, Bristol, United Kingdom, **6** UMRS 592, Institut de la Vision, Paris, France

Abstract

Injury to the glomerular podocyte is a key mechanism in human glomerular disease and podocyte repair is an important therapeutic target. In Fabry disease, podocyte injury is caused by the intracellular accumulation of globotriaosylceramide. This study identifies in the human podocyte three endocytic receptors, mannose 6-phosphate/insulin-like growth II receptor, megalin, and sortilin and demonstrates their drug delivery capabilities for enzyme replacement therapy. Sortilin, a novel α-galactosidase A binding protein, reveals a predominant intracellular expression but also surface expression in the podocyte. The present study provides the rationale for the renal effect of treatment with α-galactosidase A and identifies potential pathways for future non-carbohydrate based drug delivery to the kidney podocyte and other potential affected organs.

Editor: Jean-Claude Dussaule, INSERM, France

Funding: The work was supported in part by the Danish Medical Research Council, Novo Nordisk Foundation and Arvid Nilsson's Foundation, the European Commission EUNEFRON (FP7, GA#201590), Aarhus University, and Genzyme Corporation. The funders had no role in study design, data collection and analysis, decision to publish, or preparation of the manuscript.

Competing Interests: TP's salary is paid by one third Genzyme, one third Danish Medical Council, and one third Aarhus University. UFR has received unrestricted research grants from Genzyme and Shire and serves at Advisory Boards in both Genzyme and Shire. This does not alter the authors' adherence to all the PLoS ONE policies on sharing data and materials.

* E-mail: eic@ana.au.dk

Introduction

Fabry disease is an X-linked lysosomal disorder that results from mutations of the gene (*GLA*) that encodes α-galactosidase A (α-Gal A) [1,2,3]. The enzymatic defect leads to progressive lysosomal accumulation of globotriaosylceramide (GL-3) and related glycosphingolipids in the kidney and other tissues [3]. Glycosphingolipid accumulates over time leading to kidney failure, cerebrovascular manifestations, and heart failure, and eventually premature death [4].

Nephropathy is a dominant feature in Fabry disease and impairment of renal function occurs due to progressive accumulation of GL-3 in a variety of renal cells [3,5,6,7,8]. End-stage renal failure usually occurs in the third to fifth decade of life, when the lysosomal GL-3 accumulation becomes irreversible [7,9] and patients are in need of dialysis or renal transplantation [9,10]. The podocytes are the renal cells with the most abundant glycosphingolipid deposits [3,8,11,12,13] and this accumulation appears to be central for the development of nephropathy in Fabry disease [14,15].

Lysosomal storage diseases in general [16], including Fabry disease, can now be treated with enzyme replacement therapy (ERT) [12,17,18,19,20,21,22,23,24,25]. ERT reduces GL-3 deposits in podocytes [12,22,26] and can stabilize kidney function in patients with Fabry nephropathy [27]. Furthermore, for ERT to be maximally effective, it must be initiated early, before irreversible renal damage occurs [28,29,30].

Therapeutic effectiveness of α-Gal A is dependent on endocytosis by recognition of mannose 6-phosphate (M6P) residues on the enzyme by the widely distributed M6P/insulin-like growth II (IGF-II) receptor [31,32,33]. We previously showed that megalin, a multiligand receptor, binds α-Gal A and takes up α-Gal A in proximal tubule cells by receptor-mediated endocytosis [34]. However, the mechanism for the uptake in mouse podocytes in the same study was not investigated.

We have identified M6PR, but also megalin and sortilin as α-Gal A binding proteins important for α-Gal A accumulation in human podocytes by use of different biochemical and morphological approaches, including affinity chromatography, surface plasmon resonance analysis, laser microdissection, and immunocytochemistry to analyze human podocytes in culture and renal tissue from Fabry patients. On the basis of these data, we suggest a new and complex mechanism of α-Gal A cellular internalization in podocytes involving the sorting and endocytic receptors M6PR and sortilin and the high molecular weight endocytic receptor megalin.

Results

Podocytes take up recombinant α-Gal A

We have previously shown that endogenous α-Gal A is not detectable in normal human podocytes [34]. However in α-Gal A knockout mice, the enzyme was found in lysosomes of mouse podocytes 2 h after intravenous injection of recombinant α-Gal A [34]. To study if this was also the case in humans, we investigated a renal biopsy from a male Fabry patient infused with α-Gal A. Two hours after infusion of recombinant α-Gal A, the enzyme was localized in the podocytes (Figure 1A). For comparison, a renal biopsy from a male Fabry patient who was not infused with recombinant α-Gal A demonstrated no detectable α-Gal A in the podocytes (Figure 1B). Furthermore, the treated male Fabry patient showed no detectable endogenous α-Gal A in the collecting ducts (compare Figure 1C to Figure 1D from normal human kidney with normal expression).

To study in detail the podocyte uptake of α-Gal A, we used an already established human podocyte cell culture model [35]. Recombinant α-Gal A is also taken up by these conditionally immortalized podocytes showing time-dependent uptake (Figure 1E). The endocytosed enzyme was localized to the lysosomes as confirmed by colocalization of LysoTracker-Red with Alexa-Fluor-488 conjugated α-Gal A (Figure 1F).

Isolation and identification of M6PR, megalin, and sortilin as α-Gal A-interacting proteins in podocytes

The receptor-mediated uptake of lysosomal hydrolases in podocytes has so far not been investigated. To identify receptors involved in the uptake of α-Gal A in podocytes, we employed an affinity-chromatography approach. A detergent-soluble extract of cultured podocytes was passed over recombinant α-Gal A affinity resin, and, following extensive washing, the resin bound proteins were eluted using pH 3 Glycine buffer. Fractions were collected and analyzed by SDS-PAGE and silver staining (Figure 2A). A sample of the same extract was also passed over a control resin to monitor nonspecific background binding of proteins to the resin. Comparison of the eluates from the two columns revealed that three protein bands with apparent masses of 600, 250 and 100 kDa were present in the fractions eluted from the α-Gal A resin but not the control resin (Figure 2A). To determine the identity of the proteins, the eluted fractions from the α-Gal A resin with the highest protein content were run on SDS-PAGE gel followed by immunoblotting. The proteins were identified as megalin, M6PR, and sortilin using the corresponding antibodies (Figure 2B).

^{125}I-labeled α-Gal A uptake in human podocytes

The endocytic activity of megalin, M6PR, and sortilin expressed by cultured human podocytes was investigated by their ability to mediate uptake of ^{125}I-labeled α-Gal A (both cell association and degradation) (Figure 3). M6P, a ligand for M6PR, inhibited the α-Gal A uptake by approximately 26% after 12 h ($P<0.001$). RAP, a ligand for both megalin and sortilin, inhibited 19% ($P<0.001$), and

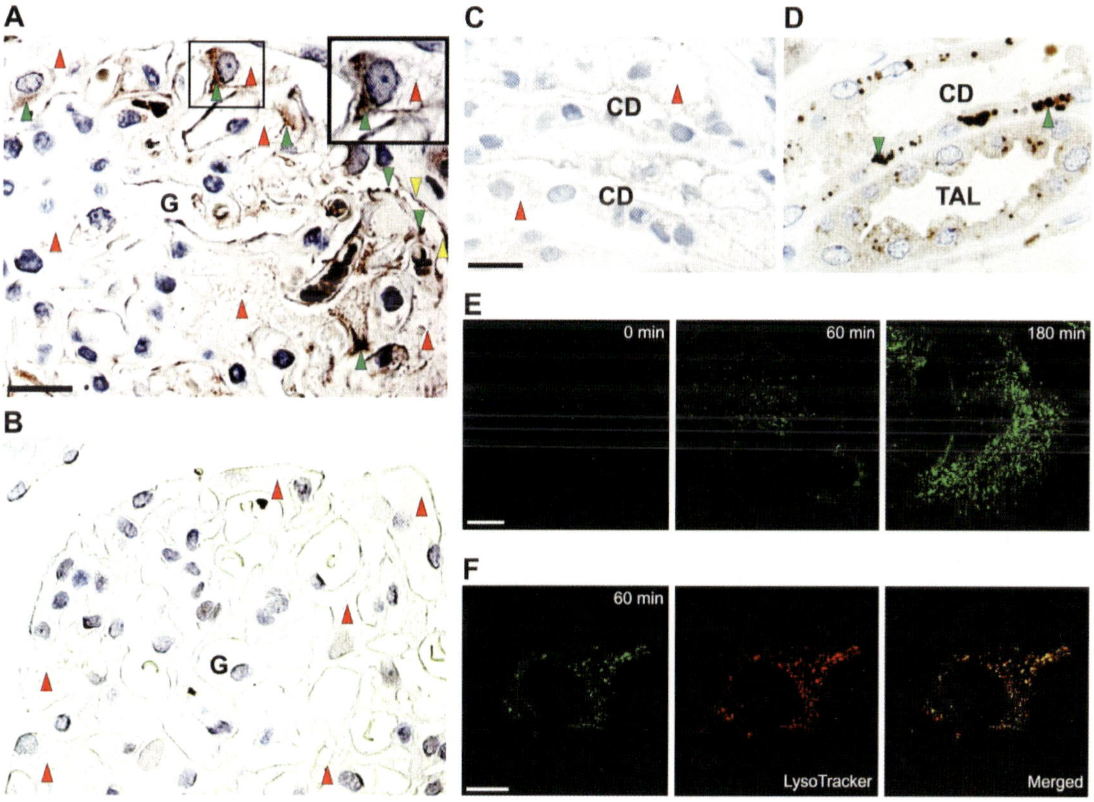

Figure 1. Uptake of recombinant α-Gal A by human podocytes. (A) Peroxidase immunohistochemistry for α-Gal A in a biopsy from a male Fabry patient using anti-human α-Gal A antibody. The patient was intravenously infused with α-Gal A 2 h before the biopsy was taken. Labeling of a human glomerulus (G) showing α-Gal A localization in the podocytes (indicated with green arrowheads) and GL-3 inclusions seen as vacuoles (indicated with red arrowheads). Staining is also seen in parietal epithelial cells (indicated with yellow arrows). Scale bar, 25 µm. A high-power view of a portion of the glomerulus (top-right) demonstrates the localization of infused recombinant α-Gal in the podocyte. (B) For comparison, no α-Gal A labeling is seen in the podocytes in a biopsy from an untreated male Fabry patient. (C) The treated male Fabry patient shows no detectable labeling of endogenous α-Gal A in the collecting ducts (CD). Red arrowheads indicate heavy GL-3 inclusions. Scale bar, 25 µm. (D) A normal individual shows labeling of endogenous α-Gal A (green arrowheads) in both thick ascending limbs of Henle (TAL) and in CD. Scale bar, 25 µm. (E) Immunofluorescent demonstration of Alexa-Fluor 488-labeled α-Gal A uptake in human podocytes as a function of time at 37°C. At the indicated times, the cells were fixed and analyzed by confocal microscopy. Scale bar, 10 µm. (F) For colocalization of α-Gal A (green) and lysosomes (red) a merged image is shown. The yellow color illustrates colocalization. Scale bar, 5 µm.

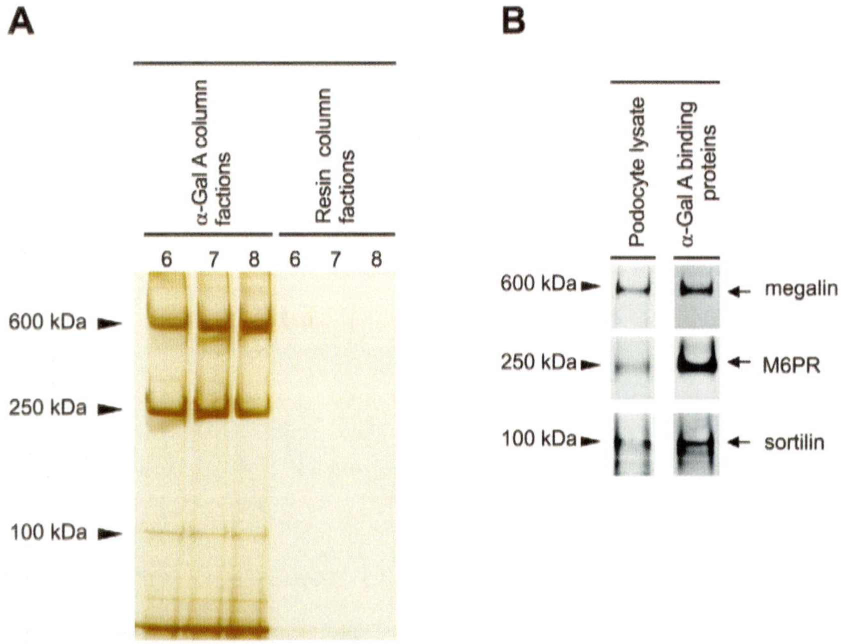

Figure 2. Megalin, M6PR and sortilin bind specifically to recombinant α-Gal A in podocytes. (A) Affinity chromatography: the arrowheads indicate the migration of the different α-Gal A binding proteins. (B) Western blot analysis demonstrated that the three bands were megalin, M6PR, and sortilin as indicated with arrows. Lysate from human podocyte culture was used as a positive control.

sortilin propeptide, a specific sortilin ligand that is known to inhibit the binding/uptake of sortilin ligands [36], inhibited 7% after 12 h (not significant). Finally, the inhibition by all three ligands combined was tested, and the uptake of ^{125}I-α-Gal A was inhibited 39% after 12 h ($P<0.001$).

Sortilin, a new receptor for α-Gal A

Surface plasmon resonance (SPR) analysis for megalin binding to α-Gal A was shown previously [34] with a K_d of 600 nM. Biacore analysis of α-Gal A binding to M6PR has already been shown in previous experiments [37]. We then focused on sortilin, SPR analysis showed binding of α-Gal A to purified and immobilized sortilin (Figure 4A). Using the BIAevaluation program, K_d was estimated to 400 nM. We next examined if neurotensin (NT), a neuropeptide with high affinity for sortilin [38], inhibited the binding of α-Gal A to sortilin. At 20 μM, NT markedly inhibited the binding of α-Gal A to sortilin (Figure 4A) indicating that NT and α-Gal A bind to sortilin at the same binding site as the sortilin propeptide. Other members of the Vps10p (vacuolar protein sorting 10 protein)-domain family [39], sorLA and sorCS3, did not show significant binding to α-Gal A (data not shown), and neither did the low density lipoprotein related protein (LRP). These results further substantiated that sortilin specifically binds α-Gal A.

Thus we had clear evidence that α-Gal A bound sortilin in order to demonstrate the ability of sortilin to take up α-Gal A. We developed a system in which sortilin is expressed in absence of megalin. We therefore used HEK293 cells stably transfected with sortilin to demonstrate α-Gal A binding to sortilin and uptake (Figure 4B). The transfectants expressed full-length sortilin in contrast to the wild-type cells. When cells were incubated in the presence of 5 mM M6P uptake by the M6PRs were totally inhibited in HEK293 wild-type but uptake was still present in the sortilin transfected HEK293 cells (Figure 4B). Next, we inhibited with NT and M6P, as shown in Figure 4B. NT at 20 μM essentially eliminated the binding and uptake of α-Gal A demonstrating the ability of sortilin to take up α-Gal A.

Cultured human podocytes express megalin, sortilin and M6PR

We next examined the surface expression of megalin, M6PR, and sortilin in cultured human podocytes by immunofluorescent studies under non-permeabilized conditions. It appears that megalin was predominantly expressed on the cell-surface, whereas M6PR and sortilin were mainly expressed intracellularly with some cell-surface expression (Figure 5). The expression of megalin, M6PR, and sortilin was also studied in permeabilized cells, where all three receptors demonstrated intracellular labeling (Figure 5). The phenotype of podocytes was characterized by using podocyte-specific antibodies to podocin and nephrin under permeabilized conditions (Figure 5). Controls incubated with serum or IgG fractions revealed no significant labeling.

Expression of megalin, sortilin, and M6PR in human glomerular podocytes

To study the expression of megalin, sortilin, and M6PR, we isolated human glomeruli by laser capture microdissection and evaluated if the receptors' mRNAs could be identified by RT-PCR. In order to avoid contamination with especially proximal tubule cells only the largest cross sections of the glomeruli from the 10 μm thick cryosections were chosen in order to be close to the equator, and furthermore the dissection was performed with safe distance to the glomerular parietal epithelium. To confirm, that the isolated glomeruli are not contaminated with proximal tubule, we demonstrate that the proximal tubule marker aminopeptidase N (APN) [40] is not present in the laser dissected glomeruli (Figure 6A). The expression of mRNA for megalin, M6PR, sortilin, podocin and nephrin is shown in the isolated human

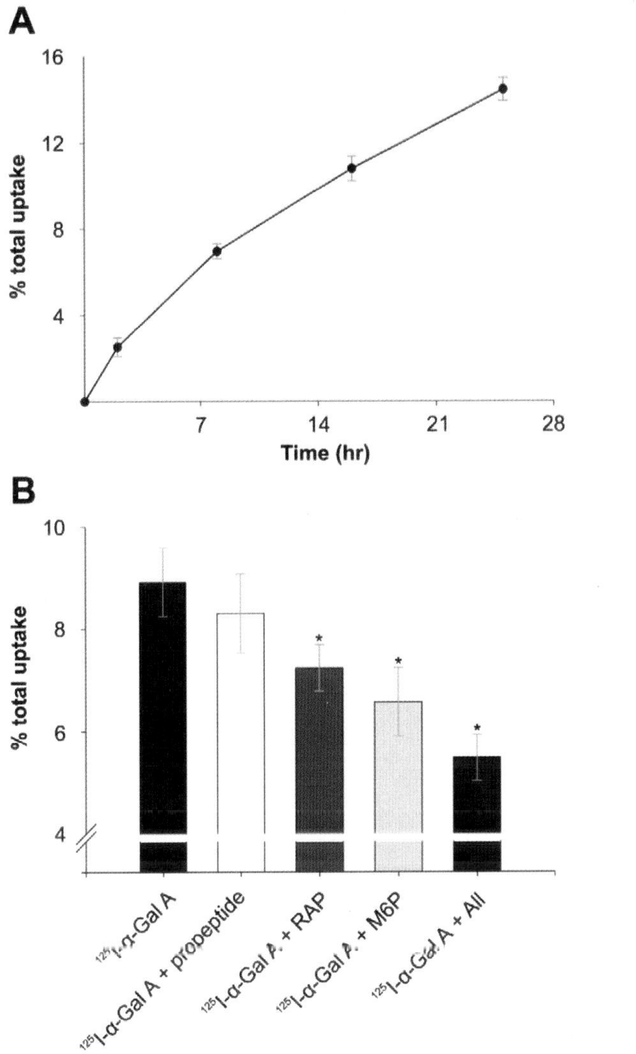

Figure 3. Uptake of ^{125}I-labeled α-Gal A by human podocytes. (A) Human podocytes were incubated with ^{125}I-α-Gal A for different times. (B) Podocytes incubated with ^{125}I-α-Gal A for 12 h in the presence or absence of RAP, sortilin propeptide, M6P, and with all three ligands combined at 37°C. Uptake was assayed as described in the method section of the paper. Values are means of triplicate experiments with standard deviations (SD). The addition of sortilin propeptide shows no significant inhibition, however the addition of M6P, RAP or a combination of all three inhibitors show significant reductions (* indicate P<0.001) in the α-Gal A uptake after 12 h.

glomeruli and human kidney cortex in Figure 6A. No expression was observed in the negative controls.

To further confirm that the receptors were indeed expressed in the human glomerular podocytes, we performed immunohistochemistry studies on human kidney sections. We used three well characterized polyclonal antibodies to megalin, sortilin, and M6PR described in the literature. Immunoperoxidase staining using the three antibodies showed the presence of the receptors in the glomeruli and in the tubule segments (Figure 6B). This labeling was specific, as established by preabsorption of the three antibodies with their respective antigens (Figure 6B). We performed dual immunofluorescence using the three antibodies and a specific podocyte marker antibody against the Wilms' tumor 1 (WT1) protein to study the expression of the receptors in the podocytes of the human glomeruli. By immunolocalization, we detected megalin, sortilin, and M6PR localization to podocytes as demonstrated by colocalization with the podocyte cytoplasmic marker WT1 protein (Figure 6C). The receptors were present predominantly in podocyte cell bodies as seen on the merged high-power views of the glomeruli (Figure 6C).

Discussion

In the present study, we have identified megalin, sortilin, and M6PR in human podocytes as endocytic receptors required for the delivery of recombinant α-Gal A to lysosomes. The M6PR mediated pathway has been very well characterized as the major route for the delivery of lysosomal enzymes; however, the mechanism for delivery of α-Gal A to lysosomes in human podocytes has been unclear until now. The heterogeneity of the uptake system of α-Gal A offers new perspectives to improve ERT for Fabry disease.

ERT given to Fabry patients has been shown to reduce GL-3 deposits in the podocytes [12,22,26], the principal affected cells in the progress of nephropathy in Fabry disease [3,5,6,7]. The glomerular filtration barrier allows macromolecules such as albumin [41], transferrin, 80 kDa [42], and a pancreatic lipase, 110 kDa [43], to be filtered. Recently we have shown that there is a limited but significant glomerular filtration of recombinant α-Gal A in α-Gal A-deficient mice and Fabry patients [34]. These findings supported the hypothesis that ERT have an effect on podocytes, which has now been enforced by demonstration of uptake of recombinant α-Gal A by podocytes in a kidney from a Fabry disease patient (Figure 1A). The uptake of α-Gal A in the glomerular endothelial and the mesangial cells is currently under investigation and future studies will in detail reveal the uptake in these cells and the receptors involved.

We show here for the first time that megalin, sortilin, and M6PR are expressed in the human glomerular podocytes. Using laser capture microdissection to isolate human glomeruli, we show that mRNA transcripts of megalin, sortilin, and M6PR are expressed in human kidney cortex and in purified human glomeruli. Immunoperoxidase staining identified a specific glomerular staining with a pattern highly suggestive of podocyte labeling in the human kidney. Extraglomerular labeling was also present in tubule segments. Dual immunofluorescence study demonstrated that megalin, sortilin, and M6PR were all expressed in the podocytes as verified by perfect colocalization with WT1 and labeling was confirmed to the cell body of the podocytes. Furthermore, we also show that the expression of these receptor proteins can be detected by immunofluorescence and Western blot in human cultured podocytes.

Previous studies have described the presence of M6PR in the proximal tubule and glomeruli [44,45]. Uptake of α-Gal A in podocytes was reduced by more than 25% with the addition of excess amounts of M6P. This was expected as the M6P residues on the recombinant α-Gal A are targeting the signal for the high-efficiency uptake by M6PR [32,33]. M6PR is primarily (90–95%) localized in the intracellular compartments, particularly in the trans-Golgi network (TGN) and endosomes, with 5–10% of the receptor present on the cell surface [46]. The primary function of M6PR is to sort and transport M6P-bearing glycoproteins from TGN to endosomes/lysosomes [46]. In addition, M6PR can bind extracellular ligands and mediate endocytosis [47]. A small proportion of M6PR was localized on the cell surface in podocytes, and most of the M6PR was observed in intracellular compartments.

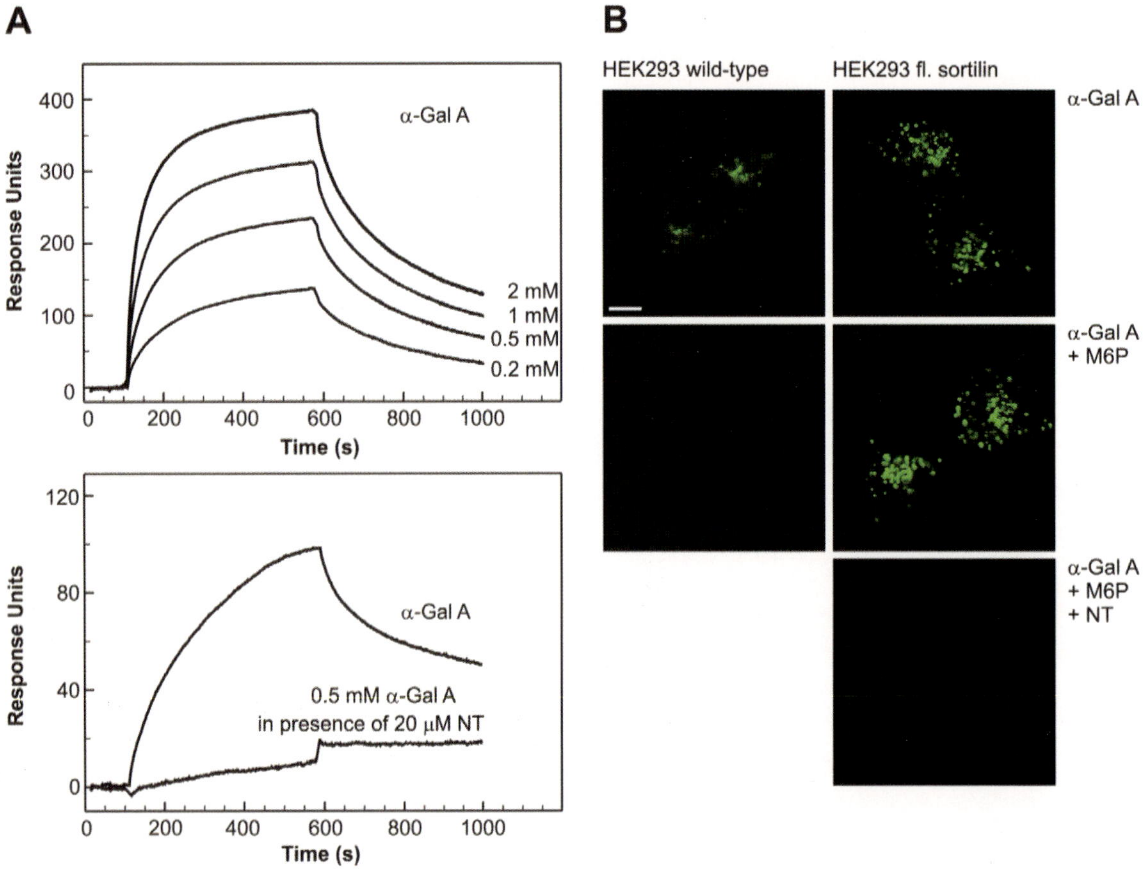

Figure 4. Binding and uptake of α-Gal A by sortilin. (A) SPR analysis of α-Gal A binding to purified human sortilin and inhibition of binding by NT. The lower binding curve was corrected for the binding of NT itself to sortilin. (B) Uptake of Alexa-Fluor 488-labeled α-Gal A by wild-type and full-length sortilin transfected HEK293 cells in the presence or absence of M6P or M6P and NT for 60 min at 37°C. At the given time, cells were fixed, and analyzed by confocal microscopy. Scale bar, 10 μm.

In our study we have shown that alternative M6PR-independent mechanisms exist for the uptake of α-Gal A. We expressed full-length sortilin in sortilin negative HEK293 cells. These transfected cells accumulated α-Gal A in intracellular compartments, and the uptake was inhibited with NT, a high affinity ligand for sortilin. These results demonstrated that sortilin is a multifunctional receptor that binds recombinant α-Gal A and, when expressed on the surface, mediates endocytosis. Sortilin is a multifunctional receptor belonging to the Vps10p-domain family receptors [38,48] and strongly homologous to that of the M6PR [48]. Sortilin is like the M6PR mainly located in the Golgi compartment and vesicles [38,48], but is also expressed on the cell surface. Sortilin has been shown to co-localize with the M6PR, both intracellularly and on the plasma membrane [49]. Thus, like the M6PR, sortilin has the potential of functioning both as a sorting receptor in the Golgi compartment and as a clearance receptor on the cell surface. Our studies demonstrated that sortilin like M6PR is located on the cell surface and in intracellular compartments in human podocytes. Uptake and degradation studies of ^{125}I-labeled α-Gal A in human podocytes demonstrate that sortilin and M6PR participate in the endocytosis of α-Gal A. Our results show that sortilin could be a new receptor for α-Gal A endocytosis in podocytes.

Megalin, a multiligand endocytic receptor, binds many of the same ligands as sortilin, and is expressed in the renal tubular epithelium and in many other organs [50,51]. Our results showed that megalin is present in human podocytes, and takes part in the uptake of α-Gal A. Megalin has previously not been described in human podocytes; however, it has been described and located in glomerular podocytes of rats [52], and also recently in cultured mouse podocytes [53]. The affinity of α-Gal A for binding to megalin is less than for sortilin [34]. Previous studies have shown that cubilin do not bind α-Gal A [34], and we did not find binding of α-Gal A to LRP (data not shown). These findings are consistent with our previous results showing that megalin is the receptor responsible for the proximal tubular accumulation of α-Gal A [34]. It has been shown that apolipoprotein B (apoB) and apoE rich lipoproteins are taken up by a receptor-mediated pathway in primary podocytes isolated from a human carcinoma kidney [54], and recently albumin was shown to be endocytosed by human podocytes in vitro and in vivo [55]. The uptake of these and other ligands could very well be facilitated by megalin, which is a receptor for apoB, apoE and albumin [50,56,57].

The contribution of each of the receptors in vivo is difficult to estimate based on our studies. RAP is a ligand for both megalin and sortilin and it binds to megalin with a higher affinity (8 nM) than for sortilin (78 nM) [58,59]. Thus, the inhibition of ^{125}I-labeled α-Gal A uptake with RAP may be due to the inhibition of both megalin and sortilin receptors.

The expression of megalin, sortilin, and M6PR in human podocytes is of general interest in the understanding of the rapidly progressing podocyte physiology. In addition, the expression of

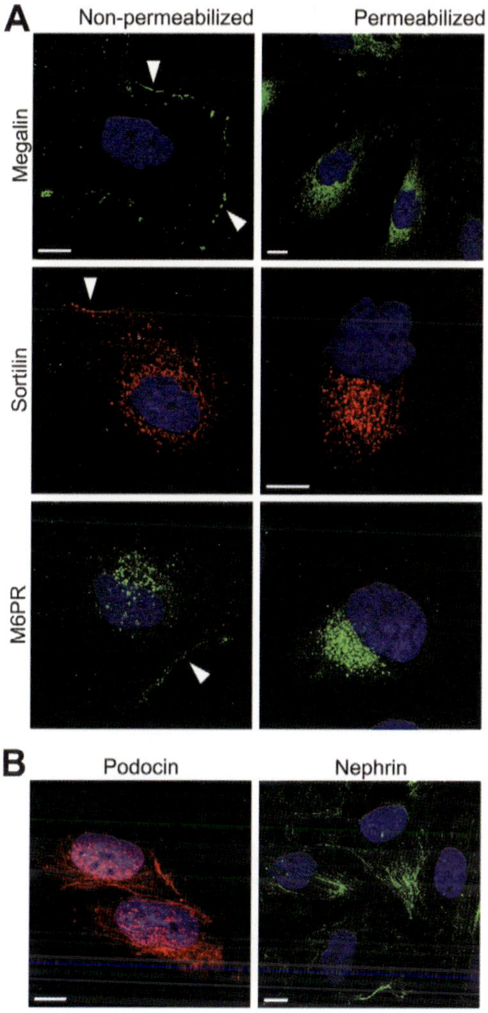

Figure 5. Megalin, sortilin, and M6PR are expressed in cultured podocytes. (A) Immunofluorescent demonstration of megalin, sortilin, and M6PR in cultured human podocytes and (B) specific podocyte-markers podocin and nephrin. Cells were fixed, stained with the appropriate antibodies and detected with Alexa-Fluor-conjugated secondary antibodies. Controls were incubated with serum and detected with same secondary antibodies (data not shown). Nuclei (blue) were stained with DAPI. Scale bars, 5 µm. White arrows indicate potential cell surface labeling of the different receptors in the human podocytes.

megalin may be of significance in immune-pathology. Megalin was initially discovered in 1982 as a pathogenic antigen of Heymann Nephritis in rats [60]. Our findings suggest that also in human, megalin may act as a pathogenic antigen for membranous glomerulonephritis. In the context of Fabry disease identification of two novel receptors on the podocyte opens new pathways of investigations to improve even further ERT.

In Fabry disease the effective targeting of recombinant α-Gal A depends on the M6P residues recognized by M6PR [31,32,33]. The limiting factor to this system includes the extent to which the recombinant enzyme is modified with M6P and the distribution of M6PR in different tissues. New approaches rely on the uptake mechanisms different from the M6P-based using protein-based mechanisms. Recently, a non-carbohydrate targeting platform for lysosomal proteins was evaluated [61]. The authors described that a fusion protein of β-glucuronidase with IGF-II, a high-affinity M6PR ligand, improved the targeting to podocytes in Mucopolysacccharidosis VII, another lysosomal disorder, where the podocyte is the most severely-affected kidney cell-type [62]. They also showed that α-Gal A modified with attachment of either apoE or IGF-II peptides increased the half-life by ~20-fold in animal models, and that the in vitro uptake of these modified enzymes was not competed by M6P. Recent data have shown that fusion proteins between lysosomal enzymes and RAP were efficiently endocytosed by fibroblasts and other cell types from patients with lysosomal storage disorders. The uptake exceeded that of the phosphorylated enzyme and was presumably mediated by megalin and other members of low-density lipoprotein receptor (LDLR) family [63]. Since sortilin and megalin bind RAP, a fusion protein between α-Gal A and RAP could be used for a more efficient cellular delivery of α-Gal A using other pathways than M6PR. However, this will also target the other members of LDLR family, thus sortilin provides an alternative pathway using a fusion protein between α-Gal A and sortilin propeptide [36], and may deliver the therapeutic enzyme specifically via a sortilin mediated pathway.

In conclusion, we have identified M6PR, sortilin, and megalin as the receptors responsible for the lysosomal delivery of α-Gal A in human podocytes. Sortilin and megalin provide two M6P independent uptake systems for the delivery of the recombinant α-Gal A to the lysosomes in podocytes in Fabry disease patients. These findings are important steps in developing a rationale for ERT in Fabry disease.

Materials and Methods

Antibodies and proteins

Recombinant α-Gal A (Fabrazyme) and affinity-purified rabbit polyclonal anti-human α-Gal A were provided by Genzyme Corp. (Framingham, MA, USA). Sheep anti-rat megalin has been described earlier [64]. A specific polyclonal rabbit anti-human megalin was a kind gift from Dr. S. Moestrup, Aarhus University, Aarhus, DK. This antibody gave a specific band for megalin when tested by Western blot on human kidney homogenate. Recombinant receptor-associated protein (RAP) was provided by Novo Nordisk A/S (Bagsværd, DK) and Dr. S. Moestrup, Aarhus University, Aarhus, DK. Affinity purified rabbit polyclonal anti-sortilin was generated against the ectodomain of human sortilin, as previously described [36]. Polyclonal rabbit anti-sortilin (ab16640) and sortilin peptide (ab16686) were purchased from Abcam. Recombinant GST-sortilin propeptide were expressed in *Escherichia coli* and purified as previously described [36]. A specific affinity purified rabbit polyclonal anti-IGF-II/M6PR was generated against the full-length bovine IGF-II/M6PR as previously described [65]. Polyclonal rabbit anti-rat IGF-II/M6PR 3637 was a kind gift from Dr. W. Kiess, Hospital for Children and Adolescence, University of Leipzig, Leipzig, DE. Recombinant human IGF-II receptor (2447-GR) was purchased from R & D systems (Minneapolis, MN, USA). The mannose 6-phosphate (M6P; M3655), neurotensin (NT; N6383), affinity purified rabbit polyclonal anti-podocin (P0372) were purchased from Sigma Aldrich (Saint Louis, MO, USA). Monoclonal mouse anti-nephrin IgG1 was a kind gift from Dr. K. Tryggvason, Karolinska Institute, Stockholm, SE. Monoclonal mouse anti-human Wilms' tumor 1 (WT1; clone 6F-H2) protein and peroxidase-conjugated secondary antibodies were purchased from DAKO A/S (Glostrup, DK). Fluorescence-conjugated secondary antibodies were purchased from Molecular Probes (Eugene, OR, USA). Controls for unspecific binding were performed with nonspecific rabbit, mouse, or sheep IgG from DAKO.

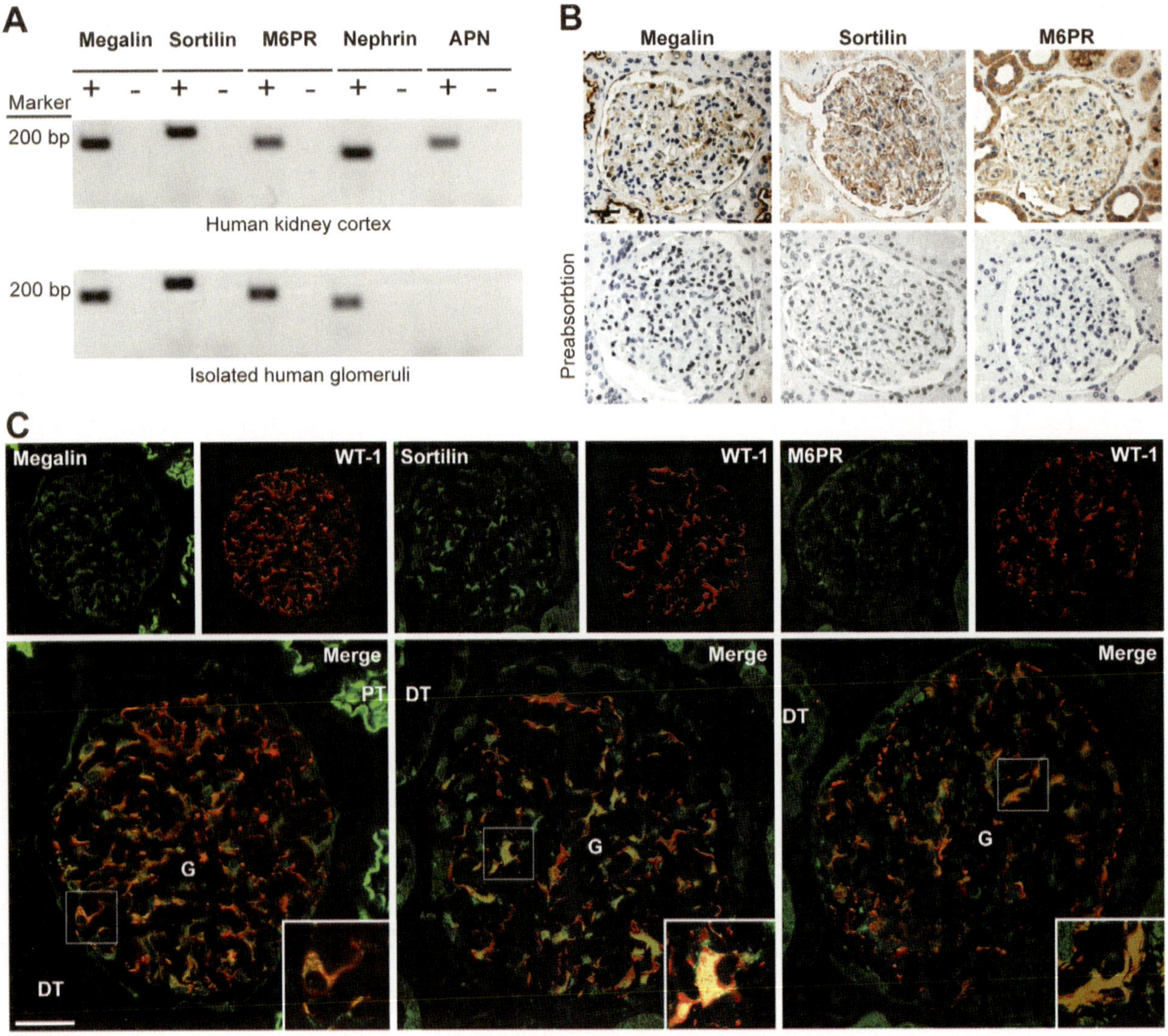

Figure 6. Expression of megalin, sortilin, and M6PR in human glomeruli. (A) Expression of megalin, M6PR, sortilin, podocin, nephrin, APN mRNAs by RT-PCR (+). Negative controls (−) run without RT enzyme. The marker used was 100 bp ladder. (B) Immunoperoxidase labeling of paraffin sections from a normal human kidney incubated with antibodies to megalin, M6PR, and sortilin show that the brush borders of proximal tubules (PT) are heavily stained. The distal tubules (DT) are unstained for megalin, but stained for sortilin and M6PR. The glomeruli (G) show staining for megalin, sortilin and M6PR. Preabsorption of the antibodies with the respective antigens show loss of immunoreactivity, demonstrating antibody specificity. Tubular and podocyte staining was blocked by preincubation. Controls that included only the secondary antibody showed no labeling (data not shown). Scale bar, 50 μm. (C) Dual immunofluorescence and confocal microscopy with monoclonal anti-WT1 antibody (red) and polyclonal antibodies (green) against megalin, sortilin, and M6PR. The respective merge images are shown in both low and high magnifications. Megalin, sortilin, and M6PR are localized in the glomerular podocytes and co-localizes with WT-1 as seen by the merged images indicated with white arrow-heads. High-power views of a portion of a glomerulus show merged images of the receptors and WT1 demonstrating that megalin, sortilin, and M6PR localize primarily to the podocyte cell bodies. Scale bar, 50 μm.

Cells

The human podocyte cell line conditionally immortalized by introducing temperature-sensitive SV40-T antigen by transfection has previously been characterized in detail [35]. The podocyte cell line (passages 12 to 25) was maintained in RPMI 1640 (R-8758) medium supplemented with insulin, transferrin, selenite (ITS; I-3146), 10% FBS (F7524) all from Sigma Aldrich, at 33°C in 5% CO_2. Podocyte differentiation was induced under nonpermissive conditions by thermo shifting the cells to 37°C for 14 days. HEK 293 cells were obtained from Invitrogen (Carlsbad, CA, USA) and maintained in DMEM (LONZA, BE) supplemented with 10% FBS (GIBCO, Paisley, UK), at 37°C in 5% CO_2. The human cDNA construct encoding full-length sortilin [66] was expressed using the mammalian expression vector pcDNA3.1/zeo (Invitrogen, Groningen, NL). Cells were transfected with pcDNA3.1/zeo using FUGENE 6 (Roche, CH), and a stably transfected clone was selected in medium containing 150 μg/ml zeocin. All cell culture media were supplemented with 100 U/ml penicillin, and 100 μg/ml streptomycin (LONZA). The media was renewed every second day, and cells were split at confluence approximately once a week using a trypsin-EDTA solution (LONZA). Experiments were carried out with confluent monolayers of cells cultured in 24-well plates (Nagle Nunc International, Hereford, UK) with or without cover slips for uptake studies, and in 75 cm^2 culture flasks (Corning

Incorporated, Corning, NY, USA) for the affinity purification experiment. Podocytes were only used after they were differentiated under non-permissive conditions for 14 days at 37°C.

Biopsy preparation

Renal biopsies were obtained from A) a kidney from a male Fabry patient, 37 years of age, 2 h after enzyme replacement infusion, 0.2 mg/kg body wt recombinant α-Gal A and B) an untreated male Fabry patient, 38 years of age. The biopsies were prepared for paraffin-embedding by routine methodology. Ethical approval for the human studies was granted by the Copenhagen Local Research Ethics Committee and informed consent was obtained from the patient.

Immunofluorescence microscopy of cell cultures

Uptake of Alexa Fluor 488-labeled α-Gal A in cultured human podocytes. Recombinant α-Gal A was labeled with Alexa Fluor 488 according to the instructions of the manufacturer (Molecular Probes). Podocytes, parental and full-length sortilin HEK293 cells were incubated with Alexa Fluor 488-labeled α-Gal A at 37°C at indicated times with or without inhibitors, and fixed with 4% paraformaldehyde for 10 min at room temperature. LysoTracker Red DND-99 (L-7528; Molecular Probes) was used as described by the manufacturer. Cells were counterstained with LysoTracker Red for 15 min before fixation.

Localization of proteins in podocytes. Immunofluorescence on human podocytes was performed as described previously [35] at room temperature. In brief, cover slips were fixed with 2% paraformaldehyde, 4% sucrose in PBS for 10 min and permeabilized with 0.3% Triton X 100 (Sigma Aldrich) in PBS for 10 min. Nonspecific binding sites were blocked with 4% FBS+0.1% Tween 20 (Sigma Aldrich) in PBS for 60 min. Primary and secondary antibodies were applied at the appropriate dilutions according to standard techniques.

Cell surface localization of proteins in podocytes. For surface labeling of proteins, cover slips were fixed with 2% paraformaldehyde, 4% sucrose in phosphate-buffered saline and incubated with primary antibodies over night at 4°C. After this, they were incubated with Alexa Fluor conjugated antibodies for 1 h at room temperature, and nuclei-stained with DAPI (Molecular Probes) according to the directions from manufacturer.

All cover slips were mounted on glass slides in DAKO Fluorescent Medium. Staining was analyzed by confocal laser scanning microscope (LSM510; Carl Zeiss, DE). Images were acquired using the software from the manufacturer and processed with Adobe Photoshop CS3 software. Controls for nonspecific binding were performed with nonspecific serum and IgG fractions.

Protein extraction

Cell proteins were extracted by addition of modified RIPA buffer (R-0278; Sigma Aldrich) containing 50 mmol/L Tris-HCL, 150 mmol/L NaCl, 1% Triton X-100, 1 mmol/L ethylenediaminetetraacetic acid, 1 mmol/L phenylmethyl sulfonyl fluoride, 1 μg/mL aprotinin, 1 μg/mL leupeptin, 1 μg/mL pepstatin, 1 mmol/L Na vanadate; and complete protease inhibitor (Roche Diagnostics, Mannheim, DE; 1 tablet per 50 ml of solution) at 4°C. The suspension was centrifuged at 14000×g for 15 min at 4°C, and the supernatant containing cellular protein was collected. Total protein was quantified using Pierce BCA Protein Assay kit (Pierce, Rockford, IL, USA) according to the manufacturer.

Affinity purification of α-Gal A binding proteins

Purified recombinant α-Gal A covalently coupled using the AminoLink Plus Immobilization Kit (Pierce) following the guidelines from the manufacturer. Affinity purification was done following the Pierce instructions. Briefly, differentiated podocytes were lysed with RIPA buffer as described before. The cell lysate was diluted in PBS binding buffer (pH 7.4) at a ratio of at least 1:4 and recirculated over the column three times at room temperature. The column was extensively washed in wash solution (1 M NaCl, 0.05% NaN_3) followed by elution of bound proteins with 0.2 M glycine·HCl buffer (pH 2.5). Fractions (300 μl) were collected, subjected to SDS-PAGE, and stained by silver staining using SilverSNAP Stain Kit II (Pierce). Additional gels were blotted onto PVDF membranes for further protein identification by Western blotting.

SDS-PAGE and Western blotting

Eluted α-Gal A binding protein fraction with the highest protein content and podocyte lysates were loaded on the SDS-PAGE gels. The samples were mixed with NuPAGE LDS sample buffer (Invitrogen, Carlsbad, CA) with 2.5% SDS, and the proteins were separated by SDS-PAGE and electrophoretically transferred to PVDF membranes (Millipore Corporation; Bedford, MA, USA) for Western blot. Blots were blocked with 5% milk in PBS-T (80 mM Na_2HPO_4, 20 mM NaH_2PO_4, 100 mM NaCl, and 0.1% Tween 20 [pH 7.5]) for 1 h and incubated overnight at 4°C with primary antibody in PBS-T with 1% BSA. After washing in PBS-T, the blots were incubated for 1 h with horseradish peroxidase-conjugated secondary antibody (DAKO). After a final wash, antibody binding was visualized using ECL system (Amersham International, Bucks, UK).

Surface plasmon resonance analysis

For the surface plasmon resonance (SPR) analyses, BIAcore sensor chips (type CM5; Biacore, Uppsala, SE) were activated with a 1:1 mixture of 0.2 M *N*-ethyl-N′-(3-dimethylaminopropyl) carbodiimide and 0.05 M *N*-hydroxysuccinimide in water according to the manufacturer. Sortilin was immobilized as previously described [36]. The SPR signal from immobilized sortilin generated BIAcore resonance units (RU) that were equivalent to 66 $fmol/mm^2$. The flow cells were regenerated with 20 μl of 1.5 M glycine-HCl (pH 3.0). The flow buffer was 10 mM HEPES, 150 mM NaCl, 1.5 mM $CaCl_2$, and 1 mM EGTA (pH 7.4). The binding data was analyzed using the BIAevaluation program. The number of ligands bound per immobilized receptor was estimated by dividing the ratio RU ligand/mass ligand with RU receptor/mass receptor. The K_d for binding was estimated using a BIA evaluation program.

^{125}I-labeled α-Gal A uptake by podocytes

Lysosomal α-Gal A was iodinated with the use of the chloramine-T method [67] to a specific activity of approximately 217,000 cpm/μg protein. Human podocytes were incubated with 10 nM ^{125}I-α-Gal A in the presence or absence of 1 μM RAP, 10 μM M6P, 1 μM sortilin propeptide, and all three ligands at 37°C in 5% CO2/95% air for 4, 8, and 12 h. Incubation with ^{125}I-α-Gal A was carried out in serum-free medium (RPMI1640) containing 0.1% BSA (Sigma Aldrich), and stopped by aspiration of the medium. Cells were washed in PBS and collected by trypsinization with 150 μl of Trypsin-EDTA. The samples were counted in a γ-counter (Cobra 5003, Packard, Meriden, CT, USA). Degradation was measured by precipitation of the medium in 10% TCA and the TCA-soluble fraction, defined as the degraded fraction. To correct for liberation *per se* of iodine from ^{125}I-α-Gal A during the experiment, the medium in control wells was incubated without cells. Degradation was calculated as the TCA-soluble fraction in the incubation medium minus the TCA-soluble fraction in the medium from control wells. Cell-associated ^{125}I-α-Gal A was measured by counting the cells after trypsinization. Total uptake was defined as the sum of degraded and cell-associated fraction divided by the total amount of tracer added in each well. The medium from control wells contained a TCA-soluble fraction of approximately 10%.

Tissue Preparation and LCM

Human kidneys were obtained from renal carcinoma patients. Ethical approval for the human studies was granted by the Local Research Ethics Committee and informed consent was obtained from the patients. Immediately after surgical removal, carcinoma free parts of the kidneys were excised, embedded in Tissue-Tek OCT Compound, and immediately snap-frozen, placed on dry ice and stored at −80°C until use. Tissues were cryosectioned into 10 µm thick sections at −20°C using a cryostat. Cryosections were then attached to RNase-free glass slides (Arcturus, Mountain View, CA, USA). The slides were processed with an RNase-free technique. The slides were thawed at room temperature for 30 sec and then dehydrated in 75% ethanol for 1 min, 95% ethanol for 1 min, and 100% ethanol for 1 min. Finally, sections were incubated in xylene for 5 min and air dried for 5 min.

Immediately after dehydration LCM was performed using the automated VERITAS™ Microdissection Instrument (Arcturus). The laser beams were adjusted to cut and capture the visualized glomeruli. Dissection was performed at room temperature and was limited to 30 min to prevent RNA degradation. CapSure HS LCM caps (Arcturus) were used to capture the glomeruli, ensuring precise capture and preventing contamination from the surrounding tissue while microdissecting. Furthermore, CapSure HS LCM caps together with ExtracSure devices (Arcturus) enabled the highly sensitive extraction of glomeruli. For RNA extraction, a total of 200 glomeruli were captured.

RNA Isolation and RT-PCR

Total human glomerular- and cortex RNA were extracted using the PicoPure RNA Isolation Kit (Arcturus) as described by the manufacturer. DNase treatment was performed on PicoPure column with a RNase-free DNase set (Qiagen, Hilden, DE). Total RNA was estimated using a NanoDrop 2000 (Thermo Scientific, Wilmington, DE, USA), showing that each sample yielded 3–8 ng/µl.

Reverse transcription was performed for 60 minutes at 42°C in a volume of 20 µl using Sensiscript RT (Qiagen) and respective buffer. This was performed in the presence of 0.5 mM deoxyribonucleoside triphosphates (dATP, dTTP, dGTP, dCTP) (Qiagen), 1 µM of a 16mer d(T) oligonucleotide primer (Perkin Elmer, USA), 0.5 unit/µl RNase inhibitor (Perkin Elmer), 1 µl Sensiscript RT and purified RNA (25 ng). A reaction without RT enzyme was made in parallel with purified RNA to ascertain that the amplification occurred on RNA and not DNA.

PCR was performed in a volume of 10 µl using a HotStarTaq Master Mix Kit (Qiagen) following the protocol from manufacturer. This was performed with 5 µl HotStarTaq Master Mix, 2.5 µl cresol, 5 pmol of sense and antisense primers (Table 1) and 1 µl of the RT-product. The PCR program was as follows: denaturation 15 min 94°C and 35 cycles of: 1 min 94°C, 30 sec 58°C, 1 min 72°C. After cycling the reaction ended with 10 min at 72°C. After the PCR reaction the products were visualized by running a 1.5% agarose gel stained with ethidium bromide (0.5 µg/ml) and developed using Fluor-S™ MultiImager (BIO RAD, USA).

Immunohistochemistry

Renal sections were obtained from paraffin-embedded Fabry disease kidneys or normal human kidneys (autopsy materials). For light microscope immunohistochemistry, 2-µm tissue paraffin sections were cut on a Leica RM 2165 microtome (Leica, Wetzlar, Germany). Sections were dried at 60°C in an oven for 1 h, placed in xylene overnight, rehydrated in graded alcohols, heated in TEG buffer (Tris-EGTA buffer, pH 9) at approximately 100°C in a microwave oven for 20 min, cooled at room temperature for 30 min, incubated for 30 min in 50 nM NH_4Cl in 0.01 M PBS. Sections were permeabilized with 0.05% saponin (1% BSA, 0.2% gelatine, 0.05% saponin in 0.01 M PBS) and blocked for endogenous peroxidase before incubation with the primary antibody. Sections were incubated with a primary antibody in 0.01 M PBS, 0.1% BSA and 0.02 M NaN_3, followed by incubation with HRP-conjugated secondary antibody. For the preabsorption experiments, primary polyclonal rabbit anti-megalin, anti-sortilin and anti-M6PR antibodies were incubated with affinity purified megalin, sortilin, and M6PR respectively for 2 h at room temperature before incubating the preincubated antibody and antigen mixture on the tissue-slide. Megalin was purified from human cortical membranes on RAP affinity column, using the AminoLink Plus Immobilization Kit and human cortical membranes were obtained from human kidneys and prepared as previously described [68]. Sortilin and M6PR were purchased

Table 1. Primers for RT-PCR.

Transcript	GenBank accession #	Primer pair	Product size *bp*
Megalin	NM_004525.2	5′-AGCCTCTGGAGTTGGACAGA-3′ (forward) 5′-ACAGTGCGGTTAGACCCATC-3′ (reverse)	189
M6PR	NM_000876.2	5′-AGTGGAAGGGGACAACTGTG-3′ (forward) 5′-ACATGAGGAGACCACCTTGG-3′ (reverse)	184
Sortilin	NM_002959.4	5′-TCCTGGGTTGGAGATAGCAC-3′ (forward) 5′-TTCCTCCAGACACCTCTGCT-3′ (reverse)	232
Podocin	NM_014625.1	5′-TGGGGAATCAAAGTGGAGAG-3′ (forward) 5′-GAATCTCAGCTGCCATCCTC-3′ (reverse)	169
Nephrin	NM_004646.1	5′-GACCCAGCTTCCCATCACTA-3′ (forward) 5′-GCATTGGAGAGGAGCAGAAG-3′ (reverse)	150
Aminopeptidase N	NM_001150.2	5′-CAGGGGCCTGTACGTTTTTA-3′ (forward) 5′-CCACCAGCTCAGTCTTGTCA-3′ (reverse)	179

from Abcam and R&D systems, respectively. Sections were counterstained with Meier's haematoxylin stain and peroxidase labeling was visualized by incubation with diaminobenzidine and H_2O_2 for 10 min.

For dual immunofluorescence labeling mouse anti-WT1 and rabbit anti-megalin (antiserum), anti-sortilin (immunopurified polyclonal antibody to human sortilin), or anti-M6PR (immunopurified polyclonal antibody to bovine M6PR) antibodies were applied followed by Alexa Fluor conjugated anti-mouse and anti-rabbit IgG. All incubations with primary antibodies were done overnight at 4°C and secondary incubations were done at room temperature for 1 hour. Sections were subsequently examined in a Leica DMR microscope equipped with a Leica DFC320 camera or a Zeiss LSM510 Meta laser confocal microscope. Images were transferred by a Leica TFC Twain 6.1.0 program and processed using Adobe Photoshop 8.0. Negative controls were performed by replacing the primary antibody with the normal serum of the species in which the primary antibody was raised or without the primary antibody.

Statistical analysis

The results of ^{125}I- α-Gal A uptake experiments are presented as means ± SD, and the t test was used to test for significant differences. P values<0.05 were considered significant.

Acknowledgments

The skillful technical assistance by Christian Jacobsen, Anne Marie Bundsgaard, Maj Margrethe Kjærgaard, Pia Nielsen, Inger B. Kristoffersen, and Hanne Sidelmann is gratefully acknowledged.

Author Contributions

Conceived and designed the experiments: TP RN PJV EIC. Performed the experiments: TP RN JVL SSS UF-R CMP PJV EIC. Analyzed the data: TP RN JVL SSS UF-R MAS CMP PJV EIC. Contributed reagents/materials/analysis tools: TP RN JVL SSS UF-R MAS CMP PJV EIC. Wrote the paper: TP.

References

1. Brady RO, Gal AE, Bradley RM, Martensson E, Warshaw AL, et al. (1967) Enzymatic defect in Fabry's disease. Ceramidetrihexosidase deficiency. N Engl J Med 276: 1163–1167.
2. Kint JA (1970) Fabry's disease: alpha-galactosidase deficiency. Science 167: 1268–1269.
3. Desnick RJ, Ioannou YA, Eng CM (2006) α-Galactosidase A deficiency: Fabry disease. In: Scriver CRBA, Sly WS, Valle D, eds. The Metabolic and Molecular Bases of Inherited Disease. 8 ed. New York, NY.: McGraw-Hill. pp 3733–3774.
4. Mehta A, Ricci R, Widmer U, Dehout F, Garcia de Lorenzo A, et al. (2004) Fabry disease defined: baseline clinical manifestations of 366 patients in the Fabry Outcome Survey. Eur J Clin Invest 34: 236–242.
5. Colley JR, Miller DL, Hutt MS, Wallace HJ, De Wardener HE (1958) The renal lesion in angiokeratoma corporis diffusum. Br Med J 1: 1266–1268.
6. Meroni M, Sessa A, Battini G, Tazzari S, Torri Tarelli L (1997) Kidney involvement in Anderson-Fabry disease. Contrib Nephrol 122: 178–184.
7. Branton MH, Schiffmann R, Sabnis SG, Murray GJ, Quirk JM, et al. (2002) Natural history of Fabry renal disease: influence of alpha-galactosidase A activity and genetic mutations on clinical course. Medicine (Baltimore) 81: 122–138.
8. Najafian B, Svarstad E, Bostad L, Gubler MC, Tondel C, et al. (2011) Progressive podocyte injury and globotriaosylceramide (GL-3) accumulation in young patients with Fabry disease. Kidney Int 79: 663–670.
9. Thadhani R, Wolf M, West ML, Tonelli M, Ruthazer R, et al. (2002) Patients with Fabry disease on dialysis in the United States. Kidney Int 61: 249–255.
10. Ojo A, Meier-Kriesche HU, Friedman G, Hanson J, Cibrik D, et al. (2000) Excellent outcome of renal transplantation in patients with Fabry's disease. Transplantation 69: 2337–2339.
11. Gubler MC, Lenoir G, Grunfeld JP, Ulmann A, Droz D, et al. (1978) Early renal changes in hemizygous and heterozygous patients with Fabry's disease. Kidney Int 13: 223–235.
12. Thurberg BL, Rennke H, Colvin RB, Dikman S, Gordon RE, et al. (2002) Globotriaosylceramide accumulation in the Fabry kidney is cleared from multiple cell types after enzyme replacement therapy. Kidney Int 62: 1933–1946.
13. Tondel C, Bostad L, Hirth A, Svarstad E (2008) Renal biopsy findings in children and adolescents with Fabry disease and minimal albuminuria. Am J Kidney Dis 51: 767–776.
14. Alroy J, Sabnis S, Kopp JB (2002) Renal pathology in Fabry disease. J Am Soc Nephrol 13 Suppl 2: S134–138.
15. Meehan SM, Junsanto T, Rydel JJ, Desnick RJ (2004) Fabry disease: renal involvement limited to podocyte pathology and proteinuria in a septuagenarian cardiac variant. Pathologic and therapeutic implications. Am J Kidney Dis 43: 164–171.
16. Hers HG (1965) Inborn Lysosomal Diseases. Gastroenterology 48: 625–633.
17. Schiffmann R, Murray GJ, Treco D, Daniel P, Sellos-Moura M, et al. (2000) Infusion of alpha-galactosidase A reduces tissue globotriaosylceramide storage in patients with Fabry disease. Proc Natl Acad Sci U S A 97: 365–370.
18. Schiffmann R, Kopp JB, Austin HA, 3rd, Sabnis S, Moore DF, et al. (2001) Enzyme replacement therapy in Fabry disease: a randomized controlled trial. JAMA 285: 2743–2749.
19. Eng CM, Banikazemi M, Gordon RE, Goldman M, Phelps R, et al. (2001) A phase 1/2 clinical trial of enzyme replacement in fabry disease: pharmacokinetic, substrate clearance, and safety studies. Am J Hum Genet 68: 711–722.
20. Schiffmann R, Ries M, Timmons M, Flaherty JT, Brady RO (2006) Long-term therapy with agalsidase alfa for Fabry disease: safety and effects on renal function in a home infusion setting. Nephrol Dial Transplant 21: 345–354.
21. Schiffmann R, Askari H, Timmons M, Robinson C, Benko W, et al. (2007) Weekly enzyme replacement therapy may slow decline of renal function in patients with Fabry disease who are on long-term biweekly dosing. J Am Soc Nephrol 18: 1576–1583.
22. Germain DP, Waldek S, Banikazemi M, Bushinsky DA, Charrow J, et al. (2007) Sustained, long-term renal stabilization after 54 months of agalsidase beta therapy in patients with Fabry disease. J Am Soc Nephrol 18: 1547–1557.
23. Banikazemi M, Bultas J, Waldek S, Wilcox WR, Whitley CB, et al. (2007) Agalsidase-beta therapy for advanced Fabry disease: a randomized trial. Ann Intern Med 146: 77–86.
24. West M, Nicholls K, Mehta A, Clarke JT, Steiner R, et al. (2009) Agalsidase alfa and kidney dysfunction in Fabry disease. J Am Soc Nephrol 20: 1132–1139.
25. Mehta A, Beck M, Elliott P, Giugliani R, Linhart A, et al. (2009) Enzyme replacement therapy with agalsidase alfa in patients with Fabry's disease: an analysis of registry data. Lancet 374: 1986–1996.
26. Eng CM, Guffon N, Wilcox WR, Germain DP, Lee P, et al. (2001) Safety and efficacy of recombinant human alpha-galactosidase A–replacement therapy in Fabry's disease. N Engl J Med 345: 9–16.
27. Fervenza FC, Torra R, Warnock DG (2008) Safety and efficacy of enzyme replacement therapy in the nephropathy of Fabry disease. Biologics 2: 823–843.
28. Breunig F, Weidemann F, Strotmann J, Knoll A, Wanner C (2006) Clinical benefit of enzyme replacement therapy in Fabry disease. Kidney Int 69: 1216–1221.
29. Vedder AC, Linthorst GE, Houge G, Groener JE, Ormel EE, et al. (2007) Treatment of Fabry disease: outcome of a comparative trial with agalsidase alfa or beta at a dose of 0.2 mg/kg. PloS ONE 2: e598.
30. Oqvist B, Brenner BM, Oliveira JP, Ortiz A, Schaefer R, et al. (2009) Nephropathy in Fabry disease: the importance of early diagnosis and testing in high-risk populations. Nephrol Dial Transplant 24: 1736–1743.
31. Dahms NM, Lobel P, Kornfeld S (1989) Mannose 6-phosphate receptors and lysosomal enzyme targeting. J Biol Chem 264: 12115–12118.
32. Sando GN, Neufeld EF (1977) Recognition and receptor-mediated uptake of a lysosomal enzyme, alpha-l-iduronidase, by cultured human fibroblasts. Cell 12: 619–627.
33. Kaplan A, Achord DT, Sly WS (1977) Phosphohexosyl components of a lysosomal enzyme are recognized by pinocytosis receptors on human fibroblasts. Proc Natl Acad Sci U S A 74: 2026–2030.
34. Christensen EI, Zhou Q, Sorensen SS, Rasmussen AK, Jacobsen C, et al. (2007) Distribution of alpha-galactosidase A in normal human kidney and renal accumulation and distribution of recombinant alpha-galactosidase A in Fabry mice. J Am Soc Nephrol 18: 698–706.
35. Saleem MA, O'Hare MJ, Reiser J, Coward RJ, Inward CD, et al. (2002) A conditionally immortalized human podocyte cell line demonstrating nephrin and podocin expression. J Am Soc Nephrol 13: 630–638.
36. Munck Petersen C, Nielsen MS, Jacobsen C, Tauris J, Jacobsen L, et al. (1999) Propeptide cleavage conditions sortilin/neurotensin receptor-3 for ligand binding. EMBO J 18: 595–604.
37. Lee K, Jin X, Zhang K, Copertino L, Andrews L, et al. (2003) A biochemical and pharmacological comparison of enzyme replacement therapies for the glycolipid storage disorder Fabry disease. Glycobiology 13: 305–313.
38. Mazella J, Zsurger N, Navarro V, Chabry J, Kaghad M, et al. (1998) The 100-kDa neurotensin receptor is gp95/sortilin, a non-G-protein-coupled receptor. J Biol Chem 273: 26273–26276.
39. Willnow TE, Petersen CM, Nykjaer A (2008) VPS10P-domain receptors - regulators of neuronal viability and function. Nat Rev Neurosci 9: 899–909.

40. Rahmoune H, Thompson PW, Ward JM, Smith CD, Hong G, et al. (2005) Glucose transporters in human renal proximal tubular cells isolated from the urine of patients with non-insulin-dependent diabetes. Diabetes 54: 3427–3434.
41. Brenner BM, Baylis C, Deen WM (1976) Transport of molecules across renal glomerular capillaries. Physiol Rev 56: 502–534.
42. Kozyraki R, Fyfe J, Verroust PJ, Jacobsen C, Dautry-Varsat A, et al. (2001) Megalin-dependent cubilin-mediated endocytosis is a major pathway for the apical uptake of transferrin in polarized epithelia. Proc Natl Acad Sci U S A 98: 12491–12496.
43. Comte B, Franceschi C, Sadoulet MO, Silvy F, Lafitte D, et al. (2006) Detection of bile salt-dependent lipase, a 110 kDa pancreatic protein, in urines of healthy subjects. Kidney Int 69: 1048–1055.
44. Cui S, Flyvbjerg A, Nielsen S, Kiess W, Christensen EI (1993) IGF-II/Man-6-P receptors in rat kidney: apical localization in proximal tubule cells. Kidney Int 43: 796–807.
45. Haskell JF, Pillion DJ, Meezan E (1988) Specific, high affinity receptors for insulin-like growth factor II in the rat kidney glomerulus. Endocrinology 123: 774–780.
46. Kornfeld S (1992) Structure and function of the mannose 6-phosphate/insulinlike growth factor II receptors. Annu Rev Biochem 61: 307–330.
47. Oka Y, Rozek LM, Czech MP (1985) Direct demonstration of rapid insulin-like growth factor II Receptor internalization and recycling in rat adipocytes. Insulin stimulates 125I-insulin-like growth factor II degradation by modulating the IGF-II receptor recycling process. J Biol Chem 260: 9435–9442.
48. Petersen CM, Nielsen MS, Nykjaer A, Jacobsen L, Tommerup N, et al. (1997) Molecular identification of a novel candidate sorting receptor purified from human brain by receptor-associated protein affinity chromatography. J Biol Chem 272: 3599–3605.
49. Morris NJ, Ross SA, Lane WS, Moestrup SK, Petersen CM, et al. (1998) Sortilin is the major 110-kDa protein in GLUT4 vesicles from adipocytes. J Biol Chem 273: 3582–3587.
50. Christensen EI, Birn H (2002) Megalin and cubilin: multifunctional endocytic receptors. Nat Rev Mol Cell Biol 3: 256–266.
51. Verroust PJ, Birn H, Nielsen R, Kozyraki R, Christensen EI (2002) The tandem endocytic receptors megalin and cubilin are important proteins in renal pathology. Kidney Int 62: 745–756.
52. Kerjaschki D, Farquhar MG (1983) Immunocytochemical localization of the Heymann nephritis antigen (GP330) in glomerular epithelial cells of normal Lewis rats. J Exp Med 157: 667–686.
53. Yamazaki H, Saito A, Ooi H, Kobayashi N, Mundel P, et al. (2004) Differentiation-induced cultured podocytes express endocytically active megalin, a heymann nephritis antigen. Nephron Exp Nephrol 96: e52–58.
54. Grone HJ, Walli AK, Grone E, Kramer A, Clemens MR, et al. (1990) Receptor mediated uptake of apo B and apo E rich lipoproteins by human glomerular epithelial cells. Kidney Int 37: 1449–1459.
55. Eyre J, Ioannou K, Grubb BD, Saleem MA, Mathieson PW, et al. (2007) Statin-sensitive endocytosis of albumin by glomerular podocytes. Am J Physiol Renal Physiol 292: F674–681.
56. Willnow TE, Goldstein JL, Orth K, Brown MS, Herz J (1992) Low density lipoprotein receptor-related protein and gp330 bind similar ligands, including plasminogen activator-inhibitor complexes and lactoferrin, an inhibitor of chylomicron remnant clearance. J Biol Chem 267: 26172–26180.
57. Stefansson S, Chappell DA, Argraves KM, Strickland DK, Argraves WS (1995) Glycoprotein 330/low density lipoprotein receptor-related protein-2 mediates endocytosis of low density lipoproteins via interaction with apolipoprotein B100. J Biol Chem 270: 19417–19421.
58. Kounnas MZ, Argraves WS, Strickland DK (1992) The 39-kDa receptor-associated protein interacts with two members of the low density lipoprotein receptor family, alpha 2-macroglobulin receptor and glycoprotein 330. J Biol Chem 267: 21162–21166.
59. Tauris J, Ellgaard L, Jacobsen C, Nielsen MS, Madsen P, et al. (1998) The carboxy-terminal domain of the receptor-associated protein binds to the Vps10p domain of sortilin. FEBS Lett 429: 27–30.
60. Kerjaschki D, Farquhar MG (1982) The pathogenic antigen of Heymann nephritis is a membrane glycoprotein of the renal proximal tubule brush border. Proc Natl Acad Sci U S A 79: 5557–5561.
61. Stefano JE, Hou L, Honey D, Kyazike J, Park A, et al. (2009) In vitro and in vivo evaluation of a non-carbohydrate targeting platform for lysosomal proteins. J Control Release 135: 113–118.
62. LeBowitz JH, Grubb JH, Maga JA, Schmiel DH, Vogler C, et al. (2004) Glycosylation-independent targeting enhances enzyme delivery to lysosomes and decreases storage in mucopolysaccharidosis type VII mice. Proc Natl Acad Sci U S A 101: 3083–3088.
63. Prince WS, McCormick LM, Wendt DJ, Fitzpatrick PA, Schwartz KL, et al. (2004) Lipoprotein receptor binding, cellular uptake, and lysosomal delivery of fusions between the receptor-associated protein (RAP) and alpha-L-iduronidase or acid alpha-glucosidase. J Biol Chem 279: 35037–35046.
64. Moestrup SK, Nielsen S, Andreasen P, Jorgensen KE, Nykjaer A, et al. (1993) Epithelial glycoprotein-330 mediates endocytosis of plasminogen activator-plasminogen activator inhibitor type-1 complexes. J Biol Chem 268: 16564–16570.
65. Nykjaer A, Christensen EI, Vorum H, Hager H, Petersen CM, et al. (1998) Mannose 6-phosphate/insulin-like growth factor-II receptor targets the urokinase receptor to lysosomes via a novel binding interaction. J Cell Biol 141: 815–828.
66. Nielsen MS, Madsen P, Christensen EI, Nykjaer A, Gliemann J, et al. (2001) The sortilin cytoplasmic tail conveys Golgi-endosome transport and binds the VHS domain of the GGA2 sorting protein. EMBO J 20: 2180–2190.
67. Greenwood FC, Hunter WM, Glover JS (1963) The Preparation of I-131-Labelled Human Growth Hormone of High Specific Radioactivity. Biochem J 89: 114–123.
68. Birn H, Fyfe JC, Jacobsen C, Mounier F, Verroust PJ, et al. (2000) Cubilin is an albumin binding protein important for renal tubular albumin reabsorption. J Clin Invest 105: 1353–1361.

6

Two Years after Molecular Diagnosis of Familial Hypercholesterolemia: Majority on Cholesterol-Lowering Treatment but a Minority Reaches Treatment Goal

Roeland Huijgen[1]*, Iris Kindt[2], Sjoerd B. J. Verhoeven[1], Eric J. G. Sijbrands[3], Maud N. Vissers[1], John J. P. Kastelein[1], Barbara A. Hutten[4]

1 Department of Vascular Medicine, Academic Medical Center (AMC), Amsterdam, The Netherlands, **2** Foundation for the Identification of Persons with Inherited Hypercholesterolemia, Amsterdam, The Netherlands, **3** Department of Cardiovascular Genetics and Department of Pharmacology, Vascular and Metabolic Diseases, Erasmus Medical Center, Rotterdam, The Netherlands, **4** Department of Clinical Epidemiology, Biostatistics and Bioinformatics, Academic Medical Center (AMC), Amsterdam, The Netherlands

Abstract

Background: The risk of premature cardiovascular disease in patients with familial hypercholesterolemia (FH) can be profoundly reduced by cholesterol-lowering therapy, and current guidelines for FH advocate ambitious low-density lipoprotein cholesterol (LDL-C) goals. In the present study, we determined whether these goals are reflected in current clinical practice once FH has been diagnosed.

Methodology/Principal Findings: In 2008, we sent questionnaires to all subjects (aged 18–65 years) who were molecularly diagnosed with FH in the year 2006 through the screening program in the Netherlands. Of these 1062 subjects, 781 completed the questionnaire (46% males; mean age: 42±12 years; mean LDL-C at molecular diagnosis (baseline): 4.1±1.3 mmol/L). The number of persons that used cholesterol-lowering therapy increased from 397 (51%) at baseline to 636 (81%) after diagnosis. Mean treated LDL-C levels decreased significantly to 3.2±1.1 mmol/L two years after diagnosis. Only 22% achieved the LDL-C target level of ≤2.5 mmol/L.

Conclusions/Significance: The proportion of patients using cholesterol-lowering medication was significantly increased after FH diagnosis through genetic cascade screening. The attained LDL-C levels were lower than those reported in previous surveys on medication use in FH, which could reflect the effect of more stringent lipid target levels. However, only a minority of the medication users reached the LDL-C target.

Editor: Pieter H. Reitsma, Leiden University Medical Center, The Netherlands

Funding: J.J.P.K. received grant support from AstraZeneca, Pfizer, Roche, Novartis, Merck, Merck-Schering-Plough, Isis, Genzyme, and Sanofi-Aventis; lecture fees from AstraZeneca, GlaxoSmithKline, Pfizer, Novartis, Merck-Schering-Plough, Roche, Isis, and Boehringer Ingelheim; and consulting fees from AstraZeneca, Abbott, Pfizer, Isis, Genzyme, Roche, Novartis, Merck, Merck-Schering-Plough, and Sanofi-Aventis. The FH screening program itself is financed by the Ministry of Health of the Dutch Government. Although no specific additional funding was required for the author's survey, the authors state that the funders of the screening program had no role in the study design, data collection and analysis, decision to publish, or preparation of the manuscript.

Competing Interests: No competing interest was declared for R.H., I.K., S.B.J.V., E.J.G.S., M.N.V., B.A.H..

* E-mail: r.huijgen@amc.uva.nl

Introduction

Familial hypercholesterolemia (FH) is an inherited disorder of lipid metabolism that predisposes to severe premature cardiovascular disease (CVD).[1,2] Cholesterol-lowering therapy can prevent or delay the onset of CVD and premature death in these individuals.[3,4]

Although FH is relatively common (1:400 in The Netherlands), many patients are not diagnosed at all or they are identified only after symptomatic onset of CVD.[5] Therefore, a molecular screening program was set up to actively identify all FH patients in the Netherlands.[6] During the last five years, approximately 9000 FH mutation carriers were identified. However, the success of this national screening program in preventing CVD depends also on the acceptance of physicians and patients to start preventive measures, including foremost cholesterol-lowering medication.

In 2001, we demonstrated that 38% of the participants used cholesterol-lowering therapy before the screening compared to 86% two years after the molecular diagnosis.[7] In the years after this survey, new evidence was presented on the benefit of statin treatment. In fact, two large meta-analyses demonstrated a linear relationship between LDL-C levels and the occurrence of coronary heart disease in both primary and secondary prevention of CVD.[8,9] Additionally, more aggressive treatment was shown to further decrease CVD risk.[10,11] New treatment options as well as the growing awareness among physicians of the beneficial effect of aggressive LDL-C lowering have resulted in the development of ambitious treatment targets for persons with FH.[12,13] Dutch guidelines now recommend a LDL-C treatment target of ≤2.5 mmol/L (97 mg/dL) for subjects with FH.[13] These new insights and guidelines may have changed the treatment of FH patients compared to the setting of the previous survey in 2001.[7]

In the present study, we therefore assessed whether the molecular screening program has improved the preventive care for FH. In addition, we analyzed the determinants that predict the decisions about cholesterol-lowering medication once a molecular diagnosis of FH is made.

Methods

Ethics Statement

We recruited subjects from the database of the nation-wide cascade screening program for FH in the Netherlands.[6] This program was instituted by the Dutch government and approved and financed by the Ministry of Health. All subjects who consented to participate in the screening for the FH mutation were also asked for written consent for additional scientific studies. For our survey we only approached those who gave written informed consent for additional studies. We received approval to perform such a questionnaire follow-up study by the Medical Ethical Committee of the Academic Medical Center of the University of Amsterdam.

Patient Selection and Recruitment

Subjects between 18 and 65 years of age were potentially eligible if they were visited in 2006 by a genetic fieldworker, a functional FH mutation was identified, and the lipid profile was assessed. We excluded patients if their address information was incorrect or unavailable or if they had declared that they did not want to be approached for scientific research. All probands with whom family screening was initiated were excluded as well.

We sent a questionnaire by surface mail to all selected FH patients in May 2008. Two months after the questionnaire had been distributed, we sent a reminder to the subjects who had not returned the questionnaire. If we had not received the questionnaire after six months, we contacted a random sample of the non-responder population by telephone in order to elucidate the medication use at follow-up, and inquired after their reasons for non-response. We selected these non-responders per month in which they were diagnosed, and we choose the months January, April, July, and October in 2006. We subsequently phoned until 25 consecutively diagnosed individuals in each period had consented to participate, which resulted in an additional number of 100 participants.

Data on demographics, CVD risk factors, lipid profile and medication use at baseline were extracted from the database of the screening organization.

Outcome Measures

The primary endpoints were attained LDL-C levels and the difference of the proportions treated persons at molecular diagnosis ('at baseline') and on average two years after the molecular diagnosis ('at follow-up'). The secondary endpoints were the differences in CVD risk factors and lipid profiles between the individuals who were treated or had been treated with cholesterol-lowering drugs and those who were never treated.

When untreated LDL-C levels or recent on-treatment levels were not available, we imputed these LDL-C levels by means of the estimated LDL-C lowering potency of a specific lipid-lowering drug and dose. These potency scores were summarized in a supplementary table (**table S1**). Potency scores for statins were derived from Walma et al.[13] We estimated the potency of ezetimibe as 1.20 based on the approximately 17% additional LDL-C lowering when added to statins.[14] The potency of a resin was estimated as 1.11 and that of fibrates and nicotinic acid derivatives 1.05.[3] We calculated the age and sex specific percentiles for the LDL-C levels for each subject based on reference values of a Caucasian population.[15]

Statistical Analyses

Differences in continuous and binary variables between subgroups were compared by linear or logistic regression analyses with generalized estimating equations (GEE) in the SAS procedure GENMOD accounting for correlations within families. The association between initiation of treatment since molecular diagnosis and demographics, clinical characteristics, and lipids, was analyzed with logistic regression (GEE) for all individuals who were treatment naïve at baseline. We assessed the relation between treatment potency of the drug regimen used after the molecular diagnosis and demographic, clinical, and lipid characteristics by linear regression analyses (GEE) for all persons that had been treated at baseline and/or during follow-up. We used paired t-tests to compare LDL-C levels and potency of prescribed medication within persons over time, e.g. at baseline and after on average two years of follow-up. Variables with a skewed distribution were log-transformed before analysis. A $p\text{-value}<0.05$ was considered significant. Statistical analyses were performed with the SAS package version 9.1 (SAS Institute Inc, Cary, NC, USA).

Results

Study Population

During 2006, a pathogenic LDLR or apolipoprotein B (ApoB) mutation was identified in 341 probands with a clinical diagnosis of FH. In the same period, a total of 4228 relatives aged between 18 and 65 years were screened for the presence of the specific mutation that was identified in the proband. Such a mutation was identified in 1328 of these relatives. Of these mutation carriers, 458 (34%) were first, 257 (19%) were second, 276 (21%) were third and 312 (23%) were fourth or further degree relatives of the proband, and for 25 (2%) we could not retrieve the distance from the proband.

We excluded 266 patients with FH: 134 had not given written informed consent for additional studies at the time of molecular diagnosis and of 132 we lacked up-to-date contact information. Of the remaining 1062 persons, 781 (74%) completed the questionnaire of whom 100 completed it upon a telephone call. The two main reasons for not returning the questionnaire by surface mail were that they had not received the two mailings ($n = 33$) or that they had been too busy ($n = 30$).

The 781 participants had a mean age (± standard deviation (SD)) of 42±12 years and a mean LDL-C level at diagnosis of 4.1±1.3 mmol/L and 359 (46%) were male (**table 1**). The overall prevalence of CVD was 10% ($n = 77$). Most participants had a LDL-receptor mutation ($n = 681$; 87%). Of the 100 participants with an ApoB mutation, 85 had the R3500Q mutation.[16]

The 281 non-participants, i.e. those who did not respond to the questionnaires and could not be reached by telephone, were significantly younger (36 vs. 42 years of age; $p<0.001$), had a lower prevalence of CVD (4% vs. 10%; $p = 0.003$), were more often smokers (56% vs. 42%; $p<0.001$) and used less cholesterol-lowering medication at baseline (37% vs. 51%; $p<0.001$) than the 781 participants.

Use of Cholesterol-Lowering Medication

At baseline, 397 of the 781 subjects (51%) already used cholesterol-lowering medication and 239 of 384 initially untreated persons (62%) started cholesterol-lowering treatment during follow-up (**figure 1**). Hence, the total number of treated persons increased from 397 (51%) at baseline to 636 (81%) during follow-up ($p<0.001$). As expected, the group that initiated treatment

Table 1. aracteristics of treated and untreated FH patients.

	Treated n = 636	Untreatedn = 145	p-value
Demographic and clinical			
Age *years*	44±12	35±12	<0.001
Male gender - *n (%)*	297 (47)	62 (42)	0.27
History of CVD - *n (%)*	76 (12)	1 (1)	0.002
Diabetes mellitus - *n (%)*	20 (3)	0 (0)	0.02
Hypertension - *n (%)*	75 (12)	2 (1)	<0.001
Body mass index *kg/m²*	25±4.4	24±3.8	<0.001
Current smoker (at diagnosis) - *n (%)*	277 (44)	52 (35)	0.05
Mutation			
LDLR or ApoB – *n (LDLR)/n (ApoB)*	560/76	121/24	0.10
Lipids ***mmol/L***			
Untreated LDL-C[#]	6.1±2.1	3.9±1.3	<0.001
Percentile untreated LDL-C[#]	92±13	68±29	<0.001
Cholesterol at baseline			
- TC	6.0±1.4[*]	5.7±1.4	0.04
- LDL-C	4.2±1.3[*]	3.9±1.3	0.08
- HDL-C	1.2±0.35[*]	1.3±0.34	0.18
- Triglycerides - *median [IQR]*	1.1 [0.76–1.7][*]	1.0 [0.64–1.4]	0.006
Reported TC at follow-up	5.2±1.1[a]	5.3±1.3[b]	0.45
Reported LDL-C at follow-up	3.2±1.1[c]	3.4±1.1[d]	0.36
Treatment			
Potency of medication at baseline[e]	1.84±0.34[c]	–	–
Potency of medication at follow-up	1.90±0.35	–	–

Data are expressed as mean ± standard deviation unless otherwise indicated. Variables are based on information at time of molecular FH diagnosis in 2006 (baseline) unless otherwise indicated. Follow-up is at completion of the questionnaire in 2008.
ApoB = apolipoprotein B; CVD = cardiovascular disease; HDL-C = high-density lipoprotein cholesterol; IQR = interquartile range; LDL-C = low-density lipoprotein cholesterol; LDLR = LDL-receptor; TC = total cholesterol. [#]Estimated LDL-C with correction for treatment potency at diagnosis when applicable; [*]Based on mean LDL-C of treated (n = 397) and untreated (n = 239) levels; [a]n = 441; [b]n = 51; [c]n = 262; [d]n = 35, [e]n = 397.

before the molecular diagnosis maintained treatment much better compared to those starting during follow-up (97% vs. 81%, respectively; $p<0.001$). During follow-up, a total of 55 patients discontinued medication for various reasons: adverse events (n = 25; 45%); physician's advice (n = 14; 25%); intention to become pregnant, pregnancy or to breastfeed (n = 13; 24%); and own choice (n = 3; 5%).

Nearly one fifth (n = 145) of the 781 participants never started medication. The main reasons were physicians' advice (n = 82; 56%); own choice (n = 56; 39%); intention to become pregnant, pregnancy or to breastfeed (n = 7; 5%).

LDL-C Levels at Molecular Diagnosis and Two Years after Diagnosis

After two years of follow-up, the mean LDL-C level (± SD [interquartile range (IQR)]) of all participants, was significantly reduced by 22% as compared with the level at baseline (3.2±1.1 [2.6–3.8] vs. 4.1±1.3 [3.2–4.9] mmol/L, respectively; $p<0.001$). In the group of 239 treatment naïve persons that started cholesterol-lowering medication after diagnosis the mean LDL-C level (± SD) was decreased with 44% from 5.1±1.3 at baseline to 2.8±0.80 mmol/L ($p<0.001$) two years later. The mean additional reduction in patients who were already treated at baseline was 8%: from 3.5±0.9 to 3.2±0.9 mmol/L ($p<0.001$).

The mean baseline LDL-C levels ± SD [IQR] differed significantly between 239 treatment naïve subjects at diagnosis who started medication during follow-up and 145 subjects who did not initiate treatment (5.1±1.3 [4.2–5.7] vs. 3.9±1.3 [3.0–4.8] mmol/L, respectively; $p<0.001$). The mean age and sex specific percentiles of the untreated LDL-C levels were considerably higher in the subjects that initiated medication after the molecular diagnosis than those who did not (88th vs 68th percentile, respectively; $p<0.001$).

Characteristics of Treated and Untreated Individuals

The 636 persons, who already used medication at baseline or started during follow-up (i.e. 'treated'), were older (44±12 vs. 35±12 years; $p<0.001$) than those 145 persons, who had never used medication (i.e. 'untreated') (see **table 1**). As expected, the treated patients had a higher prevalence of cardiovascular risk factors than untreated patients, such as history of CVD, diabetes mellitus, hypertension and history of smoking.

The proportion of ApoB mutation carriers among treated subjects did not differ significantly from the proportion among untreated subjects at follow-up (12% vs. 17%, respectively; $p = 0.10$). The four most prevalent LDLR mutations that had been reported to result in a severe LDL-C and CVD phenotype, i.e. V408M (exon 9), 1359-1 (intron 9), 313+1/2 (intron 3) and W23X (exon 2), were more prevalent in the treated than in the untreated group (97/636 = 15% vs. 7/145 = 5%; $p<0.001$).[17] The treated carriers were more often first degree relatives of the proband as compared to the non-treated carriers (231/636 = 36% vs. 40/145 = 28%, $p<0.001$).

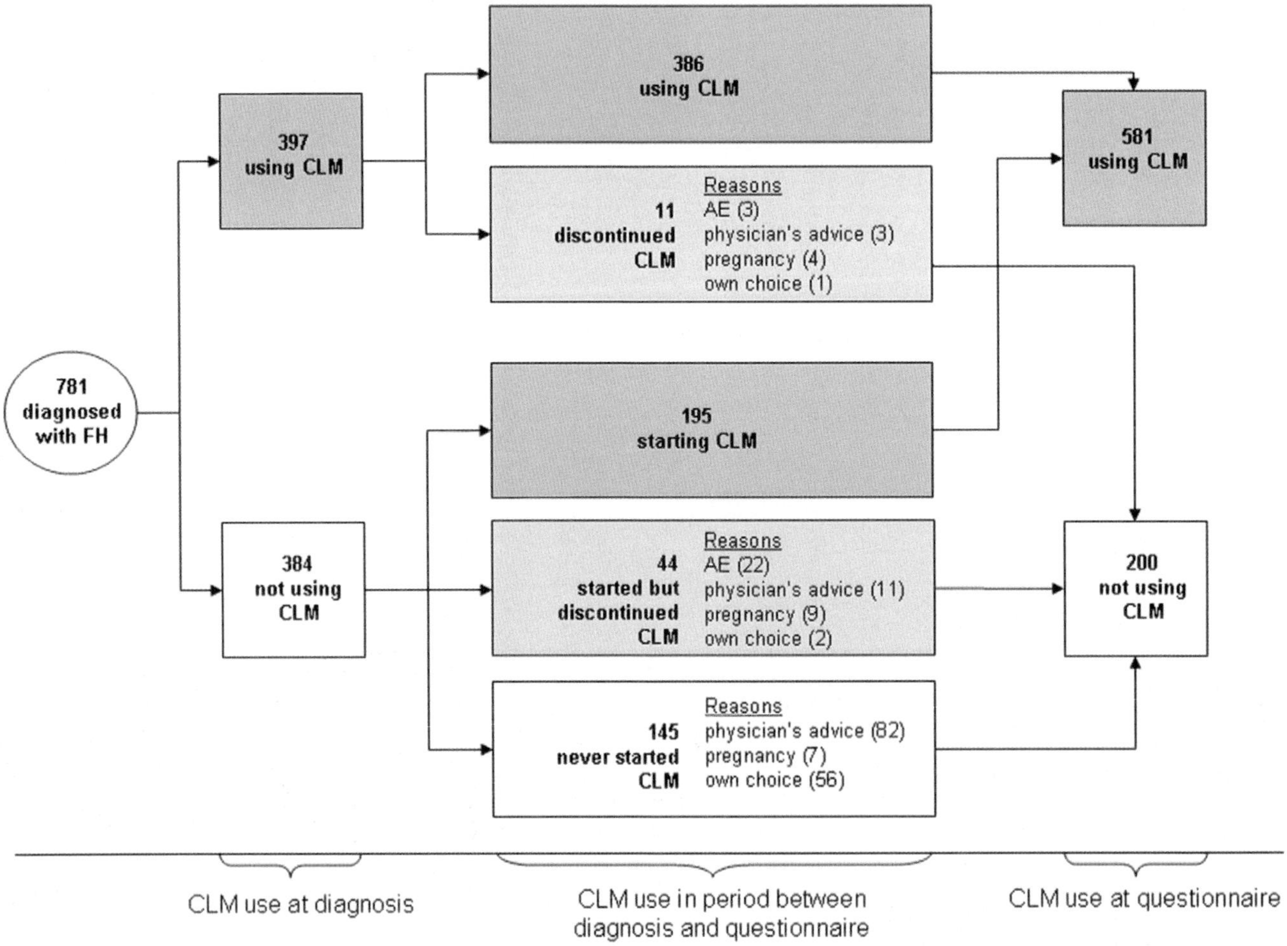

Figure 1. Use of cholesterol-lowering medication between molecular diagnosis of FH and completion of questionnaire. Molecular diagnosis of FH was made in 2006 and the questionnaire was send and completed in 2008. AE = adverse events related to CLM; FH = familial hypercholesterolemia; CLM = cholesterol-lowering medication; pregnancy = no use of medication due to pregnancy, intention to become pregnant or breastfeeding.

Treated patients (n = 581) had more frequently been referred to a specialist than untreated patients: 312 (54%) visited an internist and/or a cardiologist, whereas 26 of the 145 untreated patients (18%) had visited a specialist. In fact, 65 (45%) of the untreated patients responded that they did not visit a doctor at all with regard to FH treatment.

Predictors of Initiation of Treatment

Among the 384 untreated subjects at baseline, increased age, body mass index (BMI), LDL-C and triglycerides levels and low levels of high-density lipoprotein cholesterol (HDL-C) were associated with the start of medication after molecular diagnosis in univariate analyses. After stepwise multivariate regression analysis, age, LDL-C, and HDL-C independently predicted the start of medication (**table 2**).

Characteristics of Used Cholesterol-Lowering Treatment

The mean potency of the medication of the 636 treated patients was 1.90±0.35. For the 397 subjects that already used cholesterol-lowering medication at baseline, the LDL-C lowering capacity was increased after the identification of their mutation from 1.84±0.34 to 1.99±0.36 ($p<0.001$). A total of 265 (34%) participants used dairy products enriched with sterols and stanols, with a similar proportion in those did or did not use cholesterol-lowering medication (34% vs. 33%, respectively; $p = 0.92$).

Predictors of Potency of Treatment

For the 636 persons that used cholesterol-lowering medication during follow-up, a number of variables were significantly associated in the univariate analyses with the potency of the drug regimen after diagnosis: increased age and BMI, history of CVD, presence of diabetes or hypertension, smoking status at diagnosis, high pre-treatment LDL-C and triglycerides, and low HDL-C. After stepwise multivariate regression analysis, untreated LDL-C levels, age, history of CVD, and diabetes were independent predictors of the potency of the drug regimen used after the molecular diagnosis (**table 3**).

LDL-C Target Attainment

Of the 781 participants, 297 (38%) persons could report a LDL-C level at the end of follow-up: the target level of ≤2.5 mmol/L was achieved in 65 (22%) persons. Based on the mean potency of the current medication (1.90), we expected that 25% of the 636 treated patients would attain the target LDL-C level. In total, 492 of the 636 (77%) subjects that used cholesterol-lowering medication after diagnosis did not achieve LDL-C levels ≤2.5 mmol/L.

Table 2. Association of CVD risk factors with initiation of cholesterol-lowering medication in FH patients that were untreated at diagnosis (n = 384).

	Univariate		Multivariate	
	OR [95% CI]	p-value	OR [95% CI]	p-value
Age *years*	1.03 [1.01–1.05]	0.0060	1.02 [1.0009 – 1.05]	0.041
Male gender	1.30 [0.88–1.92]	0.18	–	–
History of CVD	1.07 [0.09–13.4]	0.96	–	–
Hypertension	3.11 [0.81–12.0]	0.10	–	–
Body Mass Index *kg/m²*	1.07 [1.01–1.12]	0.017	–	–
Smoker at diagnosis	1.29 [0.90–1.83]	0.16	–	–
LDL-C *mmol/L*	2.11 [1.65–2.71]	<0.001	2.03 [1.60–2.58]	<0.001
HDL-C *mmol/L*	0.48 [0.27–0.86]	0.014	0.45 [0.22–0.93]	0.031
Triglycerides# *mmol/L*	1.69 [1.19–2.40]	0.0033	–	–

CVD = cardiovascular disease; HDL-C = high-density lipoprotein cholesterol; LDL-C = low-density lipoprotein cholesterol; OR = odds ratio. #log-transformed before analyses.

Of these, 176 (36%) did achieve a reduction of 50% or more in LDL-C levels. Of the 145 subjects that remained untreated, 15 (10%) already had LDL-C levels ≤2.5 mmol/L at screening.

Discussion

In the current study, we found that mean LDL-C levels of individuals, who were untreated at baseline, decreased by 44% with treatment in the two years after molecular diagnosis. This means that cascade screening by molecular diagnosis not only leads to identification of FH but also supports the decision to treat these new FH patients. The decision whether or not to initiate lipid-lowering treatment was found to be dependent on age, and HDL-C and LDL-C levels. The proportion of individuals on cholesterol-lowering medication increased from 51% to 81% during follow-up. In contrast, one fifth of the identified FH subjects never started cholesterol-lowering medication. In the majority of these cases the general practitioner advised to refrain from medication because their untreated LDL-C levels were not so severely increased, i.e. on average at the 68th percentile, compared to the treated persons, whose levels were at the age and sex specific 92nd percentile before initiation of cholesterol-lowering drugs.

The achieved LDL-C level in all participants two years after molecular diagnosis was significantly lower than the achieved level in a similar survey in 2001: 3.2 mmol/L in 2008 vs. 4.2 mmol/L in 2001.[7] This is likely a consequence of the more stringent LDL-C targets for the FH population. Thus, ambitious goals and treatment possibilities for patients with FH indeed seem to be reflected by current clinical practice.

Surveys with a similar topic have also been performed in Norway and the United Kingdom. The survey in Norway focussed on medication use after molecular FH diagnosis among first degree relatives of probands.[18] The proportion of treated adult subjects increased from 67.5% at the time of genetic testing to 86.0% after six months. The decrease in LDL-C was 13.9% for the entire group with a mean achieved LDL-C level of 4.3±1.4 mmol/L at 6 months follow-up. By contrast, in our survey, we found significant lower achieved LDL-C levels (mean 3.2±1.1 mmol/L). This difference may be explained by a lower baseline LDL-C level in our cohort, a longer follow-up period to up-titrate the treatment and a more potent treatment regimen than in the Norwegian survey.

Audits on management of FH patients in outpatient clinics specifically were recently performed in the United Kingdom (UK) and the Netherlands. In the UK, Hadfield and colleagues showed that the proportion of patients on cholesterol-lowering medication ranged between of 88-94% with on-treatment LDL-C levels between 3.0 and 3.7 mmol/L.[19] Similarly, Pijlman and colleagues found mean achieved LDL-C levels of 3.2±1.1 mmol/L with 96% of the patients being on statin treatment for those visiting outpatient clinics in the Netherlands since 2006. [20] In our study, the percentage of subjects on lipid-lowering medication who visited a specialist amounted 93%, which is rather similar to the percentages found by Pijlman et al. and Hadfield et al. and much higher than the average percentage (81%) in our entire cohort. Taken together, one

Table 3. Association of CVD risk factors with the potency of cholesterol-lowering drug regimen in all treated FH patients (n = 636).

	Univariate		Multivariate	
	B [95% CI]	p-value	B [95% CI]	p-value
Age *years*	0.0058 [0.10; 0.15]	<0.001	0.0030 [0.0009; 0.0052]	0.0057
Male gender	0.016 [−0.034; 0.066]	0.53	–	–
History of CVD	0.22 [0.14; 0.31]	<0.001	0.098 [0.02; 1.2]	0.019
Diabetes	0.23 [0.06; 0.41]	0.008	0.16 [0.02; 0.30]	0.030
Hypertension	0.16 [0.08;0.25]	<0.001	–	–
Body Mass Index *kg/m²*	0.0091 [0.003; 0.015]	0.0031	–	–
Smoker at diagnosis	0.070 [0.02;0.12]	0.0089	–	–
Untreat. LDL-C *mmol/L*	0.071 [0.056; 0.086]	<0.001	0.066 [0.054; 0.078]	<0.001
HDL-C *mmol/L*	−0.089 [−0.17; −0.013]	0.022	–	–
Triglycerides# *mmol/L*	0.053 [0.001; 0.10]	0.046	–	–

Untreat. LDL-C = LDL-C level at FH diagnosis, when applicable corrected for lipid- lowering therapy use to calculate a pre-treatment value. CVD = cardiovascular disease; HDL-C = high-density lipoprotein cholesterol; LDL-C = low-density lipoprotein cholesterol. #log-transformed before analyses.

could argue that patients with a molecular diagnosis are better off when referred to a specialized clinic. On the other hand, the FH population that remained at the general practitioner's office clearly had a different phenotype with less raised LDL-C and fewer risk factors.

In general, management of FH patients is not successful when measured against the new guideline targets. In fact, a sizable subset of persons with FH does not get pharmacological treatment at all and the treatment target of LDL-C levels ≤2.5 mmol/L is achieved only in 22% of the treated patients.[13] This failure to meet LDL-C targets may be partly due to the hesitation of some physicians and patients to use most potent available drug regimens. This notion is supported by the findings of Pijlman and colleagues, who conducted a cross-sectional study in five large outpatient lipid clinics in The Netherlands. The main reason why treating physicians did not prescribe maximum therapy to FH patients despite an LDL-C >2.5 mmol/L, was because they accepted that higher LDL-C level.[20] Another reason for not reaching target levels is that some patients may not have been able to due to extremely high LDL-C levels. In our study we found that, of all treated patients who were not on target (LDL-C≤2.5 mmol/L), 36% had LDL-C levels that were reduced by more than 50%. Nonetheless, LDL-C levels could have been further reduced, since only a minority (5%) of all participants was treated with potent dual therapy with the highest dose of atorvastatin or rosuvastatin in combination with ezetimibe. The estimated percentage of subjects that would have achieved an LDL-C level ≤2.5 mmol/L would be 61% based on that most potent lipid-lowering strategy. Thus, even with the most potent dual treatment regimens, in some cases the Dutch target level can not be reached. More potent options are needed.

One fifth of individuals with a molecular diagnosis of FH did not use cholesterol-lowering medication at all. Almost half of the untreated patients had not consulted a physician, which is unexpected, since genetic field workers encouraged all subjects who were found to have dyslipidemia at screening to visit their physician. Moreover, those with confirmed molecular diagnosis were explicitly urged to seek for medical consultation. The other half did not start treatment even though they had consulted a physician, which is remarkable. However, the FH patients who remained untreated had on average few cardiovascular risk factors and above all, absence of severe dyslipidemia. Whether this group of FH 'patients' should receive medication based on mutation carriership or not, is of scientific and clinical importance, and should be further elucidated.[21,22]

It is intriguing to observe that a relatively large group of subjects had a molecular diagnosis of FH but lacked a severe dyslipidemia phenotype. One of the explanations could be a high prevalence in this group of mild mutations such as ApoB mutations, which in general result in a less severe FH phenotype than LDLR mutations.[23] Indeed, we observe a non-significant trend towards a higher prevalence of ApoB among those without severe dyslipidemia in our study population. Conversely, the LDLR mutations reported to result in a severe FH phenotype, are less common in this group.[17] We further speculate that some sequence variants, which were used in the cascade screening programme in 2006 and assumed to cause FH, may not be pathogenic after all. This could have explained the lack of dyslipidemia in some subjects identified with molecular FH in 2006. An ongoing project aims to correctly label such sequence variants as non-pathogenic.[24] A final possible explanation is that other genetic variants counterbalanced the effect of the FH mutation, such as concurrent ApoB or loss-of-function PCSK9 mutations that usually result in hypobetalipoproteinemia.[25–27] We aim to perform additional studies in the near future to find out whether the proposed putative explanations hold true.

One drawback of our approach is the possible bias inflicted by non-participation. Based on the characteristics of the 281 patients who did not participate, i.e. lower proportion of cholesterol-lowering medication use at baseline, younger age and lower prevalence of CVD as compared to the 781 participants, one could reason that the proportion of treated subjects at follow-up will be an overestimation. However, LDL-C levels and the proportion of subjects that used of cholesterol-lowering medication at follow-up did not differ between the 681 participants that returned the questionnaire by surface mail and the 100 subjects that completed the questionnaire by telephone. Assuming that these 100 participants by telephone contact are a random sample of the source population of which the 281 non-participants are a part, we expect the impact of potential selection bias to be modest.

In conclusion, the molecular diagnosis of FH leads to an increased proportion of patients that start or intensify cholesterol-lowering medication, and consequently, to a robust decrease in LDL-C levels. The attained LDL-C levels are lower than those reported in a previous survey which could reflect the effect of more stringent lipid target levels. However, only a minority of the patients was treated with a potent drug regimen to reach set targets.

Supporting Information

Table S1 Potency scoring for several cholesterol-lowering drugs. *Potency scores for statins were derived from Walma Ned Tijdschr Geneeskd 2006;150:18–23, who based the scores themselves on Law BMJ 2003;326:1423-7. #Correction factor for ezetimibe was based on 17% additional decrease in LDL-C (100%/(100%-17%) = 1.20) when added to statins (Kastelein NEJM 2008; 358: 1431-43). Our study population used relative low doses of bile acid sequestrants and these were estimated to have only a modest effect on LDL-C levels. Even lower potency scores were applied for fibrates and nicotinic acid, which influence primarily triglyceride and HDL-cholesterol levels respectively and have a modest effect on LDL-C levels (Huijgen Expert Rev Cardiovasc Ther 2008;6:567-81).

Acknowledgments

The authors thank the Foundation for the Identification of Persons with Inherited Hypercholesterolaemia (StOEH), the Rijksinstituut voor Volksgezondheid en Milieu (RIVM), Ministry of Health and the Dutch Government for executing the screening program. We also are indebted to the participants of this survey.

Author Contributions

Conceived and designed the experiments: RH IK JJPK. Performed the experiments: RH IK SBJV. Analyzed the data: RH EJGS MNV BAH. Contributed reagents/materials/analysis tools: RH IK SBJV EJGS MNV JJPK BAH. Wrote the paper: RH IK SBJV EJGS MNV JJPK BAH.

References

1. Goldstein JL, Hobbs HH, Brown SM (2001) The metabolic and molecular bases of inherited disease. New York: McGraw-Hill. pp 2863–2913.
2. Slack J (1969) Risks of ischaemic heart-disease in familial hyperlipoproteinaemic states. Lancet 2: 1380–1382.

3. Huijgen R, Vissers MN, Defesche JC, Lansberg PJ, Kastelein JJ, et al. (2008) Familial hypercholesterolemia: current treatment and advances in management. Expert Rev Cardiovasc Ther 6: 567–581.
4. Versmissen J, Oosterveer DM, Yazdanpanah M, Defesche JC, Basart DC, et al. (2008) Efficacy of statins in familial hypercholesterolaemia: a long term cohort study. BMJ 337: a2423.
5. Neil HA, Hammond T, Huxley R, Matthews DR, Humphries SE (2000) Extent of underdiagnosis of familial hypercholesterolaemia in routine practice: prospective registry study. BMJ 321: 148.
6. Umans-Eckenhausen MA, Defesche JC, Sijbrands EJ, Scheerder RL, Kastelein JJ (2001) Review of first 5 years of screening for familial hypercholesterolaemia in the Netherlands. Lancet 357: 165–168.
7. Umans-Eckenhausen MA, Defesche JC, van Dam MJ, Kastelein JJ (2003) Long-term compliance with lipid-lowering medication after genetic screening for familial hypercholesterolemia. Arch Intern Med 163: 65–68.
8. Baigent C, Keech A, Kearney PM, Blackwell L, Buck G, et al. (2005) Efficacy and safety of cholesterol-lowering treatment: prospective meta-analysis of data from 90,056 participants in 14 randomised trials of statins. Lancet 366: 1267–1278.
9. Robinson JG, Smith B, Maheshwari N, Schrott H (2005) Pleiotropic effects of statins: benefit beyond cholesterol reduction? A meta-regression analysis. J Am Coll Cardiol 46: 1855–1862.
10. Josan K, Majumdar SR, McAlister FA (2008) The efficacy and safety of intensive statin therapy: a meta-analysis of randomized trials. CMAJ 178: 576–584.
11. Smilde TJ, van Wissen S, Wollersheim H, Trip MD, Kastelein JJ, et al. (2001) Effect of aggressive versus conventional lipid lowering on atherosclerosis progression in familial hypercholesterolaemia (ASAP): a prospective, randomised, double-blind trial. Lancet 357: 577–581.
12. Wierzbicki AS, Humphries SE, Minhas R (2008) Familial hypercholesterolaemia: summary of NICE guidance. BMJ 337: a1095.
13. Walma EP, Visseren FL, Jukema JW, Kastelein JJ, Hoes AW, et al. (2006) The practice guideline 'iagnosis and treatment of familial hypercholesterolaemia'of the Dutch Health Care Insurance Board. Ned Tijdschr Geneeskd 150: 18–23.
14. Kastelein JJ, Akdim F, Stroes ES, Zwinderman AH, Bots ML, et al. (2008) Simvastatin with or without ezetimibe in familial hypercholesterolemia. N Engl J Med 358: 1431–1443.
15. Gotto AM Jr, Bierman EL, Connor WE, Ford CH, Frantz ID Jr, et al. (1984) Recommendations for treatment of hyperlipidemia in adults. A joint statement of the Nutrition Committee and the Council on Arteriocslerosis. Circulation 69: 1065A–1090A.
16. Fouchier SW, Kastelein JJ, Defesche JC (2005) Update of the molecular basis of familial hypercholesterolemia in The Netherlands. Hum Mutat 26: 550–556.
17. Umans-Eckenhausen MA, Sijbrands EJ, Kastelein JJ, Defesche JC (2002) Low-density lipoprotein receptor gene mutations and cardiovascular risk in a large genetic cascade screening population. Circulation 106: 3031–3036.
18. Leren TP, Finborud TH, Manshaus TE, Ose L, Berge KE (2008) Diagnosis of familial hypercholesterolemia in general practice using clinical diagnostic criteria or genetic testing as part of cascade genetic screening. Community Genet 11: 26–35.
19. Hadfield SG, Horara S, Starr BJ, Yazdgerdi S, Bhatnagar D, et al. (2008) Are patients with familial hypercholesterolaemia well managed in lipid clinics? An audit of eleven clinics from the Department of Health Familial Hypercholesterolaemia Cascade Testing project. Ann Clin Biochem 45: 199–205.
20. Pijlman AH, Huijgen R, Verhagen SN, Imholz BP, Liem AH, et al. (2009) Evaluation of cholesterol lowering treatment of patients with familial hypercholesterolemia: a large cross-sectional study in The Netherlands. Atherosclerosis. In press.
21. Souverein OW, Defesche JC, Zwinderman AH, Kastelein JJ, Tanck MW (2007) Influence of LDL-receptor mutation type on age at first cardiovascular event in patients with familial hypercholesterolaemia. Eur Heart J 28: 299–304.
22. Neil HA, Seagroatt V, Betteridge DJ, Cooper MP, Durrington PN, et al. (2004) Established and emerging coronary risk factors in patients with heterozygous familial hypercholesterolaemia. Heart 90: 1431–1437.
23. Fouchier SW, Defesche JC, Kastelein JJ, Sijbrands EJ (2004) Familial defective apolipoprotein B versus familial hypercholesterolemia: an assessment of risk. Semin Vasc Med 4: 259–264.
24. Huijgen R, Kindt I, Fouchier SW, Defesche JC, Hutten BA, et al. (2009) Non-functionality of three *LDL-R* and *APOB* gene mutations that were assumed to cause familial hypercholesterolemia. Atherosclerosis Supplement 2009 10: P841.
25. Abifadel M, Rabes JP, Jambart S, Halaby G, Gannage-Yared MH, et al. (2009) The molecular basis of familial hypercholesterolemia in Lebanon: Spectrum of LDLR mutations and role of PCSK9 as a modifier gene. Hum Mutat 30: E682–691.
26. Fouchier SW, Huijgen R, Vis K, Defesche JC, Kastelein JJ (2009) Identification of *APOB* and *PCSK9* mutations causing a non-autosomal dominant hypercholesterolemia (ADH) phenotype in molecular diagnosed ADH patients. Atherosclerosis Supplement 2009 10: P870.
27. van der Graaf A, Fouchier SW, Vissers MN, Defesche JC, Wiegman A, et al. (2008) Familial defective apolipoprotein B and familial hypobetalipoproteinemia in one family: two neutralizing mutations. Ann Intern Med 148: 712–714.

7

Metabolomics of Dietary Fatty Acid Restriction in Patients with Phenylketonuria

Ulrike Mütze[1]*, Skadi Beblo[1], Linda Kortz[2,3], Claudia Matthies[4], Berthold Koletzko[4], Mathias Bruegel[5], Carmen Rohde[1], Joachim Thiery[2], Wieland Kiess[1], Uta Ceglarek[2,3]

1 Department of Women and Child Health, Hospital for Children and Adolescents, University Hospital, University of Leipzig, Leipzig, Germany, **2** Clinical Chemistry and Molecular Diagnostics, Institute of Laboratory Medicine, University Hospital, University of Leipzig, Leipzig, Germany, **3** LIFE – Leipzig Research Center for Civilization Diseases, University Leipzig, Leipzig, Germany, **4** Division Metabolic Diseases and Nutritional Medicine, Dr. von Hauner Children's Hospital, Ludwig-Maximilians-University of Munich, Munich, Germany, **5** Institute of Laboratory Medicine, Ludwig-Maximilians-University of Munich, Munich, Germany

Abstract

Background: Patients with phenylketonuria (PKU) have to follow a lifelong phenylalanine restricted diet. This type of diet markedly reduces the intake of saturated and unsaturated fatty acids especially long chain polyunsaturated fatty acids (LC-PUFA). Long-chain saturated fatty acids are substrates of mitochondrial fatty acid oxidation for acetyl-CoA production. LC-PUFA are discussed to affect inflammatory and haemostaseological processes in health and disease. The influence of the long term PKU diet on fatty acid metabolism with a special focus on platelet eicosanoid metabolism has been investigated in the study presented here.

Methodology/Principal Findings: 12 children with PKU under good metabolic control and 8 healthy controls were included. Activated fatty acids (acylcarnitines C6–C18) in dried blood and the cholesterol metabolism in serum were analyzed by liquid chromatographic tandem mass spectrometry (LC-MS/MS). Fatty acid composition of plasma glycerophospholipids was determined by gas chromatography. LC-PUFA metabolites were analyzed in supernatants by LC-MS/MS before and after platelet activation and aggregation using a standardized protocol. Patients with PKU had significantly lower free carnitine and lower activated fatty acids in dried blood compared to controls. Phytosterols as marker of cholesterol (re-) absorption were not influenced by the dietary fatty acid restriction. Fatty acid composition in glycerophospholipids was comparable to that of healthy controls. However, patients with PKU showed significantly increased concentrations of y-linolenic acid (C18:3n-6) a precursor of arachidonic acid. In the PKU patients significantly higher platelet counts were observed. After activation with collagen platelet aggregation and thromboxane B_2 and thromboxane B_3 release did not differ from that of healthy controls.

Conclusion/Significance: Long-term dietary fatty acid restriction influenced the intermediates of mitochondrial beta-oxidation. No functional influence on unsaturated fatty acid metabolism and platelet aggregation in patients with PKU was detected.

Editor: Michael Müller, Wageningen University, The Netherlands

Funding: Junior research grant by the Medical Faculty, University of Leipzig, Germany. This publication is supported by LIFE – Leipzig Research Center for Civilization Diseases, Universität Leipzig. This project was funded by means of the European Social Fund and the Free State of Saxony. Further support was received from the Commission of the European Communities, specific RTD Programme "Quality of Life and Management of Living Resources", within the 7th Framework Programme NUTRIMENTHE, FP7-212652. This manuscript does not necessarily reflect the views of the Commission and in no way anticipates the future policy in this area. The funders had no role in study design, data collection and analysis, decision to publish, or preparation of the manuscript.

Competing Interests: The authors have declared that no competing interests exist.

* E-mail: Ulrike.Muetze@medizin.uni-leipzig.de

Introduction

Phenylketonuria (PKU; OMIM 261600) is one of the most common inborn metabolic diseases, approximately affecting one in 8000 newborns in Western Europe [1]. It is caused by deficient activity of phenylalanine hydroxylase. Children with untreated PKU suffer from severe physical and mental disability. Postnatal diagnosis by newborn screening, early treatment with a lifelong protein restricted diet and substitution of a phenylalanine free amino acid formula result in a normal cognitive development [2]. Since protein-rich foods such as meat, milk products, eggs, and fish are the predominant nutritional sources of animal fat, especially of saturated fatty acids and long chain polyunsaturated fatty acids (LC-PUFA), patients with PKU have a low dietary LC-PUFA intake [3,4]. Reduced LC-PUFA concentrations in plasma and erythrocytes have been found previously [4–7]. LC-PUFA, as arachidonic acid (AA; 20:4n-6), docosahexaenoic acid (DHA; 22:6n-3) and eicosapentaenoic acid (EPA; 20:5n-3), are discussed to affect inflammatory and haemostaseological processes in health and disease [8–11]. AA, the precursor of eicosanoids, plays a central role in proinflammatory response and haemostasis [8–10].

There is some evidence that the reduced LC-PUFA intake may influence hemostaseological processes in PKU-patients. Decreased concentrations of AA and its metabolite, thromboxane B_2 (TXB_2), have been found in serum [5]. In addition, the low nutritional intake of saturated fatty acids seems to influence the concentrations of intermediates (acylcarnitines) of mitochondrial beta-oxidation of fatty acids. Patients with PKU showed a lower concentration of free carnitine (C0) [12–15] and lower concentrations of the activated fatty acids (acylcarnitines) octanoylcarntine (C8) and decanoylcarnitine (C10) in dried whole blood compared to controls [15]. Furthermore, cholesterol concentrations in plasma are described to be lower in patients with PKU under good metabolic control [16–18].

We studied the metabolic pathways of saturated and unsaturated fatty acids in patients with PKU and in controls, because these pathways are suspected, to be influenced by the long-term strict PKU diet. The aim was to get an overview of long term fatty acid metabolome in children with PKU under strict diet and to investigate for the first time the possible functional influences on homeostasis using a standardized non-invasive cell-model.

Materials and Methods

Participants

Patients with diagnosed classical PKU were eligible for inclusion if they were under good metabolic control; i.e. a documented average phenylalanine concentration in dried blood spots was below 360 μmol/L for patients <10 years, below 900 μmol/l for patients >10 years, determined at least monthly over the previous six months. Patients with PKU followed their usual treatment consisting of protein-restricted diet and supplementation of a phenylalanine free amino acid formula containing also vitamins and trace elements. Prior study entry, a diet record over three days was performed.

Healthy controls were recruited before elective surgery (n = 4, remove of orthopedic material) or before endocrinological testing (n = 4, arginine test, only patients with normal test results were included) and if they followed an omnivore Western diet. No patient or volunteer received additional medication; especially no cyclooxygenase inhibitors during the last 14 days prior study entry, or over the counter nutritional supplements. Study samples were collected while blood withdrawal for diagnostic reasons after fasting for 4 to 6 hours.

For standardization of platelet activation experiments, 10 healthy adult volunteers (age 23–37 years, 5 females, 5 males) were included after informed consent. All of them were on a omnivore Western diet, without medication, especially no cyclooxygenase inhibitors during the last 14 days prior blood withdrawal.

Blood (10 ml) was drawn without occluding the vein from each participant using multifly needle sets and polypropylene monovettes with and without anticoagulants (Ethylenediaminetetraacetic acid (EDTA), citrate and lithium-heparinate) obtained from Sarstedt (Nümbrecht, Germany). EDTA whole blood was dropped on filter paper (grade 903; GE Health Care, Germany).

Procedures and Investigations

Baseline-parameters - clinical chemistry and routine analysis. Blood count parameters were measured on the Sysmex XE 2100 (Norderstedt, Germany). Coagulation parameters (activated partial thromboplastin time (aPTT), prothrombin time, fibrinogen, and antithrombin III (AT III) were measured on the BCS System (Siemens, Munich, Germany). Alanine aminotransferase, aspartate aminotransferase, gamma-glutamyl transferase, triglycerides, cholesterol, free fatty acids, creatinine, albumin, serum proteins, c-reactive protein, sodium, potassium, and calcium, folic acid, vitamin B12, and ferritin in serum were measured on the Modular Analytics system from Roche (Mannheim, Germany). Amino acids in plasma were analyzed by ion exchange chromatography (IEC) and ninhydrine derivatisation.

Analysis of acylcarnitines in dried blood. Acylcarnitines in dried blood spots were measured as formerly described by liquid chromatography/tandem mass spectrometry (LC-MS/MS) [19]. Briefly, 3.0 mm diameter punches (containing approx. 3 μL) of the dropped-on filter paper were placed into 96-well polypropylene micro titer plates and extracted with 100 μL of a methanol solution, containing isotope labelled amino acid and acylcarnitine internal standards (NSK-A, NSK-B, Cambridge Isotope Laboratories, Andover, USA), for 30 min by gentle shaking at room temperature. After evaporation at 70°C for 40 min, 60 μL of 3n butanolic-HCL was added for derivatisation at 65°C. After a second evaporation step the samples were reconstituted with 150 μL of the mobile phase (1/1 v/v isopropanol/water) and analysed by flow injection analysis (FIA)-MS/MS using a API 2000 triple quadrupole mass spectrometer (AB SCIEX, Darmstadt, Germany).

Analysis of sterols in serum. Serum concentrations of brassicasterol, campesterol, stigmasterol, beta-sitosterol, cholesterol, lanosterol and desmosterol were measured by our formerly described LC-MS/MS method using a API 3000 triple quadrupole mass spectrometer with photospray ionization (AB SCIEX, Darmstadt, Germany) [20]. 10 μL of human serum were diluted with 490 μL of 50/50 v/v methanol/acetonitrile. After centrifugation, free and esterified beta-sitosterol, campesterol, and brassicasterol were simultaneously analyzed by LC-MS/MS.

Fatty acid composition of plasma glycerophospholipids. The analysis of plasma glycerophospholipid composition was performed by a sensitive and precise high-throughput method recently described [21]. In brief, 100 μl of serum, 100 μl of internal standard (1,2-dipentadecanoyl-sn-glycero-3-phosphocholine dissolved in methanol) and 0.6 ml methanol (precooled to 5°C) were combined in glass tubes and shaken for 30 s. Samples were centrifuged and the supernatant was transferred into another glass tube. Sodium methoxide solution (25 μl) was added, tubes were shaken, and synthesis of methyl esters proceeded at room temperature. The reaction was stopped after 3 minutes by adding 75 μl methanolic HCl. Fatty acid methyl ester (FAME) were extracted twice by adding 300 μl hexane at a time. Extracts were combined and dried under nitrogen flow at room temperature and taken up in 50 μl hexane (containing 2 g/l BHT) for gas chromatographic (GC) analysis. Individual FAMEs were quantified by GC with flame ionization.

Eicosanoid analysis in plasma and supernatants. Eicosanoids in EDTA plasma and supernatants after activation of platelet rich citrate-plasma were analyzed by LC-MS/MS [22]. Solid phase extraction (SPE) was used for extraction and concentration of the eicosanoids [23]. 150 μl of the platelet supernatants or EDTA plasma were spiked with 50 μl 1/1 v/v methanol/water containing 0.2 μg/ml of arachidonic acid-d8 (AA-d8) and 0.02 μg/ml of prostaglandin $F_{2\alpha}$-d4 ($PGF_{2\alpha}$-d4), prostaglandin E_2-d4 (PGE_2-d4), leukotriene B_4-d4 (LTB_4-d4), and 5-S-hydroxyeicosatetraenoic acid-d8 (5-HETE-d8), thromboxane B_2-d4 (TxB_2-d4), eicosapentaenoic acid-d5 (EPA-d5), and docosahexaenoic acid-d5 (DHA-d5). The samples were extracted using Strata X SPE columns (Phenomenex, Aschaffenburg, Germany). Samples were dried under nitrogen and stored at −80°C until analysis. After elution 10 μl of each aliquot were injected into the LC-MS/MS system. Chromatographic separation was performed based on the protocols by Deems et al [23]. A triple quadrupole mass spectrometer (API 5500 QTrap, SCIEX Toronto, Canada) using electrospray ionization (ESI) was used in negative ion mode. Analytes were quantified in multiple reaction monitoring transitions (MRMs) using the corresponding labeled internal standards [22]. Table S1 shows the analyzed metabolites.

Platelet function analysis. In a first step a standardized protocol for reproducible platelet activation with collagen and analysis of subsequent eicosanoid release was developed.

For standardization TXB_2 release after platelet activation was used. The measured metabolite TXB_2 is a stable, biologically inert metabolite formed from the non-enzymatic hydrolysis of TXA_2 [24]. The latter has a half-life of approximately 30 seconds [24]. TXB_2 in plasma and urine reflects platelet TXA_2 synthesis [25]. Thromboxane B_3 (TXB_3) is the equivalent metabolite metabolized competitively by the same enzymes from omega-3 LC-PUFA (i.e. EPA) [8].

Platelet-rich plasma (150 Gpt/l ±15) of freshly drawn citrate-blood from five healthy adult volunteers was activated with collagen. After 10 minutes of platelet activation (compared to 1 and 5 minutes) with collagen a plateau of TXB_2 release was found. Variability for TXB_2 release after platelet activation with collagen was tested. Intra-assay variability, activation three times consecutively, was ≤6.2%. Between-day variability, at three consecutive days, blood withdrawal at noon, was ≤8.7%. Circadian variability was ≤14.8%. Therefore, platelet activation from five healthy subjects was performed after blood withdrawal once in the morning, at noon and in the afternoon at three consecutive days. Interindividual variability of TXB_2 release after platelet activation with collagen was 15.6%.

From this data the following standardized protocol was established: 225 µl platelet-rich plasma (150 Gpt/l ±15 Gpt/l) from freshly drawn citrate-blood was transferred to three micro glass silicon tubes with magnetic stirrers on Platelet Aggregation Profiler 4 (PAP 4, mölab, Langenfeld, Germany). In two samples platelet activation was performed with bovine collagen (25 µl, 1.9 g/l) for 10 minutes, registered by the PAP 4 (mölab, Langenfeld, Germany). The third sample remained inactivated for 10 minutes. Afterwards, stirrers were removed, plasma transferred to 0.5 ml tubes (Eppendorf, Hamburg, Germany) and centrifuged at 5260 g for 10 minutes (20°C) to remove platelets and cell detritus. The supernatants were stored at −80°C under nitrogen to avoid oxygen-induced radical formation until analysis.

Ethics

The study protocol was approved by the local ethics committee of the Medical Faculty of the University of Leipzig (Leipzig, Germany; registration number 021-09-180808). The trial was performed in accordance with the Declaration of Helsinki/ Somerset West and followed ICH-GCP guidelines. Informed written consent was obtained from all patients and/or parents.

Statistical Methods

All statistical analyses were performed using PASW statistic 18 (Chicago, IL, USA). For descriptive reasons we displayed the median and minimum/maximum of all data. Wilcoxon-test, for paired samples, or Mann-Whitney-U-test, for independent samples, was used. A probability value of $p<0.05$ was considered significant.

For initial analysis the study population was divided in groups regarding age (patients <10 years, patients >=10 years) or regarding diet (phenylalanine consumption <300 mg/day, 300–400 mg/day, >400 mg/day). This did not influence the results. Therefore, final analysis was performed using the entire sample.

Results

Participants

12 (6 females, 6 males) early treated children and adolescents with classical PKU aged 5–14 years and 8 healthy controls (5 females, 3 males) aged 5–17 years were included in the study.

Age, height, weight, body mass index (BMI) and Tanner stages did not differ significantly between the two groups (Table S2).

Diet Records and Basic Laboratory Parameters

The results of the diet records of patients with PKU were compared to the regular daily allowance, recommended for the German speaking countries [26] as shown in table 1. The overall energy intake was just below the recommended amount. None of the 12 PKU-patients had signs of over- or undernutrition with a median BMI SDS of 0.6 (−1.24–1.51; Table S2). Nevertheless, the patients reached only about 75% of the recommended fat intake under the strict PKU diet. Median fat intake from vegetable sources was 56.9% (45.1–91.8%; predominant vegetable oil) and from animal sources was 42.7% (8.2–55.1%, predominant butter). Although fat intake was under the recommended amount, the precursors of AA and DHA, linoleic acid and alpha-linolenic acid, respectively, were consumed as recommended (Table 1).

Carbohydrate intake was slightly below the recommended amount and the intake of protein was sufficient under substitution of amino acid formula [26] (Table 1).

Basic liver and kidney parameters, electrolytes, lipids, infection parameters, and coagulation parameters were within the normal range in both groups without significant differences. In PKU patients, essential amino acid concentrations in plasma were within the normal range except from the elevated phenylalanine concentrations (Table S2).

Patients with PKU showed a significant higher median platelet count (329 Gpt/l, range 257–435 Gpt/l) compared to controls (271.5 Gpt/l, range 197–330 Gpt/l) ($p<0.05$). Platelet volume in patients with PKU was 10.2 fL (7.8–11.8 fL) compared to controls

Table 1. Analysis of three-day diet record of patients with phenylketonuria (PKU).

	Patients with PKU (n = 12) median (range)
Energy intake [kcal/day]	1678.0 (919–2075)
% DACH RDA	98 (66–131)
Carbohydrates [g/day]	232.6 (148.4–367.5)
% DACH RDA	93 (69–127)
Proteine [g/day]	41.1 (22.5–78.3)
% DACH RDA	197 (132–321)
Fat [g/day]	47.3 (18–65)
% DACH RDA	75 (28–125)
Phenylalanine [mg/day]	338 (254–690)
Linoleic acid [mg/day]	4536 (876–10866)
% DACH RDA	110 (67–240)
alpha-linolenic acid [mg/day]	805 (219–1461)
% DACH RDA	96 (22–182)

% DACH RDA: percentage of regular daily allowance, recommended for the German speaking countries [26].

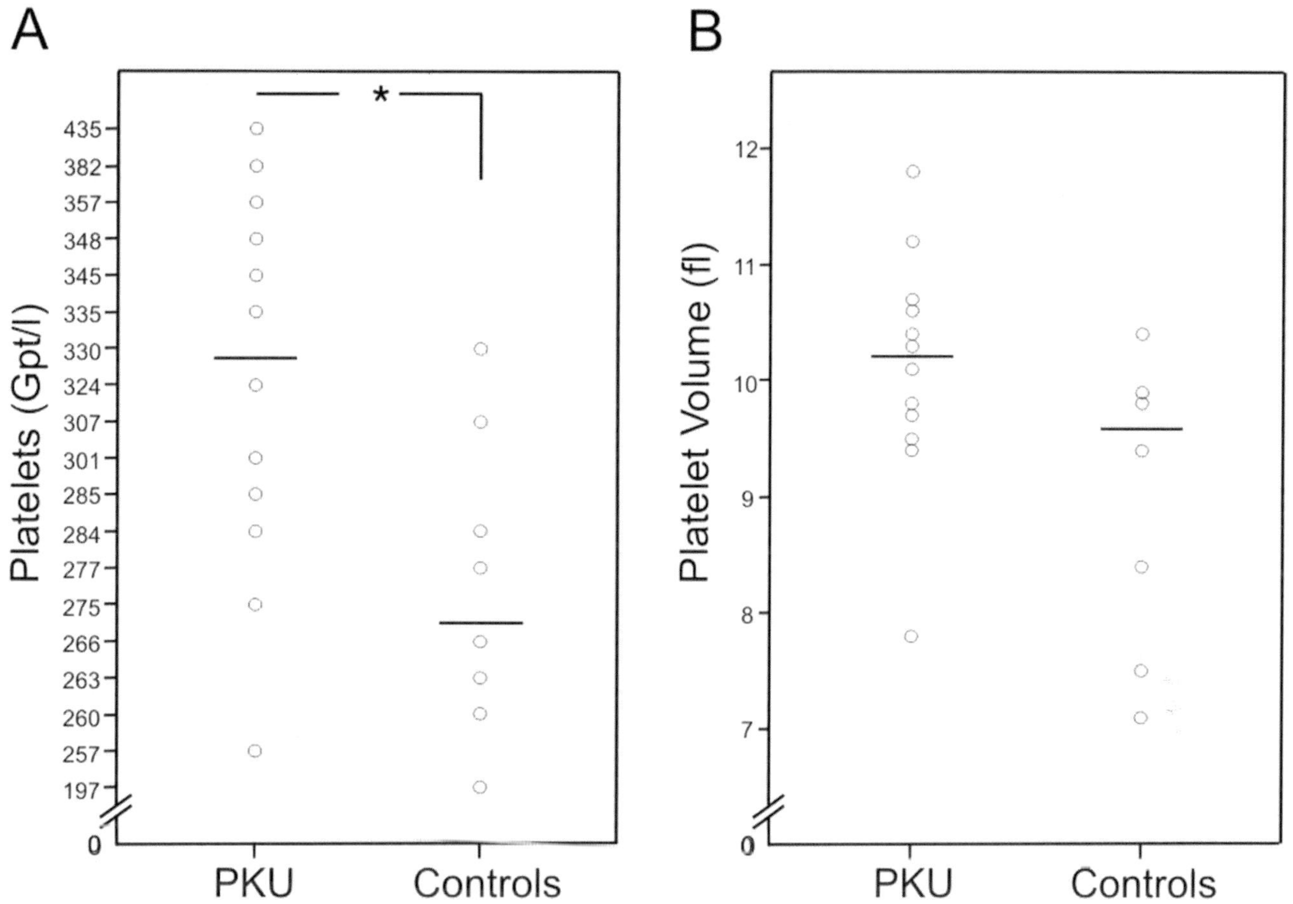

Figure 1. Platelet count and platelet volume. Data of patients with phenylketonuria (PKU) (n = 12) and healthy controls (n = 8). **A** platelet count (* $p<0.05$) and **B** platelet volume. The stripe marks the median.

9.6 fL (7.1–10.4 fL) ($p = 0.063$) (Figure 1, Table S2). Plasma concentrations of folic acid ($p<0.01$), vitamin B12 ($p<0.01$), and ferritin ($p<0.05$) in patients with PKU were significantly higher than in controls (Table S2).

Investigations of Saturated Fatty Acid Metabolism, Mitochondrial Beta-oxidation, Cholesterol Adsorption and Synthesis

Patients with PKU had significantly lower concentrations of free carnitine (C0) ($p<0.01$), total acylcarnitines ($p<0.001$) and of activated fatty acids of the different chain-lengths ($p<0.001$: C2, C3, C18, C18OH, C18:1), ($p<0.01$: C4–0H, C5, C8), ($p<0.05$: C6, C10:1, C14:1, C16:1, C18:2) compared to the healthy controls (Figure 2, Table S3).

Serum concentrations of cholesterol absorption markers brassicasterol, campesterol, stigmasterol, beta-sitosterol, and lanosterol as marker for cholesterol synthesis did not differ significantly between both groups. Also the cholesterol concentration and the relative non-cholesterol concentrations showed no significant differences (Table S3).

Investigation of Unsaturated Fatty Acid Metabolism

Patients with PKU showed significant higher concentrations of y-linolenic acid (C18:3n-6) (2.1 mg/l, range 1.0–5.1 mg/l versus 1.1 mg/l, range 0.6–2.4 mg/l; $p<0.01$) and a trend to higher concentrations of di-homo-y-linolenic acid (C20:3n-6) (43.3 mg/l, range 33.0–60.0 mg/l versus 36.2 mg/l, range 30.0–52.8 mg/l; $p = 0.069$) in plasma glycerophospholipids (Table S3, Figure 3). Both are precursors in endogenous AA synthesis. For other fatty acids of plasma glycerophospholipids no differences between patients with PKU and controls were found (Table S3).

There was no difference for TXB_2 (derived from AA) plasma concentrations in the study groups. However, TXB_3 (derived from EPA) plasma concentrations were significantly lower in patients with PKU (0.01 ng/ml, range 0.00–0.12 ng/ml) compared to controls (0.10 ng/ml, range 0.03–0.25 ng/ml; $p<0.005$; Table S3).

Functional Investigations of Platelet Activation Induced Eicosanoid Release

Platelet activation with collagen for 10 minutes induced a significant release of AA, TXB_2, TXB_3, prostaglandin E_2 (PGE_2), prostaglandin D_2 (PGD_2), 11-S-hydroxyeicosatetraenoic acid (11-HETE), and 12-S-hydroxyeicosatetraenoic acid (12-HETE) in patients with PKU and controls (Table 2). The concentrations of TXB_2, TXB_3, PGE_2, PGD_2, 11-HETE, and 12-HETE after platelet activation with/without collagen did not differ significantly between the two groups. To assure reproducibility of analysis of eicosanoid release after platelet activation we validated a standardized protocol for the activation experiments.

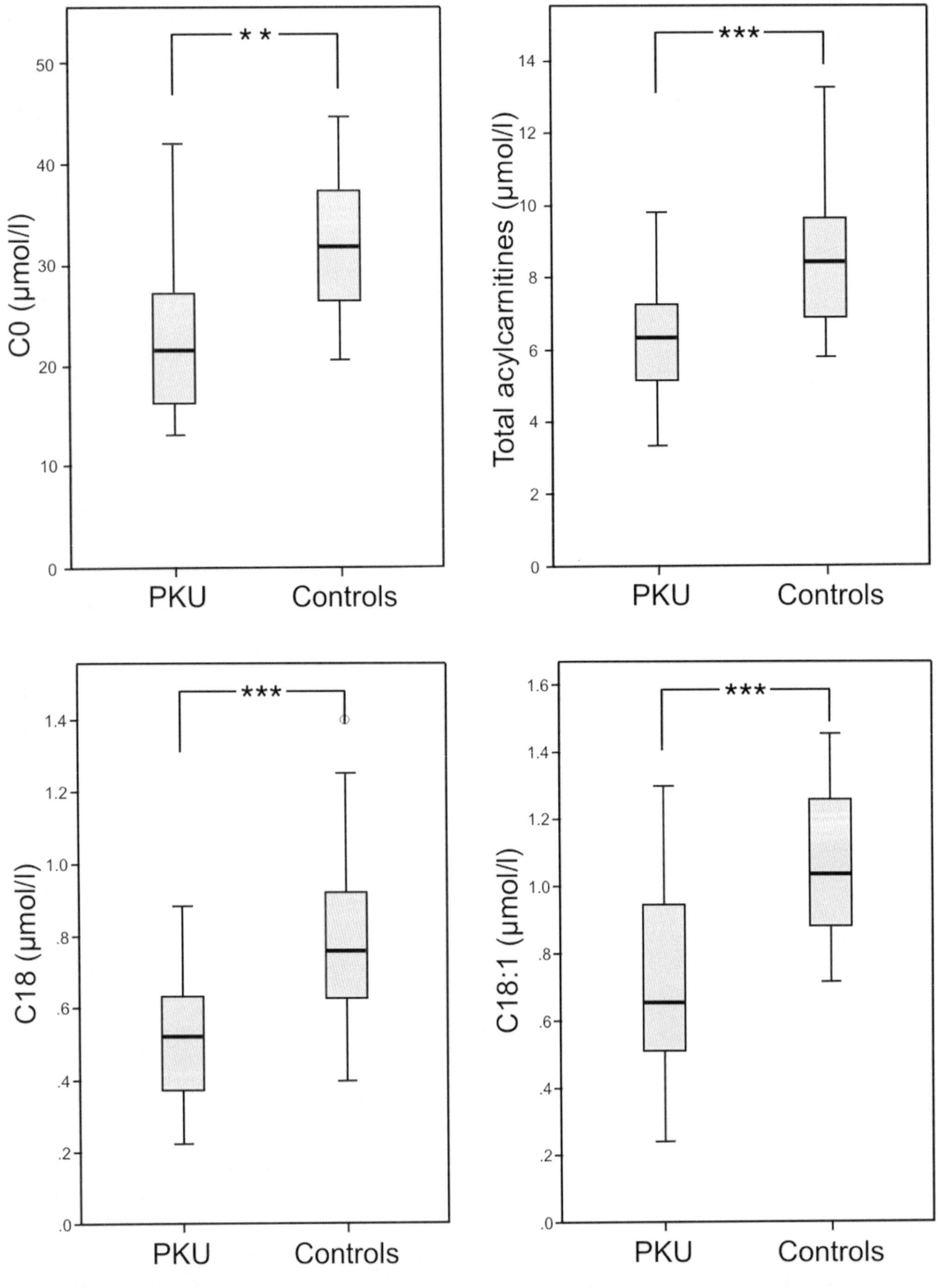

**
C0 (μmol/l)
50
40
30
20
10
0
PKU
Controls
***
Total acylcarnitines (μmol/l)
14
12
10
8
6
4
2
0
PKU
Controls
***
C18 (μmol/l)
1.4
1.2
1.0
.8
.6
.4
.2
.0
PKU
Controls
***
C18:1 (μmol/l)
1.6
1.4
1.2
1.0
.8
.6
.4
.2
.0
PKU
Controls

Figure 2. Free carnitine and acylcarnitines. Data of patients with phenylketonuria (PKU) (n = 12) and healthy controls (n = 8); measured by liquid chromatography/tandem mass spectrometry (LC-MS/MS). **A** Free carnitine (C0) in dried blood (**p<0.01). **B** Total acylcarnitines in dried blood (***p<0.001). **C** Octadecanoylcarnitine (C18) in dried blood (***p<0.001). **D** Octadecenoylcarnitine (C18:1) in dried blood (***p<0.001).

Discussion

PKU-patients have to undergo a livelong phenylalanine restricted diet beginning in the first weeks of life, which is associated with a long-term restriction of saturated and non-saturated fatty acids compared to a regular western diet [5,7,13–15,17,18,27].

As may be expected, the investigated PKU patients had only 75% (median 47,3 g per day) of the age related recommended fat intake [26]. Similar results have been found previously [18,27,28]. Moreover, an inverse relation of animal to vegetable fat was observed in our PKU group (42.7% animal fat/56.9% vegetable fat). In contrast healthy German children 6–11 years/12–17 years consume 62.5 g/100.5 g fat per day, including 65.7% animal fat and 34.3% vegetable fat [29]. However, the intake of the essential fatty acids linoleic acid and alpha-linolenic acid, precursors for endogenous AA and DHA synthesis, was in the recommended range [26].

The influence of the restricted intake of saturated fatty acids with the PKU diet was found to be evident in both, the metabolism of C0 and the intermediates of mitochondrial ß-oxidation [15]. We observed significantly lower C0 and acylcarnitine concentrations in dried whole blood of PKU patients, although free fatty acids in serum were comparable between PKU patients and controls. Lower C0 concentrations in patients with PKU on a strict diet have been described previously as possible consequence of the low nutritional carnitine intake [14] or the reduced endogenous synthesis due to the lower plasma concentrations of the essential substrates methionine and lysine [15]. Additionally phenylacetic acid, a pathological metabolite found in serum and urine of PKU-patients, was found to be capable of inhibiting the endogenous carnitine synthesis [30]. However concentrations of C0 are not as low as in other inborn

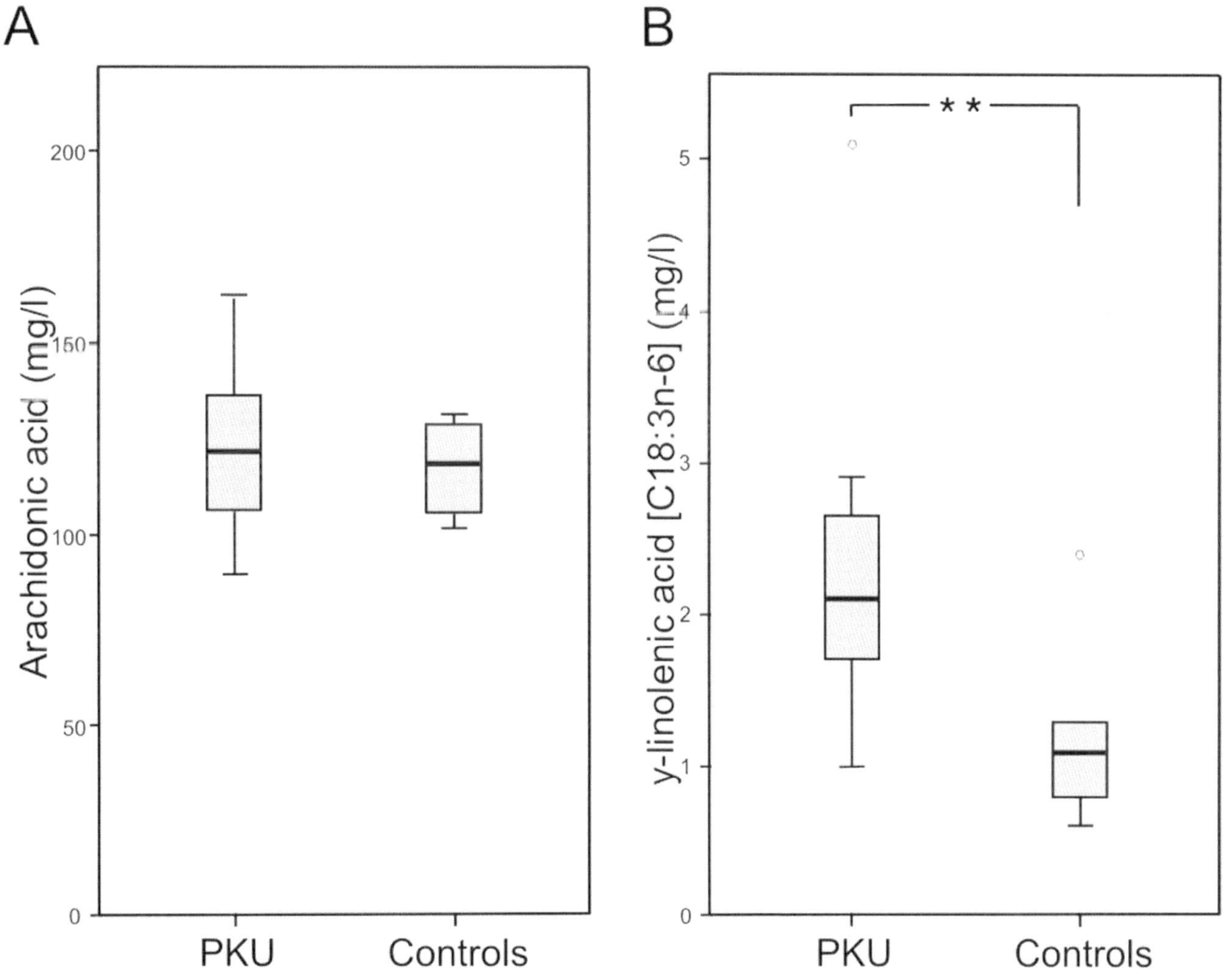

Figure 3. Arachidonic acid and y-linolenic acid concentrations in plasma glycerophospholipids. Data of patients with phenylketonuria (PKU) (n = 12) and healthy controls (n = 8). **A** Arachidonic acid in plasma glycerophospholipids. **B** y-linolenic acid in plasma gylcerophospholipis (** p<0.01).

Table 2. Eicosanoid concentrations in supernatants after 10 minutes of activation of platelet rich plasma (225 µl; 150±15 Gpt/l) with/without collagen in patients with phenylketonuria (PKU) and healty controls.

	PKU (n = 11) median (Range)		Controls (n = 8) median (Range)	
	Without collagen	With collagen	Without collagen	With collagen
AA [ng/ml]	1470 (948–2470)	3720 (2880–5520)	1520 (1070–2610)	3830 (3400–5130)
TXB2 [ng/ml]	6.0 (2.7–21.8)	390 (252–502)	3.9 (2.2–10.2)	351 (262–534)
TXB3 [ng/ml]	0.17 (0–0.46)	2.56 (0.77–4.28)	0.1 (0–0.4)	2.59 (1.57–3.59)
PGE2 [ng/ml]	0.24 (0.1–2.65)	11.5 (6.0–15.5)	0.20 (0–0.33)	11.2 (5.9–17.6)
PGD2 [ng/ml]	0.08 (0.02–0.24)	1.56 (0.51–4.38)	0.03. (0.01–0.08)	1.0 (0.51–1.97)
11-HETE [ng/ml]	1.64 (0.84–2.36)	44.4 (26.2–58)	1.45 (0.96–3.14)	38.3 (29.6–366)
12-HETE [ng/ml]	9.03 (4.18–15.6)	299 (120–425)	7.37 (3.71–11.5)	279 (209–411)

AA = arachidonic acid, TXB_2, = thromboxane B_2, TXB_3 = thromboxane B_3, PGE_2 = prostaglandin E_2, PGD_2 = prostaglandin D_2, 11-HETE = 11-S-hydroxyeicosatetraenoic acid, 12-HETE = and 12-S-hydroxyeicosatetraenoic acid.

metabolic diseased like carnitine transporter defects known to show clinical symptoms, as (cardio-) myopathy. However, up to now, there is no data of long-term follow up in adult PKU patients available. Interestingly, carnitine substitution in amino acid formula appears not to affect carnitine and acylcarnitine status in patients with PKU [15]. We could confirm these findings, as the carnitine substitution (mean 27 mg/d, 10–48 mg/day per person) of four PKU patients of our study group did not affect their carnitine and acylcarnitine status (data not shown).

Next to reduced C8 und C10 concentrations in dried whole blood in PKU patients, as already being described in a previous study [15], also decreased concentrations of the C16- and C18-fatty acids as substrates of mitochondrial beta-oxidation as well as their intermediates (C14–C6) were found. The reduced concentrations of C18 acylcarnitine and of the intermediates may reflect the reduced fat intake, a diminished mobilization of fatty acids from fat tissue, and a lower energy production by ß-oxidation in patients with PKU. Furthermore: as result acetyl-CoA (measured as acetylcarnitine C2), the central metabolite in the energy metabolism and the link between carbohydrate, amino acid, and fatty acid metabolism, was significant lower in PKU patients compared to controls. However, no association to lower phospholipids, free fatty acids, ketone bodies, or cholesterol concentrations could be revealed.

Because of the lower total fat intake and the higher amount of nutritional fat intake as vegetable oil in the PKU diet [28], we initially suspected that serum cholesterol might be lower and the cholesterol synthesis might be higher in PKU patients compared to controls. In our study cohort, serum cholesterol concentrations did not differ between patients with PKU and healthy controls. These findings are in contrast to previous studies revealing lower serum cholesterol concentrations in patients with PKU [16,17,27], especially while under good metabolic control [18], and also compared to patients with a protein-restricted diet due to other inborn errors of amino acid metabolism [27]. Other studies showed a possible inhibition of cholesterol synthesis in vitro [31] and in animal models of PKU [32]. Colomé et al. [27] detected an inverse correlation of phenylalanine and cholesterol concentrations in serum and hypothesized high plasma phenylalanine concentrations to inhibit cholesterol synthesis. We could not confirm these results, because the marker for cholesterol synthesis lanosterol and the lanosterol/cholesterol ratio did not differ significantly between the two groups, who were comparable in BMI and Tanner stages.

LC-PUFA play an important role in neuronal development and cognitive function [33–37]. The imbalanced PKU diet with nearly absence of animal proteins and markedly reduced fatty acids of animal sources is known to result in lower plasma and cell membrane concentrations of LC-PUFA [4–7]. We could not confirm reduced LC-PUFA levels in the PKU study group. AA, EPA and DHA in plasma glycerophospholipids, a good biomarker for dietary fatty acid intake and body status [21], were comparable in both study groups and adequate regarding reference values of serum glycerophospholipids in children [38,39]. This may be caused by a higher endogeneous LC-PUFA synthesis in our patients supported by the fact that we found higher concentrations of AA precursors y-linolenic acid (C18:3n-6) and di-homo-y-linolenic acid (C20:3n-6) in plasma glycerophospholipids. In addition, intake of the essential fatty acids linoleic acid and a-linolenic acid was as recommended. Former studies reported that even an enhanced dietary intake of a-linolenic acids was not sufficient to increase DHA-phosholipid concentrations in infants [40–42].

Reactive thrombocytosis was described to be associated with metabolic diseases in children [43,44]. The PKU patients studied here had higher platelet count and a trend to higher platelet volume compared to controls, but showed no other signs leading to reactive thrombocytosis (e.g. no infection, iron, cobalamin, and folic acid deficiency). These results were reproduced in a bigger PKU cohort of our outpatient clinic (n = 49, data not shown).

Plasma AA and TXB_2 concentrations did not differ between both groups. In contrast, Agostoni and colleagues found reduced serum TXB_2 and AA concentrations [5]. However, plasma concentrations of TXB_3, metabolite of EPA, were significantly lower in PKU patients compared to the control group. This may indicate a reduced omega-3 LC-PUFA metabolism in PKU patients, although, the amount of EPA and DHA in plasma glycerophospholipids was adequate regarding reference values [38,39].

Based on the fact that we found more and larger platelets which are known to contain more granules producing higher amounts of vasocative and prothombotic factors [45–47] and the hypothesis that the dietary restriction of fatty acids, especially LC-PUFA, affects the platelet function, we established a well standardized protocol for platelet activation and eicosanoid release. Collagen was chosen for activation of the cyclooxygenase and lipoxygenase pathway. No differences between the two groups concerning aggregation and platelet eicosanoid release were found, neither analysing TXB_2, nor TXB_3. The same was true for total eicosanoid concentrations with or without activation and for the percental increase of eicosanoid concentrations after activation. This is an important finding, as it shows that although PKU patients follow a strict diet, which influences LC-PUFA status, cellular eicosanoid metabolism seems not to be affected as it were shown for platelet aggregation. Nevertheless, we found more than 15% interindividual variability of TBX_2 release. The number of study subjects in each group maybe therefore too small to answer this question definitely.

In conclusion, fat is an essential part of nutrition. It affects many different metabolic pathways. We applied a LC-MS/MS approach to some of these pathways to analyze the influence of the moderate long-term fatty acid restriction in PKU patients on the metabolome of saturated and unsaturated fatty acids and found for the first time the diet to influence the complete mitochondrial ß-oxidation pathway and energy metabolism, but not cholesterol metabolism. In our newly established cellular experiment, patients with PKU were found to have more large platelets, but the aggregation and platelet eicosanoid release was not different from healthy controls. To assess the value of these findings for the possible resulting comorbidities, the long-term outcome of PKU patients, and potential therapeutic approaches further studies with bigger cohorts and older PKU patients should be investigated.

Supporting Information

Table S1 Eicosanoids and long chain polyunsaturated fatty acids (LC-PUFA) measured in plasma by liquid chromatography/tandem mass spectrometry (LC-MS/MS) [22].

Table S2 Baseline data of patients with phenylketonuria (PKU) (n = 12) and healthy controls (n = 8).

Table S3 Concentrations of activated fatty acids (acylcarnitines), sterols, and plasma glycerophospholipids composition in patients with phenylketonuria (PKU) and healthy controls.

Acknowledgments

We are indebted to the patients and healthy volunteers/controls for their participation in the study. We are grateful to Babette Niescher for her laboratory assistance. We thank the Institute of Clinical Chemistry and Laboratory Medicine, University Hospital Carl Gustav Carus, Dresden, Germany for the amino acid analyses.

Author Contributions

Conceived and designed the experiments: UM SB MB JT WK UC. Performed the experiments: UM LK CM. Analyzed the data: UM UC SB. Contributed reagents/materials/analysis tools: UM JT WK LK UC CM BK CR MB. Wrote the paper: UM SB LK JT WK CR UC BK.

References

1. Loeber JG 2007. Neonatal screening in Europe; the situation in 2004. J Inherit Metab Dis 30: 430–438.
2. Scriver CR, Kaufman S, Eisensmith RC, Woo SLC (1998) The hyperphenylalaninemias. In: Scriver RC, Beaudet AL, Sly WS, Valle D, editors. The metabolic and molecular basis of inherited disease. New York: Mc Graw-Hill. 1015–75.
3. Koletzko B, Sauerwald T, Demmelmair H, Herzog M, von Schenck U, et al. (2007). Dietary long-chain polyunsaturated fatty acid supplementation in infants with phenylketonuria: a randomized controlled trial. J Inherit Metab Dis. 30: 326–32.
4. Pöge AP, Bäumann K, Müller E, Leichsenring M, Schmidt H, et al. (1998) Long-chain polyunsaturated fatty acids in plasma and erythrocyte membrane lipids of children with phenylketonuria after controlled linoleic acid intake. J Inherit Metab Dis. 21: 373–81.
5. Agostoni C, Marangoni F, Riva E, Giovannini M, Galli C (1997) Plasma arachidonic acid and serum thromboxane B2 concentrations in phenylketonuric children negatively correlate with dietary compliance. Prostaglandins Leukot Essent Fatty Acids 56: 219–22.
6. Galli C, Agostoni C, Mosconi C, Riva E, Salari PC, et al. (1991) Reduced plasma C-20 and C-22 polyunsaturated fatty acids in children with phenylketonuria during dietary intervention. J Pediatr 119: 562–7.
7. Moseley K, Koch R, Moser AB (2002) Lipid status and long-chain polyunsaturated fatty acid concentrations in adults and adolescents with phenylketonuria on phenylalanine-restricted diet. J Inherit Metab Dis 25: 56–64.
8. Calder PC (2006) N-3 polyunsaturated fatty acids, inflammation and inflammatory diseases. Am J Clin Nutr 83: 1505S–1519S.
9. Calder PC (2008) The relationship between the fatty acid composition of immune cells and their function. Prostaglandins Leukot Essent Fatty Acids 79: 101–108.
10. Russo GL (2009) Dietary n-6 and n-3 polyunsaturated fatty acids: from biochemistry to clinical implications in cardiovascular prevention. Biochemical Pharmacology 77: 937–946.
11. Riediger ND, Othman RA, Suh M, Moghadasian MH (2009) A systemic Review of the roles of n-3 Fatty Acids in Health and Disease. J Am Diet Assoc 109: 668–679.
12. Böhles H, Ullrich K, Endres W, Behbehani AW, Wendel U (1991) Inadequate iron availability as a possible cause of low serum carnitine concentrations in patients with phenylketonuria. Eur J Pediatr 150: 425–8.
13. Schulpis KH, Nounopoulos C, Scarpalezou A, Bouloukos A, Missiou-Tsagarakis S (1990) Serum carnitine level in phenylketonuric children under dietary control in Greece. Acta Paediatr Scand 79: 930–934.
14. Vilaseca MA, Briones P, Ferrer I, Campistol J, Riverola A, et al. (1993) Controlled diet in phenylketonuria may cause serum carnitine deficiency. J Inherit Metab Dis 16: 101–104.
15. Weigel C, Kiener C, Meier N, Schmid P, Rauh M, et al. (2008) Carnitine status in early-treated children, adolescents and young adults with phenylketonuria on low phenylalanine diets. Ann Nutr Metab. 53: 91–95.
16. Acosta PB, Alfin-Slater RB, Koch R (1973) Serum lipids in children with phenylketonuria (PKU). J Am Diet Assoc 63: 631–635.
17. Galluzzo CR, Ortisi MT, Castelli L, Agostoni C, Longhi R (1985) Plasma lipid concentrations in 42 treated phenylketonuric children. J Inherit Metab Dis Suppl 2: 129.
18. Schulpis KH, Karakonstantakis T, Bartzeliotou A, Karikas GA, Papassotiriou I (2004) The association of serum lipids, lipoproteins and apolipoproteins with selected trace elements and minerals in phenylketonuric patients on diet. Clin Nutr. 23: 401–407.
19. Brauer R, Leichtle A, Fiedler GM, Thiery J, Ceglarek U (2011) Preanalytical standardization of amino acid and acylcarnitine metabolite profiling in human blood using tandem mass spectrometry. Metabolomics 7: 344–353.
20. Lembcke J, Ceglarek U, Fiedler GM, Baumann S, Leichtle A, et al. (2005). Rapid quantification of free and esterified phytosterols in human serum using APPI-LC-MS/MS. J Lipid Res 46; 21–26.
21. Glaser C, Demmelmair H, Koletzko B (2010) Hight-throughput analysis of fatty acid composition of plasma gylcerophospholids. J lipid Res. 51: 216–221.
22. Kortz L, Geyer R, Ludwig U, Planert M, Bruegel M, et al. (2009) Simultaneous eicosanoid profiling and identification by liquid chromatography and hybrid triple quadrupole-linear ion trap mass spectrometry for metabolomic studies in human plasma. J Lab Med 33, 341–348.
23. Deems R, Buczynski MW, Bowers-Gentry R, Harkewicz R, Dennis EA (2007) Detection and quantitation of eicosanoids via high performance liquid chromatography-electrospray ionization-mass spectrometry. Methods Enzymol. 432: 59–82.
24. Needleman P, Moncada S, Bunting S, et al. (1976) Identification of an enzyme in platelet microsomes which generates thromboxane A_2 from prostaglandin endoperoxides. Nature 261: 558–560.
25. Lawson JA, Patrono C, Ciabattoni G, et al. (1986) Long-lived enzymatic metabolites of thromboxane B_2 in the human circulation. Anal Biochem 155: 198–205.
26. Deutsche Gesellschaft für Ernährung e.V.(DGE), Österreichische Gesellschaft für Ernährung (ÖGE), Schweizerische Gesellschaft für Ernährungsforschung (SGE), Schweizerische Vereinigung für Ernährung (DACH). Referenzwerte für die Nährstoffzufuhr (German). Anon. 2000. 1st ed. Frankfurt am Main: Umschau/Braus.

27. Colomé C, Artuch R, Lambruschini N, Cambra FJ, Campistol J, et al. (2001) Is there a relationship between plasma phenylalanine and cholesterol in phenylketonuric patients under dietary treatment? Clin Biochem 34: 373–6.
28. Rohde C, Mütze U, Weigel JF, Ceglarek U, Thiery J, et al. (2012) Unrestricted consumption of fruits and vegetables in phenylketonuria: no major impact on metabolic control. Eur J Clin Nutr. [Epub ahead of print] 2012 Feb 8.
29. Mensink GBM, Heseker H, Richter A, Stahl A, Vohmann C (2007) Ernährungsstudie als KiGGS-Modul (EsKiMo). Forschungsbericht. Robert Koch-Insitut, Berlin, Universität Paderborn. p.100.
30. Fischer GM, Nemeti B, Farkas V, Debreceni B, Laszlo A, et al. (2000) Metabolism of carnitine in phenylacetic acid-treated rats and in patients with phenylketonuria. Biochim Biophys Acta. 1501: 200–10.
31. Castillo M, Zafra MF, Garcia-Peregrin E (1988) Inhibition of brain and liver 3-hydroxy-3-methylglutaryl-CoA reductase and mevalonate-5-pyrophosphate decarboxylase in experimental hyperphenylalaninemia. Neurochem Res. 13: 551–5.
32. Shefer S, Tint GS, Jean-Guillaume D, Daikhin E, Kendler A, et al. (2000) Is there a relationship between 3-hydroxy-3-methylglutaryl coenzyme a reductase activity and forebrain pathology in the PKU mouse? J Neurosci Res. 61: 549–63.
33. Beblo S, Reinhardt H, Demmelmair H, Muntau AC, Koletzko B (2007) Effect of fish oil supplementation on fatty acid status, coordination, and fine motor skills in children with phenylketonuria. J Pediatr 150: 479–84.
34. Birch EE, Hoffman DR, Uauy R, Birch DG, Prestidge C (1998) Visual acuity and the essentiality of docosahexaenoic acid and arachidonic acid in the diet of term infants. Pediatr Res. 44: 201–9.
35. Birch EE, Garfield S, Hoffman DR, Uauy R, Birch DG. (2000) A randomized controlled trial of early dietary supply of long-chain polyunsaturated fatty acids and mental development in term infants. Dev Med Child Neurol. 42: 174–81.
36. Salem N Jr, Litman B, Kim HY, Gawrisch K (2001) Mechanisms of action of docosahexaenoic acid in the nervous system. Lipids. 36: 945–59.
37. Beblo S, Reinhardt H, Muntau AC, Mueller-Felber W, Roscher AA, Koletzko B. Fish oil supplementation improves visual evoked potentials in children with phenylketonuria. Neurology 2001;57: 1488–1491.
38. Decsi T, Koletzko B (1994) Fatty acid composition of plasma lipid classes in healthy subjects from birth to young adulthood. Eur J Pediatr. 153: 520–5.
39. Glaser C, Demmelmair H, Sausenthaler S, Herbarth O, Heinrich J, et al. (2010) Fatty acid composition of serum glycerophospholipids in children. J Pediatr.157: 826–31.
40. Martinez M (1992) Tissue levels of polyunsaturated fatty acids during early human development. J Pediatr 120: S129–S138.
41. Koletzko B, Rodriguez-Palmero M (1999) Polyunsaturated fatty acids in human milk and their role in early infant development. J mammary Gland Biol Neoplasia 4: 269–284.
42. Koletzko B, Sinclair AJ (1999) Long-chain polyunsaturated fatty acids in diets for infants: choices for recommendingand regulating bodies annd for manufacturers of dietary products. Lipids 34: 215–220.
43. Sutor AH (1999) Thrombozytosis. In: Lilleyman JS, Hann IM, Blanchette VS, editors. Pediatric Hematology Churchil Livingstone, London, Edinburgh, New York, Philadelphia, Sydney, Toronto 455–464.
44. Dame C, Sutor AH (2005) Primary and secondary thrombocytosis in childhood. Br J Haematol. 129: 165–77.
45. Bath PM, Butterworth RJ (1996) Platelet size: measurement, physiology and vascular disease. Blood Coagul Fibrinolysis. 7: 157–61.
46. Thompson CB, Jakubowski JA, Quinn PG, Deykin D, Valeri CR (1983) Platelet size as a determinant of platelet function. J Lab Clin Med 101: 205–13.
47. Vizioli L, Muscari S, Muscari A (2009) The relationship of mean platelet volume with the risk and prognosis of cardiovascular diseases. Int J Clin Pract. 63: 1509–15.

Genome-Wide Linkage Scan of a Pedigree with Familial Hypercholesterolemia Suggests Susceptibility Loci on Chromosomes 3q25-26 and 21q22

Xu Wang[1], Xin Li[2]**, Yong-Biao Zhang[2], Feng Zhang[2], Liyuan Sun[1], Jie Lin[1], Duen-Mei Wang[2], Lu-Ya Wang[1]***

1 The Key Laboratory of Remodeling-related Cardiovascular Diseases, Capital Medical University, Ministry of Education, and Beijing Institute of Heart Lung and Blood Vessel Diseases, Beijing Anzhen Hospital of the Capital University of Medical Sciences, Beijing, People's Republic of China, 2 CAS Key Laboratory of Genome Sciences and Information, Beijing Institute of Genomics, Chinese Academy of Sciences, Beijing, People's Republic of China

Abstract

Background: Familial hypercholesterolemia (FH) is a heritable disorder that can increase the risk of premature coronary heart disease. Studies suggest there are substantial genetic heterogeneities for different populations. Here we tried to identify novel susceptibility loci for FH in a Chinese pedigree.

Methodology/Principal Findings: We performed a SNP-based genome-wide linkage scan with the Chinese FH pedigree. Two suggestive linkage loci not previously reported were identified on chromosomes 3q25.1-26.1 (NPL = 9.01, nominal $P<0.00001$, and simulated occurrence per genome scan = 1.08) and 21q22.3 (NPL = 8.95, nominal $P<0.00001$, and simulated occurrence per genome scan = 1.26). In the interaction analysis with a trimmed version of the pedigree, we obtained a significantly increased joint LOD score (2.70) compared with that obtained when assuming the two loci uncorrelated, suggesting that more than one locus was involved in this pedigree. Exon screening of two candidate genes *ABCG1* and *LSS* from one of the suggestive region 21q22 didn't report any causative mutations.

Conclusions/Significances: These results confirm complex etiologies and suggest new genetic casual factors for the FH disorder. Further study of the two candidate regions is advocated.

Editor: Ralf Krahe, University of Texas MD Anderson Cancer Center, United States of America

Funding: This study was supported by grants from the National Natural Science Foundation of China (No. 30771986) and Beijing Natural Science Foundation (No. 7112022). The funders had no role in study design, data collection and analysis, decision to publish, or preparation of the manuscript.

Competing Interests: The authors have declared that no competing interests exist.

* E-mail: wangluya@126.com (L-YW)

These authors contributed equally to this work.

Introduction

Familial hypercholesterolemia (FH) is a heritable disorder characterized by high concentration of total cholesterol and low density lipoprotein cholesterol in serums. Elevated levels of cholesterol can give rise to xanthomas, a deposit of cholesterol in peripheral tissues, accelerating atherosclerosis, and therefore increase the risk of premature coronary heart disease (CHD) [1]. The FH phenotype is affected by both environmental and genetic factors [2].

The majority of FH cases are transmitted in an autosomal-dominant manner, known as autosomal dominant hypercholesterolemia (ADH or FH, MIM ID #143890). Three genes identified in autosomal dominant FH disorder are the low density lipoprotein receptor gene (*LDLR*) on chromosome 19 [3], the apolipoprotein B gene (*APOB*) on chromosome 2 [4], and the proprotein convertase subtilisin/kexin type 9 gene (*PCSK9*) on chromosome 1 [5]. Other FH loci currently listed in OMIM include 1q21-q23, 9q22-q31, 8p21-p12, 7p15, 5p13-p12, 3p21.2-p14.1, and 19p13.2 (MIM ID #143890). Autosomal recessive inheritance, referred to as autosomal recessive hypercholesterolemia (ARH, MIM ID #603813), was also observed in some pedigrees. Thus far only one ARH locus, 1p36-35 [6,7], is listed in OMIM, although two other loci for ARH, located on 13q22-32 [7] and 15q25-26 [8], have also been reported.

Genetic heterogeneity for FH among different populations provides the possibility of uncovering other uncharacterized genes that may be involved in the pathogenesis of the disease. For example, in a Mexican population, no *PCSK9* mutations were found in one large FH family that showed positive linkage to the 1p34.1-32 locus; this indicates genes other than *PCSK9* in the locus may be involved [9]. In addition, a Portuguese FH study found only 48% of its total received cases with clinical diagnosis of FH had genetic defects on *LDLR*, *APOB* or *PCSK9*, leaving the other 52% of FH cases with possible undiscovered gene mutations [10].

To identify novel FH loci in Chinese individuals, we performed a genome-wide linkage analysis of a Chinese pedigree without the known FH mutations in *LDLR*, *APOB*, and *PCSK9*, using an Illumina Human Linkage-12 panel, which contains 6,090 SNP markers with an average spacing of 0.58 cM. A two-locus linkage (assuming two disease loci) analysis was performed to identify linkage signals and potential locus interaction.

Results

Plasma lipid concentrations and clinical characteristics

Lipid levels and clinical features including xanthoma and coronary heart disease (CHD) for the pedigree members are shown in Table 1. Without lipid-lowering drug therapy, the plasma total cholesterol levels of these patients ranged from 226.9 to 817.2 mg/dl and the levels of LDL cholesterol ranged from 122.6 to 761.1 mg/dl. Clinical manifestations of the proband are shown in Figure 1. Patient 209 died of coronary heart disease at 45 years old and patients 2 and 34 developed coronary heart disease. The remaining members of the pedigree showed no abnormal signs of related diseases, such as coronary heart disease, diabetes mellitus, thyroid disorder, or hepatorenal disease. All pedigree members had undergone a bland diet without smoking or drinking alcohol.

Genome-wide linkage analysis

The nonparametric genome-wide scan revealed two prominent signals with nonparametric linkage (NPL) scores of 9.01 (nominal $P<0.00001$, and simulated occurrence per genome scan = 1.08) and 8.95 (nominal $P<0.00001$, and simulated occurrence per genome scan = 1.26) on chromosomes 3q25-26 and 21q22, respectively (Figure 2), while no other genomic regions showed NPL scores greater than 5. The significance levels of these two NPL signals were of proximity to the standard of suggestive linkage proposed by Lander & Kruglyak [11], where suggestive linkage is statistical evidence that would be expected to occur one time at random in a genome scan. The two highest LOD scores (both were 1.45) of parametric genome-wide linkage analysis coincided with the two NPL peak regions on chromosomes 3q25-26 and 21q22.

No linkage signals were found in those previously reported regions for either autosomal dominant or recessive FH. The two regions with prominent linkage signal, chromosomes 3q25-26 and 21q22, were used for further interaction analysis.

Haplotype analysis

To define the minimal co-segregating intervals on chromosomes 3q25-26 and 21q22 in our affected individuals, haplotypes were constructed in the relevant genomic regions. The centromeric boundary of the interval on 3q25-26 was defined by a recombination event between SNP markers rs1920395 and rs325762, which was observed in individual 7. The telomeric boundary of this interval corresponded to a historic recombination event between rs17782339 and rs1369276 in individual 2. These recombination events defined the linkage signal on 3q25-26 to a 7.42 cM interval (160.00–167.42 cM; 152.45–165.64 Mb) between rs1920395 and rs1369276 (Figure 3A). On chromosome 21q22, the centromeric boundary was defined by recombination events between rs220271 and rs876498 in individuals 7 and 37. Thus, a 20-cM interval (59.28 cM-telomere; 42.36–46.90 Mb) on chromosome 21 from rs220271 to the q telomere was defined (Figure 3B). All the affected members shared both of the disease linked haplotypes on 3q25-26 and 21q22. With these data from our FH pedigree, we refined the linkage signals of the two susceptibility loci to 3q25.1-26.1 and 21q22.3, respectively.

Notably, the disease linked haplotype on either locus was also shared among some unaffected individuals. On chromosome 3q25-26, those individuals were 27, 28, and 21 (Figure 3A). On chromosome 21q22, they were 1, 28, and 22 (Figure 3B). This phenomenon suggests a possible incomplete penetrance of either susceptibility locus.

Two-locus linkage analysis

The two-locus linkage analyses on 3q25-26 and 21q22 further improved the linkage scores in both parametric and nonparametric

Table 1. Plasma lipid concentrations and clinical characteristics.

ID	Sex	Age (years)	TC (mg/dl)	TG (mg/dl)	LDL-C (mg/dl)	HDL-C (mg/dl)	ApoAI (g/L)	ApoB (g/L)	Xanthomas	CHD	FH diagnosis
1	Female	46	141.6	224.8	45.5	51.1	1.17	0.69	no	no	unaffected
2	Female	54	226.9	132.4	141	59.4	1.31	0.87	no	yes	affected
3	Male	56	146.7	132.4	62.6	57.6	1.28	0.71	no	no	unaffected
7	Female	28	290.6	270.3	166.5	70	1.47	0.68	no	no	affected
21	Male	33	102	129.4	31.4	44.7	1.24	0.55	no	no	unaffected
22	Male	32	148	134.8	60	61.1	1.55	0.62	no	no	unaffected
24	Female	57	317.9	195.6	220	58.8	1.04	0.79	no	no	affected
27	Male	32	146.1	100.9	62.1	63.8	1.35	0.58	no	no	unaffected
28	Female	26	104.2	65.5	29.1	62	1.25	0.46	no	no	unaffected
34	Male	50	260.2	262.6	152.1	55.6	1.27	1.04	no	yes	affected
35	Male	25	228.2	92.4	133.3	76.4	1.09	0.51	no	no	affected
36	Male	33	241.8	212.7	122.6	36.7	1.19	1.21	no	no	affected
37	Female	30	356.6	83.2	285.9	54.1	1.13	1.24	no	no	affected
38	Male	5	817.2	113.2	761.1	33.5	0.77	0.99	yes	no	affected
40	Female	48	290.6	148.6	176.2	84.7	1.49	0.85	no	no	affected
41	Male	22	241.2	129.4	58.2	157.1	1.29	0.94	no	no	affected
45	Female	30	285.6	123.9	186.4	74.4	1.18	0.89	no	no	affected

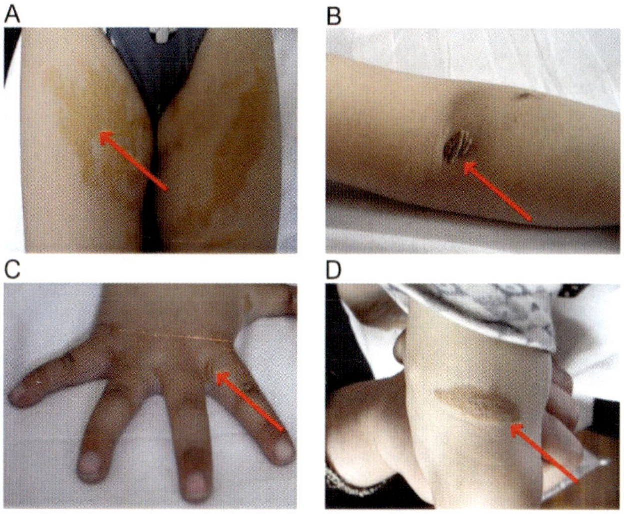

Figure 1. Clinical manifestations of the proband that had a typical FH phenotype (top panel). (A) Cutaneous xanthomas of buttocks, (B) Cutaneous xanthomas on elbow region, (C) Tendinous xanthomas and small cutaneous xanthomas of the hands, (D) Achilles tendon xanthomas.

analyses over those from single-locus analyses. The two-locus linkage analysis using a trimmed version of the pedigree (without individuals 35, 40, and 41) under a multiplicative model yielded a maximum joint LOD score of 2.70. This was a significant increase over the single-locus LOD scores of 1.10 and 1.14 on chromosomes 3q25-26 and 21q22, respectively, with the same trimmed pedigree structure. It was also observed that, the parametric two-locus linkage analyses using a heterogeneous and an additive model yielded LOD scores of 1.17 and 1.19, respectively, which are no better than the single-locus LOD scores with the same trimmed pedigree structure. Therefore, the interaction between these two regions was better modeled by the multiplicative model. This interaction was further supported by a joint NPL score (6.47; $P = 0.000565$) that was higher than those from single-locus analysis on chromosomes 3q25-26 and 21q22 (4.09 and 4.47, respectively).

Candidate gene sequencing

We sequenced all the exons and intron-exon boundaries of two most likely candidate genes *ABCG1* and *LSS* on 21q22.3, using DNA samples from 8 selected individuals of the pedigree. Five SNPs were detected in the exons of *LSS*, including 2 synonymous SNPs, rs11558754 and rs2254522, and 3 nonsynonymous SNPs, rs2254524, rs34115287, and rs2839158. No SNPs were observed in the exons of *ABCG1*, however 6 SNPs were detected in the introns of *ABCG1*. No *de novo* mutations or indels were found in the sequenced regions of these genes. None of the observed SNPs was related to the FH phenotype or was reported from HapMap to be associated with diseases.

Discussion

Based on a genome-wide linkage scan of a Chinese pedigree using SNP markers, we identified two suggestive linkage loci for

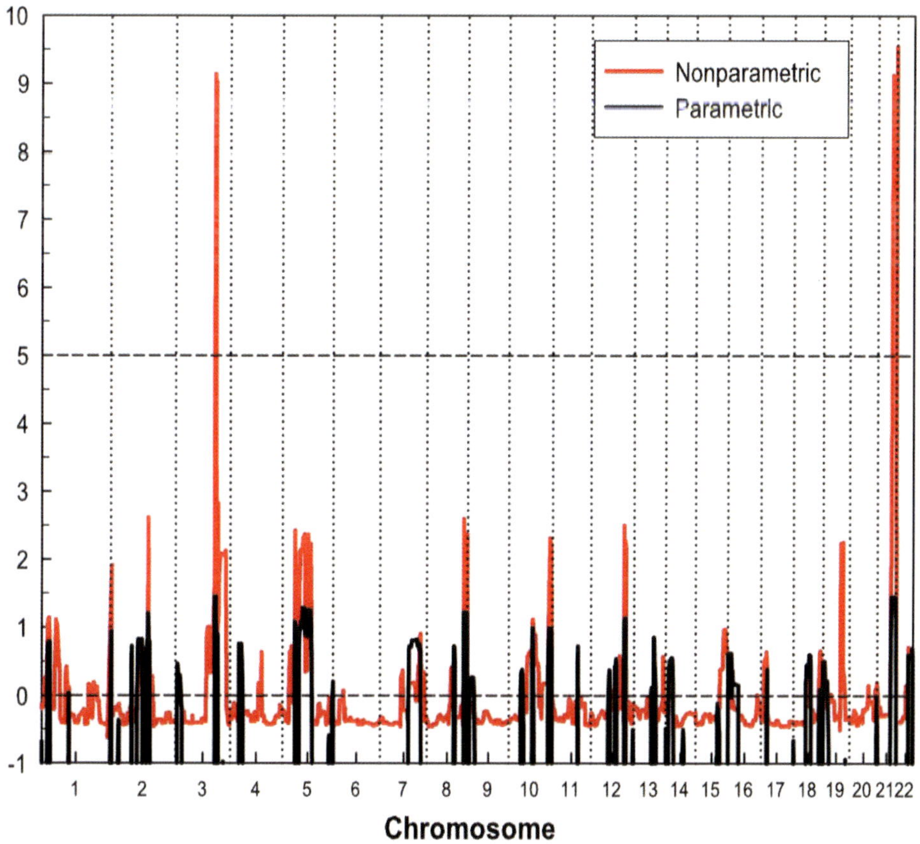

Figure 2. Genome-wide parametric and nonparametric linkage results of the FH pedigree. In the parametric linkage analysis, an autosomal dominant model with a risk allele penetrance of 0.2 and a phenocopy rate of 0.0001 was assumed.

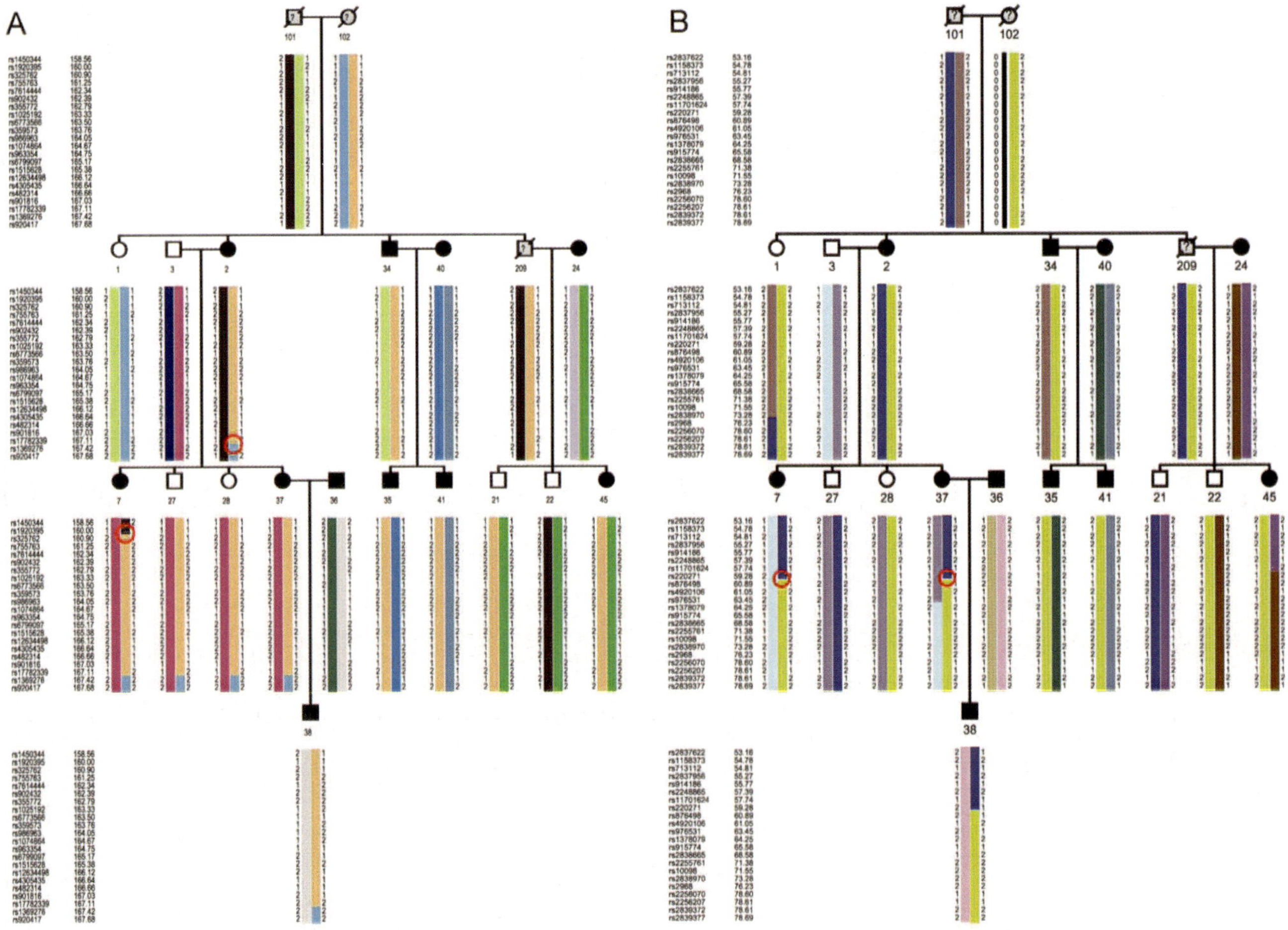

Figure 3. The most likely haplotypes of the FH pedigree on chromsomes 3q25-26 (A) and 21q22 (B). The black symbols indicated the affected individuals. The red circles indicated critical recombinations. Marker names and their positions (cM) are listed on the left side.

FH. One locus was mapped to 3q25.1-26.1 in a 7.42-cM interval (13.19 Mb) between rs1920395 and rs1369276, and the other was mapped to 21q22.3 in a 20-cM interval (4.54 Mb) from rs220271 to the q telomere. Both regions are distinct from the previously reported candidate regions for both autosomal dominant and recessive FH. Although the parametric linkage scores for both loci were not significant, the nonparametric scores were suggestively significant for both loci (nominal $P<0.00001$, with an occurrence of about 1 time per genome scan). The main reason for the insignificance of the parametric linkage score was the difficulty in defining an accurate mode of inheritance. Incomplete penetrances, phenocopies, or polygenic inheritance may also lead to loss of power in single-locus parametric linkage mapping [12]. Nonparametric linkage analysis has been described as a powerful approach that can account for the possibility of alternative modes of inheritance, and has been referred to as the method of choice for pedigree studies of complex traits [13].

The two-locus model can greatly improve the power to detect linkage for traits governed by two or more loci. The interaction between the two uncovered loci on chromosomes 3q25-26 and 21q22 was suggested by both parametric and nonparametric two-locus linkage analyses. Two-locus linkage analysis has been successfully used to detect susceptibility loci for familial hypercholesterolemia [7] and other complex traits, such as familial combined hyperlipidemia [14], high factor VIII (FVIII) levels in blood [15] and bipolar affective disorder [16]. In these studies, the superiority of the two-locus linkage scores compared to the single-locus scores was considered as evidence of genetic interaction. It is regarded that the greater scores of two-locus linkage yields, the stronger interaction between the examined loci. Our two-locus linkage analysis supported the two linkage signals, and suggested a multiplicative interaction between the two loci. The observed haplotype transmission was also in agreement with the assumption of two disease loci, because it reduced the number of unaffected disease-linked haplotype carriers from 3 for single locus (either 3q25-26 or 21q22) to 1 for two loci (Figure 3). Thus, the genome-wide linkage scan indicated a different and complex genetic basis of FH for this pedigree compared with those previously reported.

There are 92 and 113 genes in the candidate regions of chromosomes 3q25.1-26.1 and 21q22.3, respectively. We selected the two most likely candidate genes *ABCG1* and *LSS* for a preliminary mutation screening. Both genes are located on 21q22.3. *ABCG1* is a key gene involved in both cholesterol efflux to HDL and tissue lipid homeostasis [17]. ABCG1 and ABCG4 act in concert with ABCA1 to maximize the removal of excess cholesterol from cells and to generate cholesterol-rich lipoprotein particles [18]. *LSS* encodes an enzyme that catalyzes the first step of cholesterol biosynthesis, the conversion of (S)-2, 3 oxidosqualene to lanosterol. Exon screening of both genes failed to identify any mutation that co-segregated with the disease trait in this pedigree. This result was not unexpected, because more than one gene was implied in the pedigree according to our results. It is more probable that a few common variants, each with mild effect rather than a single causative mutation, may contribute to FH. Nevertheless, detailed screening for molecular variants in the candidate genes should be carried out, perhaps with increased screening size in a case-control design, and including extended screening regions beyond exons. Indeed, recently a novel *ABCG1* −257T>G promoter polymorphism that influences CHD severity in Japanese males has been found [19].

In this study, the proband had a characteristic FH phenotype with extremely high levels of plasma TC (817.2 mg/dl) and LDL-C (761.1 mg/dl) and tendinous xanthomas, while the other affected members had a relatively mild phenotype. Because both parents were affected, one possibility was that the proband may inherit two sets of pathogenic mutations (i.e., the maternal and paternal mutations) in one gene or in different genes. Previous clinical observations revealed that patients with compound heterozygote *LDLR* mutations can exhibit a more severe FH phenotype than their parents who carried only a single mutation [20]. Unfortunately, the proband's paternal family members were unavailable for the linkage study. An intensive study of the family members with next-generation sequencing technology should be helpful in indentifying the molecular basis of the phenotype.

In summary, the SNP-based genome-wide linkage scan with a Chinese FH pedigree revealed two suggestive linkage signals on chromosomes 3q25.1-26.1 and 21q22.3. Both loci are distinct from previously reported FH regions. Interaction analysis assuming two disease loci suggested the involvement of more than one locus in this pedigree. *ABCG1* and *LSS* were identified as plausible candidate genes in one of the candidate regions. Our findings revealed new and complex genetic etiology for the disease. Further research is advocated to identify the susceptibility genes in these newly discovered candidate regions.

Materials and Methods

Ethics Statement

The study complies with the Declaration of Helsinki. All participants provided written consent, and the ethics committee of the Beijing Anzhen Hospital of the Capital University of Medical Sciences approved all studies. Separate informed consent was obtained to publish the photographs in Figure 1 from the guardian of the proband.

Pedigree ascertainment and description

A 5-year-old boy with cutaneous vegetations on bilateral elbows, knees, and buttocks was identified as the proband. A further examination at the Beijing Anzhen Hospital found multiple cutaneous and tendinous xanthomas in the boy (Figure 1). The concentrations of plasma total cholesterol (TC) and LDL-cholesterol (LDL-C) of the proband were 817.2 mg/dl and 761.1 mg/dl, respectively. Doppler ultrasound revealed increased intima-media thickness and multiple atherosclerotic plaques in the common carotid artery, right subclavian artery, abdominal aorta, and femoral artery of the proband, especially in bifurcate region and posterior walls of arteries.

An extended four-generation pedigree of the proband with 17 available members from Henan Province, China was obtained for this study. All individuals had their lipoprotein measurements recorded and general information such as gender, age, history of smoking, dietary habits, personal history, and family history were collected at the same time (Table 1). None of the parents were in a consanguineous marriage. Individuals were evaluated clinically by at least two cardiologists. In total, 11 individuals (5 males and 6 females) were diagnosed as FH-affected. All the affected individuals, except individual 2, meet the criteria suggested by Williams [21]. Individual 2 was diagnosed as "affected," based on her borderline high TC concentration (226.9 mg/dl), family history, and positive status of CHD.

Serum lipids measurements

Venous blood samples were drawn from the pedigree members after overnight fasting for 12 to 14 hours. The concentrations of total plasma cholesterol, triglycerides, and high-density lipoprotein cholesterol (HDL-C) were measured by applying standard enzymatic techniques. The LDL-C concentration was calculated by applying the Friedewald formula [22]. Levels of Apo AI and Apo B100 were measured by ELISA.

Genotyping

Genomic DNA was extracted from venous blood of the 17 available pedigree members using a phenol-chloroform method. Prior to the linkage scan, we excluded the possibility that any known mutations from the three FH genes, *LDLR*, *APOB*, and *PCSK9*, caused the FH phenotype of this pedigree. The *LDLR* gene was examined by sequencing, whereas the *APOB* and *PCSK9* loci were examined by genotyping locus-linked microsatellite markers.

The genome-wide linkage scan was then conducted using the Illumina Human Linkage-12 panel. The panel contains 6,090 single nucleotide polymorphism (SNP) markers that are well spaced. Reactions were performed according to the manufacturer's protocols. Fluorescent signals were scanned using Illumina's BeadStation; genotypes were called with Illumina BeadStudio Software v3.1.8.

Genome-wide linkage analysis

Mendelian inconsistencies of the genotype data were investigated with PEDCHECK v1.1 [23]. Unlikely double recombinants were identified with the genotype error option of the linkage software MERLIN v1.01. In our linkage analyses, either monomorphic or non-Mendelian transmitted markers were removed before analysis. Of the 6090 SNPs gentoyped, 5170 informative autosomal markers were used for linkage analysis. The average genetic and physical distances between these markers were 0.69 cM and 557 kb, respectively. Both parametric and non-parametric linkage analyses were performed using the linkage software MERLIN v1.01 [24]. Parametric linkage analysis was under an autosomal-dominant model with the following parameters: a risk allele frequency of 0.001, an incomplete penetrance of 0.2 for genotypes with 1 or 2 copies of the risk allele, and a phenocopy rate of 0.0001. The low penetrance 0.2 was chosen for the following two reasons: (i) the model with a penetrance of 0.2 gave higher LOD scores than the other tested models for both the NPL-peak regions of the genome; and (ii) the disease transmission patterns in the pedigree, including the existence of affected marry-ins, unaffected offspring sharing putative disease-locus-linked haplotype, and unknown affection status for deceased individuals, indicated a low penetrance. The critical recombination events of the pedigree members were determined through haplotype construction in MERLIN v1.01.

Power estimation and simulation

The pedigree used in our study contained 17 genotyped individuals with 11 affected and 6 unaffected members. Power calculation was performed with SLINK [25], assuming an autosomal-dominant model with penetrance of 0.95 and a phenocopy rate of 0.001. The power to detect LOD scores greater than 1 and 2 were 80% and 51%, respectively.

To determine the genome-wide significance level of the linkage signal, we performed simulation studies of 1000 replicates generated with the gene-dropping approach implemented in MERLIN. In each simulation, marker allele frequencies, genetic distances, pedigree structures, and missing data patterns were retained. The number of simulations exhibiting equal or greater linkage scores was used to calculate the frequency of the observed linkage signal occurring by chance.

Two-locus linkage analysis

To test for an interaction between two putative loci on different chromosomes, GENEHUNTER-TWOLOCUS software was used to perform parametric and nonparametric linkage analysis under two disease loci [26]. Three classes of interaction models (heterogeneity, multiplicative, and additive) were tested according to the method described by Strauch et al. The heterogeneity model assumes that a mutation at either locus can cause the phenotype by itself ("or" condition). The multiplicative model assumes that only mutations at both loci can cause the phenotype ("and" condition). As for the additive model, penetrances of a single locus are simply added and rescaled to form two-locus penetrances. Table 2 shows the two-locus penetrance we used in this analysis. Because the two-locus analysis is computationally-intense, to speed up the interaction test, the pedigree was trimmed by removing the least-informative individuals 35, 40, and 41.

Table 2. Penetrance for two-locus linkage analysis.

Model	risk genotype for single locus	risk genotype for both loci
Heterogeneity	0.1997	0.3597
Multiplicative	0.0005	1.0000
Additive	0.1996	0.3995

Candidate gene sequencing

Five affected and 3 unaffected pedigree members, including the proband, his parents, his maternal uncles and aunts, and his maternal grandparents, were selected for sequencing of the candidate gene. All exons and intron-exon boundaries of the two candidate genes, *ABCG1* (15 exons) and *LSS* (23 exons) were amplified with PCR and sequenced on ABI Prism 3730xl DNA Analyzer.

Acknowledgments

We gratefully acknowledge the support of the pedigree members and cardiologists who participated in this study.

Author Contributions

Conceived and designed the experiments: D-MW L-YW. Performed the experiments: XL FZ Y-BZ JL. Analyzed the data: XL. Contributed reagents/materials/analysis tools: LS. Wrote the paper: XL XW.

References

1. Soutar AK, Naoumova RP (2007) Mechanisms of disease: genetic causes of familial hypercholesterolemia. Nat Clin Pract Cardiovasc Med 4: 214–225.
2. Bhatnagar D (2006) Diagnosis and screening for familial hypercholesterolaemia: finding the patients, finding the genes. Ann Clin Biochem 43: 441–456.
3. Goldstein JL, Schrott HG, Hazzard WR, Bierman EL, Motulsky AG (1973) Hyperlipidemia in coronary heart disease. II. Genetic analysis of lipid levels in 176 families and delineation of a new inherited disorder, combined hyperlipidemia. J Clin Invest 52: 1544–1568.
4. Innerarity TL, Weisgraber KH, Arnold KS, Mahley RW, Krauss RM, et al. (1987) Familial defective apolipoprotein B-100: low density lipoproteins with abnormal receptor binding. Proc Natl Acad Sci U S A 84: 6919–6923.
5. Abifadel M, Varret M, Rabes JP, Allard D, Ouguerram K, et al. (2003) Mutations in PCSK9 cause autosomal dominant hypercholesterolemia. Nat Genet 34: 154–156.
6. Eden ER, Naoumova RP, Burden JJ, McCarthy MI, Soutar AK (2001) Use of homozygosity mapping to identify a region on chromosome 1 bearing a defective gene that causes autosomal recessive homozygous hypercholesterolemia in two unrelated families. Am J Hum Genet 68: 653–660.
7. Al-Kateb H, Bahring S, Hoffmann K, Strauch K, Busjahn A, et al. (2002) Mutation in the ARH gene and a chromosome 13q locus influence cholesterol levels in a new form of digenic-recessive familial hypercholesterolemia. Circ Res 90: 951–958.
8. Ciccarese M, Pacifico A, Tonolo G, Pintus P, Nikoshkov A, et al. (2000) A new locus for autosomal recessive hypercholesterolemia maps to human chromosome 15q25-q26. Am J Hum Genet 66: 453–460.
9. Robles-Osorio L, Huerta-Zepeda A, Ordonez ML, Canizales-Quinteros S, Diaz-Villasenor A, et al. (2006) Genetic heterogeneity of autosomal dominant hypercholesterolemia in Mexico. Arch Med Res 37: 102–108.
10. Medeiros AM, Alves AC, Francisco V, Bourbon M, investigators of the Portuguese FH Study (2010) Update of the Portuguese Familial Hypercholesterolaemia Study. Atherosclerosis 212(2): 553–558.
11. Lander E, Kruglyak L (1995) Genetic dissection of complex traits: guidelines for interpreting and reporting linkage results. Nat Genet 11(3): 241–247.
12. Strauch K, Fimmers R, Baur MP, Wienker TF (2003) How to model a complex trait. 1. General considerations and suggestions. Hum Hered 55: 202–210.
13. Kruglyak L, Daly MJ, Reeve-Daly MP, Lander ES (1996) Parametric and nonparametric linkage analysis: a unified multipoint approach. Am J Hum Genet 58: 1347–1363.
14. Coon H, Myers RH, Borecki IB, Arnett DK, Hunt SC, et al. (2000) Replication of linkage of familial combined hyperlipidemia to chromosome 1q with additional heterogeneous effect of apolipoprotein A-I/C-III/A-IV locus. The NHLBI Family Heart Study. Arterioscler Thromb Vasc Biol 20: 2275–2280.
15. Berger M, Mattheisen M, Kulle B, Schmidt H, Oldenburg J, et al. (2005) High factor VIII levels in venous thromboembolism show linkage to imprinted loci on chromosomes 5 and 11. Blood 105: 638–644.
16. Abou Jamra R, Fuerst R, Kaneva R, Diaz GO, Rivas F, et al. (2007) The first genomewide interaction and locus-heterogeneity linkage scan in bipolar affective disorder: Strong evidence of epistatic effects between loci on chromosomes 2q and 6q. Am J Hum Genet 81: 974–986.
17. Kennedy MA, Barrera GC, Nakamura K, Baldan A, Tarr P, et al. (2005) ABCG1 has a critical role in mediating cholesterol efflux to HDL and preventing cellular lipid accumulation. Cell Metab 1: 121–131.
18. Vaughan AM, Oram JF (2006) ABCA1 and ABCG1 or ABCG4 act sequentially to remove cellular cholesterol and generate cholesterol-rich HDL. J Lipid Res 47: 2433–2443.
19. Furuyama S, Uehara Y, Zhang B, Baba Y, Abe S, et al. (2009) Genotypic Effect of ABCG1 gene promoter −257T>G polymorphism on coronary artery disease severity in Japanese men. J Atheroscler Thromb 16: 194–200.
20. Wang L, Lin J, Liu S, Cao S, Liu J, et al. (2009) Mutations in the LDL receptor gene in four Chinese homozygous familial hypercholesterolemia phenotype patients. Nutr Metab Cardiovasc Dis 19: 391–400.
21. Williams RR, Hunt SC, Schumacher MC, Hegele RA, Leppert MF, et al. (1993) Diagnosing heterozygous familial hypercholesterolemia using new practical criteria validated by molecular genetics. Am J Cardiol 72: 171–176.
22. Friedewald WT, Levy RI, Fredrickson DS (1972) Estimation of the concentration of low-density lipoprotein cholesterol in plasma, without use of the preparative ultracentrifuge. Clin Chem 18: 499–502.
23. O'Connell JR, Weeks DE (1998) PedCheck: a program for identification of genotype incompatibilities in linkage analysis. Am J Hum Genet 63: 259–266.
24. Abecasis GR, Cherny SS, Cookson WO, Cardon LR (2002) Merlin-rapid analysis of dense genetic maps using sparse gene flow trees. Nat Genet 30: 97–101.
25. Ott J (1989) Computer-simulation methods in human linkage analysis. Proc Natl Acad Sci U S A 86: 4175–4178.
26. Strauch K, Fimmers R, Baur MP, Wienker TF (2003) How to model a complex trait. 2. Analysis with two disease loci. Hum Hered 56: 200–211.

9

Low Bone Strength Is a Manifestation of Phenylketonuria in Mice and Is Attenuated by a Glycomacropeptide Diet

Patrick Solverson[1], Sangita G. Murali[1], Suzanne J. Litscher[2,3], Robert D. Blank[2,3], Denise M. Ney[1]*

1 Department of Nutritional Sciences, University of Wisconsin, Madison, Wisconsin, United States of America, **2** Geriatrics Research, Education, and Clinical Center, William S. Middleton Veterans Hospital, Madison, Wisconsin, United States of America, **3** Division of Endocrinology, Diabetes and Metabolism, Department of Medicine, University of Wisconsin, School of Medicine and Public Health, Madison, Wisconsin, United States of America

Abstract

Purpose: Phenylketonuria (PKU), caused by phenylalanine (phe) hydroxylase loss of function mutations, requires a low-phe diet plus amino acid (AA) formula to prevent cognitive impairment. Glycomacropeptide (GMP), a low-phe whey protein, provides a palatable alternative to AA formula. Skeletal fragility is a poorly understood chronic complication of PKU. We sought to characterize the impact of the PKU genotype and dietary protein source on bone biomechanics.

Procedures: Wild type (WT; $Pah^{+/+}$) and PKU ($Pah^{enu2/enu2}$) mice on a C57BL/6J background were fed high-phe casein, low-phe AA, and low-phe GMP diets between 3 to 23 weeks of age. Following euthanasia, femur biomechanics were assessed by 3-point bending and femoral diaphyseal structure was determined. Femoral *ex vivo* bone mineral density (BMD) was assessed by dual-enengy x-ray absorptiometry. Whole bone parameters were used in prinicipal component analysis. Data were analyzed by 3-way ANCOVA with genotype, sex, and diet as the main factors.

Findings: Regardless of diet and sex, PKU femora were more brittle, as manifested by lower post-yield displacement, weaker, as manifested by lower energy and yield and maximal loads, and showed reduced BMD compared with WT femora. Four principal components accounted for 87% of the variance and all differed significantly by genotype. Regardless of genotype and sex, the AA diet reduced femoral cross-sectional area and consequent maximal load compared with the GMP diet.

Conclusions: Skeletal fragility, as reflected in brittle and weak femora, is an inherent feature of PKU. This PKU bone phenotype is attenuated by a GMP diet compared with an AA diet.

Editor: Marlon R. Schneider, University of Munich, Germany

Funding: This work was supported by the National Phenylketonuria Alliance, United States Department of Agriculture HATCH Grant WIS01517, and National Institutes of Health Grant R01- AR-54753. This material is based upon work supported by the Office of Research and Development, Biomedical Laboratory R&D Service, Department of Veterans Affairs (RDB) and performed in part in the Geriatrics Research, Education, and Clinical Center at the William S. Middleton Memorial Veterans Hospital. The funders had no role in study design, data collection and analysis, decision to publish, or preparation of the manuscript.

Competing Interests: DMN is a co-inventor on United States Patent Application US-2010-0317597, entitled "Glycomacropeptide (GMP) medical foods for nutritional management of phenylketonuria (PKU) and other metabolic disorders," which is held by the Wisconsin Alumni Research Foundation and licensed to Cambrooke Foods, LLC. A percentage of all royalty payments is awarded to the inventors. This does not alter the authors' adherence to all the PLOS ONE policies on sharing data and materials.

* E-mail: ney@nutrisci.wisc.edu

Introduction

Phenylketonuria (PKU; OMIM 261600) is a recessive genetic disease of amino acid (AA) metabolism caused by loss of function mutations of the gene encoding phenylalanine hydroxylase (EC 1.14.16.1, *PAH* in humans and *Pah* in mice), resulting in an inability to convert phenylalanine (phe) to tyrosine [1]. PKU results in gross elevations of phe concentrations in tissue and blood, with downstream cytotoxicity, culminating in profound cognitive impairment if left untreated. Fortunately, this can be averted with lifelong adherence to a low-phe diet that excludes all high protein foods and requires an AA formula to meet nutrient needs [2]. With implementation of newborn screening for PKU in 1960–1970, there are an estimated 50,000 individuals worldwide with treated PKU and a normal range of cognitive function. Skeletal fragility in early adulthood has emerged as a chronic complication of PKU treated with a low-phe AA diet [3,4,5,6,7,8,9,10,11]. Because a low-phe AA diet is the standard of care and is instituted shortly after birth, it remains unknown whether bone fragility in PKU is inherent to the PKU genotype or secondary to its essential dietary management [3].

Compliance with the low-phe diet is often poor after early childhood owing to limited food choices and the bitter taste and strong odor of AA formulas [12,13,14,15]. Moreover, a number of suboptimal outcomes in patients with PKU treated with diet have been identified [16]. Glycomacropeptide (GMP), a whey protein produced during cheese making, provides an alternative to AA formula because pure GMP contains no phe and can be made into a variety of low-phe, high protein foods and beverages for those with PKU [17]. Studies in humans with PKU indicate that GMP improves protein retention, phe concentrations, and palatability of the low-phe diet compared with AA formula [18,19,20]. Long term studies in the PKU mouse model (*Pah*^{enu2}) demonstrate that a GMP diet supports similar growth and accretion of lean body mass and attenuates indices of metabolic stress compared with an AA diet [21,22]. The evidence suggests that the GMP diet provides an acceptable, physiologic source of low-phe dietary protein that may also impact bone development for PKU.

In order to distinguish the contributions of the PKU genotype itself and dietary treatment of the disease, we have conducted a factorial experiment in PKU (*Pah*$^{enu2/enu2}$) and wild type (WT, *Pah*$^{+/+}$) mice fed casein, AA and GMP diets. The objective was to characterize the impact of the PKU genotype and dietary protein source on bone biomechanical performance. We assessed the femora by 3 point bending, allowing us to obtain information regarding bone strength (load and stress) and brittleness (displacement and strain), distinct mechanical properties that both contribute to fracture susceptibility [23]. Measuring the bones after testing allowed us to assess the contribution of cross-sectional bone geometry to mechanical performance. This is the first report to rigorously establish the separate contributions of genotype and diet to skeletal fragility in PKU.

Materials and Methods

Animals and Experimental Design

The University of Wisconsin-Madison Institutional Animal Care and Use Committee approved the facilities and protocols used in this study. A breeding colony of PKU mice was used to produce experimental animals by breeding C57BL/6J mice heterozygous for the *Pah*^{enu2} mutation to yield homozygous PKU mice and WT control mice [21,24]. Experimental mice were genotyped for the presence of the *Pah*^{enu2} mutation as described previously [22]. The experiment controlled for three main effects and their interactions in a 2×2×3 factorial design: genotype (WT or PKU), sex (male or female), and diet (low-phe GMP, low-phe AA, or high-phe casein) with casein serving as a control diet, **Figure 1A**. Mice were randomized to diet, separated by sex and housed within their litters at the time of weaning (21d) in shoe-box cages. Mice had free access to food and water and the facility was maintained at 22°C on a 12:12-h light-dark cycle.

Mice were fed the experimental diets from weaning through young adulthood (3–25 weeks of age), which resulted in mice being fed diet for 20.4±0.11 weeks on average (range 17–22 weeks of feeding, n = 217 mice). The casein, AA and GMP diets were isoenergetic and the source of protein was the only variable manipulated (Harlan Teklad, Madison, WI; TD.09667 - TD.09669), as previously reported [22]. The casein diet included 20% (wt/wt) casein plus 0.3% L-cystine, the AA diet included 17.5% free AAs [25] and the GMP diet included 20% GMP (BioPURE GMP, Davisco Foods International, LeSueur, MN) plus 1.5 times the NRC requirement (equivalent to a total supplementation of 2.8% AA) for 5 limiting AA in order to provide a complete source of protein. The AA profile of the diets was previously reported [22]. All three diets were supplemented with approximately 10% more than NRC requirements for calcium, phosphorus and magnesium to optimize bone growth.

Dual-energy x-ray absorptiometry (DXA) with PIXImus software version 2.10 (GE/Lunar Corp, Madison, WI) was performed to obtain in vivo whole body bone mineral density (BMD) and bone mineral content (BMC) at the end of the experiment. Mice were anesthetized with isoflurane with an anesthesia machine (IsoFlo, Abbott Laboratories, North Chicago, IL) and placed prone on the DXA scanner bed with their tail and appendages fully extended. Each mouse received one scan at the completion of the study. Handling of the data obtained from the DXA scan was performed by a single scientist blinded to the treatment groups and subsequent statistical analysis of the densitometry data was performed by the authors. Once mice completed the feeding study, they were placed under anesthesia using an isoflurane anesthesia machine and euthanized by exsanguination via cardiac puncture. Following euthanasia, both femora were dissected free of soft tissue, wrapped in phosphate buffered saline-saturated gauze, and stored at −80°C. Specimens were subjected to two freeze thaw cycles, one prior to DXA, and the second prior to biomechanical testing. Using DXA we measured areal BMD of isolated femura twice with repositioning, as previously described [26]. Prior to biomechanical analysis, femora were gradually warmed by placing them at 4°C for at least 12 hours, and then allowing them to come to room temperature prior to analysis. Bones were broken in two different sessions. Prior to bone fracture femur length of the second block of femora (n = 78 mice) was measured using Vernier calipers measuring the distance between the greater trochanter and the medial condyle.

Biomechanical Testing

We tested femoral diaphysis biomechanical performance by quasi-static 3-point bending under displacement control at a rate of 0.3 mm/sec, with a support span of 7.5 mm as previously described, **Figure 1B**. [27]. This produces a mid-diaphyseal fracture directly below the crosshead. By using the femoral condyles and the 3rd trochanter as anatomical landmarks to position bones consistently, the testing protocol produces highly reproducible fractures. We obtained the periosteal perimeter, cortical cross-sectional area, outer and inner major and minor axis lengths, shape factor (ratio of outer major axis length to outer minor axis length), and cross-sectional moment of inertia in the fracture plane from digital photographs [27]. We used the geometric properties and the whole bone mechanical testing data to calculate the material properties of the bone tissue according to the standard beam theory equations [23], using the averages of both femora for further analysis:

Stress (σ), (MPa) = $FLc/4I$ with F = force, L = length, c = outer radius in the plane of bending, and I = cross-sectional moment of inertia in the plane of bending.

Strain (ε), (mm/mm) = $12cd/L^2$ with c = outer radius in the plane of bending, d = displacement, L = length.

Young's Modulus (E), (MPa) = $(F/d)(L^3/48I)$ with F = force, L = length, and I = cross sectional moment of inertia in the plane of bending.

Principal Component Analysis

The following input variables were included in principal component analysis (PCA): Body mass, femoral BMD, post-yield deflection, total deflection, yield load, maximum load, energy, stiffness, femoral cross-sectional area, femoral periosteal perimeter, femoral inner major and minor axis lengths, femoral outer major and minor axis lengths, femoral diaphyseal shape factor, and femoral diaphyseal cross-sectional moment of inertia. The PCA was performed with the SAS function "proc princomp" (SAS Institute, Cary, NC) [28,29,30]. We performed further analysis of the principal components (PCs) with Eigenvalues ≥1. PC values for each animal were calculated by multiplying each PC's Eigenvector by the animal's parameter vector.

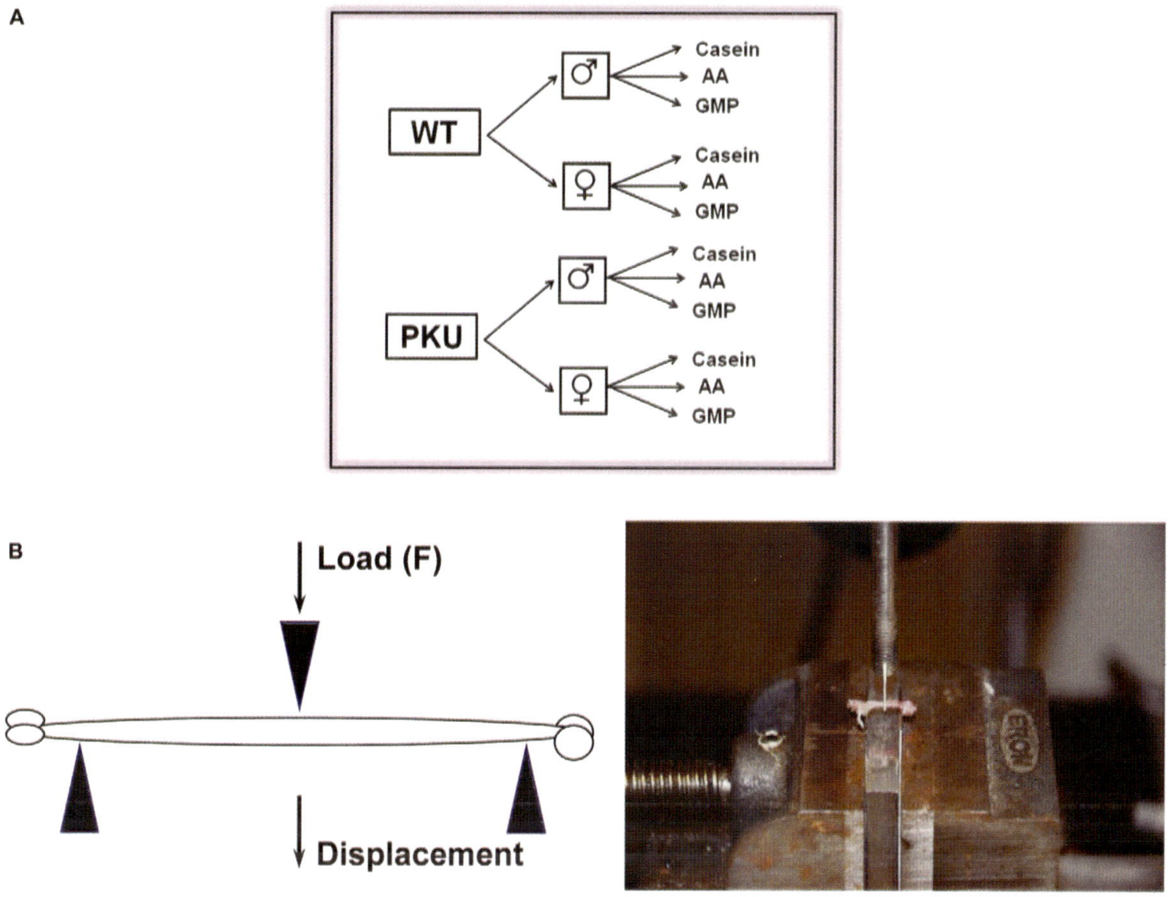

Figure 1. Experimental design and three-point bending test. The experiment utilized a 2×2×3 factorial design with a total of 12 groups (A). A cartoon of the three-point bending test of a mouse femur and a representative photograph (B).

Statistical Analysis

Data were analyzed by three-way ANOVA or ANCOVA using "proc mixed". Femoral biomechanical testing was performed on two different days due to the large number of femora, thus a random effect of time as a blocking factor was included in the model. The three-way ANCOVA tested for main effects of genotype, sex, and diet as well as their two and three way interactions. Femoral cross section measurements and biomechanical data were adjusted for the animal's body mass by including body mass as a covariate. When body mass wasn't a significant predictor for a parameter the term was removed and results from a subsequent three-way ANOVA are presented. Data presented are raw data or actual measurements, and the statistical significance shown represents the analysis adjusted for body weight based on ANCOVA where appropriate. Differences between treatment groups were detected using a protected Fisher's Least Significant Difference (LSD) test (SAS Institute, 2007, Cary, NC). Data transformations were performed where appropriate to fit assumptions of normality and equal variance prior to statistical analysis. If data transformations failed, a respective non-parametric ANCOVA or ANOVA was performed on ranked data. Untransformed data are presented in the tables. Data are analyzed per animal; biomechanical data are an average of the right and left femora. Data are presented as mean ± SE. P-values <0.05 are considered significant. Where there was no significant interaction, data were pooled into treatment groups by their respective significant main effects.

Results

Growth and Whole Body Bone Mineral Density

The low-phe AA and GMP diets significantly reduced plasma phe concentration in both WT and PKU mice, **Table 1.** In spite of restricting dietary phe to the minimum needed to support nearly normal growth, plasma phe concentration in PKU mice remained abnormally elevated, approximately 14-fold higher in PKU compared with WT mice. Regardless of diet, whole body BMD was significantly lower in PKU compared with WT mice. Regardless of sex, femur length was significantly shorter in WT mice fed the AA diet compared with the GMP and casein diets, and not significantly different from PKU mice. Plasma phe concentration did not predict femur length, whole body BMD or BMC.

Femora of PKU Mice Have Decreased Strength and Increased Brittleness

The 3-point bending test produces mid-diaphyseal fractures under controlled loading conditions (Figure 1B). The primary analysis of the test measures 3 elements of biomechanical performance: displacement (the amount the bone bends), strength (load, or the force applied to the bone), and absorbed energy (the area under the load-displacement curve), as summarized in **Figure 2A and Table 2**. Representative load-displacement curves for a WT and PKU femur are shown in **Figure 2B**. Following fracture, specimen geometry in the plane of the fracture

Table 1. In vivo measurements.

	Wild Type Mice						PKU Mice					
	Males			Females			Males			Females		
Variable	Casein	AA	GMP	Casein	AA	GMP	Casein	AA	GMP	Casein	AA	GMP
N	17 (10)	18 (7)	19 (7)	23 (9)	16 (4)	22 (10)	18 (7)	16 (5)	14 (6)	19 (6)	20 (4)	13 (3)
Body Mass (g)[a,b,c,e,g]	31.1±0.8	28.5±0.5	28.1±0.8	22.5±0.3	22.5±0.3	21.9±0.4	26.2±0.4	29.5±1.0	26.8±0.7	21.4±0.4	22.0±0.3	21.5±0.5
[r]Plasma phe (μmol/L)[a,c,e]	51.5±4.5	38.5±7.0	41.0±9.0	50.2±1.6	34.3±6.1	41.9±2.2	2026±151	726±61	745±26	2206±76	719±19	786±24
BMC (mg)[a,c,d,f]	574±13	533±12	528±13	533±18	527±15	602±14	571±16	504±14	555±15	489±16	495±11	542±8
BMD (mg/cm^2)[a,b,f]	51.4±0.3	50.7±0.4	50.2±0.6	51.6±0.6	51.4±0.6	52.2±0.4	49.8±0.3	50.1±0.7	48.2±0.6	48.5±0.5	50.4±0.3	49.9±0.6
Length (mm)[a,b,e]	16.91± 0.01	16.86± 0.02	16.91± 0.01	16.89± 0.02	16.84± 0.02	16.88± 0.01	16.86± 0.01	16.84± 0.03	16.85± 0.01	16.83± 0.01	16.87± 0.02	16.81±0.01

Values are means ± SE; *N*, no of mice for measurement of body mass; BMC, whole-body bone mineral content; BMD, whole-body bone mineral density.
[r]Data analyzed by 3 way ANOVA on ranked data.
[a]genotype effect,
[b]sex effect,
[c]diet effect,
[d]gt*sex effect,
[e]gt*diet effect,
[f]sex*diet effect,
[g]gt*sex*diet effect.
Body mass: WT female mice weighed more than PKU female mice. WT males fed casein and PKU males fed AA weighed the most. There was no difference in body mass between WT males fed AA and WT or PKU males fed GMP, and PKU males fed casein weighed the least.
Plasma phe: PKU mice had higher plasma phe than WT mice. Among PKU mice, there was a significant reduction in plasma phe with the GMP or AA diet. Among WT mice, there was also a significant reduction in plasma phe with the GMP or AA diet.
BMC: Females fed GMP and males fed casein had the highest BMC. There was no difference between females fed casein and males or females fed AA, but males fed GMP had a higher BMC than females fed AA. There was a significant reduction in BMC in PKU females compared to either WT females or WT and PKU males.
BMD: PKU animals had a lower BMD compared to WT animals. Males fed GMP had a lower BMD compared to females fed GMP or AA and males fed casein. Females fed casein had a lower BMD than females fed GMP.
Length: Males had longer femurs than female mice. WT mice fed AA had a significant reduction in femur length compared to WT mice fed GMP and casein. Moreover, PKU mice fed casein, AA and GMP had significantly shorter femurs than WT mice fed GMP and casein, but were not different from WT mice fed AA. Numbers in parenthesis indicate sample size from femur length analysis.

is assessed (**Table 3**), allowing calculation of the corresponding tissue-level mechanical properties (**Table 4)** from standard beam equations, as described in the methods section. The raw data reflect the biomechanical performance of the actual bone, while the tissue level or material properties (i.e., tissue properties and material properties are synonyms) reflect the performance of an idealized sample of the bone tissue, independent of its size and shape.

Regardless of sex or diet, the PKU genotype was associated with reduced femoral biomechanical properties assessed by three-point bending **Figure 2B–H**. Yield load, or the force required to elicit permanent damage to the femur, and the maximum load achieved before fracture were significantly lower in PKU mice. Total displacement, or the total amount of deformation by the femur before fracture, was also reduced in PKU compared with WT mice. The post-yield displacement, a measurement of ductility, was significantly lower with PKU, thus the femora of PKU mice are more brittle (i.e., the opposite of ductile) and yield sooner than WT femora. The stiffness of PKU bones was lower than WT bones. Additionally, the energy required to fracture the bone, measured as the area under the load-displacement curve, was significantly reduced in PKU femora. These measures of whole bone biomechanical performance are paralleled by the tissue level analysis of the stress-strain relationship (Table 4). This suggests an inherent disturbance in the biomechanical performance of PKU bone tissue, independent of size. Moreover, decreases in mineralization are supported by *ex vivo* DXA data. Both areal BMD as well as BMC of femora (Table 3) are significantly reduced in PKU mice compared with WT mice. In summary, the femora in PKU mice display global deficits of biomechanical performance, and are more brittle, weaker, less stiff, and absorb less energy than those of WT mice.

We sought evidence regarding whether plasma phe levels are related to bone status. We found no significant relationship between plasma phe and any biomechanical or BMD outcomes (data not shown).

Dietary Protein Source Modifies the PKU Bone Phenotype

Regardless of genotype and sex, the AA diet reduced femoral size, as manifested in a significant reduction in femoral cross sectional area (CSA) and in the femoral perimeter, compared with the casein and GMP diets (**Figure 3A)**. Femoral size expressed as the cross sectional moment of inertia (CSMI), a measure of the distribution of material around a neutral axis, was also significantly lower in PKU mice fed the AA diet compared with the casein and GMP diets (Table 3). Consequent to the reduction in femoral size, both WT and PKU mice fed an AA diet tolerated a lower maximum load compared with the GMP diet, **Figure 3B**. Tissue level analysis across diet treatments provides supporting evidence that the AA diet yields a more brittle and weaker bone compared to the GMP diet in that it decreases yield strain, total strain, and maximum stress in PKU mice (**Table 4**). In summary, the reduction in both femoral size and maximum load in mice fed the low-phe AA diet suggests that providing dietary protein from GMP rather than AA attenuates the PKU bone phenotype.

Principal Components Analysis

The bone properties we measured in this study are not mutually independent. For example, yield load and maximum load are

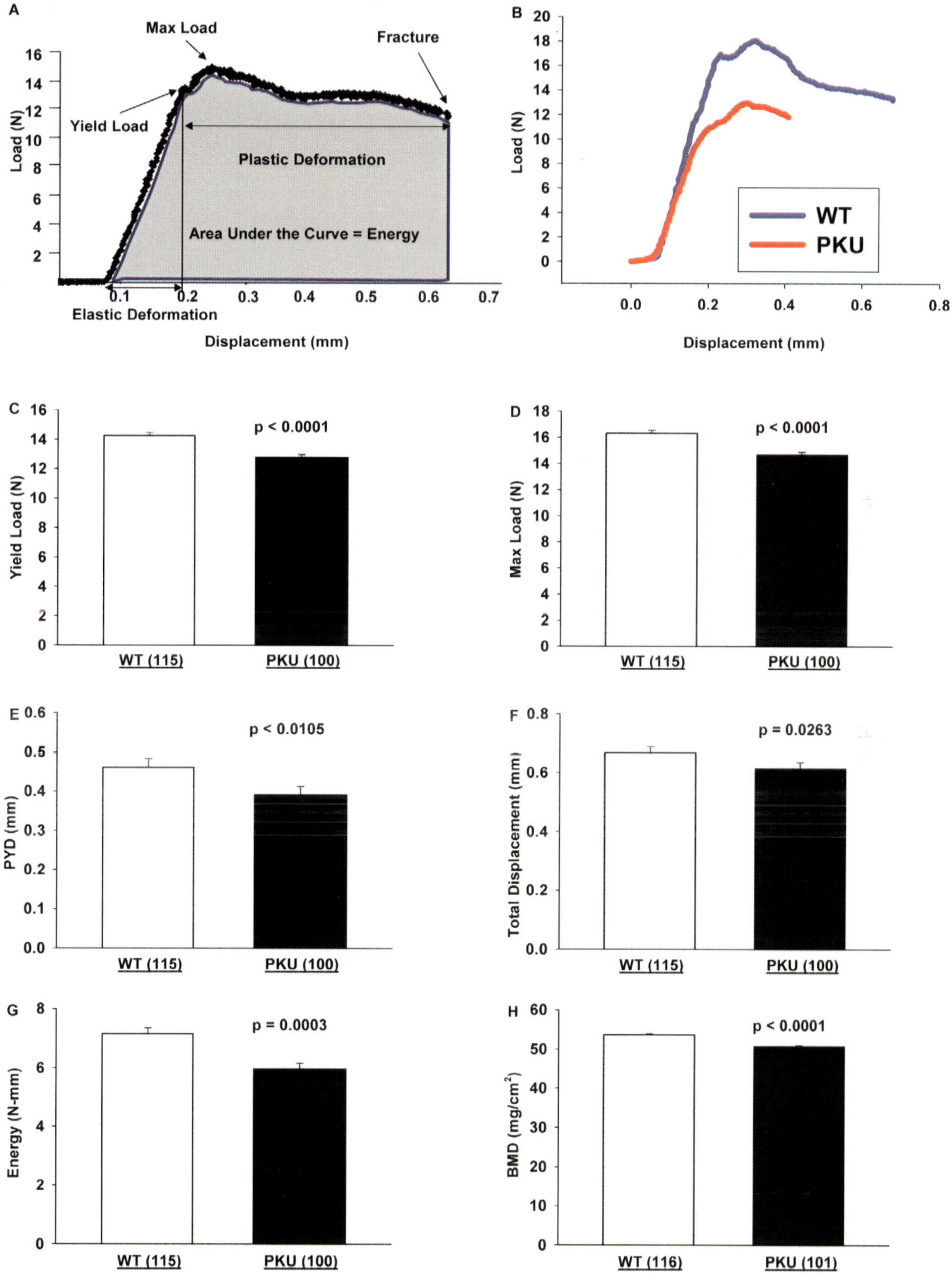

Figure 2. Force-displacement curve analysis of WT and PKU mice. Schematic of a load-displacement curve generated from the three-point bending test from which the yield point, maximum load, elastic and plastic deformation, and energy to failure (shaded area under the curve) are

obtained (A). Representative load-displacement curves for WT and PKU mice (B). Effects in WT and PKU mice for yield load (C), maximum load (D), post-yield displacement (PYD) (E), total displacement (F), energy to failure (G), and femoral bone mineral density (BMD) (H). Values are means ± SE; p-values represent main effect of genotype. Sample size is shown in parenthesis. All values for femoral biomechanical performance had a significant main effect for genotype, WT >PKU.

highly correlated with an R of 0.85 (**Table 5**). Furthermore, with so many properties measured, one might ask which are most important. PCA provides a linear transformation of the raw data to an equal number of mutually orthogonal PCs, each of which is a linear function of the raw data [31,32]. By established convention, further analysis is limited to those PCs with Eigenvalues exceeding 1. The goal of the analysis is to explain the experimental variation while reducing the dimensionality of the data and maintaining the statistical independence of the PCs. PCA of 16 whole bone femoral measurements yielded four PCs with Eigenvalues >1, which collectively accounted for 87% of the variance (**Table 6**).

The PCs are composites of all the measured parameters, but can be interpreted on the basis of the coefficients for each, as summarized in the Eigenvectors (**Table 7**). PC1 is "size-like," with cross-sectional area, perimeter, inner major axis, outer minor axis, outer major axis, and cross-sectional moment of inertia contributing most to it. PC2 is "strength-like," but at the material rather than the whole-bone level, with large contributions from stiffness, yield and maximum load, and BMD, but with negative contributions from multiple size parameters. PC3 is "ductility-like," with post-yield deflection, total deflection, and energy to failure prominent contributors. PC4 is the most difficult to interpret, with body mass, cross-sectional area, shape factor, and areal BMD of femora having large coefficients. Regardless of their interpretation, it is notable that there are significant genotype-dependent differences in all 4 PCs, indicating that the bone phenotype in PKU mice represents a global deficit in biomechanical performance (**Table 8**).

Discussion

Success in managing the neurological manifestations of PKU by dietary phe restriction has allowed many patients to enjoy a greatly improved prognosis, spared of devastating cognitive impairment. Because of their improved function, other, more subtle deficits have become apparent [16]. Chief among these is skeletal fragility, as noted by multiple independent research groups [3,4,5,6,7,8,9,10,11]. However, since dietary phe restriction is initiated within days of birth, it has previously not been possible to distinguish whether skeletal fragility is a manifestation of PKU

Table 2. Force-displacement curve analysis showing whole bone biomechanical performance.

	Wild Type Mice						PKU Mice					
	Males			Females			Males			Females		
Variable	Casein	AA	GMP	Casein	AA	GMP	Casein	AA	GMP	Casein	AA	GMP
N	17	18	19	23	16	22	18	16	14	19	20	13
[t]PY disp (mm)[a,b]	0.48± 0.04	0.51± 0.07	0.55± 0.08	0.38± 0.04	0.45± 0.04	0.40± 0.03	0.47± 0.05	0.43± 0.06	0.46± 0.07	0.38± 0.05	0.31± 0.03	0.30± 0.04
[t]Total disp (mm)[a,b]	0.69± 0.04	0.74± 0.07	0.78± 0.07	0.57± 0.04	0.65± 0.04	0.61± 0.04	0.69± 0.05	0.65± 0.06	0.70± 0.06	0.61± 0.05	0.51± 0.03	0.55± 0.04
*[r]Stiffness (N/mm)[a,b,d,e]	87±4	80±2	78±4	110±5	94±5	102±3	78±4	74±4	79±7	75±2	89±3	81±3
*[r]Yield load (N)[a,b]	13.7± 0.6	13.5± 0.3	12.9± 0.4	15.2± 0.5	14.8± 0.4	15.2± 0.4	11.7± 0.4	12.3± 0.4	12.6± 0.4	13.0± 0.5	13.2± 0.4	14.3± 0.5
*[r]Max load (N)[a,b,c,d]	15.8± 0.5	15.0± 0.3	14.6± 0.4	18.1± 0.5	16.6± 0.4	17.6± 0.4	14.1± 0.4	14.1± 0.4	14.6± 0.6	14.8± 0.4	15.3± 0.3	16.2± 0.4
*[t]Energy (N-mm)[a]	7.54± 0.37	7.01± 0.55	7.15± 0.61	6.87± 0.44	7.09± 0.39	7.33± 0.46	6.61± 0.50	5.86± 0.50	6.56± 0.65	5.90± 0.53	5.31± 0.30	5.71± 0.37

Values are means ± SE of raw data; *N*, no of mice; PY, post-yield; disp, displacement; N, newtons.
*Data analyzed using ANCOVA with a covariate of body mass.
[t]Data transformed to satisfy assumptions of normality and variance.
[r]Non-transformable data was ranked.
[a]genotype effect,
[b]sex effect,
[c]diet effect,
[d]gt*sex effect,
[e]gt*sex*diet effect.
PY disp: Males had a greater PY disp than females. WT mice had a greater PY disp than PKU mice.
Total disp: Males had a greater total disp than females. WT mice had a greater total disp than PKU mice.
Stiffness: All female groups except PKU females fed GMP or casein had stiffer bones than males. Among female groups WT females fed casein and GMP had the stiffest bones. There was no difference between female mice fed AA diet and female PKU mice fed GMP, however PKU females fed casein had a significant reduction in stiffness. Among male mice the only significant difference was a reduction in stiffness in male PKU mice fed AA compared to WT males fed casein.
Yield load: Female mice tolerated a higher load at the yield point than male mice. WT mice tolerated a higher load at the yield point compared to PKU mice.
Max Load: Females had a greater maximum load before fracture compared to males. Moreover, WT females had a greater max load than PKU females, however there were no difference between genotypes for the males. Mice fed the GMP diet had a significant increase in maximum load compared to mice fed the AA diet, but there was no difference between mice fed the GMP and casein diets, additionally there was no difference between mice fed the casein and AA diets.
Energy: It required more energy to fracture the femurs of WT mice than it did to fracture the femurs of PKU mice.

Table 3. Size, shape, and content of mice femora.

	Wild Type Mice						PKU Mice					
	Males			Females			Males			Females		
Variable	Casein	AA	GMP	Casein	AA	GMP	Casein	AA	GMP	Casein	AA	GMP
N	17	18	19	23	16	22	18	16	14	19	20	13
*^{t}CSA (mm^2)^{b,c,d}	1.07± 0.04	0.97± 0.03	0.97± 0.02	1.01± 0.02	0.98± 0.04	0.96± 0.02	0.96± 0.02	0.95± 0.03	1.00± 0.04	0.90± 0.02	0.91± 0.02	0.94± 0.02
*^{r}Perimeter (mm)^{b,c}	6.07± 0.12	5.78± 0.12	5.80± 0.10	5.60± 0.05	5.47± 0.08	5.37± 0.04	5.80± 0.07	5.60± 0.09	5.72± 0.12	5.49± 0.07	5.34± 0.06	5.38± 0.07
*^{r}Inner Minor Axis (mm)^{a,b,c,e}	0.93± 0.03	0.90± 0.02	0.91± 0.02	0.89± 0.01	0.85± 0.01	0.84± 0.01	0.92± 0.01	0.88± 0.02	0.87± 0.01	0.93± 0.01	0.86± 0.01	0.88± 0.02
*^{t}Inner Major Axis (mm)^{c,e}	1.68± 0.05	1.60± 0.05	1.64± 0.04	1.48± 0.02	1.46± 0.02	1.41± 0.02	1.62± 0.03	1.54± 0.03	1.49± 0.04	1.49± 0.03	1.41± 0.02	1.41± 0.03
*^{r}Outer Minor Axis (mm)^{b,c,e}	1.34± 0.03	1.27± 0.02	1.29± 0.02	1.32± 0.01	1.27± 0.02	1.27± 0.01	1.29± 0.01	1.25± 0.02	1.27± 0.02	1.31± 0.01	1.24± 0.01	1.28± 0.02
*^{t}Outer Major Axis (mm)^{c}	2.25± 0.05	2.11± 0.05	2.11± 0.03	2.02± 0.02	1.97± 0.03	1.93± 0.02	2.11± 0.03	2.06± 0.04	2.10± 0.05	1.95± 0.03	1.90± 0.03	1.92± 0.02
*Shape Factor (unitless)^{b}	1.68± 0.02	1.66± 0.03	1.64± 0.02	1.54± 0.02	1.55± 0.02	1.52± 0.01	1.64± 0.02	1.65± 0.03	1.65± 0.02	1.49± 0.01	1.53± 0.02	1.50± 0.02
*^{t}CSMI (mm^4)^{b,c,e}	0.19± 0.01	0.16± 0.01	0.17± 0.01	0.17± 0.01	0.16± 0.01	0.15± 0.00	0.16± 0.01	0.15± 0.01	0.16± 0.01	0.16± 0.01	0.14± 0.00	0.15± 0.01
^{t}BMD (mg/cm^2)^{a,b,d}	54.0± 0.7	51.9± 0.6	51.8± 0.7	55.0± 0.8	54.1± 0.9	55.0± 0.5	50.8± 0.6	50.5± 0.9	51.1± 0.8	49.8± 0.7	51.2± 0.4	51.3± 0.7
BMC (mg)^{a,b}	29.2± 0.6	27.3± 0.5	27.0± 0.6	27.8± 0.6	27.1± 0.5	27.5± 0.4	26.0± 0.5	25.5± 0.8	25.6± 0.7	23.3± 0.6	24.6± 0.3	24.4± 0.7

Values are means ± SE of raw data; *N*, no of mice; CSA, cross sectional area; CSMI, cross sectional moment of inertia; BMD, areal bone mineral density; BMC, bone mineral content.
*Data analyzed using ANCOVA with a covariate of body mass.
^{t}Data transformed to satisfy assumptions of normality and variance.
^{r}Non-transformable data was ranked.
^{a}genotype effect,
^{b}sex effect,
^{c}diet effect,
^{d}gt*sex effect,
^{e}gt*diet effect.
CSA: WT females had a greater CSA than PKU females, both of which were greater than the males per unit body weight. A main effect of diet demonstrated a significant reduction in CSA in mice fed the AA diet.
Perimeter: Females had a larger perimeter than males. Mice fed casein had the greatest perimeter, followed by GMP, and then AA.
Inner minor axis (IMA): Females had a larger IMA than males. PKU mice fed casein had the largest IMA. There was no difference between WT mice fed casein and WT or PKU mice fed GMP. Mice fed GMP were also not different from mice fed AA, however PKU mice fed AA had a significantly smaller IMA compared to WT mice fed casein.
Inner Major Axis (IMAJA): Mice fed the casein diet had the greatest IMAJA.
Outer minor axis (OMA): Females had a greater OMA than males. PKU mice fed casein had the longest OMA and PKU mice fed AA had the shortest.
Outer major axis (OMAJA): Mice fed casein had a larger OMAJA than mice fed either GMP or AA diet.
Shape factor (SF) = OMAJA/OMA: Females had a more circular cross section than males.
CSMI: Females had a larger CSMI compared to males after correction for body weight. PKU mice fed casein had the greatest CSMI. There was no difference in CSMI between WT mice fed casein, WT and PKU mice fed GMP and WT mice fed AA, however there was a significant reduction in CSMI in PKU mice fed AA. There also was no difference between WT and PKU mice fed casein or GMP.
BMD: WT females had a higher BMD than WT males, both of which were higher than the BMD of PKU mice, where there were no differences due to gender or diet.
BMC: Male mice had a greater BMC than females. WT mice had a greater BMC than PKU mice.

itself, or of its dietary treatment. The availability of an animal model of PKU, harboring an ENU-induced point mutation of the murine *Pah* gene allowed this uncertainty to be resolved experimentally [21].

Our data show that PKU mice have impaired bone biomechanical performance, regardless of the effects of sex or diet. The biomechanical deficit is complex, encompassing strength, stiffness, and ductility. PCA reveals a genotype effect for all 4 PCs, confirming the principal findings of the whole bone biomechanics. Bone is a composite tissue composed of a protein matrix, containing primarily type 1 collagen, and precipitated mineral, containing primarily calcium and phosphate in the form of apatite [33]. The protein elements of bone matrix contribute tensile strength and ductility to the composite, while the mineral provides compressive strength and stiffness [34,35]. These are distinct properties, both of which are needed to resist fracture. In our study, strength, stiffness, and ductility are reduced in PKU mice relative to WT mice. The finding that all 4 PCs of biomechanical performance differ significantly between genotypes further supports the inference that multiple aspects of bone function are impaired in the PKU mice relative to WT mice.

While our data clearly support the existence of deficits in bone strength and ductility in PKU mice, the present data are insufficient to identify the biochemical, cellular, and physiological

Table 4. Stress-strain curve analysis showing tissue level biomechanical performance.

	Wild Type Mice						PKU Mice					
	Males			Females			Males			Females		
Variable	Casein	AA	GMP	Casein	AA	GMP	Casein	AA	GMP	Casein	AA	GMP
N	17	18	19	23	16	22	18	16	14	19	20	13
*[t]Yield strain (unitless)[c,e]	0.030± 0.002	0.031± 0.002	0.031± 0.002	0.028± 0.001	0.028± 0.001	0.028± 0.001	0.031± 0.002	0.029± 0.002	0.032± 0.002	0.031± 0.001	0.026± 0.001	0.034± 0.003
[t]PY strain (unitless)[a,b]	0.068± 0.005	0.070± 0.011	0.076± 0.012	0.053± 0.005	0.061± 0.005	0.054± 0.005	0.064± 0.007	0.058± 0.008	0.061± 0.009	0.054 ±0.008	0.041± 0.004	0.041± 0.006
*[t]Total strain (unitless)[e]	0.098± 0.006	0.101± 0.011	0.107± 0.011	0.080± 0.006	0.089± 0.006	0.083± 0.005	0.095± 0.007	0.087± 0.008	0.093± 0.008	0.085± 0.008	0.067± 0.003	0.075± 0.005
*Modulus (MPa)[a,c,d,e,g]	4184± 256	4543± 234	4305± 231	5670± 202	5374± 223	6017± 184	4236± 253	4386± 173	4520± 274	4314± 145	5768± 234	4915± 281
*[r]Yield stress (MPa)[a,b,c]	92±3	102±4	96±3	111±3	115±4	121±3	86±2	98±2	98±3	103±3	112±4	117±4
*[t]Max stress (MPa)[a,b,c,e,f]	105±3	113±4	109±3	131±3	129±4	141±3	104±2	112±2	113±3	118±3	130±3	133±4
[t]Toughness (MPa)[a]	7.14± 0.29	6.97± 0.40	7.19± 0.51	6.95± 0.43	7.51± 0.47	7.87± 0.45	6.74± 0.50	6.13± 0.45	6.84± 0.63	6.39± 0.49	5.95± 0.31	6.39± 0.45
*[t]Failure stress (MPa)[e]	80±4	76±7	72±6	99±5	91±5	105±3	76±5	84±5	82±4	92±5	104±4	106±5

Values are means ± SE of raw data; *N*, no of mice; PY, post-yield; MPa, megapascals.
*Data analyzed using ANCOVA with a covariate of body mass.
[t]Data transformed to satisfy assumptions of normality and variance.
[r]Non-transformable data was ranked.
[a]genotype effect,
[b]sex effect,
[c]diet effect,
[d]gt*sex effect,
[e]gt*diet effect,
[f]sex*diet effect,
[g]gt*sex*diet effect.

Yield strain: PKU mice fed GMP and casein had the highest strain at their yield point and PKU mice fed AA had the lowest. There was no difference between WT mice fed the three diets and PKU mice fed AA. Additionally, there was no difference between WT mice fed GMP and AA with PKU mice fed casein.
PY strain: Males had a greater strain after yielding than females. WT mice had a greater strain after yielding than PKU mice.
Total strain: PKU mice fed AA had a significant reduction in total strain and there was no difference across all other groups.
Modulus: The three way interaction demonstrated that females tended to have bones with a higher intrinsic stiffness than males; WT females fed GMP and PKU females fed AA had a higher modulus than WT and PKU males fed GMP as well as PKU males fed casein. Additionally, WT females fed casein or AA had a higher modulus than PKU males fed casein. Among females, PKU mice fed casein had a significant reduction in intrinsic stiffness, moreover WT females fed all three diets and PKU females fed AA had a higher modulus than PKU females fed GMP. Among males, PKU mice fed casein had a significant reduction in modulus compared to male mice fed AA and there was no difference across the other five groups.
Yield stress: Wild type mice tolerated more stress before yielding compared to PKU mice. Female mice tolerated more stress before yielding compared to male mice. Mice fed AA and GMP tolerated more stress before yielding compared to mice fed casein.
Max stress: Female groups fed GMP and AA had a higher max stress before fracture compared to male groups and female mice fed casein had a higher max stress than males fed casein. Among females, groups fed GMP had the highest max stress, followed by AA and then casein. Among males, groups fed AA had a higher max stress than males fed casein, but males fed GMP were not different from the other two. PKU mice fed casein had a significant reduction in max stress compared to WT and PKU mice fed GMP and AA as well as WT mice fed casein.
Toughness: WT mice had tougher bones than PKU mice, as measured by area under the stress strain curve.
Failure stress: PKU mice fed AA had a higher stress at fracture compared to WT mice fed AA and PKU mice fed casein. WT mice fed casein and PKU mice fed GMP also had a higher stress at fracture compared to PKU mice fed casein.

mechanisms underlying them. The organic components of bone matrix are produced by osteoblasts and these are mineralized following secretion into the extracellular space [34,36]. Matrix synthesis is a complex, hierarchically organized process, so that abnormalities at early stages will have cascading effects at higher levels of structure [35,37]. Increased brittleness could arise as a consequence of a primary abnormality of type 1 collagen, its cross-linking, its assembly, abnormalities of other matrix proteins, disorganization of matrix assembly, or a combination of these [34,38,39]. Decreased strength reflects a quantitative deficit of mineralization, as suggested by our observation of decreased BMD in PKU mice, but changes in the composition or crystal structure could also contribute to reduced strength.

It is important to recall that bone is known to model in response to its usual loading environment, and bone size and strength therefore vary as a function of body size and activity [33,40]. PKU mice are smaller than WT mice, resulting in lower loads if activity were equivalent in the 2 genotypes. We adjusted our data for body mass prior to comparison of biomechanical performance, so our results have accounted for differential growth. However, our experiment did not assess cage activity while the mice were living. It is possible that neurological damage arising from phe toxicity leads to reduced activity, and that the activity difference contributes to the observed differences in skeletal phenotypes. Assessing whether PKU bones respond similarly to WT bones to defined loading conditions *in vivo* remains an important question for future research.

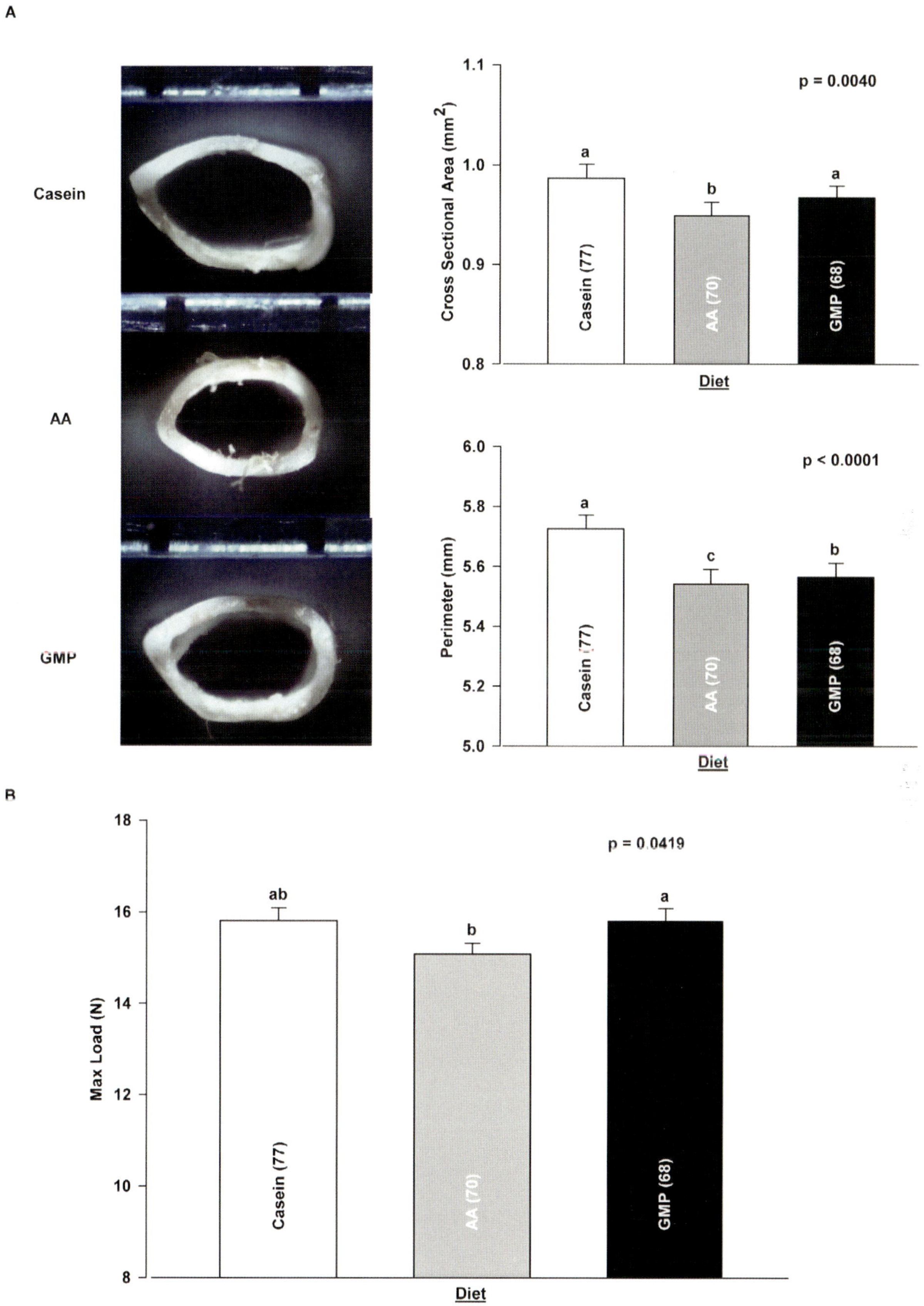

Figure 3. Diet modifies femoral size and strength in WT and PKU mice. Representative photographs of femoral cross-sectional geometry in mice fed casein, AA, and GMP diets from which measurements of cross-sectional area and perimeter are obtained (A). Diet effect on maximum load derived from load-displacement curve analysis (B). Values are means ± SE; p-values represent main effect of diet. Sample size is shown in parenthesis. Groups with different letter superscripts are significantly different ($p<0.05$).

Table 5. Correlations among phenotypes.

	Mass	CSA	Perim	InMin	InMaj	OutMin	OutMaj	SF	CSMI	PYD	TD	Stiff	YLoad	MLoad	Energy	fBMD
Mass	–	0.45	0.63	0.30	0.56	0.29	0.67	0.61	0.47	0.27	0.29	−0.15	−0.08	−0.10	0.22	0.14
CSA		–	0.73	0.23	0.33	0.65	0.71	0.36	0.85	0.23	0.24	0.39	0.44	0.51	0.40	0.64
Perim			–	0.67	0.80	0.74	0.97	0.61	0.87	0.30	0.33	−0.01	0.11	0.10	0.29	0.31
InMin				–	0.70	0.78	0.58	0.09	0.65	0.10	0.10	−0.07	−0.01	0.01	0.03	0.06
InMaj					–	0.53	0.82	0.60	0.64	0.34	0.36	−0.16	−0.08	−0.12	0.22	0.11
OutMin						–	0.63	−0.04	0.91	0.13	0.14	0.25	0.33	0.40	0.22	0.42
OutMaj							–	0.75	0.79	0.31	0.35	−0.02	0.08	0.06	0.30	0.31
SF								–	0.25	0.29	0.33	−0.22	−0.17	−0.25	0.19	0.05
CSMI									–	0.26	0.27	0.28	0.35	0.42	0.36	0.53
PYD										–	0.98	0.00	−0.05	−0.02	0.86	0.11
TD											–	−0.10	−0.02	−0.05	0.84	0.09
Stiff												–	0.46	0.73	0.20	0.68
YLoad													–	0.85	0.30	0.67
MLoad														–	0.36	0.76
Energy															–	0.39
fBMD																–

Phenotypes are Mass, body mass; CSA, cortical cross-sectional area; Perim, periosteal perimeter; InMin, inner minor axis; InMaj, inner major axis; OutMin, outer minor axis; OutMaj, outer major axis; SF, shape factor; CSMI, cross-sectional moment of inertia; PYD, post-yield deflection; TD, total deflection; Stiff, stiffness; YLoad, yield load; MLoad, maximum load; Energy, energy to failure; fBMD, BMD by ex vivo DXA. Each cell shows R.

Our data also demonstrate that dietary protein source consistently affects both size and strength in WT and PKU mice. The AA diet impairs the radial growth of the femur, affecting all diaphyseal dimensions relative to casein (Table 3). The GMP and casein diets yielded larger femoral dimensions than the AA-based diet. This occurs in both WT and PKU mice, and is important because biomechanical performance at the whole bone is highly dependent on radial size [41]. Insufficient amounts of AA that are abundant in type 1 collagen, such as glutamic acid, arginine, lysine and proline, is one possible reason for this. Type 1 collagen comprises approximately 90% of the protein in bone matrix, and during skeletal growth, it is synthesized and degraded at a rapid rate. Subtle deficiency of amino acids that are abundant in collagen might therefore be manifested by reduced skeletal modeling. This possibility is attractive because it can account for reduced bone growth in mice fed the AA diet. A second possibility, applicable only to the AA diet, is that the acid load imposes a metabolic burden that restricts skeletal modeling. We previously showed that PKU mice fed the AA diet experience metabolic stress as evidenced by an increase in food and water intake, and renal hypertrophy compared to mice fed a GMP diet [22]. Moreover, PKU mice fed the AA diet had an increase in energy expenditure not different from the elevation observed in PKU mice fed casein. The experiments reported here do not address whether these mechanisms contribute to restricted radial bone growth, but are readily testable.

The work reported here can only be compared to prior studies in limited ways. A prior experiment reported that 8 weeks of phe restriction improved bone status in PKU mice [42]. However, the technical quality of the bone characterization was inferior to our methods, and the work was conducted in a BTBR/J rather than a C57BL/6J background. The human literature includes several reports addressing the relationship between plasma phe and BMD. The data are equivocal on this point, with some showing a negative correlation [7,9,10] while other studies do not [3,4,6,43]. A human cohort study reported that low BMD is apparent in patients with PKU from an early age and that the deficit remains stable over time [3]. However, since all subjects were prescribed low-phe AA diets, the contributions of genotype and diet could not be resolved. Human work has primarily been cross-sectional and the bone characterization has been limited to clinical fractures, BMD, and serum markers of bone turnover [3,4,5,6,7,8,9,10,43,44,45,46]. Use of a mouse model allowed us to overcome these limitations. We recently reported an increase in systemic inflammation as evidenced by significant splenomegaly and increases in inflammatory cytokines in PKU mice fed AA or casein diets; this response was normalized with the GMP diet [22]. Our observations parallel findings in human PKU. Roato et al. reported that activated T-cells, a major source of tumor necrosis factor alpha, induced spontaneous osteoclastogenesis which was associated with decreased bone status in human PKU [47].

Our experiment featured several notable strengths. Use of a uniform C57BL/6J genetic background eliminated possible confounding due to the segregation of genes other than *Pah*, and sample sizes were adequate to power main effect comparisons of all important biomechanical endpoints [48]. The biomechanical characterization of the bones was comprehensive and used robust

Table 6. Principal Component Analysis.

	PC1	PC2	PC3	PC4
Eigenvalue	6.68	3.57	2.39	1.29
Difference	3.11	1.19	1.09	0.72
r^2	0.418	0.223	0.149	0.081
Cumulative r^2	0.418	0.641	0.79	0.871

Difference is subtraction of subsequent PC from former PC.

Table 7. Eigenvectors of Principal Components 1–4.

	PC1	PC2	PC3	PC4
Body mass	0.239	−0.205	−0.026	0.318
Cross-sectional area	0.316	0.161	−0.025	0.227
Perimeter	0.358	−0.125	−0.147	0.040
Inner minor axis	0.234	−0.111	−0.296	−0.474
Inner major axis	0.289	−0.242	−0.116	−0.077
Outer minor axis	0.302	0.107	−0.230	−0.375
Outer major axis	0.350	−0.153	−0.112	0.171
Shape factor	0.194	−0.282	0.053	0.538
CSMI	0.358	0.081	−0.143	−0.122
Post-yield deflection	0.183	−0.125	0.518	−0.203
Total deflection	0.189	−0.147	0.507	−0.186
Stiffness	0.083	0.409	0.036	0.074
Yield load	0.123	0.407	0.028	0.071
Max load	0.136	0.468	0.035	0.027
Energy	0.209	0.063	0.506	−0.116
Femoral BMD	0.209	0.362	0.051	0.202

CSMI, cross-sectional moment of inertia; BMD, bone mineral density.

methods. Lastly, diets were isoenergetic allowing the animals' growth and metabolism to be characterized in detail [22].

Several limitations of our work must also be acknowledged. The C57BL/6 background is inbred, and therefore not reflective of the varied, outbred genetic backgrounds encountered in human PKU. The 3 point bending test, while robust and reproducible, produces experimental fractures in the mid-diaphysis of the femur, a site that is not generally susceptible to clinical fracture. Moreover, this is a skeletal site that is composed of cortical bone, so our data do not address the consequences of PKU on trabecular bone. Mice, because of their small size, do not have the osteonal structure characteristic of human cortical bone. The diets were only started at 3 weeks of age, when mice are weaned. This is distinct from PKU management in humans, which features dietary restriction beginning in the first week following birth. However, since long bones in mice undergo extensive linear and radial growth between weaning and young adulthood, most, if not all the femoral diaphyseal bone present at the time of testing was synthesized during the course of study. Finally, while our study was adequately powered to detect genotype, diet, and sex differences in all aspects of biomechanical performance at the main effect level, the sample sizes were insufficient to detect the impact of interactions on energy, post-yield displacement, and their material level correlates.

In summary, the data reported here demonstrate that skeletal fragility is an intrinsic feature of PKU in mice. The biomechanical defects are complex, affecting both strength and ductility. In mice, an AA diet exacerbates skeletal fragility by limiting radial bone growth, which is attenuated by a GMP diet. As an AA diet is presently the standard of care, this finding suggests that there is a need to determine whether improved diets can improve bone health in patients with PKU. The mechanisms by which PKU causes bone fragility and the AA-based diet impairs radial bone growth remain unknown, illustrating the need for further work to fully define the skeletal pathophysiology of PKU and its treatment.

Acknowledgments

We thank Dr. Adam Brinkman for his assistance with tissue processing and review of the manuscript, graduate student Emily Sawin for assistance with data analysis, undergraduate students Wing Pun and Jennifer Mallon for their assistance with the PKU mouse colony, and Peter Crump for assistance with statistical models.

Table 8. Principal component phenotypes of WT and PKU mice fed casein, AA, and GMP diets.

	Wild Type Mice						PKU Mice					
	Males			Females			Males			Females		
Variable	Casein	AA	GMP	Casein	AA	GMP	Casein	AA	GMP	Casein	AA	GMP
N	17	18	19	23	16	22	18	16	14	19	20	13
[t]PC1[a,c,d]	25.1±0.6	23.4±0.4	23.1±0.6	24.8±0.6	23.2±0.5	23.9±0.4	22.2±0.5	22.4±0.6	22.5±0.8	20.7±0.4	21.8±0.3	21.4±0.4
[t]PC2[a,b,d,e]	40.8±1.7	38.2±1.1	37.0±2.0	53.7±2.4	46.3±2.1	50.5±1.5	36.4±1.9	34.3±1.7	37.4±3.1	37.2±1.1	43.1±1.1	40.9±1.4
[t]PC3[a,b]	5.75±0.23	5.41±0.36	5.42±0.47	6.58±0.35	6.20±0.20	6.65±0.30	5.04±0.36	4.47±0.38	5.12±0.53	4.75±0.34	4.94±0.23	4.93±0.25
[t]PC4[a,b,d]	17.3±0.4	15.9±0.2	15.6±0.4	16.4±0.4	15.1±0.4	15.5±0.3	14.9±0.4	15.8±0.5	15.3±0.6	13.3±0.3	14.7±0.2	14.0±0.4

Values are means ± SE; *N*, no of mice; PC, principal component.
[t]Data transformed to satisfy assumptions of normality and variance.
[a]genotype effect,
[b]sex effect,
[c]gt*sex,
[d]gt*diet effect,
[e]gt*sex*diet effect.
PC1: WT mice fed Casein had a significant increase in their calculated PC1 values compared to WT mice fed GMP or AA. PKU mice on the three diets had significantly lower values than WT mice. Additionally, PKU males and females had lower values than WT males and females of which PKU female values were the lowest.
PC2: WT males fed GMP had reduced values compared to WT males fed casein, but were not different from WT males fed AA. There were no differences within the PKU male groups on the three diets, however PKU males fed AA had lower values than WT males fed AA or casein. There were no differences between the values within the WT females groups, however WT females fed AA were not different from PKU females fed GMP or AA, whereas WT females fed GMP or casein were significantly higher. PKU females fed casein had a significant reduction compared to PKU females fed AA, but not GMP. Additionally, WT females had higher values than WT males, and PKU females had higher values than PKU males with the exception of PKU females fed casein.
PC3: WT mice had greater values than PKU mice, and females had greater values than males.
PC4: WT mice fed casein had greater values than WT mice fed GMP or AA. PKU mice fed the three diets had a significant reduction in values compared to WT mice; however PKU mice fed AA were not different from WT mice fed GMP or AA. Male mice had greater values than female mice.

Author Contributions

Conceived and designed the experiments: PS SGM RDB DMN. Performed the experiments: PS SGM SJL RDB DMN. Analyzed the data: PS SGM RDB DMN. Contributed reagents/materials/analysis tools: SJL RDB DMN. Wrote the paper: PS RDB DMN.

References

1. NIH (2000) Phenylketonuria (PKU): screening and management. NIH Consensus Statement 17: 1–33.
2. MacLeod EL, Ney DM (2010) Nutritional management of phenylketonuria. Ann Nestle 68: 58–69.
3. de Groot MJ, Hoeksma M, van Rijn M, Slart RH, van Spronsen FJ (2012) Relationships between lumbar bone mineral density and biochemical parameters in phenylketonuria patients. Mol Genet Metab 105: 566–570.
4. Perez-Duenas B, Cambra FJ, Vilaseca MA, Lambruschini N, Campistol J, et al. (2002) New approach to osteopenia in phenylketonuric patients. Acta Paediatr 91: 899–904.
5. Greeves LG, Carson DJ, Magee A, Patterson CC (1997) Fractures and phenylketonuria. Acta Paediatr 86: 242–244.
6. Zeman J, Bayer M, Stepan J (1999) Bone mineral density in patients with phenylketonuria. Acta Paediatr 88: 1348–1351.
7. McMurry MP, Chan GM, Leonard CO, Ernst SL (1992) Bone mineral status in children with phenylketonuria–relationship to nutritional intake and phenylalanine control. Am J Clin Nutr 55: 997–1004.
8. Allen JR, Humphries IR, Waters DL, Roberts DC, Lipson AH, et al. (1994) Decreased bone mineral density in children with phenylketonuria. Am J Clin Nutr 59: 419–422.
9. Schwahn B, Mokov E, Scheidhauer K, Lettgen B, Schonau E (1998) Decreased trabecular bone mineral density in patients with phenylketonuria measured by peripheral quantitative computed tomography. Acta Paediatr 87: 61–63.
10. Al-Qadreh A, Schulpis KH, Athanasopoulou H, Mengreli C, Skarpalezou A, et al. (1998) Bone mineral status in children with phenylketonuria under treatment. Acta Paediatr 87: 1162–1166.
11. Koura HM, Abdallah Ismail N, Kamel AF, Ahmed AM, Saad-Hussein A, et al. (2011) A long-term study of bone mineral density in patients with phenylketonuria under diet therapy. Arch Med Sci 7: 493–500.
12. Koch R, Burton B, Hoganson G, Peterson R, Rhead W, et al. (2002) Phenylketonuria in adulthood: a collaborative study. J Inherit Metab Dis 25: 333–346.
13. MacDonald A (2000) Diet and compliance in phenylketonuria. Eur J Pediatr 159 Suppl 2: S136–141.
14. Macdonald A, Daly A, Davies P, Asplin D, Hall SK, et al. (2004) Protein substitutes for PKU: what's new? J Inherit Metab Dis 27: 363–371.
15. Walter JH, White FJ, Hall SK, MacDonald A, Rylance G, et al. (2002) How practical are recommendations for dietary control in phenylketonuria? Lancet 360: 55–57.
16. Enns GM, Koch R, Brumm V, Blakely E, Suter R, et al. (2010) Suboptimal outcomes in patients with PKU treated early with diet alone: revisiting the evidence. Mol Genet Metab 101: 99–109.
17. Laclair CE, Ney DM, MacLeod EL, Etzel MR (2009) Purification and use of glycomacropeptide for nutritional management of phenylketonuria. J Food Sci 74: E199–206.
18. Ney DM, Gleason ST, van Calcar SC, Macleod EL, Nelson KL, et al. (2009) Nutritional management of PKU with glycomacropeptide from cheese whey. J Inherit Metab Dis 32: 32–39.
19. Van Calcar SC, Macleod EL, Gleason ST, Etzel MR, Clayton MK, et al. (2009) Improved nutritional management of phenylketonuria by using a diet containing glycomacropeptide compared with amino acids. Am J Clin Nutr 89: 1068–1077.
20. Van Calcar SC aND (2012) Food Products Made with Glycomacropeptide, a Low-Phenylalanine Whey Protein, Provide a New Alternative to Amino Acid-Based Medical Foods for Nutrition Management of Phenylketonuria Journal of the Academy of Nutrition and Dietetics In press.
21. McDonald JD, Bode VC, Dove WF, Shedlovsky A (1990) Pahhph-5: a mouse mutant deficient in phenylalanine hydroxylase. Proc Natl Acad Sci U S A 87: 1965–1967.
22. Solverson P, Murali SG, Brinkman AS, Nelson DW, Clayton MK, et al. (2012) Glycomacropeptide, a low-phenylalanine protein isolated from cheese whey, supports growth and attenuates metabolic stress in the murine model of phenylketonuria. Am J Physiol Endocrinol Metab 302: E885–895.
23. Turner CH, Burr DB (1993) Basic biomechanical measurements of bone: a tutorial. Bone 14: 595–608.
24. Harding CO, Gillingham MB, Hamman K, Clark H, Goebel-Daghighi E, et al. (2006) Complete correction of hyperphenylalaninemia following liver-directed, recombinant AAV2/8 vector-mediated gene therapy in murine phenylketonuria. Gene Ther 13: 457–462.
25. Rogers QR, Harper AE (1965) Amino acid diets and maximal growth in the rat. J Nutr 87: 267–273.
26. Lopez Franco GE, O'Neil TK, Litscher SJ, Urban-Piette M, Blank RD (2004) Accuracy and precision of PIXImus densitometry for ex vivo mouse long bones: comparison of technique and software version. J Clin Densitom 7: 326–333.
27. Saless N, Litscher SJ, Lopez Franco GE, Houlihan MJ, Sudhakaran S, et al. (2009) Quantitative trait loci for biomechanical performance and femoral geometry in an intercross of recombinant congenic mice: restriction of the Bmd7 candidate interval. Faseb J 23: 2142–2154.
28. Becker RA, Chambers JM, Wilks AR (1988) The New S Language. Monterey, CA: Wadsworth and Brooks/Cole Advanced Books & Software. 702 p.
29. Mardia KV, Kent JT, Bibby JM (1979) Multivariate Analysis. London: Academic Press. 521 p.
30. Venables WN, Ripley BD (2002) Modern Applied Statistics with S. New York: Springer. 515 p.
31. Saless N, Litscher SJ, Vanderby R, Demant P, Blank RD (2011) Linkage mapping of principal components for femoral biomechanical performance in a reciprocal HCB-8 × HCB-23 intercross. Bone 48: 647–653.
32. Pearson K (1901) On lines and planes of closest fit to systems of points in space. Philos Mag 2: 559–572.
33. Frost HM (2001) From Wolff's law to the Utah paradigm: Insights about bone physiology and its clinical applications. Anatomical Record 262: 398–419.
34. Robey PG, AL B (2008) The Composition of Bone. In: CJ R, editor. Primer on the Metabolic Bone Diseases and Disorders of Bone and Mineral Metabolism. 7th ed. Washington, DC: American Society for Bone and Mineral Research. 32–38.
35. Fratzl P (2008) Collagen: an Introduction. In: Fratzl P, editor. Collagen: Structure and Mechanics. New York: Springer. 1–13.
36. Stein GS, Lian JB (1993) Molecular mechanisms mediating proliferation/differentiation interrelationships during progressive development of the osteoblast phenotype. Endocr Rev 14: 424–442.
37. Lakes R (1993) Materials with Structural Hierarchy Nature 361: 311–315.
38. Blank RD, AL B (2008) Genetic Collagen Diseases. In: Fratzl P, editor. Collagen: Structure and Mechanics. New York: Springer. 447–474.
39. Marini JC, Forlino A, Cabral WA, Barnes AM, San Antonio JD, et al. (2007) Consortium for osteogenesis imperfecta mutations in the helical domain of type I collagen: regions rich in lethal mutations align with collagen binding sites for integrins and proteoglycans. Hum Mutat 28: 209–221.
40. Sievanen H, Kannus P, Jarvinen TL (2007) Bone quality: an empty term. PLoS Med 4: e27.
41. Bonadio J, Jepsen KJ, Mansoura MK, Jaenisch R, Kuhn JL, et al. (1993) A murine skeletal adaptation that significantly increases cortical bone mechanical properties. Implications for human skeletal fragility. J Clin Invest 92: 1697–1705.
42. Yannicelli S, Medeiros DM (2002) Elevated plasma phenylalanine concentrations may adversely affect bone status of phenylketonuric mice. J Inherit Metab Dis 25: 347–361.
43. Modan-Moses D, Vered I, Schwartz G, Anikster Y, Abraham S, et al. (2007) Peak bone mass in patients with phenylketonuria. J Inherit Metab Dis 30: 202–208.
44. Ambroszkiewicz J, Gajewska J, Laskowska-Klita T (2004) A study of bone turnover markers in prepubertal children with phenylketonuria. Eur J Pediatr 163: 177–178.
45. Millet P, Vilaseca MA, Valls C, Perez-Duenas B, Artuch R, et al. (2005) Is deoxypyridinoline a good resorption marker to detect osteopenia in phenylketonuria? Clin Biochem 38: 1127–1132.
46. Nagasaka H, Tsukahara H, Takatani T, Sanayama Y, Takayanagi M, et al. (2011) Cross-sectional study of bone metabolism with nutrition in adult classical phenylketonuric patients diagnosed by neonatal screening. J Bone Miner Metab 29: 737–743.
47. Roato I, Porta F, Mussa A, D'Amico L, Fiore L, et al. (2010) Bone impairment in phenylketonuria is characterized by circulating osteoclast precursors and activated T cell increase. PLoS One 5: e14167.
48. Leppanen OV, Sievanen H, Jarvinen TL (2008) Biomechanical testing in experimental bone interventions–May the power be with you. J Biomech 41: 1623–1631.

Subjects with Molecularly Defined Familial Hypercholesterolemia or Familial Defective apoB-100 Are Not Being Adequately Treated

Trond P. Leren*, Knut Erik Berge

Medical Genetics Laboratory, Department of Medical Genetics, Oslo University Hospital Rikshospitalet, Oslo, Norway

Abstract

Objectives: To study whether subjects with a molecular genetic diagnosis of familial hypercholesterolemia (FH) or familial defective apoB-100 (FDB) are being adequately treated.

Design: A questionnaire regarding medical history was sent to 2611 subjects who had been provided with a molecular genetic diagnosis of FH or FDB, and a blood sample was obtained for lipid measurements.

Results: 956 (36.6%) of the 2611 subjects participated. The mean age for starting lipid-lowering therapy was 33.4 (±12.1) years. Among those below 18 years of age, only 20.4% were on lipid-lowering drugs, whereas 89.1% of those aged 18 and above were on lipid-lowering drugs. The mean levels of total serum cholesterol and LDL-cholesterol were 5.7 (±1.5) mmol/l and 3.9 (±1.3) mmol/l, respectively. Among those who were on lipid-lowering drugs, 29.0% and 12.2% had levels of LDL cholesterol below 3.0 mmol/l and 2.6 mmol/l, respectively. Only 47.3% of the 956 subjects were considered as being adequately treated largely due to a failure to titrate their drug regimens. From the use of cholesterol-years score, lipid-lowering therapy must start before the age of 20 in order to prevent the subjects from contracting premature coronary heart disease.

Conclusion: The majority of FH/FDB subjects are being diagnosed late in life and are not being adequately treated. In order to prevent them from contracting premature coronary heart disease, it is key that levels of LDL cholesterol are normalized from a young age and that sufficient doses of lipid-lowering drugs are being used.

Editor: Jos Verbeek, Finnish Institute of Occupational Health, Finland

Funding: This study was funded by Extrastiftelsen Helse og Rehabilitering. The funder had no role in study design, data collection and analysis, decision to publish, or preparation of the manuscript.

Competing Interests: The authors have declared that no competing interests exist.

* E-mail: trond.leren@rikshospitalet.no

Introduction

Familial hypercholesterolemia (FH) is an autosomal dominant disorder caused by mutations in the low density lipoprotein (LDL) receptor gene [1]. As a result of defective cell-surface LDL receptors, clearance of LDL from plasma is reduced leading to increased plasma levels of LDL cholesterol and total cholesterol [1]. Those who are heterozygotes have values for total serum cholesterol in the range of 7 to 15 mmol/l, whereas those who are homozygotes have values for total serum cholesterol in the range of 20 to 25 mmol/l [1]. As a result of the increased cholesterol levels, FH subjects are at an increased risk of contracting premature coronary heart disease (CHD) [1,2]. FH is one of the most common genetic disorders with a prevalence of heterozygotes of approximately 1/500 in most western countries [3,4]. Thus, FH has a significant impact on public health and it has been estimated that FH heterozygotes constitute approximately 5% of those with premature CHD [5,6].

However, efficient lipid-lowering therapy is available for FH heterozygotes which may normalize their levels of total serum cholesterol and LDL cholesterol [7]. The general experience, however, is that too few patients are being treated, and those who are being treated, are not being adequately treated [8–13]. Moreover, lipid-lowering therapy generally starts late in life at a time when advanced atherosclerosis has already developed [13]. It is believed that a major cause for these treatment failures is difficulties in diagnosing FH by the use of the clinical diagnostic criteria consisting of autosomal dominant hypercholesterolemia and presence of premature CHD and xanthomas [1,14–16]. The sensitivity of these criteria is particularly low in children/adolescents who do not have manifest CHD nor xanthomas. In contrast to the relatively vague clinical criteria, a specific diagnosis can be obtained by identifying a mutation in the LDL receptor gene by molecular genetic methods [1,10,16].

Two genocopies of FH have been identified. One is familial defective apoB-100 (FDB) which is caused by mutation R3500Q in the apoB-100 gene [17], and the other is FH3 which is caused by gain-of-function mutations in the proprotein convertase subtilisin/kexin type 9 (PCSK9) gene [18]. Among subjects provided with a molecular genetic diagnosis of autosomal dominant hypercholesterolemia in Norway, 95% are FH heterozygotes, 3% are FDB heterozygotes and 2% are FH3 heterozygotes (unpublished data).

To study whether a molecular genetic diagnosis of autosomal dominant hypercholesterolemia secures that the subjects become adequately treated, we have performed a questionnaire-based study and performed lipid measurements among subjects who have been provided with a molecular genetic diagnosis of FH or FDB during a 10-year period in Norway.

Materials and Methods

Subjects

During the period 1998–2008, 2611 subjects have been provided with a molecular genetic diagnosis of FH or FDB in our laboratory. This had been done by the use of various mutations detection methods to screen for mutations in the LDL receptor gene (NG_009060) and apoB-100 gene (NG_011793), respectively. The subjects were invited to participate in a follow-up study to have their current therapies evaluated. Thus, the main aim of the study was to secure that subjects who had been diagnosed with FH or FDB, were being adequately treated. In order to participate, the subjects would have to answer a questionnaire for assessment of their risk profile and to have a non-fasting blood sample drawn for lipid analyses. The blood samples were sent to Department of Medical Biochemistry, Oslo University Hospital Rikshospitalet for analysis, and the report was sent to us. Values for LDL cholesterol were obtained by direct measurement and not calculated according to the formula of Friedewald et al. [19]. Thus, measurements of values for LDL cholesterol were not dependent on fasting blood samples. Because, the goal of this initiative was to secure that patients were being adequately treated, it did not need approval of an ethics committee as confirmed by a statement of August 30, 2006 from Regional Committee for Research Ethics in Southern Norway. Thus, the ethics committee specifically waived the need to collect written informed consent.

Evaluation of the adequacy of the current lipid-lowering therapy

Evaluation of the adequacy of the current lipid-lowering therapy was based upon assessment of the subject's global risk for CHD from medical and family histories obtained at the time of genetic testing and from information in the questionnaire. Several factors were considered for this evaluation such as age of the subject, family history, lipid levels before lipid-lowering therapy was started, age for start of lipid-lowering therapy, number of years on lipid-lowering therapy, lipid profile on lipid-lowering therapy, presence of manifest CHD such as myocardial infarction or angina pectoris and the presence of additional risk factors such as smoking and hypertension. Based upon the subject's risk profile which was established by the two authors who are well experienced with genetic lipid disorders, the current lipid profile was evaluated and the lipid-lowering therapy was classified as being adequate or not. No defined algorithm was being used for this classification, as there is no validated algorithm that considers all relevant parameters for assessing the global risk for CHD in FH/FDB heterozygotes. However, with respect to the lipid profile the values for total serum cholesterol and LDL cholesterol should generally be below 5 mmol/l and 3 mmol/l, respectively for the therapy to be considered adequate.

Results

Of the 2611 subjects with a molecular genetic diagnosis of FH or FDB who had been invited to participate, 956 (36.6%) actually answered the questionnaire and had a blood sample drawn for lipid measurements. Descriptive statistics of the participants are given in Table 1. There were 534 females and 422 males and there was a clear tendency towards relative more females in the higher age groups. This probably reflects that females develop CHD later in life than males. The mean age of the subjects was 44.3 (±17.0) years. The youngest was 5 and the oldest was 77 years old. Molecular genetic testing with respect to FH or FDB had been performed at a mean age of 39.8 (±17.3) years, and 35 subjects were heterozygous for the R3500Q mutation in the apoB-100 gene and 921 were heterozygous for one of 88 different mutations in the LDL receptor gene. 266 (27.8%) subjects were index patients and 690 (72.2%) had been diagnosed by cascade genetic screening.

Table 1. Characteristics of subjects with FH or FDB of different age groups who participated in the follow-up study to evaluate their treatment status.

Age groups	All	5–14	15–24	25–34	35–44	45–54	55–64	>65
N (males/females)	422/534	29/21	54/54	37/64	94/100	82/117	158/226	50/169
Age (years)	44.3 (±17.0)	12.2 (±2.1)	18.7 (±2.9)	29.9 (±3.1)	39.8 (±2.8)	49.2 (±2.8)	54.1 (±5.8)	69.1 (±3.3)
Age of molecular genetic testing (years)	39.8 (±17.3)	8.8 (±2.9)	13.7 (±3.7)	25.4 (±4.0)	35.1 (±3.5)	44.3 (±3.8)	49.4 (±6.6)	65.4 (±4.0)
Index patients (%)	27.8	12.0	10.2	29.7	35.1	34.5	33.6	18.5
Age for measurement of total serum cholesterol without lipid-lowering therapy (years)	27.4 (±13.3)	6.5 (±3.1)	8.9 (±4.8)	18.8 (±6.0)	24.5 (±7.3)	29.4 (±8.8)	33.0 (±10.0)	41.0 (±12.2)
Value for total serum cholesterol without lipid-lowering therapy (mmol/l)	10.5 (±2.5)	8.2 (±1.5)	8.5 (±1.6)	9.1 (±1.8)	10.1 (±2.5)	11.0 (±2.4)	11.1 (±2.4)	11.9 (±2.4)
Age for starting lipid-lowering drugs (years)	33.4 (±12.1)	10.5 (±1.1)	15.4 (±3.1)	22.0 (±5.1)	29.5 (±6.5)	33.7 (±8.3)	37.4 (±9.7)	45.3 (±11.7)
Manifest CHD# (%)	16.1	0	0	1.0	9.8	14.7	20.2	42.7
Current smoker (%)	13.5	0	9.3	9.0	13.9	20.8	19.3	7.6
Hypertension (%)	12.1	0	1.9	3.2	5.3	11.2	15.2	35.1

#Myocardial infarction, angina pectoris, coronary artery bypass graft or percutaneous coronary intervention.

The mean age for the first measurement of total serum cholesterol without lipid-lowering therapy was 27.4 (±13.3) years, and the reported value for total serum cholesterol was 10.5 (±2.5) mmol/l (Table 1). The relationship between age and levels of total serum cholesterol before lipid-lowering therapy was started, is shown in Fig. 1. 84.8% of the subjects had used lipid-lowering drugs, and the mean age for starting lipid-lowering therapy was 33.4 (±12.1) years (Table 1). 16.1% reported that they had manifest CHD, 13.5% were current smokers and 12.1% had hypertension.

At the follow-up, 82.3% were on lipid-lowering drugs (Table 2). However, among those below age 18, only 20.4% were on lipid-lowering drugs, whereas 89.1% of those aged 18 and above were on lipid-lowering drugs. Among the subjects aged 30 and below or 40 and below, 45.3% and 62.9%, respectively were on lipid-lowering drugs.

The levels of total serum cholesterol and LDL cholesterol measured at the follow-up for the 956 subjects, were 5.7 (±1.5) mmol/l and 3.9 (±1.3) mmol/l, respectively (Table 2). Thus, compared to the reported levels of total serum cholesterol before lipid-lowering therapy were started, a reduction in the levels of total serum cholesterol of 45.7% had been achieved. The mean value for total serum cholesterol in the 772 subjects who were on lipid-lowering therapy, was 5.4 (±1.2) mmol/l (LDL cholesterol: 3.6 (±1.2) mmol/l), and these subjects had achieved a reduction in levels of total serum cholesterol of 49.5%. Among the 772 subjects who were on lipid-lowering therapy, 34.9% were on atorvastatin monotherapy with a mean dosis of 53 mg, and 29.3% were on simvastatin monotherapy with a mean dosis of 43 mg. 22.5% were on combination therapy with atorvastatin and ezetimibe, 4.8% were on combination therapy with simvastatin and ezetimibe and 3.7% were on combinatation therapy with three or more lipid-lowering drugs.

Among those who were on lipid-lowering therapy, only 29.0% had an LDL cholesterol value below 3.0 mmol/l, and only 12.2% had an LDL cholesterol value below 2.6 mmol/l. Among all 956 subjects, 52.7% were considered as being inadequately treated (Table 2). The levels for total serum cholesterol and LDL cholesterol among those whose lipid-lowering therapies were considered as being inadequate, were 6.6 (±1.4) mmol/l and 4.7 (±1.3) mmol/l, respectively. These levels were significantly higher than the corresponding levels of 4.9 (±1.1) mmol/l ($p<0.0001$) and 3.1 (±0.9) mmol/l ($p<0.0001$), respectively in those whose therapy was considered as being adequate.

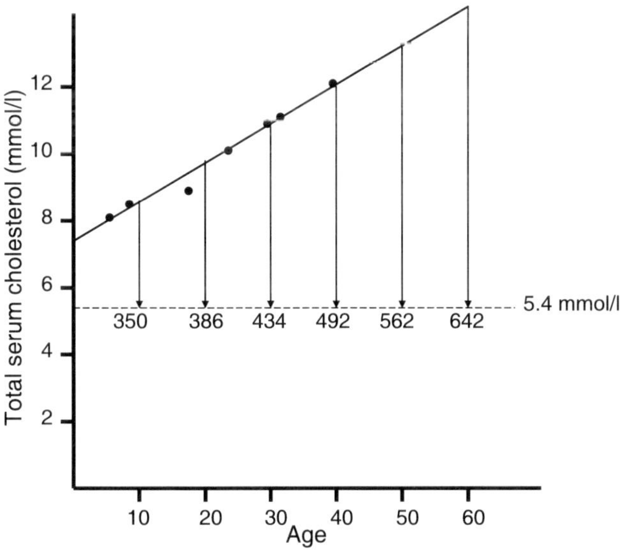

Figure 1. Cholesterol-years score in FH/FDB heterozygotes. Levels of total serum cholesterol in FH/FDB heterozygotes in different age groups before lipid-lowering therapy is started are plotted against age of the subjects (data from Table 1). Linear regression ($y = 0.111x + 7.408$) has been used to generate the relationship between levels of total serum cholesterol and age from birth until the age of 60. Cholesterol-years scores for subjects who are put on lipid-lowering therapy at different decades and achieved a total serum cholesterol level of 5.4 mmol/l, are indicated.

There was a wide variation regarding the age both for diagnosis and for the start of lipid-lowering therapy (Table 1). Some had been diagnosed and put on lipid-lowering therapy in their first or second decades, whereas others had not been diagnosed and put on lipid-lowering therapy until their sixth or seventh decades. The later in life lipid-lowering therapy starts, and the higher the total serum cholesterol level, the more atherosclerosis is present [20]. The cholesterol-years score can be used as a measurement of the atherosclerosis burden [21]. To determine the cholesterol-years score, the value for total serum cholesterol is multiplied by the age of the subject to generate the "area under the curve" in Fig. 1.

If the mean value for total serum cholesterol in the 772 subjects who were on lipid-lowering therapy at the follow-up of 5.4 (±1.2) mmol/l, is being used as a fixed value for total serum cholesterol on lipid-lowering therapy, the data in Fig. 1 can be used to calculate the cholesterol-years score for subjects who start lipid-lowering therapy at different ages until the seventh decade. Whereas, a non-FH/FDB subject with a value for total serum cholesterol of 5.4 mmol/l until the age of 60 will have a cholesterol-years score of 324 mmol years/l, an FH/FDB subject who does not start lipid-lowering therapy before the age of 60, will have a cholesterol-years score of 642 mmol years/l (Fig. 1). However, an FH/FDB subject who starts lipid-lowering therapy at the age of 10 and achieves a total serum cholesterol level of 5.4 mmol/l, will have a cholesterol-years score of 350 mmol years/l at the age of 60 (Fig. 1). For subjects who starts lipid-lowering therapy at the age of 10 or 20 years, treatment values for total serum cholesterol must be 4.9 mmol/l or 3.9 mmol/l, respectively in order to achieve a cholesterol-years score of 324 mmol years/l at the age of 60.

Discussion

In this study we have determined the treatment status of FH/FDB patients provided with a molecular genetic diagnosis during the period 1998–2008 in Norway. The main finding was that even though the subjects had obtained a specific molecular genetic diagnosis, only 47.3% were considered as being adequately treated. This finding reflects that submaximal doses of lipid-lowering drugs were used with mean doses of atorvastatin and simvastatin monotherapies of 53 mg and 43 mg, respectively. Thus, there is a need to educate physicians in order to improve the lipid-lowering therapy in FH/FDB patients. Moreover, our study has shown that lipid-lowering therapy had been started late in life at a mean age of 33.4 (±12.1) years. This partly reflects that the mean age for the first measurement of total serum cholesterol was 27.4 (±13.3) years and that the mean age for the molecular genetic diagnosis was 39.8 (±17.3) years. Thus, there is a need to diagnose these subjects earlier in life.

However, some caution should be exerted when interpreting our findings since only 36.6% of those who were invited to participate, actually did participate. The participants could therefore in theory represent a selected group of patients who could be particularly well or particularly poorly treated. Moreover, because information regarding medical history was obtained from the patients themselves through a questionnaire, and not extracted from medical files, some uncertainties may exist regarding the quality of this information.

Among those aged 18 and above, 89.1% were on lipid-lowering drugs. For comparison 96% of adult Dutch FH patients were on

Table 2. Lipid-lowering therapy in subjects with FH or FDB of different age groups at the follow-up.

Age groups	All	5–14	15–24	25–34	35–44	45–54	55–64	>65
Number on lipid-lowering therapy (%)	82.3	16.0	46.6	78.8	85.8	96.4	95.8	95.8
Total serum cholesterol (mmol/l)	5.7 (±1.5)	6.7 (±1.3)	6.0 (±1.7)	5.9 (±1.8)	5.6 (±1.5)	5.5 (±1.4)	5.6 (±1.4)	5.6 (±1.4)
HDL cholesterol (mmol/l)	1.4 (±0.4)	1.3 (±0.3)	1.3 (±0.3)	1.4 (±0.4)	1.3 (±0.4)	1.4 (±0.4)	1.4 (±0.4)	1.5 (±0.5)
Triglycerides (mmol/l)	1.0 (±0.6)	0.9 (±0.4)	1.0 (±0.7)	1.0 (±0.7)	1.0 (±0.6)	1.1 (±0.6)	1.1 (±0.6)	1.1 (±0.6)
LDL cholesterol (mmol/l)	3.9 (±1.3)	4.8 (±1.2)	4.1 (±1.4)	4.0 (±1.6)	3.8 (±1.3)	3.7 (±1.2)	3.7 (±1.2)	3.7 (±1.3)
Reduction in levels of total serum cholesterol (%)	45.7	18.3	29.4	35.2	44.6	50.0	49.5	52.9
Achieved levels of LDL cholesterol <3 mmol/l (%)	29.0	0	27.1	33.3	31.9	27.8	29.6	26.3
Therapy considered adequate (%)	52.7	36.0	56.5	52.5	47.4	57.0	54.4	59.7

lipid-lowering drugs [22]. This minor difference may partly reflect that the Dutch patients were treated at specialized out-patient clinics, whereas the majority of the Norwegian patients were being treated by general practitioners. Among the Norwegian patients who were on lipid-lowering drugs, 29.0% and 12.2% had levels of LDL cholesterol below 3.0 mmol/l and 2.6 mmol/l, respectively. Thus, the majority of Norwegian FH/FDB subjects are being diagnosed late in life and are not being adequately treated. 16% of the subjects in our study had a history of CHD which is similar to that of 17% found among Dutch FH heterozygotes [22].

The American Academy of Pediatrics has recommended that screening for FH should be performed at an age of 2–10 years, and that lipid-lowering therapy may start from the age of 8 [23]. These recommendations reflect that the atherosclerotic lesions are largely reversible before the age of 10 in contrast to the calcified lesions seen in untreated middle-aged FH/FDB subjects. Moreover, it has been well documented that lipid-lowering therapy from late childhood/adolescence is effective, safe and well tolerated [24].

The cholesterol-years score in Fig. 1 illustrates the importance of starting lipid-lowering therapy at a young age. This score has been found to be a predictor of aortic stenosis [25,26] and is correlated with the severity of atherosclerosis in carotid arteries in FH heterozygotes [27,28]. It also correlates well with the severity of calcific atherosclerosis and angina pectoris in FH homozygotes with an apparent threshold for calcific atherosclerosis at a cholesterol-years score of 182 mmol l/years [21]. If lipid-lowering therapy starts at the age of 10, and a realistic treatment value for total serum cholesterol of 4.9 mmol/l is achieved, the cholesterol-years score until the age of 60 is 324 mmol year/l. This score is identical to that of a non-FH/FDB subject who has had a total serum cholesterol level of 5.4 mmol/l during the same periode. For comparison, the median levels of total serum cholesterol in the Nordic countries for subjects in their fourth, fifth and sixth decades are 4.8 mmol/l, 5.2 mmol/l and 5.6 mmol/l, respectively [www.furst.no/norip/]. If lipid-lowering therapy starts at the age of 20, a total serum cholesterol value of 3.9 mmol/l is required to achieve a cholesterol-years score of 324 mmol year/l at the age of 60. Such a cholesterol value will probably only be achievable in a minority of FH/FDB patients. If lipid-lowering therapy starts after the second decade, it is not realistic to achieve sufficiently low levels of total serum cholesterol and LDL cholesterol to achieve a risk of CHD at the age of 60 similar to that of a non-FH/FDB subject. Thus, for subjects diagnosed after the age of 20, maximum tolerated doses of combination therapies should be prescribed in order to reduce the risk of CHD.

The question then is how secure that patients with FH/FDB are being diagnosed early in life. Several strategies have been discussed, including population-based cholesterol screening of children which has not been recommended by any pediatric organizations [29]. Because lipid measurements do not have the required sensitivity and specificity and because clinical characteristics such as xanthomas and premature CHD do not occur in children, the diagnosis should preferentially be based on molecular genetic testing [16]. Our recommendation which is in line with the NICE guidelines [30] is that cholesterol screening is made common in young adults in order to select index patients for molecular genetic screening. Once the underlying mutation has been identified, cascade genetic screening, which is the most cost-effective strategy to diagnose FH/FDB patients [31-33], is being used to diagnose children and other family members. However, our study clearly illustrates the need for educating physicians in order to improve the lipid-lowering therapy even in FH/FDB patients with a molecular genetic diagnosis.

Author Contributions

Conceived and designed the experiments: TPL KEB. Performed the experiments: TPL KEB. Analyzed the data: TPL. Contributed reagents/materials/analysis tools: TPL. Wrote the paper: TPL KEB.

References

1. Goldstein JL, Hobbs HH, Brown MS (2001) Familial hypercholesterolemia. In: Scriver CR, Baudet AL, Sly WS, Valle D, eds. The metabolic basis of inherited disease. New York: McGraw-Hill. pp 2863–2913.
2. Slack J (1969) Risks of ischaemic heart disease in familial hyperlipoproteinaemic states. Lancet ii: 1380–1382.
3. Heiberg A, Berg K (1976) The inheritance of hyperlipoproteinemia with xanthomatosis. A study of 132 kindreds. Clin Genet 9: 203–233.
4. Slack J (1979) Inheritance of familial hypercholesterolemia. In: Paoletti R, Gotto AM, eds. Atheroscl Rev New York. Raven Press. pp 35–66.
5. Williams RR, Hopkins PN, Hunt SC, Wu LL, Hasstedt SJ (1990) Population-based frequency of dyslipidemia syndromes in coronary-prone families in Utah. Arch Intern Med 150: 582–588.
6. Koivisto UM, Hämäläinen L, Taskinen MR, Kettunen K, Kontula K (1993) Prevalence of familial hypercholesterolemia among young north Karelian

patients with coronary heart disease: a study based on diagnosis by polymerase chain reaction. J Lipid Res 34: 269–277.
7. Huigen R, Vissers MN, Defesche JC, Lansberg PJ, Kastelein JJ, et al. (2008) Familial hypercholesterolemia: current treatment and advances in management. Expert Rev Cardiovasc 6: 567–581.
8. Williams RR, Hamilton-Craig I, Kostner GM, Hegele RA, Hayden MR, et al. (1996) MED PED: An integrated genetic strategy for preventing early deaths. In: Berg K, Boulyjenkov V, Christen Y, eds. Genetic approaches to noncommunicable diseases Berlin. Springer Verlag. pp 35–46.
9. Neil HAW, Hammond T, Huxley R, Matthews DR, Humphries SE (2000) Extent of underdiagnosis of familial hypercholesterolemia in routine practice: prospective registry study. BMJ 321: 148.
10. Maarle MCV, Stouthard MEA, Mheen JMVD, Klazinga NS, Bonsel GJ (2002) Follow up after a family based screening programme for familial hypercholesterolemia: is screening alone enough? BMJ 324: 1367–1368.
11. Umans-Eckenhausen MAW, Defesche JC, Sijbrands EJG, Scheerder RLJM, Kastelein JJP (2001) Review of the first 5 years of screening for familial hypercholesterolemia in the Netherlands. Lancet 357: 165–168.
12. Umans-Eckenhausen MAW, Defesche JC, van Dam MJ, Kastelein JJP (2003) Long-term compliance with lipid-lowering medication after genetic screening for familial hypercholesterolemia. Am Med Ass 163: 65–68.
13. Leren TP, Finborud TH, Manshaus TE, Ose L, Berge KE (2008) Diagnosis of familial hypercholesterolemia in general practice using clinical diagnostic criteria or genetic testing as part of cascade genetic screening. Community Genet 11: 26–35.
14. Scientific Steering Committee on behalf of the Simon Broome Register Group (1991) Risk of fatal coronary heart disease in familial hypercholesterolemia. BMJ 303: 893–896.
15. Defesche J (2000) Familial hypercholesterolemia. In: Betteridge DJ, ed. Lipids and vascular disease London. Martin Dunitz Ltd. pp 65–76.
16. Leren TP, Berge KE (2009) Comparison of clinical and molecular genetic criteria for diagnosing familial hypercholesterolemia. Clin Lipidol 4: 303–310.
17. Soria LF, Ludwig EH, Clarke HRG, Vega GL, Grundy SM, et al. (1989) Association between a specific apolipoprotein B mutation and familial defective apolipoprotein B-100. Proc Natl Acad Sci USA 86: 587–591.
18. Mousavi SA, Berge KE, Leren TP (2009) The unique role of proprotein convertase subtilisin/kexin 9 in cholesterol homeostasis. J Intern Med 266: 507–519.
19. Friedewald WT, Levy RI, Fredrickson DS (1972) Estimation of the concentration of low density lipoprotein cholesterol in plasma, without use of preparative ultracentrifuge. Clin Chem 18: 499–502.
20. Law MR, Wald NJ (1995) An ecological study of serum cholesterol and ischaemic heart disease between 1950 and 1990. Eur J Clin Nutr 49: 221–224.
21. Hoeg J, Feuerstein IM, Tucker EE (1994) Detection and quantitation of calcific atherosclerosis by ultrafast computed tomography in children and young adults with homozygous familial hypercholesterolemia. Arterioscler Thromb 14: 1066–1074.
22. Pijlman AH, Huigen R, Verhagen SN, Imholz BP, Liem AH, et al. (2010) Evaluation of cholesterol lowering treatment of patients with familial hypercholesterolemia: A large cross-sectional study in The Netherlands. Atherosclerosis 209: 189–194.
23. Daniels SR, Greer FR (2008) Lipid screening and cardiovascular health in childhood. Pediatrics 122: 198–208.
24. Vuorio A, Kuoppala J, Kovanen PT, Humphries SE, Strandberg T, et al. (2010) Statins for children with familial hypercholesterolemia. Cochrane Database Syst Rev 7: CD006401.
25. Nozue T, Kawashiri M, Higashikata T, Nohara A, Inazu A, et al. (2006) Cholesterol-years score is associated with development of senile degenerative aortic stenosis in heterozygous familial hypercholesterolemia. J Atheroscler Thromb 13: 323–328.
26. Rallidis L, Naoumova RP, Thompson GR, Nihoyannopoulos P (1998) Extent and severity of atherosclerotic involvement of the aortic valve and root in familial hypercholesterolemia. Heart 80: 583–590.
27. Tonstad S, Joakimsen O, Stensland-Bugge E, Ose L, Bønaa KH, et al. (1998) Carotid intima-media thickness and plaque in patients with familial hypercholesterolaemia mutations and control subjects. Eur J Clin Invest 28: 971–979.
28. Sidhu PS, Naoumova RP, Maher VM, MacSweeney JE, Neuwirth CK, et al. (1996) The extracranial carotid artery in familial hypercholesterolaemia: relationship of intimal-medial thichness and plaque morphology with plasma lipid and coronary heart disease. J Cardiovasc Risk 3: 61–67.
29. US preventive task force (2007) Screening for lipid disorders in children: US preventive task force statement. Pediatrics 120: e215–219.
30. Wierzbicki AS, Humphries SE, Minhas R (2008) Familial hypercholesterolaemia: summary of NICE guidance. BMJ 337: 509–510.
31. Marks D, Wonderling D, Thorogood M, Lambert H, Humphries SE, et al. (2000) Screening for hypercholesterolaemia versus case finding for familial hypercholesterolaemia: a systematic review and cost-effectiveness analysis. Health Technol Assess 4: 1–123.
32. Wonderling D, Umans-Eckenhausen MA, Marks D, Defesche JC, Kastelein JJ, et al. (2004) Cost-effectiveness analysis of the genetic screening program for familial hypercholesterolemia in The Netherlands. Semin Vasc Med 4: 97–104.
33. Leren TP (2004) Cascade genetic screening for familial hypercholesterolemia. Clin Genet 66: 483–487.

11

New Splice Site Acceptor Mutation in *AIRE* Gene in Autoimmune Polyendocrine Syndrome Type 1

Mireia Mora[1,2,3], Felicia A. Hanzu[1,2,3], Marta Pradas-Juni[3,4], Gloria B. Aranda[1,2,3], Irene Halperin[1,2], Manuel Puig-Domingo[5], Sira Aguiló[6], Eduardo Fernández-Rebollo[3,4]*

1 Department of Endocrinology and Nutrition, Hospital Clinic, Barcelona, Spain, **2** Laboratory of Endocrine Disorders, Institut d'Investigacions Biomèdiques August Pi I Sunyer (IDIBAPS), Barcelona, Spain, **3** Spanish Biomedical Research Centre in Diabetes and Associated Metabolic Disorders (CIBERDEM), Barcelona, Spain, **4** Diabetes and Obesity Research Laboratory - Institut d'Investigacions Biomèdiques August Pi i Sunyer (IDIBAPS), Barcelona, Spain, **5** Department of Endocrinology and Nutrition, Hospital Germans Trias i Pujol Research Institut and Hospital, Universitat Autònoma de Barcelona, Badalona, Spain, **6** Department of Internal Medicine, Hospital Clínic, Barcelona, Spain

Abstract

Autoimmune polyglandular syndrome type 1 (APS-1, OMIM 240300) is a rare autosomal recessive disorder, characterized by the presence of at least two of three major diseases: hypoparathyroidism, Addison's disease, and chronic mucocutaneous candidiasis. We aim to identify the molecular defects and investigate the clinical and mutational characteristics in an index case and other members of a consanguineous family. We identified a novel homozygous mutation in the splice site acceptor (SSA) of intron 5 (c.653-1G>A) in two siblings with different clinical outcomes of APS-1. Coding DNA sequencing revealed that this *AIRE* mutation potentially compromised the recognition of the constitutive SSA of intron 5, splicing upstream onto a nearby cryptic SSA in intron 5. Surprisingly, the use of an alternative SSA entails the uncovering of a cryptic donor splice site in exon 5. This new transcript generates a truncated protein (p.A214fs67X) containing the first 213 amino acids and followed by 68 aberrant amino acids. The mutation affects the proper splicing, not only at the acceptor but also at the donor splice site, highlighting the complexity of recognizing suitable splicing sites and the importance of sequencing the intron-exon junctions for a more precise molecular diagnosis and correct genetic counseling. As both siblings were carrying the same mutation but exhibited a different APS-1 onset, and one of the brothers was not clinically diagnosed, our finding highlights the possibility to suspect mutations in the *AIRE* gene in cases of childhood chronic candidiasis and/or hypoparathyroidism otherwise unexplained, especially when the phenotype is associated with other autoimmune diseases.

Editor: Ruben Artero, University of Valencia, Spain

Funding: This work was sponsored by the STARTUP 01/2012 grant from IDIBAPS. MP-J is a recipient of a FPI grant BES-2011-044579 (SAF2010-19527) and EF-R is a recipient of a BIOTRACK Postdoctoral Fellowship in IDIBAPS (EC FP7/2009–2013) under the agreement no. 229673. CIBER de Diabetes y Enfermedades Metabólicas Asociadas is an initiative of ISCIII (Spanish Ministry of Science and Innovation). The funders had no role in study design, data collection and analysis, decision to publish, or preparation of the manuscript.

Competing Interests: The authors have declared that no competing interests exist.

* Email: edu.ferrebo@gmail.com

Introduction

Autoimmune polyendocrine syndrome type 1 (APS-1, OMIM 240300), previously known as Autoimmune polyendocrinopathy-candidiasis-ectodermal dystrophy (APECED), is a childhood-onset monogenic autoimmune disease [1,2]. APS-1 is highly variable clinically, genetically, and serologically, and its traditional clinical diagnosis requires the presence of at least two of three hallmark conditions: chronic mucocutaneous candidiasis, hypoparathyroidism and Addison's disease [2]. However, patients with APS-1 also may exhibit additional autoimmune diseases, including type 1 diabetes mellitus (T1D), hypothyroidism, vitiligo, alopecia, autoimmune hepatitis, pernicious anemia, and asplenism [3]. The range of these secondary autoimmune disorders is broad and variable [4].

Mutations in the autoimmune regulator (*AIRE*) gene are responsible for this rare autosomal, recessively inherited disease [5,6]. The *AIRE* gene maps to 21q22.3 and consists of 14 exons spanning approximately 13 kb of genomic DNA, which encodes a protein made up of 545 amino acids (Figure 1A and 1B). The AIRE protein contains motifs indicative of its transcription factor function, including a conserved bipartite nuclear localization signal (NLS), two Plant Homedomain (PHD) zinc-finger motifs, four LXXLL nuclear receptor binding motifs (where L is leucine and X is any amino acid), and a proline rich region (PRR) [6,7]. A SAND domain is common to AIRE and some homologous proteins and has been suggested to be a DNA binding domain [8]. The 100 NH2-terminal amino acids of AIRE form a homogenously staining region (HSR) domain also present in the Sp100 and Sp140 proteins, where it has been shown to be responsible for homodimerization and is required for their activation [7,9–11] (Figure 1B). Mutations in this transcription factor determine the development of multi-organ autoimmune disease, as the activity of this autoimmune regulator governs the expression of diverse self-antigens in the thymus, preventing the maturation of auto-reactive T cells that escape thymic negative selection [12–14].

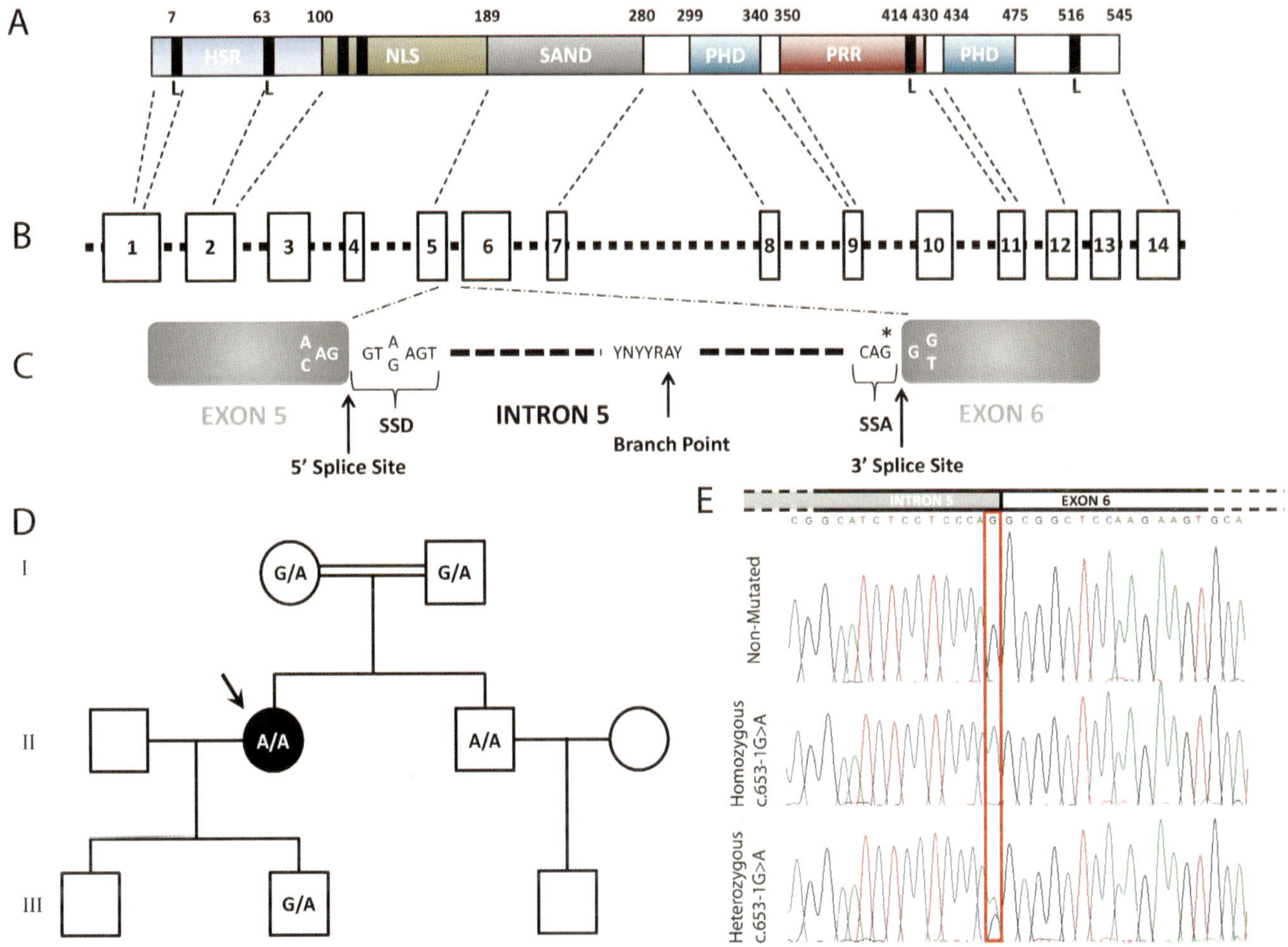

Figure 1. AIRE overview family pedigree and detection of the c.653-1G>A AIRE mutation. (A) Schematic AIRE protein representation showing the different protein domains: HSR domain (HSR), conserved bipartite nuclear localization signal (NLS), PHD zinc finger motif (PHD), proline-rich region (PRR), LXXLL motif (L), and SAND domain (SAND). (B) Schematic *AIRE* gene representation, where rectangles indicate exons and the dashed line the introns. Finally, (C) schematic representation of the consensus sequences for the 5′ splice site donor (SSD), branch site and 3′ splice site acceptor (SSA). The star indicates the mutation. (D) Pedigree of the Spanish consanguineous family. Genotypes were shown as wild-type (G/G), heterozygous (G/A) and homozygous (A/A) of the c.653-1G>A *AIRE* mutation. The arrow indicates the index case. (E) Above, the schematic representation of the junction between intron 5 and exon 6, and below, the direct sequence analysis of the *AIRE* gene identified homozygous carriers of the c.653-1G>A mutation in APS-1 patients, while heterozygous carriers were found in unaffected relatives (I-1, I-2, III-2) of the family.

To date, more than a hundred different mutations of the *AIRE* gene have been identified in APS-1 patients, but only two major mutations (p.R257X and p.L323SfsX51) are responsible for 95% of the mutant alleles in APS-1 patients [15–17]. However, it is noteworthy that few *AIRE* mutations have been thoroughly studied [18] and on the other hand, with only one previous publication about an *AIRE* mutation reported in Spain [19].

Here we report the identification of a novel splice site acceptor (SSA) mutation in intron 5 of the *AIRE* gene (c.653-1G>A) in two siblings from a Spanish consanguineous family, with a different clinical outcomes in APS-1. Moreover, *in silico* and mRNA studies showed that this mutation results in a new SSA in intron 5, which uncovers a cryptic donor splice site in exon 5, generating a truncated protein with a premature termination codon (p.A214fs67X) downstream of exon 6, losing part of the SAND domain and the PHD1, PHD2 and PRR domains completely. Finally, we explored the Nonsense-mediated decay (NMD), a mechanism that eliminates mRNAs containing premature termination codons and limits the synthesis of abnormal proteins, which helps explain if NMD accounts for the different clinical outcomes between both homozygous carriers.

Patients and Methods

Patients

The index case affected by APS-1 and her unaffected available relatives were investigated (Figure 1D). The study was approved by the Institutional Review Board (Ethics Committee of Hospital Clinic of Barcelona, Spain) and has been conducted in accordance with the guidelines established in the Declaration of Helsinki, requiring a written informed consent by all participants before the study. All participants provided written informed consent to have the details of their cases published.

Clinical data

The index case, a 52-yr-old woman (55.3 kg and 155 cm; II.1, figure 1D), was the first of two healthy children born to first cousin Spanish parents, without any previous family history for autoimmune diseases. The patient presents chronic mucocutaneous candidiasis, primary hypoparathyroidism, hypergonadotropic hypogonadism and intestinal dysfunction. Since childhood, she presented mucocutaneous and nail candidiasis, and she developed vaginal candidiasis during adulthood, as well as a chronic intestinal dysfunction. She was diagnosed with primary hypoparathyroidism at 42 years old based on paresthesias, muscle cramps and tetany, and an ionized calcium determination of 0.55 nM/l (normal range 1–1.2 nM/l) together with a parathormone (PTH) value of 10.1 pg/ml (normal range 10–65 pg/ml). During follow-up, chronic gastritis has been diagnosed with low levels of B12 vitamin and positive parietal cell antibodies. Currently, she requires 3 g of calcium carbonate, 0.75 μg of calcitriol and 1.2 g of magnesium lactate daily. She has presented several episodes of gastrointestinal dysregulation that have required modifications in the dosage of the aforementioned compounds. Recent analyses were positive for Anti-thyroid-peroxidase antibodies (TPOAb) positive (34 UI/ml in 2005 and 140 UI/ml in 2013), as well as for Anti-Glutamic acid decarboxylase antibodies (GADAb) (160 U/ml in 2013).

For his part, the brother of the index case (74.9 kg and 177 cm; II.2, figure 1D) is a 46-yr-old man with mucocutaneous and nail candidiasis since childhood and universal alopecia since his 40s. He also presents pyloric stenosis since birth, as well as hypospadia and chronic C hepatitis. Recent analyses were still negative for AcTPO antibodies, but were slightly positive for GADAb (1 U/ml in 2013).

I.1 and I.2 are first cousins, and their sons (cases II.1 and II.2) were born in Barcelona, as well as their respective sons, III.1 and III.2 from II.1, and III.3 from II.2. Cases III.1, III.2 and III.3 are healthy men of 26, 22 and 12 years old, respectively. Case I.1 is a 78-yr-old woman with type 2 diabetes and hypertension, having undergone a hysterectomy and surgical intervention for inguinal hernia. Case I.2 is an 84-yr-old man with dyslipidemia, hypertension, and ischemic cardiopathy and carries a pacemaker. Case III.2 is a healthy young man, without any clinical features suggesting APS-1. Available clinical characteristics and analytical data for all individuals are reported in table 1.

Antibody, hormonal and biochemical determinations

Main biochemical, hormonal and antibody determinations after overnight fasting were measured in serum in the laboratories of the Hospital Clínic (Barcelona, http://cdb.hospitalclinic.org) using specific standard validated assays.

Molecular studies

DNA and PCR. Genomic DNA was extracted from peripheral blood leucocytes using the QIAamp DNA Blood Midi Kit (Qiagen, Hilden, Germany). Fourteen exons and their flanking exon-intron boundaries of the *AIRE* gene were amplified by PCR, which was performed with PrimeSTAR HS DNA Polymerase (Takara Bio, Japan). The PCR products were purified using a QIAquick PCR Purification Kit (Qiagen) and sequenced by BigDye Terminator v3.1 Cycle Sequencing Kit (Applied Biosystems). Primer sequences are shown in Table S1.

Real-time quantitative PCR

RNA isolation. Total RNA from blood samples was isolated using the QIAamp RNA Blood Mini Kit (Qiagen, Hilden, Germany) according to the manufacturer's instructions.

cDNA synthesis. Reverse transcription reaction was performed using a commercially available set of High Capacity cDNA Reverse Transcription Kit (Applied Biosystems, USA). cDNA was prepared from 1 μg of mRNA, with random hexamer primers, according to the manufacturer's instructions.

Quantitative Real-time PCR (qRT-PCR) was performed on an ABI Prism 7900HT Sequence Detection System (Applied Biosystems, Foster City, CA, USA). The reaction was performed using the SYBR Premix Ex Taq (Tli RNase H Plus; Takara-Clontech), and dissociation curve analysis of the PCR products was performed at the end of amplification to verify single product amplification.

The relative quantification of gene expression in each sample was analyzed using SDS Software version 2.4 (Applied Biosystems). Relative expression of each gene to Beta Actin (β-actin) was calculated using the accurate cycle threshold method [20]. The experiment was run twice in triplicate. Primer sequences are shown in Table S1.

Mutational and *in Silico* Splicing Analyses

The mutation was identified by comparing with the reported reference sequence (NM_000383.2) and further analyzed in control individuals. Since the mutation could affect mRNA splicing, both wild-type sequence and altered sequence were analyzed *in silico* using the following splice site prediction web interfaces: SplicePort (SP: http://spliceport.cbcb.umd.edu/) [21], Human Splice Finder (HSF: http://www.umd.be/HSF/) [22] and Alternative Splice Site Predictor (ASSP: http://wangcomputing.com/assp/index.html) [23]. Predictions were made using default settings.

After carrying out the splice-site and cDNA sequence prediction *in silico*, we analyzed the putative protein sequence using Expasy software (http://web.expasy.org/translate/software), in order to predict whether this amino acid substitution affects protein function using the Protein Variation Effect Analyzer (Provean: http://provean.jcvi.org/index.php) [24].

Protein Structure Prediction

3D protein structure of mutant and normal AIRE proteins was predicted using the I-TASSER fold recognition method [25]. The predicted mutant and normal structures were superimposed and aligned using PyMol software.

Results

Identification of a new *AIRE* gene mutation and analysis of the new generated splice site

Based on the clinical features of the index case, which supported the diagnosis of APS-1, mutational screening of the *AIRE* gene was carried out including the 14 coding exons and the intronic boundaries. Direct sequencing of the *AIRE* gene revealed that not only the presumed APS-1 index case, but also her brother (cases II.1 and II.2, respectively), were homozygote for splicing mutation c.653-1G>A at the last nucleotide of intron 5 (Figure 1E), which belongs to the splice site acceptor (SSA) conserved sequence [26] (Figure 1C). The mutation was also detected in heterozygous state in the other healthy relatives examined (I.1, I.2 and III.2; Figure 1D), but was not detected in 100 healthy control subjects. This mutation has not been previously reported in the scientific literature. Surprisingly, the use of new SSA in intron 5 entails the uncovering of a cryptic exonic splice site donor (SSD) at exon 5 generating an aberrant transcript, as shown by cDNA sequencing in both homozygous and heterozygous carriers (Figure 2). These results were consistent with *in silico* analysis by Human Splicing Finder, Splicing Port and Alternative Splice Site Predictor software (Table 2).

At the amino acidic level, this mutation at the SSA generates a truncated protein, and, along these lines, the Provean software predicts that this amino acid substitution has a deleterious impact

Table 1. Clinical features and analytical data.

	I.1	I.2	II.1	II.2	III.2
Sex	**F**	**M**	**F**	**M**	**M**
Age at onset (years)	-	-	42	-	-
Age at last exam (years)	78	84	52	47	22
Candidiasis	-	-	+	+	-
Hypoparathyroidism	-	-	+	-	-
Addison's disease	-	-	-	-	-
Hypogonadism	-	-	+	-	-
IDDM	-	-	-	-	-
T2D	+	-	-	-	-
Hypothyrodism	-	-	-	-	-
Atrophic gastritis	-	-	+	-	-
Pernicious anemia	-	-	+	-	-
Autoimmune hepatitis	-	-	-	-	-
Malabsorption	-	-	+	-	-
Keratitis	-	-	-	-	-
Alopecia	-	-	-	+	-
Vitiligo	-	-	-	-	-
Enamel hypoplasia	-	-	+	+	-
***AIRE* genotype**	G/A	G/A	A/A	A/A	G/A
Calcium (8.5–10.5 mg/dl)	8.8	9	4.5	10	10
Phosphorus (2.3–4.3 mg/dl)	-	3.5	4.7	2.9	3.7
Magnesium (1.8–2.6 mg/dl)	-	2.1	1.7	2.2	2.1
PTH (10–65 pg/ml)	27	99	<2	16	40
25-hidroxi-vitaminD (30–100 ng/ml)	23.6	14.1	40.7	28	26.8
ACTH (10–60 pg/ml)	28	35	36	34	24
Basal cortisol (10–25 mcg/dl)	17.3	13.1	24	20	16.4
Anti 21-hidroxilase Ab (<1 U/ml)	<0.5	<0.5	0.7	<0.5	0.5
Anti-peroxidase Ab (<35 UI/ml)	<28	<28	32	44	32
Anti-tiroglobulin Ab (<60 UI/ml)	<15	<15	140	<15	<15
Parietal cell Antibodies	-	-	+++, 80 URF	-	-
B12 vitamine (250–1050 pg/ml)	-	-	129	424	-
Folic acid (250–1050 ng/ml)	-	-	438.9	284	-
Insulin growth factor (171–333 ng/ml)	-	-	62	87	-
Luteotropin (LH) (1.5–7.5 U/l)	-	-	49.97	1.95	-
Foliculoestimuline (FSH) (1.7–8 U/l)	-	-	113.54	2.4	-
Anti-GAD (<0.5 U/ml)	-	-	160	1	-
Anti-IA-2Ab (<0.75 U/ml)	-	-	0.3	0.2	-

Abbreviations: IDDM (Insulin-dependent Diabetes Mellitus), T2D (Type 2 Diabetes), PTH (Parathyroid hormone), ACTH (Adrenocorticotropic hormone), GAD (Glutamic acid decarboxylase), IA-2 (Islet Antigen 2) and Ab (antibodies).

(Score = −620; variants with score equal or below −2.5 are considered deleterious) on the biological function of the protein.

To assess if the generation of a premature termination codon could trigger the nonsense-mediated mRNA decay mechanism, we performed a qRT-PCR for the non-mutated (G/G) and mutated (A/A) alleles, from the index case, her brother, both parents and two healthy controls. We designed a forward primer specific for the non-mutated allele covering the junction between exon 5 and 6, another specific forward primer for the junction between the last nucleotides of the truncated exon 5 and first nucleotides from the intron 5, and finally a common reverse primer in exon 6 (Figure 3A and 3B). The relative expression of the non-mutated and mutated alleles was normalized to that of the healthy G/G control individuals. The results for the non-mutated allele showed normal expression levels for both controls, an absence of expression for the index case and her brother, and half expression levels for both heterozygous parents, as expected (Figure 3C). On the other hand, the expression results for both homozygous or the heterozygous carriers of the mutated allele were very low and even absent for the healthy controls, suggesting the activation of the NMD process in the degradation of the mRNA from the mutated allele. These results showed similar expression patterns for the mutant allele in

Table 2. Splice site prediction software output.

DESCRIPTION	ACCEPTOR/DONOR	EXON/INTRON	SPLICE SITE SEQUENCE	HSF		SP	ASSP	
				CONSENSUS VALUE	SCORE	SCORE	SCORE	CONFIDENCE
Constitutive	DONOR	EXON 5	CAGgtagac	77.32	6.89	0.48639	6.866	0.864
Cryptic	DONOR	EXON 5	CAGgtgtt	66.35	2.28	0.25713	7.430	0.512
Constitutive	ACCEPTOR	INTRON 5	cctcccagGCG	73.83	5.05	0.55301	7.595	0.822
Mutated	ACCEPTOR	INTRON 5	ctcctcccaaGCG	93.55	2.71	-0.43946	3.443	0.486
Cryptic	ACCEPTOR	INTRON 5	gccaagGCA	72.00	2.53	-2.14118	-1.914	0.941

The scores of the preprocessing models reflect the splice site strength. Abbreviations: HSF (Human Splice Finder), SP (Splice Port) and ASSP (Alternative Splice Site Predictor).

both homozygous carriers, ruling out the possibility that the NMD could account for the differences in clinical features between siblings.

Although previous *in silico* analyses have shown that this mutation encodes for a truncated protein, both proteins still share 213 amino acids, including the homodimerization and activation domain HSR, and part of the DNA binding domain SAND. We then decided to analyze the predicted protein tertiary structure based on I-TASSER, discovering that the mutated protein (score −4.9) presents a different tertiary structure (Figure 4).

Discordant clinical characteristics of APS-1 patients in a consanguineous Spanish family

In this study we examined two siblings from a consanguineous Spanish family with autosomal recessive APS-1. They were born from healthy consanguineous parents (first cousins; Figure 1D).

The index case (II.1) was a middle-aged woman who was diagnosed with severe APS-1 symptoms including chronic mucocutaneous candidiasis, primary hypoparathyroidism, hypergonadotropic hypogonadism and intestinal dysfunction at 42 years of age. Recent analyses have tested positive for both GAD and anti-peroxidase antibodies, and she has been diagnosed with atrophic gastritis.

Although her brother (II.2) also carries the same homozygous mutation, he did not present hypoparathyroidism. However, he showed early signs of mucocutaneous candidiasis, and additional symptoms appeared at adulthood, including vitiligo and alopecia. Both homozygous carriers showed normal cortisol levels and did not test positive for antibodies for 21-hidroxilase, which initially rules out Addison's disease.

Finally, although several heterozygous relatives of APS-1 patients have been reported to have various autoimmune diseases such as rheumatoid arthritis, without any of the APS-1 major syndromes [27], we did not find any APS-1 features in the relatives studied.

Discussion

Since *AIRE* was first described as the APS-1 gene in 1997, more than a hundred different mutations of the *AIRE* gene have been identified in APS-1 patients, including two major mutations (p.R257X and p.L323SfsX51) which are responsible for 95% of the mutant alleles in APS-1 patients [15–17]. The rest of the reported mutations are also other missense or nonsense mutations, while splicing mutations are less common [28].

This autosomal recessive disorder is highly prevalent in certain genetically isolated populations, such as Finns, Sardinians and Iranian Jews [28,29], but is rare in the Spanish population, as just one case with a 13 bp deletion in exon 8 has been previously described [19].

In the present study, we identified two Spanish siblings, brother and sister, who carried a new homozygous mutation of the *AIRE* gene in the SSA of intron 5. The c.653-1G>A mutation turns the trinucleotide sequence CAG into CAA, losing the consensus SSA but creating a new SSA upstream in the intron 5, as *in silico* analysis predicted and mRNA analysis demonstrated. But the c.653-1G>A mutation not only induces the use of a new SSA upstream of intron 5, but also produces the cryptic SSD activation inside the proper exon 5, as *in silico* analysis also predicted (Table 2).

This mutation at the SSA is predicted to generate a truncated protein, thus we theorized that the nonsense-mediated mRNA decay (NMD) is activated. NMD is a surveillance pathway, whose main function is to reduce errors in gene expression by abolishing

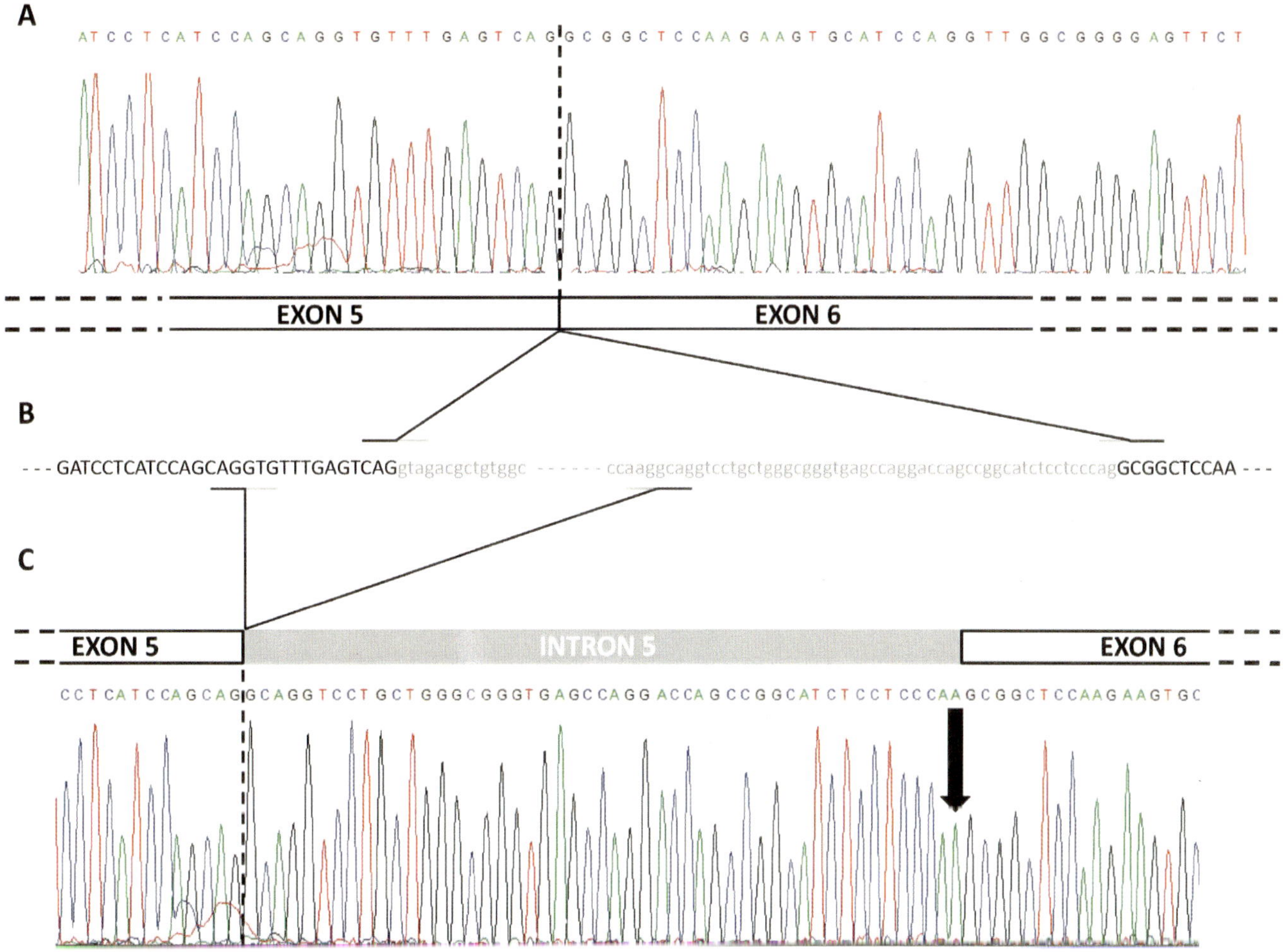

Figure 2. Sequencing representation of the cDNA analysis. (A) Chromatogram and schematic representation of the non-mutated exon 5 and 6 junction. (B) Partial gDNA sequence of exon 5, intron 5 and exon 6. Finally, (C) chromatogram and schematic representation of the mutated allele, including exon 5, part of intron 5 and exon 6. The arrow indicates the mutation.

mRNA transcripts that contain premature termination codons. This prevents the translation of aberrant transcripts and limits the synthesis of abnormal proteins [30], such as the transcripts generated from the mutated allele. Thus, NMD could take on a role as a modifier of the phenotypic and clinical consequences of the premature termination codon. This prompted us to analyze NMD in both homozygous and heterozygous carriers, studying the expression levels of the mutated and also non-mutated alleles. Our findings revealed a highly reduced expression of the mutated allele as an expected result of the activation of the NMD process (Figure 3B), but the reduced expression of the mutated allele was similar in both siblings. This suggests that the protective function of NMD contributes equally, ruling out the possibility that this mechanism was involved in the different clinical outcomes of APS-1 in these cases.

Although the expression of the mutated allele was very low and the mutation at the SSA sequence was expected to generate a truncated protein, the mutated and non-mutated proteins shared the first 213 amino acids, including the conserved bipartite nuclear localization signal domain (NLS) and the homogenously staining region (HSR) responsible for homodimerization. This made us wonder if the mutated protein could conserve in part the tertiary structure for these first domains, in which case perhaps it could exert partially its function. However, the alignment of the predicted tertiary structure for the mutated protein and the non-mutated AIRE protein (Figure 4) showed no-matching for the first domains, suggesting loss of functionality for the mutated protein.

Clinical picture of APS-1 is characterized by sequentially occurring diseases, with great variation in the severity and time course of the conditions among families and members of the family. Although candidiasis is not specific to APS-1, it is almost always present (>94% at 10 years of age and >97% at 30 years of age) [31], occurring in both homozygous members of this family. The high prevalence of candidiasis leads us to suspect APS-1, especially when clinical presentation takes place during childhood. The severity of its clinical manifestations varies widely and its most disabling feature may lead to the development of squamous cell carcinoma. However, both members of the family in question presented a less severe course, with chronic nail but intermittent oral candidiasis, since onset in childhood. Hypoparathyroidism is one of the first endocrine features of APS-1 [32] and is reported in 70–93% of the cases [33] but varies according to gender, affecting 98% of female patients, and only 71% of male patients [34]. There is no reasonable explanation for these gender differences, besides a clearly higher incidence of primary gonadal failure in females, explained by protective blood-testis barrier. Both homozygous members presented positive GADAb but negative IA-2Ab and without T1D at present. The IA-2Abs seem to be the best

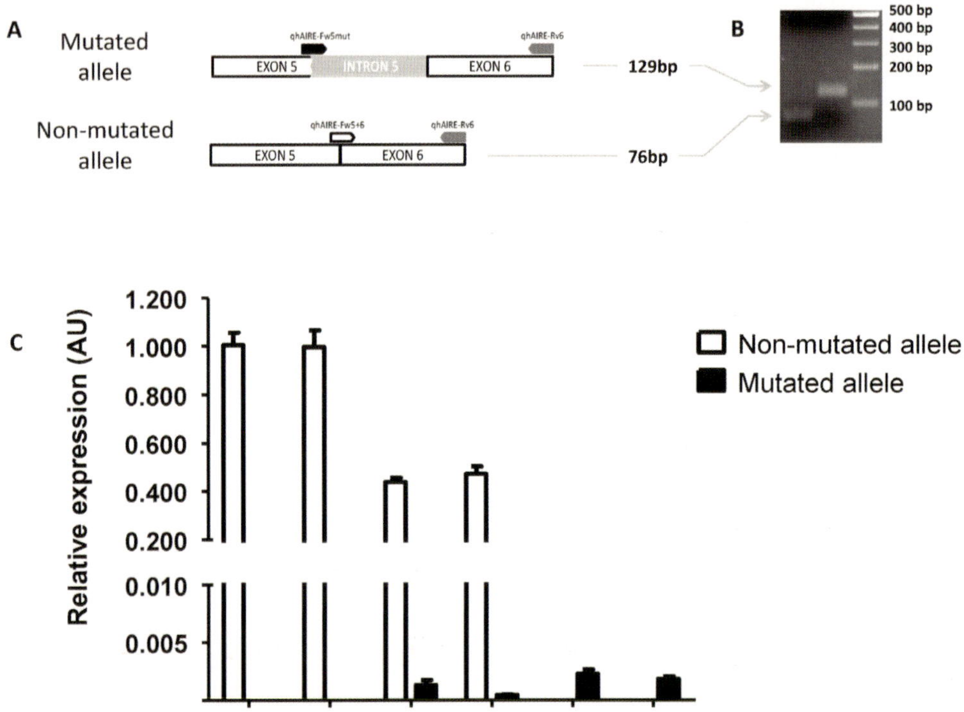

	CTRL 1 G/G		CTRL 2 G/G		I.1 G/A		I.2 G/A		II.1 A/A		II.2 A/A	
	NM	M	NM	M	NM	M	NM	M	NM	M	NM	M
MEAN	1.0040	0.0000	0.9961	0.0000	0.4371	0.0013	0.4714	0.0004	0.0000	0.0022	0.0000	0.0018
SEM	0.0539	0.0000	0.0699	0.0000	0.0184	0.0004	0.0313	0.0000	0.0000	0.0004	0.0000	0.0002

Figure 3. Nonsense pre-mRNA mediated decay analysis. (A) Schematic representation of the non-mutated and mutated allele analysis, with the specifically designed primers positions, including the non-mutated forward (white), the mutated forward (black) and the common reverse (grey). (B) Agarose gel electrophoresis of the qRT-PCR products revealed that the cDNA fragment of 76-bp corresponds to the predicted wild-type transcript, whereas the cDNA large fragment of 129-bp corresponds to the aberrant transcript. (C) Expression results of each allele normalized to that of the control G/G carriers for the individuals studied. The table below includes the mean relative expression and the standard error mean (SEM) for the non-mutated (NM) and mutated (M) alleles.

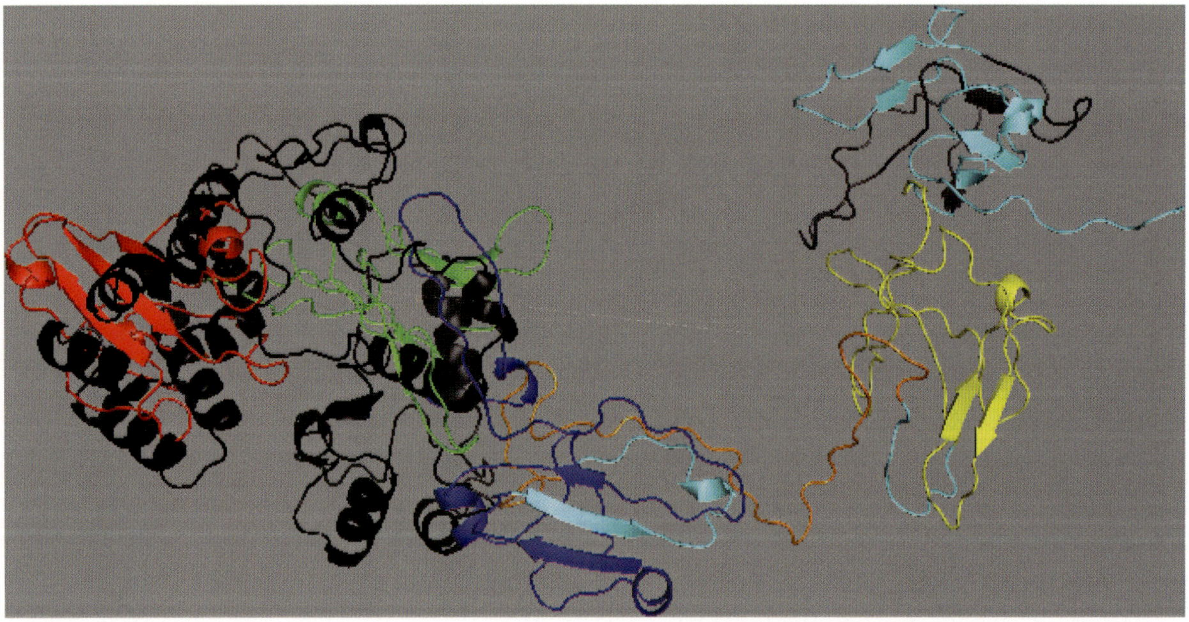

Figure 4. Tertiary schematic representation of the aligned non-mutated and mutated AIRE proteins. The non-mutated AIRE protein shows the different functional domains: HSR in red, NLS in green, SAND in blue, PHD in orange and PRR in yellow. The mutated AIRE protein, for its part, is represented in black.

predictors of T1D in APS-1, which were negative in our patients [33]; however, clinical evolution must be studied to confirm this data.

Although both siblings carried the same homozygous splicing mutation, the sister developed severe APS-1, whereas her brother presented mild symptoms. Previous reports have shown that different mutations in the *AIRE* gene lead to different phenotypes. For example, whereas most APS-1 Finnish patients present candidiasis, APS-1 Iranian Jews do not have this comorbidity and also do not show keratopathy [35]. Regarding these discrepancies, thirteen siblings from 6 families [36,37] have currently been reported to show a different phenotypic spectrum of APS-1 carrying the same mutation, emphasizing that clinical features are variable not only among patients from different families but also among affected siblings. In the consanguineous Spanish family studied, both siblings have a homozygous mutation in the last nucleotide of the SSA of intron 5; this mutation raised the hypothesis that a different degradation between siblings of the mutated mRNA by the NMD could explain, in part, the different clinical outcomes of APS-1. On the contrary, the relative expression results showed a similar degradation of the mutated mRNA for both homozygous carriers, ruling out our hypothesis. Nonetheless, we consider that NMD must be contemplated when formulating and testing hypotheses concerning heterogeneous clinical outcomes, including situations of premature termination codon mutation, in order to provide appropriate genetic counseling regarding disease prognosis.

As for the case at hand, to understand the broad clinical phenotypes involved, even though the patients carried the same mutation, we must bear in mind that the ability of the immune system to recognize a huge number of antigenic determinants ensures a comprehensive protection against invading pathogens, but at the same time distinguishes between invading pathogens and self-antigens. Positive selection of T-lymphocytes with relatively low affinity for self-antigens in the thymus is a central event of this interplay, preventing errors that could lead to autoimmune diseases, such as T1D or APS-1. On the other hand, negative selection ensures that T-cells whose receptors recognize self-antigens with a high affinity are eliminated before they are exported to the periphery [38]. At this point, *AIRE* plays a crucial role, mediating negative selection of autoreactive T-cells in the thymus and also outside, as *AIRE* expression in the periphery provides a further path for the induction of T-cell tolerance [17].

Taking all this into account, the phenotypic diversity and disease severity of APS-1 patients carrying the same mutation in the same family could be due to the failure of negative selection that occurs at different moments between siblings and/or consequence of different environmental factors, such as viral infection on T-cell immune-tolerance education in peripheral tissues.

In conclusion, we report a new homozygous splicing mutation in the *AIRE* intron 5 acceptor (c.653-1G>A, in two patients of a consanguineous Spanish family with different phenotypes of APS-1. Our findings highlight the importance of sequencing splice sites surrounding the intron-exon junctions and the need to carry out additional RNA studies to ensure precise molecular diagnosis and correct genetic counseling. On the other hand, APS-1 diagnosis should be suspected and the *AIRE* gene studied in cases of childhood chronic candidiasis and/or hypoparathyroidism that is otherwise unexplained, especially when these clinical features are associated with other autoimmune diseases.

Acknowledgments

The authors thank: Dr. Ramon Gomis from Institut d'Investigacions Biomèdiques August Pi i Sunyer (IDIBAPS) for his invaluable support and his critical review of the manuscript; Dr. Guiomar Perez de Nanclares from Hospital Universitario Araba-Txagorritxu for her helpful comments, and all patients who voluntarily collaborated on this study.

Author Contributions

Conceived and designed the experiments: MM FH EF-R. Performed the experiments. FH SA MM MP-J EF-R. Analyzed the data. MM FH MP-J GBA EF-R. Contributed reagents/materials/analysis tools: IH MPD. Contributed to the writing of the manuscript: MM EF-R. Revised the manuscript and contributed significantly to the intellectual value of the paper: FH IH GBA MPD SA.

References

1. Perheentupa J (2006) Autoimmune polyendocrinopathy-candidiasis-ectodermal dystrophy. J Clin Endocrinol Metab 91: 2843–2850.
2. Buzi F, Badolato R, Mazza C, Giliani S, Notarangelo LD, et al. (2003) Autoimmune polyendocrinopathy-candidiasis-ectodermal dystrophy syndrome: time to review diagnostic criteria? J Clin Endocrinol Metab 88: 3146–3148.
3. Michels AW, Gottlieb PA (2010) Autoimmune polyglandular syndromes. Nat Rev Endocrinol 6: 270–277.
4. Halonen M, Eskelin P, Myhre AG, Perheentupa J, Husebye ES, et al. (2002) AIRE mutations and human leukocyte antigen genotypes as determinants of the autoimmune polyendocrinopathy-candidiasis-ectodermal dystrophy phenotype. J Clin Endocrinol Metab 87: 2568–2574.
5. Aaltonen J, Horelli-Kuitunen N, Fan JB, Bjorses P, Perheentupa J, et al. (1997) High-resolution physical and transcriptional mapping of the autoimmune polyendocrinopathy-candidiasis-ectodermal dystrophy locus on chromosome 21q22.3 by FISH. Genome Res 7: 820–829.
6. Nagamine K, Peterson P, Scott HS, Kudoh J, Minoshima S, et al. (1997) Positional cloning of the APECED gene. Nat Genet 17: 393–398.
7. Mittaz L, Rossier C, Heino M, Peterson P, Krohn KJ, et al. (1999) Isolation and characterization of the mouse Aire gene. Biochem Biophys Res Commun 255: 483–490.
8. Gibson TJ, Ramu C, Gemund C, Aasland R (1998) The APECED polyglandular autoimmune syndrome protein, AIRE-1, contains the SAND domain and is probably a transcription factor. Trends Biochem Sci 23: 242–244.
9. Sternsdorf T, Grotzinger T, Jensen K, Will H (1997) Nuclear dots: actors on many stages. Immunobiology 198: 307–331.
10. Sternsdorf T, Jensen K, Reich B, Will H (1999) The nuclear dot protein sp100, characterization of domains necessary for dimerization, subcellular localization, and modification by small ubiquitin-like modifiers. J Biol Chem 274: 12555–12566.
11. Guldner HH, Szostecki C, Schroder P, Matschl U, Jensen K, et al. (1999) Splice variants of the nuclear dot-associated Sp100 protein contain homologies to HMG-1 and a human nuclear phosphoprotein-box motif. J Cell Sci 112 (Pt 5): 733–747.
12. Anderson MS, Venanzi ES, Klein L, Chen Z, Berzins SP, et al. (2002) Projection of an immunological self shadow within the thymus by the aire protein. Science 298: 1395–1401.
13. Liston A, Goodnow CC (2005) Genetic lesions in thymic T cell clonal deletion and thresholds for autoimmunity. Novartis Found Symp 267: 180–192; discussion 192–189.
14. Gardner JM, Devoss JJ, Friedman RS, Wong DJ, Tan YX, et al. (2008) Deletional tolerance mediated by extrathymic Aire-expressing cells. Science 321: 843–847.
15. Wolff AS, Erichsen MM, Meager A, Magitta NF, Myhre AG, et al. (2007) Autoimmune polyendocrine syndrome type 1 in Norway: phenotypic variation, autoantibodies, and novel mutations in the autoimmune regulator gene. J Clin Endocrinol Metab 92: 595–603.
16. Bjorses P, Halonen M, Palvimo JJ, Kolmer M, Aaltonen J, et al. (2000) Mutations in the AIRE gene: effects on subcellular location and transactivation function of the autoimmune polyendocrinopathy-candidiasis-ectodermal dystrophy protein. Am J Hum Genet 66: 378–392.

17. Akirav EM, Ruddle NH, Herold KC (2011) The role of AIRE in human autoimmune disease. Nat Rev Endocrinol 7: 25–33.
18. Mathis D, Benoist C (2009) Aire. Annu Rev Immunol 27: 287–312.
19. Martinez Lopez MM, Gonzalez Casado I, Alvarez Doforno R, Delgado Cervino E, Gracia Bouthelier R (2006) [AIRE gene mutation in polyglandular syndrome type 1]. An Pediatr (Barc) 64: 583–587.
20. Livak KJ, Schmittgen TD (2001) Analysis of relative gene expression data using real-time quantitative PCR and the 2(-Delta Delta C(T)) Method. Methods 25: 402–408.
21. Dogan RI, Getoor L, Wilbur WJ, Mount SM (2007) SplicePort–an interactive splice-site analysis tool. Nucleic Acids Res 35: W285–291.
22. Yeo G, Burge CB (2004) Maximum entropy modeling of short sequence motifs with applications to RNA splicing signals. J Comput Biol 11: 377–394.
23. Wang M, Marin A (2006) Characterization and prediction of alternative splice sites. Gene 366: 219–227.
24. Choi Y, Sims GE, Murphy S, Miller JR, Chan AP (2012) Predicting the functional effect of amino acid substitutions and indels. PLoS One 7: e46688.
25. Zhang Y (2008) I-TASSER server for protein 3D structure prediction. BMC Bioinformatics 9: 40.
26. Cartegni L, Chew SL, Krainer AR (2002) Listening to silence and understanding nonsense: exonic mutations that affect splicing. Nat Rev Genet 3: 285–298.
27. Cervato S, Mariniello B, Lazzarotto F, Morlin L, Zanchetta R, et al. (2009) Evaluation of the autoimmune regulator (AIRE) gene mutations in a cohort of Italian patients with autoimmune-polyendocrinopathy-candidiasis-ectodermal-dystrophy (APECED) and in their relatives. Clin Endocrinol (Oxf) 70: 421–428.
28. Stenson PD, Mort M, Ball EV, Shaw K, Phillips AD, et al. (2013) The Human Gene Mutation Database: building a comprehensive mutation repository for clinical and molecular genetics, diagnostic testing and personalized genomic medicine. Hum Genet.
29. Bjorses P, Aaltonen J, Vikman A, Perheentupa J, Ben-Zion G, et al. (1996) Genetic homogeneity of autoimmune polyglandular disease type I. Am J Hum Genet 59: 879–886.
30. Maquat LE (2004) Nonsense-mediated mRNA decay: splicing, translation and mRNP dynamics. Nat Rev Mol Cell Biol 5: 89–99.
31. Husebye ES, Perheentupa J, Rautemaa R, Kampe O (2009) Clinical manifestations and management of patients with autoimmune polyendocrine syndrome type I. J Intern Med 265: 514–529.
32. Kluger N, Ranki A, Krohn K (2012) APECED: is this a model for failure of T cell and B cell tolerance? Front Immunol 3: 232.
33. Weiler FG, Dias-da-Silva MR, Lazaretti-Castro M (2012) Autoimmune polyendocrine syndrome type 1: case report and review of literature. Arq Bras Endocrinol Metabol 56: 54–66.
34. Gylling M, Kaariainen E, Vaisanen R, Kerosuo L, Solin ML, et al. (2003) The hypoparathyroidism of autoimmune polyendocrinopathy-candidiasis-ectodermal dystrophy protective effect of male sex. J Clin Endocrinol Metab 88: 4602–4608.
35. Zlotogora J, Shapiro MS (1992) Polyglandular autoimmune syndrome type I among Iranian Jews. J Med Genet 29: 824–826.
36. Ishii T, Suzuki Y, Ando N, Matsuo N, Ogata T (2000) Novel mutations of the autoimmune regulator gene in two siblings with autoimmune polyendocrinopathy-candidiasis-ectodermal dystrophy. J Clin Endocrinol Metab 85: 2922–2926.
37. Pearce SH, Cheetham T, Imrie H, Vaidya B, Barnes ND, et al. (1998) A common and recurrent 13-bp deletion in the autoimmune regulator gene in British kindreds with autoimmune polyendocrinopathy type 1. Am J Hum Genet 63: 1675–1684.
38. Klein L, Hinterberger M, Wirnsberger G, Kyewski B (2009) Antigen presentation in the thymus for positive selection and central tolerance induction. Nat Rev Immunol 9: 833–844.

12

Long-Term Effect of Antibodies against Infused Alpha-Galactosidase A in Fabry Disease on Plasma and Urinary (lyso)Gb3 Reduction and Treatment Outcome

Saskia M. Rombach[1], Johannes M. F. G. Aerts[2], Ben J. H. M. Poorthuis[2], Johanna E. M. Groener[2], Wilma Donker-Koopman[2], Erik Hendriks[2], Mina Mirzaian[2], Sijmen Kuiper[2], Frits A. Wijburg[2], Carla E. M. Hollak[1], Gabor E. Linthorst[1]*

1 Department of Endocrinology and Metabolism, Division of Internal Medicine, Academic Medical Center, Amsterdam, The Netherlands, **2** Department of Medical Biochemistry, Academic Medical Center, Amsterdam, The Netherlands, **3** Department of Pediatrics, Academic Medical Center, Amsterdam, The Netherlands

Abstract

Introduction: Enzyme replacement therapy (ERT) with alpha-Galactosidase A (aGal A) may cause antibody (AB) formation against aGal A in males with Fabry disease (FD). Anti agalsidase ABs negatively influence globotriaosylceramide (Gb3) reduction. We investigated the impact of agalsidase AB on Gb3 and lysoGb3 and clinical outcome in Fabry patients on ERT.

Methods: Adult male and female patients on ERT for at least one year were included. Urinary Gb3 was measured by HPLC, plasma lysoGb3 by LC-ESI-MS/MS and AB with a neutralization assay.

Results: Of the 59 patients evaluable patients, 0/30 females and 17/29 males developed anti-agalsidase antibodies (AB+). Only 3/17 males had transient (low) titers (tolerized). All AB+ patients developed antibodies during the first year of treatment. Change of agalsidase preparation (or dose) did not induce antibody formation. AB+ males had significant less decline in plasma lysoGb3 compared to AB− males ($p = 0.04$). Urinary Gb3 levels decreased markedly in AB− but remained comparable to baseline in AB+ males ($p < 0.01$). (Lyso)Gb3 reduction in plasma and urine on ERT was correlated with LVmass reduction in females and development white matter lesions and stroke.

Conclusion: In male patients antibodies against aGal A remained present up to 10 years of ERT. The presence of these antibodies is associated with a less robust decrease in plasma lysoGb3 and a profound negative effect on urinary Gb3 reduction, which may reflect worse treatment outcome.

Editor: Rajesh Mohanraj, UAE University, Faculty of Medicine & Health Sciences, United Arab Emirates

Funding: This study was funded by The Netherlands Organization for Health Research and Development (ZON-MW). The funders had no role in study design, data collection and analysis, decision to publish, or preparation of the manuscript.

Competing Interests: GEL, FAW, JMA and CEMH have received reimbursement of expenses and honoraria for lectures on the management of from Genzyme, Actelion and Shire HGT. GEL, JMA and CEMH donated the honoraria to the Gaucher Stichting, a foundation that supports research in the field of lysosomal storage disorders. All other authors declare no conflicts of interest. This does not alter the authors' adherence to all the PLOS ONE policies on sharing data and materials.

* E-mail: g.e.linthorst@amc.nl

Introduction

The X-linked lysosomal storage disorder Fabry disease is caused by deficiency of the hydrolase alfa-galactosidase A. Due to this defect glycosphingolipids, primarily globotriaosylceramide (Gb3, also known as ceramidetrihexoside) accumulate in various cells of the body. Gb3 storage is the primary event that ultimately results in clinical symptoms that start at childhood and comprise acroparesthesia, anhidrosis, and angiokeratoma. At adult age, renal, cardiac, and cerebrovascular involvement determine the reduced life expectancy seen in this disease [1]. Both hemizygous males and heterozygous females can be affected by Fabry disease, though in females the disease course is in general milder and more protracted.

Increased levels of Gb3 can be demonstrated in organs, plasma, and urine , especially in affected Fabry males. In contrast, the majority of female Fabry patients have normal Gb3 levels in blood although most have increased levels of Gb3 in urine [2].

Clinical trials have demonstrated that biweekly infusions (enzyme replacement therapy or ERT) with two distinct aGal A preparations reduce the Gb3 content in kidney, heart and skin [3,4]. Plasma Gb3 levels decline to normal values within 3 months, while urinary Gb3 clearance is less prominent [3]. Since repeated organ biopsies are not feasible to evaluate treatment efficacy, serial measurement of plasma and urine Gb3 as a marker for treatment efficacy is advised, though the exact relevance for monitoring therapeutic efficacy of ERT has not been elucidated yet.

Emergence of antibodies towards the infused enzyme is commonly observed in Fabry males and has a negative impact on urinary Gb3 clearance [5]. A similar observation was made in skin, with recurrence of Gb3 accumulation in patients with high antibody titers [6,7]. To study the clinical impact of these antibodies on a biochemical level, renal function was used as outcome measurement in one study, in combination with clinical events (e.g. progression of disease) [6]. Analysis of patients who participated in two clinical trials and for whom long term outcome of 5 years of ERT was available did not demonstrate a difference in renal function or clinical events, but this was compared only for different titer subgroups (high, intermediate, low and no antibodies) and no direct comparison between patients with and without antibodies was made [6].

The negative effect of antibodies on Gb3 clearance is influenced by agalsidase dose. Patients who switched from agalsidase alfa or beta 0,2 mg/kg to agalsidase beta 1,0 mg/kg demonstrated an additional decrease in plasma Gb3 in AB+ patients 12 months after switch[8].

Detailed analysis of the effect of long term ERT on plasma Gb3 or urinary Gb3 in relation to the presence agalsidase antibodies is lacking. Recently de-acylated Gb3 (globotriaosylsphingosine, or lysoGb3), was shown to be highly increased in plasma of patients with Fabry disease, its relative elevation exceeding markedly that of Gb3 [9]. Plasma lysoGb3 proved to be an independent risk factor for white matter lesions in males and left ventricular hypertrophy in females [10] and was correlated with other markers of renal injury [11]. Lifetime exposure to plasma lysoGb3 tended to correlate with disease severity [10]. Enzyme replacement therapy reduced lysoGb3 levels during the first 12 months and these reductions were influenced by dose and the presence of antibodies, with higher doses resulting in a more robust lysoGb3 reduction [12] similar to the effects seen for Gb3 [8]. As lysoGb3 levels in females are more often increased than plasma Gb3 values, lysoGb3 may be a more attractive biochemical marker than Gb3 for monitoring the effect of ERT.

The aim of the current study was to analyse the impact of antibodies on long-term biochemical, and clinical outcome of ERT in Dutch Fabry patients.

Methods

Patients

Of the entire cohort of 70 adult Dutch Fabry patients only those presenting with classical manifestations of Fabry disease and treated with either agalsidase alfa or beta (ERT) for at least one year were included (n = 59). Classical Fabry disease is defined by the presence of characteristic symptoms and elevated plasma lysoGb3 and/or Gb3 in hemizygotes, and in case of heterozygotes, having a mutation known to be associated with a classical phenotype through literature or a male family member with classical symptoms [12]. Analyses were conducted until December 2010 or August 2010 in patients with dose-reductions because of a shortage of agalsidase beta [13]. In all patients plasma lysoGb3, Gb3 and urinary Gb3 were measured at baseline and for most patients also in subsequent years. In addition, antibody status was determined 6 months after start of ERT and yearly after that. Patients were treated with agalsidase alfa 0.2 mg/kg/2 weeks, with agalsidase beta 0.2 mg/kg/2 weeks as part of a previous clinical trial [14] or with agalsidase beta 1.0 mg/kg/2 weeks. Two groups were analysed: all patients and a subgroup consisting of males treated for more than five years. The latter group consisted of 8 AB+ and 9 AB− males.

Clinical evaluations were performed yearly and consisted of neurological, cardiac, and renal evaluations. The estimated glomerular filtration rate (eGFR) was calculated according to the abbreviated MDRD formula [15]. Left Ventricular Mass (LVM) was assessed by echocardiography and calculated according to Devereux [16]. Presence of (new) cerebral White Matter Lesions (WML) was determined with MRI by experienced neuro-radiologists. A complication was defined as any cardiac complication, stroke, or end stage renal disease. Cardiac complications were defined as: onset of atrial fibrillation, onset of any other rhythm disturbance needing hospitalization, pacemaker, or implantable cardiac defibrillator (ICD) implantation, cardiac congestion for which hospital admittance was needed, myocardial infarction, percutaneous coronary intervention, or coronary artery bypass graft. ESRD was defined as CKD stage 5 (a GFR<15 ml/min/1.73 m^2), starting dialysis or renal transplantation. The occurrence of a clinical event was recorded and correlated with antibody status in patients treated for five years or more. A summary of the baseline characteristics of the patients included in the study is given in Table 1.

Consent and IRB approval

Analysis of glycolipids and antibodies is part of standard of care in the treatment of Fabry disease in our expert center. A waiver from the hospital's institutional review board stating was obtained, stating that this analysis does not apply to the Medical Research Involving Human Subjects ACT (WMO) and that an official IRB approval by the institution is not required. All patients gave written consent for treatment, storage and analysis of blood samples.

Biochemical analyses

Yearly Gb3, lysoGb3 and antibody assessments were performed. Antibody (AB) analysis was performed by incubating plasma of patients with 1 ng agalsidase alfa or beta (depending on the enzyme preparation the patient was treated with). The amount of plasma needed to neutralize 50% of the enzymatic activity of 1 ng agalsidase alfa or beta was determined by titration. A sample was considered anti-agalsidase IgG negative if a sample demonstrated less than 50% neutralization at 5 µl plasma input. Previously, it was already demonstrated that the amount of neutralizing activity directly correlates with antibody titer [5]. In addition, that study also demonstrated that removal of IgG abolished the inhibitory effect of anti-agalsidase positive plasma.

Globotriaosylceramide (Gb3) and globotriaosylsphingosine (lyso-Gb3) analysis in plasma

Blood sampling in EDTA was performed for measurement of Gb3 and lyso-Gb3. Blood samples were centrifuged for 10 minutes at 3000 rpm to obtain plasma. Plasma was stored at −20°C until use. Gb3 analysis was performed by using high-performance liquid chromatography essentially as described by Groener et al [17]. Fifty µl of plasma was used and lipids were extracted according to Bligh and Dyer [18]. As internal standard C17 sphinganine was used. The intra-and interassay coefficient of variation is 4% and 14% respectively. Lyso-Gb3 concentrations in plasma samples were measured using 5,6,7,8,9 $^{13}C_5$-lysoGb3 as internal standard, extraction by a modification of the method of Bligh and Dyer, and LC-ESI-MS/MS (Gold et al, submitted). The intra- and interassay coefficient of variation is 3.5% and 6.3%, respectively.

Gb3 analysis in urine

A 50 mL urine sample was obtained from a 24 hour urine collection and stored at −20°C until Gb3 analysis was performed essentially as described for plasma with a slight modification. In short, 400 µl of urine was used and lipids were extracted according to Bligh and Dyer [19]. Instead of water, 20 mM phosphate buffer (pH 8.0) was used in the phase separation.

Table 1. Baseline characteristics of all adult classic patients treated >1 year.

	AB+males	AB−males	AB males who tolerized	Females
Number of patients	**14**	**12**	**3**	**30**
Age at start of ERT (median, range)*	41.0 (18.1–58.5)	22.8 (17.0–65.3)	41.8 (27.2–42.7)	45.6 (15.9–71.5)
LysoGb3 nmol/L (healthy controls 0.3–0.5)	85 (31–124)	74 (20–160)	102 (100–112)	8 (2.7–24)
Plasma Gb3 umol/L (healthy controls 0.45–2.46)	4.2 (1.8–7.1)	3.8 (1.5–5.7)	4.5 (3.1–5.9)	1.5 (0.5–2.8)
Urinary Gb3 nmol/24 h (healthy controls 18–90)	1885 (608–4691)	1928 (250–4494)	1689 (911–2905)	343 (20–2009)
eGFR	84.1 (24.6–130.1)	128.1 (35.5–208.3)	100.8 (38.0–151.1)	98.7 (44.7–180.5)
LVmass ($g/m^{2.7}$ per year)	53.3 (31.1–77.3)	44.5 (25.4–67.7)	53.6 (29.2–66.4)	44.1 (25.5–120.0)
Presence of white matter lesions	9/12	4/10	2/3	20/28
History of a complication	4/14	1/12	0/3	3/30

*2 males and 4 females started ERT during childhood.

Statistical analysis

Results are presented as median (range) or mean±standard deviation (SD). Chi-square was used for comparison of proportions and Mann-Whitney U to compare data between two independent groups and the Kruskal-Wallis test for more than 2 groups. Spearman's rho was used for correlation of antibody concentration (titer) and changes in (lyso)Gb3. For comparison of years of follow-up to baseline, the Wilcoxon-sign rank test was applied. Repeated measurements were used for analysis of LVMass and renal function and Cox regression to analyze time to first white matter lesions/stroke during ERT and the association with (lyso) Gb3 level.

Results were considered to be statistically significant when p-values were <0.05.

Table 2. Antibody formation in all adult male patients and the treatment received in the first year *).

		Treatment		
		Agalsidase alfa	Agalsidase beta**)	Total
Antibodies	AB neg	9	3	12
	AB pos	5	12	17
Total		14	15	29

*including those who tolerized (n = 3)
**A significant proportion (n = 5) of patients on agalsidase beta received 0,2 mg/kg as part of a clinical trial during the first years of treatment.

Results

Antibody status

Of the 59 adult patients on ERT with one year of follow-up, 29 males and 30 females received at least one year of ERT (table 1). None of the 30 female patients developed antibodies during treatment. Of the males, 17 developed antibodies, whereas 12 did not (table 2). Treatment with agalsidase alfa was associated with a lower incidence of antibody formation as compared to agalsidase beta (5/14 on agalsidase alfa vs 12/15 on agalsidase beta, p = 0.025) but in the agalsidase beta group two different dosages were used (0.2 and 1,0 mg/kg). Prevalence of antibody formation between patients treated with 0.2 mg/kg agalsidase alfa or beta did not differ significantly (5/9 versus 2/5 respectively, p = 0.18). All patients who developed antibodies did so within the first year after start of ERT. Treatment alterations after one year of treatment, i.e. an increase in dose (agalsidase beta 0.2 to 1.0 mg/kg) or a switch from agalsidase alfa to agalsidase beta, did not induce antibody formation in those who were negative after one year of treatment (data not shown).

In three patients AB's disappeared (i.e. these patients tolerized). These three patients had their highest titer already within the first year of treatment, and two of these three had the lowest titer of the 17 AB positive patients. In the other 14 patients, a maximum titer was achieved at later time points and no tolerization was observed (non-tolerized AB+ patients).

Plasma lysoGb3 and Gb3

Of the 29 males, 26 males had follow-up plasma Gb3 and lysoGb3 measurements after one year. In all classic adult male patients levels of plasma lysoGb3 decreased, but this decrease was more robust in male patients without antibodies. Baseline lysoGb3 in both groups was not different (p = 0.33). The 3 patients who tolerized were not included in the subanalysis by AB status; data of the 12 AB+ male patients were compared to 11 AB− male patients. The males in the AB+ group were treated for a median time of 7.6 (1.3–10.2) years, the AB- group for 6.1 (1.2–8.1) years, p = 0.24). At baseline, lysoGb3 in both groups was not different (p = 0.41). In the first year, lysoGb3 decreased in both the AB+ group (from 81 (31–124) to 36 (15–80) nmol/L, n = 12) as well as in the AB− group (from 73 (20–103) to 24 (6–47) nmol/L, n = 11). However during follow-up, lysoGb3 remained elevated (reference range in healthy controls: 0.3–0.5 nM) and were higher in the AB+ group compared to the AB− group (P<0.043, year 1 through 6 compared to baseline, fig 1a). Analysis of plasma Gb3 in the same patients demonstrated a similar pattern (fig 1b), but changes were less pronounced as Gb3 levels are less increased at baseline as compared to lysoGb3. Gb3 levels remained higher in het AB− group compared to the AB+ group (p<0.02). Also in females with follow-up data, both lysoGb3 (from 8 (2.7–24) to 5 (2–13), n = 27) and Gb3 (from 1.6 (0.5–2.8) to 1.1 (0.5–1.8) n = 28) declined after the first year and remained decreased after 6 years (p<0.03) (figure 2a and b) (range 2.3–11.4 nM), even though lysoGb3 did not normalize and remained elevated as compared to normal controls (0.3–0.5 nM).

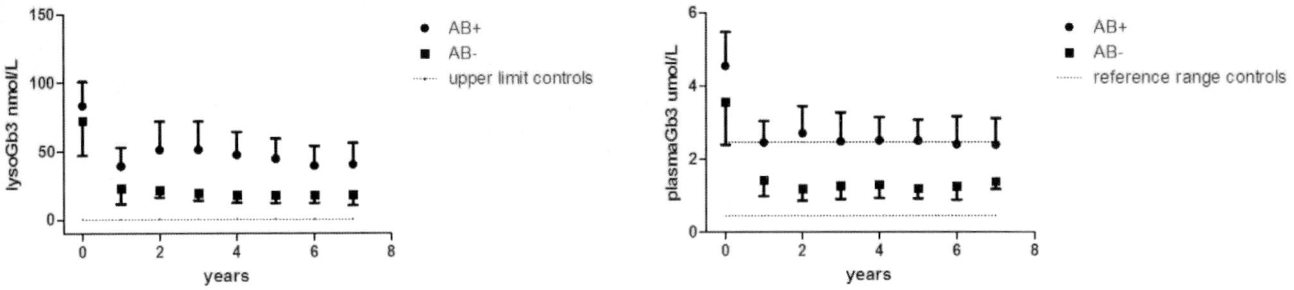

Figure 1. Plasma lysoGb3 and Gb3 in Fabry males. LysoGb3 (A) and plasma Gb3 (B) in 23 classic Fabry males, treated for at least one year (AB+ group n = 12, AB− group n = 11), depicting mean and 95% confidence intervals.

Urinary Gb3

Male patients with antibodies and those without showed a clear difference in urinary Gb3 reductions. Mean urinary Gb3 decreased from 1818 (250–4494) to 390 (68–735) nmol/24 h (p = 0.003) in all antibody negative males (n = 11) with follow-up after the first year and remained decreased after 6 years of ERT compared to baseline (range 19–387 nmol/24 hours, p = 0.028), to normal or near normal values, (healthy controls: 18–90 nmol/24 hours, fig.3a). Mean urinary Gb3 levels in patients with antibodies in patients treated for 1 year or more with follow-up (N = 11) did not decrease (from 1812 (608–4691) to 1728 (212–3619) after 1 year, p = 0.79), and remained elevated for up to 8 years of treatment (216–4547 nmol/24 hours, fig 3a). In the 25 females with urinary Gb3 data, urinary Gb3 decreased from 379 (20–2009) to 173 (17–620) nmol/24 h after the first year and remained decreased after 6 years of follow-up (28–339 nmol/24 hours, p = 0.005, fig 3b).

Effect of dose and change of preparation

In the 23 males with follow-up data (excluding the patients who tolerized), lysoGb3, plasma Gb3 and urinary Gb3 were comparable at baseline, irrespective of preparation or dose received (see table 3). After the first year of treatment, in males treated with agalsidase alfa or beta 0.2 mg/kg/2 weeks, the decrease of lysoGb3 was less pronounced compared to the AB+ group treated with 1.0 mg/kg/2 weeks ($p<0.03$) and the AB− group ($p<0.02$). Also the decline of plasma and urinary Gb3 in the AB+ group treated with agalsidase alfa 0.2 mg/kg/2 weeks was less pronounced compared to the AB+ group treated with 1.0 mg/kg ($p<0.05$) and AB− group ($p<0.01$).

In males with antibodies and treated with agalsidase beta 1.0 mg/kg/2 weeks, the decrease in lysoGb3 within the initial first year was comparable to the AB− group (p = 0.43) as well as the decrease in plasma Gb3 (p = 0.17) and urinary Gb3 (p = 0.24).

After at least one year of treatment, six AB+ males switched to a dose of 1.0 mg/kg/2 weeks. In these males, lysoGb3 declined additionally (median −13 nmol/L, range −33, −9, p = 0.028) one year after switch. Similarly, following switch plasma Gb3 declined additionally (median −0.86 (range −1.1, 0 µmol/L, p = 0.028), while urinary Gb3 declined only in a subset of males (median −216, range −1072, 576 nmol/24 hours, p = 0.75). Despite this additional decrease in lysoGb3, plasma and urinary Gb3 levels in AB+ patients who switched to agalsidase beta 1.0 mg/kg/2 weeks, these levels remained higher as compared to AB− patients ($p<0.02$).

Correlation with clinical events

To study the relation of antibodies with clinical outcome, males with antibodies were compared to males without antibodies, the 3 tolerized patients were excluded. AB+ patients were older and had more advanced disease at start of treatment, as compared to antibody negative males (see table 1). This hampers the comparison, as older patients with more advanced disease are more likely to demonstrate disease progression. Selecting only those patients treated with at least five years of ERT (8 AB+ and 9 AB− patients), again males with antibodies were older than the patients without antibodies. In this subgroup, a tendency towards a higher incidence of new complications was seen (4/9 in AB+ vs 1/8 in AB− patients), but this was not statistically significant (p = 0.18). No difference was seen in long term outcome of ERT between these small groups of male patients with regard to renal function, LVmass and the occurrence of new white matter lesions on cerebral MRI.

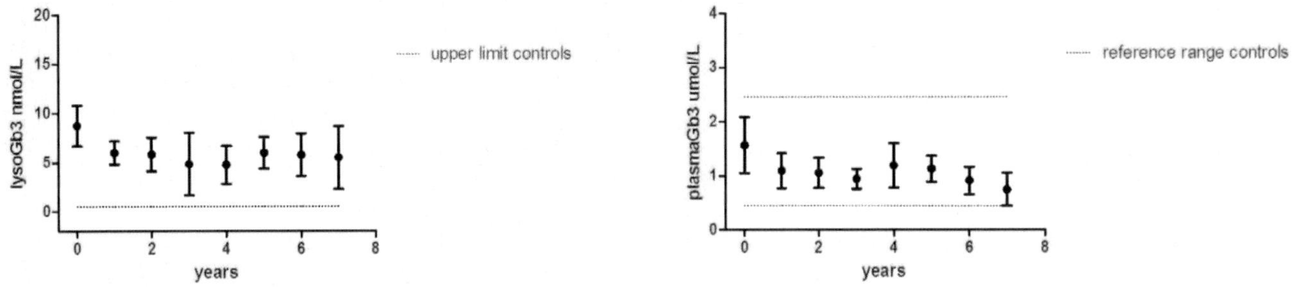

Figure 2. Plasma lysoGb3 and Gb3 in Fabry females. Plasma lysoGb3 in 27 (A) and Gb3 (B) in 28 Fabry females, treated for at least one year, depicting mean and 95% CI.

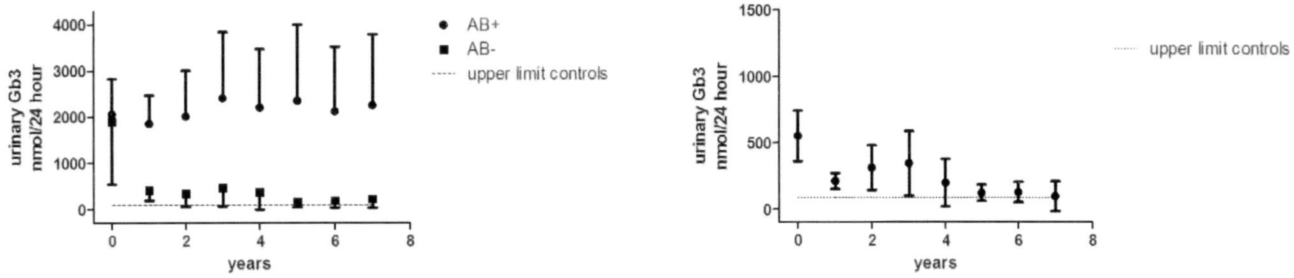

Figure 3. Urinary Gb3 in males and females. A. Urinary Gb3 in classic Fabry males, treated for at least one year (AB+ group n = 11, AB− group n = 11). **B.** Urinary Gb3 in classic Fabry females treated for at least one year (n = 28), depicting mean and 95% confidence interval. The dotted line denotes upper limit of normal in healthy controls: 18–90 nmol/24 uur.

Clinical relevance of changes in lysoGb3 and Gb3 in plasma and urine

In females (n = 29), 1 nM lysoGb3 decrease was correlated with 1.5 g/m$^{2.7}$ decrease in LVmass ($p<0.001$) independent of age or years of treatment (see figure 4). For plasma Gb3, 1 µM decrease of plasma Gb3 was correlated to 6.1 g/m$^{2.7}$ decrease in LVmass ($p = 0.005$), for urinary Gb3 100 nmol/24 h decrease was associated with 1.3 g/m$^{2.7}$ decrease in LVmass ($p<0.001$) independent of age.

For both males and females, reductions in plasma lysoGb3, plasma Gb3 and urinary Gb3 within the first year after start of ERT predicted the hazard of developing white matter lesions and stroke during ERT, while age and gender did not. The hazard ratio for developing white matter lesions and stroke was 0.74 (95%: 0.60–0.90) per 10 nM lysoGb3 decrease) during treatment ($p = 0.009$, see figure 5)). A reduction of 1 µmol/L plasma Gb3 decreased the hazard ratio to develop white matter lesions or stroke during follow-up (HR 0.54, 95% CI: 0.34–0.87) ($p = 0.012$). Similarly, a decrease of 100 nmol/24 h urinary Gb3 reduced this hazard ratio to 0.95 (95% CI: 0.92–0.99), $p = 0.018$. No correlation between the change of renal function and change of (lyso) Gb3 could be determined.

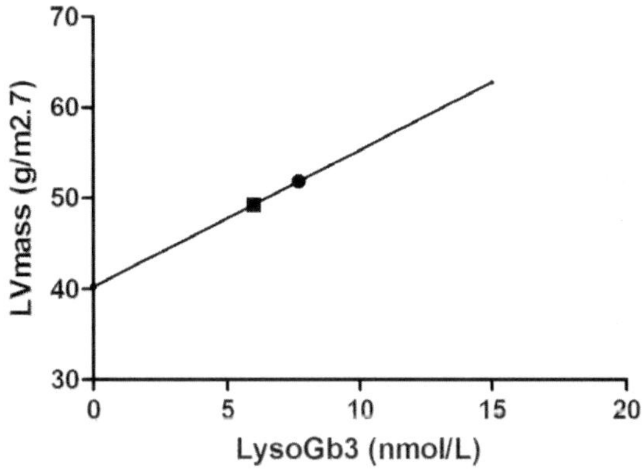

Figure 4. LVMass reduction and LysoGb3. LVMass decreases as lysoGb3 decreases. The dot represents the mean lysoGb3 and mean LVmass in females at start of ERT treatment, the square depicts mean lysoGb3 one year after start of ERT.

Discussion

Here we demonstrate the long term impact of antibody formation in male Fabry patients treated with ERT on clearance of urinary Gb3 and to a lesser extent on plasma Gb3 and lysoGb3 levels. In addition, it is also demonstrated that in both AB+ as AB− males plasma lysoGb3 levels seem to plateau after an initial decrease in the first year of treatment and do not reach normal values. While in those AB+ patients treated with 0.2 mg/kg/2 weeks a switch to a higher dose of 1.0 mg/kg/2 weeks resulted in a further reduction of lyso(Gb3), these levels still remained higher compared to AB− patients. Finally, change of lysoGb3 and plasma and urinary Gb3 levels correlate with LVMass change in females, in males with decrease of LVmass and development of

Table 3. Plasma and urinary lipids in male Fabry patients *.

Total	AB+R0.2	AB+F0.2	AB+F1.0	AB− total	*p-value (comparing all groups)*
Number	**4**	**4**	**4**	**11**	
LysoGb3 baseline (nmol/L)	91 (70–119)	79 (31–114)	76 (53–124)	73	0.68
LysoGb3 1 year ERT	65 (38–80)	36 (30–48)	17.5 (15–23)	24 (6–47)	0.003
Plasma Gb3 baseline (umol/L)	4.7 (4.0–7.1)	3.6 (1.8–5.3)	5.3(3.1–6.1)	3.7 (1.5–5.7)	0.14
Plasma Gb3 1 year ERT	3.6 (3.5–4.1)	2.1 (1.5–3.4)	2.0 (1.9–2.1)	1.2 (0.6–1.5)	0.009
Urinary Gb3 baseline (nmol/24 h)	1786 (1362–2778)	2130 (608–2979)	1790 (669–1812)	1818 (250-4494)	0.81
Urinary Gb3 1 year ERT	2442 (1714–2720)	1748 (1376–3619)	824 (212–1656)	390 (68–735)	0.003

*) including males with follow-up measurements, without the 3 males who tolerized.

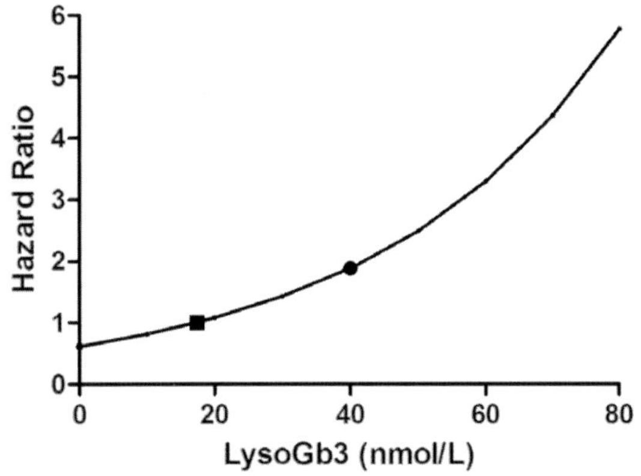

Figure 5. Risk to develop white matter lesions and LysoGb3. The hazard ratio to develop a (additional) white matter lesion or stroke decreases as the absolute value of lysoGb3 decreases. The dot represents mean lysoGb3 for males and females at start of ERT. The square depicts mean lysoGb3 level one year after start of ERT.

strokes or white matter lesions in both males and females. While it is difficult to predict the consequences of the presence of these antibodies, a potential negative effect on therapeutic effectiveness is likely [2,19,20].

Few patients in this study developed complete immune tolerance towards aGal A during prolonged treatment. This finding is consistent with a recent report of the postmarketing surveillance database on agalsidase beta. Of the 571 males treated with agalsidase beta 73% developed antibodies towards the infused enzyme, and only 11% of these tolerized, which is similar to our cohort (3/17, 18%) [21]. The continuous presence of (high) levels antibodies may also have consequences for future alternative therapies. It is conceivable that circulating anti-agalsidase antibodies may exert an effect on future second generation aGal A enzyme preparations, on treatment with chaperones that aim to promote the stability of the patient's endogenous mutated aGal A or even in gene therapeutic approaches. In other lysosomal storage disorders, most notably Pompe disease, several strategies have been proposed to reduce the levels of anti-enzyme antibodies, such as methotrexate or anti-CD20 [22]. In Fabry disease similar studies have been done in the mouse-model, but currently no studies have been performed in man [23]. The findings reported here strengthen the need to study in more detail the clinical consequences of antibody formation and approaches on treatment of patients with antibodies. One such approach may be the use of higher dosages of agalsidase as a previous study and this report demonstrate additional reduction of plasma Gb3 and urinary Gb3 following higher dosages[8]. Another possibility may be to develop immune tolerization regimes.

Previously no correlation between symptoms of Fabry disease and plasma or urinary Gb3 levels was found [2,19]. which led some to question its use as a biomarker [19,20]. However, Gb3 is believed to be pivotal in Fabry pathogenesis and clearance of accumulated Gb3 in renal capillary endothelium has been accepted as (surrogate) primary endpoint. In clinical trials reduction of plasma, urinary or organ Gb3 was considered to reflect a positive effect of ERT [3,4]. In addition, recent studies demonstrate that pre-treatment lysoGb3 levels correlated with some of the clinical features of the disease, such as white matter lesions in males and overall clinical severity and left ventricular mass in females [10]. This observation is extended as lysoGb3 response during ERT reflects change in LVmass and development of white matter lesions. In addition, there is an effect of dose: the higher dose of agalsidase beta led to more robust biochemical responses. This is in line with a study in which a lower dose of agalsidase beta (0.3 mg/kg) led to increases in Gb3 in a subset of patients [24]. A recent observation of switch to a lower dose as a result of a worldwide shortage of agalsidase beta again confirms this finding [13]. These findings once more emphasize that the debate on dose and treatment outcomes needs to be elucidated and deserves additional (clinical) studies.

However, even in those patients who do not develop antibodies, ERT resulted in a far from complete reduction to normal levels of plasma lysoGb3. After 6 years of treatment, plasma lysoGb3 in AB− Fabry patients was on average still 40-fold increased compared to normal values. The fact that decrease in lysoGb3, and in plasma and urinary Gb3 correlates with LVmass reduction upon ERT and influences the hazard of developing white matter lesions, suggests that a more robust decline of these biomarkers is probably associated with a more favourable outcome. Both the phase 4 study with agalsidase beta as well as detailed analyses of the Dutch cohort demonstrate disease progression in many patients, suggestive of a very modest effect of ERT in Fabry disease [14,25,26]. This modest treatment effect as well as the influence of end organ damage to the responsiveness of the disease [27,28] may also explain why this study and that of others [6,28] fail to demonstrate a clear effect of antibodies on treatment effectiveness. Comparing antibody positive and negative patients with regard to clinical outcome may also be hampered by the fact that patients with residual aGal A activity may not only have a lower risk for developing anti-agalsidase antibodies, but may also have a less severe course of the disease as compared to those without residual enzyme activity. The dêvelopment of anti-agalsidase antibodies may thus reflect a more severe phenotype of the disease with faster disease progression.

In this study we made some additional observations that may be of practical use in the daily care of patients on ERT. None of the females developed antibodies, which is not surprising as females have substantial residual enzyme activity (given the X-linked nature fo the disease) and the infused recombinant human enzyme is unlikely to be regarded as immunogenic. However, recently another study reported 12% of treated females developed antibodies [21]. This observed difference in antibody formation may be related to the method of antibody detection (neutralization assay vs ELISA/RIP was used in [21]). Our data suggest, that the need to monitor antibodies may be of lesser importance in females, and may be performed less frequently. In addition, in this study all patients who were antibody negative after one year of treatment remained so, irrespective of an increase in dose, or change in enzyme preparation.

Again these observations should be confirmed in larger cohorts, but may be of importance for physicians considering switching preparation or increase the dose.

Our study has some limitations. Despite covering the entire Fabry population of the Netherlands, the total number of analysed individuals remains limited, especially with regard to those on longer duration of treatment (>5 years). Moreover, during the study observation period several patients had their agalsidase dose and/or preparation changed. Our study demonstrated differences in antibody formation between the two treatment preparations, at least when given at their licensed dose. Additional analyses in larger cohorts are necessary to confirm differences between the two agalsidase preparations with regard to antibody formation or effectiveness in reducing Gb3 and lysoGb3. In addition, in this study we used a neutralizing assay to detect antibodies. While a previous study demonstrated that all patients with antibodies had an aGal A neutralizing effect in vitro[5] it is possible that a patient may develop antibodies that do not exhibit neutralizing capacity.

The lack of a uniform assay to detect and quantify agalsidase antibodies hampers direct comparison with other studies. In most studies on antibody status, antibody analyses was performed by the manufacturer of the enzyme preparation used. Subsequently, claims with respect to antibody formation cannot be extrapolated from one preparation to the other. This emphasizes the need for standardization of anti agalsidase assays and the results of a standardization initiative is eagerly awaited [29].

In conclusion, we demonstrated a negative effect of anti-agalsidase antibodies in male Fabry patients on Gb3 and lysoGb3 levels in plasma and particularly profoundly that of Gb3 in urine. Change of (lyso)Gb3 is associated with change in certain clinical parameters, such LVmass and development of white matter lesions or stroke. Thus, these results suggest a possible deleterious effect these antibodies on clinical efficacy of ERT, a finding that needs to be confirmed in a larger cohort. This emphasizes the urgent need to characterize the impact of anti-agalsidase antibodies on clinical efficacy of ERT in larger cohorts.

Acknowledgments

Els E. Ormel, Fabry specialist nurse is acknowledged for the skilful collection and handling of blood and urine samples.

Author Contributions

Conceived and designed the experiments: JMA JEG GEL BJP . Performed the experiments: WDK EH MM SK. Analyzed the data: SMR JMA BJP JEG CEMH FAW GEL. Contributed reagents/materials/analysis tools: JMA BJP JEG GEL. Wrote the paper: SMR JMA BJP JEG CEMH FAW GEL WDK EH MM SK.

References

1. Schiffmann R, Warnock DG, Banikazemi M, Bultas J, Linthorst GE et al (2009) Fabry disease: progression of nephropathy, and prevalence of cardiac and cerebrovascular events before enzyme replacement therapy. Nephrol Dial Transplant (7):2102-11.
2. Vedder AC, Linthorst GE, van Breemen MJ, Groener JEM, Bemelman FJ et al (2007) The Dutch Fabry cohort: diversity of clinical manifestations and Gb3 levels. J Inherit Metab Dis 30(1):68–78.
3. Eng CM, Guffon N, Wilcox WR, Germain DP, Lee P et al (2001) Safety and efficacy of recombinant human alpha-galactosidase A--replacement therapy in Fabry's disease. N Engl J Med 345(1):9–16.
4. Schiffmann R, Kopp JB, Austin HA, Sabnis S, Moore DF et al (2001) Enzyme replacement therapy in Fabry disease: a randomized controlled trial. JAMA 285(21):2743–2749.
5. Linthorst GE, Hollak CEM, Donker-Koopman WE, Strijland A, Aerts JMFG (2004) Enzyme therapy for Fabry disease: neutralizing antibodies toward agalsidase alpha and beta. Kidney Int 66(4):1589–1595.
6. Bénichou B, Goyal S, Sung C, Norfleet AM, Obrien F (2009) A retrospective analysis of the potential impact of IgG antibodies to agalsidase β on efficacy during enzyme replacement therapy for Fabry disease. Mol Genet Metab 96(1):4–12.
7. Hollak CEM, Linthorst GE (2009) Immune response to enzyme replacement therapy in Fabry disease: impact on clinical outcome? Mol Genet Metab. 96(1):1–3.
8. Vedder AC, Breunig F, Donker-Koopman WE, Mills K, Young E et al (2008) Treatment of Fabry disease with different dosing regimens of agalsidase: effects on antibody formation and GL-3. Mol Genet Metab. 94(3):319–325.
9. Aerts JM, Groener JE, Kuiper S, Donker-Koopman WE, Strijland A et al (2008). Elevated globotriaosylsphingosine is a hallmark of Fabry disease. Proc Natl Acad Sci 105(8):2812–2817.
10. Rombach SM, Dekker N, Bouwman MG, Linthorst GE, Zwinderman AH et al (2010) Plasma globotriaosylsphingosine: Diagnostic value and relation to clinical manifestations of Fabry disease. BBA - Molecular Basis of Disease. 9; 1–8.
11. Sanchez-Niño MD, Sanz AB, Carrasco S, Saleem MA, Mathieson PW et al (2011) Globotriaosylsphingosine actions on human glomerular podocytes: implications for Fabry nephropathy. Nephrol Dial Transplant 26(6):1797-802.
12. van Breemen MJ, Rombach SM, Dekker N, Poorthuis BJ, Linthorst GE et al (2011) Reduction of elevated plasma globotriaosylsphingosine in patients with classic Fabry disease following enzyme replacement therapy. Biochim Biophys Acta 1812(1):70–76.
13. Smid BE, Rombach SM, Aerts JM, Kuiper S, Mirzaian M et al (2011). Consequences of a global enzyme shortage of agalsidase beta in adult Dutch Fabry patients. Orphanet J Rare Dis 31;6(1):69.
14. Vedder AC, Linthorst GE, Houge G, Groener JEM, Ormel EE et al (2007). Treatment of Fabry disease: outcome of a comparative trial with agalsidase alfa or beta at a dose of 0.2 mg/kg. PLoS ONE 2(7):e598.
15. Levey AS, Bosch JP, Lewis JB, Greene T, Rogers N et al (1999) A more accurate method to estimate glomerular filtration rate from serum creatinine: a new prediction equation. Modification of Diet in Renal Disease Study Group. Ann Intern Med 130(6):461–470.
16. Devereux RB, Alonso DR, Lutas EM, Gottlieb GJ, Campo E et al (1986) Echocardiographic assessment of left ventricular hypertrophy: comparison to necropsy findings. Am J Cardiol 57(6):450–458.
17. Groener JEM, Poorthuis BJHM, Kuiper S, Helmond MTJ, Hollak CEM et al (2007) HPLC for Simultaneous Quantification of Total Ceramide, Glucosylceramide, and Ceramide Trihexoside Concentrations in Plasma. Clin Chem. 53(4):742–747.
18. Bligh EG and Dyer WJ (1959) A rapid method of total lipid extraction and purification. Can J Biochem Physiol 37(8):911–917.
19. Young E, Mills K, Morris P, Vellodi A, Lee P et al (2005) Is globotriaosylceramide a useful biomarker in Fabry disease? Acta Paediatr Suppl 94(447):51–4
20. Bekri S, Lidove O, Jaussaud R, Knebelmann B, Barbey F (2006) The role of ceramide trihexoside (globotriaosylceramide) in the diagnosis and follow-up of the efficacy of treatment of Fabry disease: a review of the literature. Cardiovasc Hematol Agents Med Chem. 4(4):289–297.
21. Wilcox WR, Linthorst GE, Germain DP, Feldt-Rasmussen U, Waldek S et al (2012) Anti-α-galactosidase A antibody response to agalsidase beta treatment: Data from the Fabry registry. Mol Genet Metab 105(3):443-9
22. Mendelsohn NJ, Messinger YH, Rosenberg AS, Kishnani PS (2009) Elimination of antibodies to recombinant enzyme in Pompe's disease. N Engl J Med. 360(2):194–195.
23. Garman RD, Munroe K, Richards SM (2004) Methotrexate reduces antibody responses to recombinant human alpha-galactosidase A therapy in a mouse model of Fabry disease. Clin Exp Immunol 137(3):496–502.
24. Lubanda J, Anijalg E, Bzdúch V, Thurberg B, Bénichou B et al (2009). Evaluation of a low dose, after a standard therapeutic dose, of agalsidase beta during enzyme replacement therapy in patients with Fabry disease. Genet Med. 11(4):256-64.
25. Banikazemi M, Bultas J, Waldek S, Wilcox WR, Whitley CB et al (2007) Agalsidase-beta therapy for advanced Fabry disease: a randomized trial. Ann Intern Med 146(2):77–86.
26. Breunig F, Weidemann F, Strotmann J, Knoll A, Wanner C (2006) Clinical benefit of enzyme replacement therapy in Fabry disease. Kidney Int 69(7):1216–1221.
27. Weideman F, Niemann M, Breunig F, Herrmann S, Beer M et al (2009) Long-Term Effects of Enzyme Replacement Therapy on Fabry Cardiomyopathy. Circulation 119(4):487–488.
28. Germain DP, Waldek S, Banikazemi M, Bushinsky DA et al (2007) Sustained, long-term renal stabilization after 54 months of agalsidase beta therapy in patients with Fabry disease. J Am Soc Nephrol. 18(5):1547–1557.
29. Schellekens H (2008) The immunogenicity of therapeutic proteins and the Fabry antibody standardization initiative. Clinical Therapeutics. 30 Suppl B:S50–1.

A Distinct Urinary Biomarker Pattern Characteristic of Female Fabry Patients That Mirrors Response to Enzyme Replacement Therapy

Andreas D. Kistler[1,2]*, Justyna Siwy[3], Frank Breunig[4], Praveen Jeevaratnam[5], Alexander Scherl[6], William Mullen[7], David G. Warnock[8], Christoph Wanner[4], Derralynn A. Hughes[5], Harald Mischak[3,9], Rudolf P. Wüthrich[1], Andreas L. Serra[1]

1 Division of Nephrology, University Hospital, Zürich, Switzerland, **2** Division of Nephrology and Hypertension, University of Miami Miller School of Medicine, Miami, Florida, United States of America, **3** Mosaiques Diagnostics and Therapeutics AG, Hannover, Germany, **4** Division of Nephrology, University Hospital, Würzburg, Germany, **5** Department of Haematology, Hampstead Campus, University College Medical School, London, United Kingdom, **6** Proteomics Core Facility, Faculty of Medicine, University of Geneva, Geneva, Switzerland, **7** School of Life Sciences, College of Medical, Veterinary and Life Sciences, University of Glasgow, Glasgow, United Kingdom, **8** Department of Medicine, University of Alabama at Birmingham, Birmingham, Alabama, United States of America, **9** BHF Glasgow Cardiovascular Research Centre, University of Glasgow, Glasgow, United Kingdom

Abstract

Female patients affected by Fabry disease, an X-linked lysosomal storage disorder, exhibit a wide spectrum of symptoms, which renders diagnosis, and treatment decisions challenging. No diagnostic test, other than sequencing of the alpha-galactosidase A gene, is available and no biomarker has been proven useful to screen for the disease, predict disease course and monitor response to enzyme replacement therapy. Here, we used urine proteomic analysis based on capillary electrophoresis coupled to mass spectrometry and identified a biomarker profile in adult female Fabry patients. Urine samples were taken from 35 treatment-naïve female Fabry patients and were compared to 89 age-matched healthy controls. We found a diagnostic biomarker pattern that exhibited 88.2% sensitivity and 97.8% specificity when tested in an independent validation cohort consisting of 17 treatment-naïve Fabry patients and 45 controls. The model remained highly specific when applied to additional control patients with a variety of other renal, metabolic and cardiovascular diseases. Several of the 64 identified diagnostic biomarkers showed correlations with measures of disease severity. Notably, most biomarkers responded to enzyme replacement therapy, and 8 of 11 treated patients scored negative for Fabry disease in the diagnostic model. In conclusion, we defined a urinary biomarker model that seems to be of diagnostic use for Fabry disease in female patients and may be used to monitor response to enzyme replacement therapy.

Editor: Iris Schrijver, Stanford University School of Medicine, United States of America

Funding: Funding for this study was supported by unrestricted research grants provided by Genzyme (to ADK, RPW and ALS), Shire (to ADK, RPW and ALS) and Amgen (to RPW) and a European Community's 7th Framework Programme grant (to HM; grant agreement HEALTH-F2-2009-241544 (SysKID)). The funders had no role in study design, data collection and analysis, or preparation of the manuscript.

Competing Interests: ADK has received travel grants from Shire HGT and honoraria from Genzyme Inc. HM is the founder and co-owner of Mosaiques Diagnostics, who developed the CE-MS technology. JS is an employee of Mosaiques Diagnostics. DAH has received research support, travel grants and honoraria for meetings and advisory boards from Genzyme Inc, Shire HGT and Amicus therapeutics. DGW is a consultant for Genzyme Corporation on Fabry disease, and has received research support from Genzyme Corporation and Amicus therapeutics. This does not alter the authors' adherence to all the PLoS ONE policies on sharing data and materials.

* E-mail: akistler@med.miami.edu

Introduction

Fabry disease (OMIM 301500) is a rare X-linked inherited lysosomal storage disorder caused by deficient enzymatic activity of α-galactosidase A (GLA). The resulting defect in the catabolism of α-D-galactosyl-containing compounds leads to intracellular accumulation of glycosphingolipids, particularly globotriaosylceramide (Gb_3), causing progressive cellular dysfunction. Main clinical manifestations include: renal disease characterized by proteinuria along with progressive decline of glomerular filtration rate (GFR), left ventricular hypertrophy, stroke, acroparesthesia, hypohidrosis, corneal opacities and angiokeratomas.

Women were previously considered to be mostly asymptomatic carriers of the disease with mild clinical features. However, it has recently become evident that some females can experience nearly all of the symptoms and signs of Fabry disease and may be as severely affected as men [1]. The high heterogeneity of the Fabry phenotype in women has been attributed, at least in part, to random inactivation of one X-chromosome during embryogenesis, which results in a mosaicism of gene expression with some cells expressing the functional enzyme and others expressing the mutated variant [2,3]. The heterogenic Fabry disease phenotype in women renders both, diagnostic testing and treatment decisions more challenging than in men.

Diagnosis of Fabry disease in adult male patients is based on reduced levels of GLA activity in plasma or leukocytes, and confirmation by genetic mutation analysis [4]. However, in heterozygous females GLA assays can be inconclusive, showing ranges of activity between low to normal levels [5]. Thus, diagnosis of Fabry disease in women requires mutation analysis based on direct sequencing of the GLA gene. Although treatment with enzyme replacement therapy (ERT) is recommended by most experts for all affected men [6,7], there is less agreement on which female patients should be treated [8]. While treating all heterozygous females is not justified given the benign disease course in many individuals and the high cost of ERT, limiting ERT to patients with end organ damage would delay therapy to a point where irreversible damage has already occurred. Lack of a reliable disease biomarker further hampers individualized therapy and current dosing recommendations for ERT are relatively arbitrary, both in men and in women.

Despite continuous efforts to identify Fabry disease biomarkers, there is still no clearly useful marker. Gb_3 accumulation in tissues and body fluids (urine and plasma) is one candidate biomarker that has been used for screening [9] and monitoring response to ERT [10,11]. However, the usefulness of plasma and urinary Gb_3 levels has been questioned [12], and in particular, it was not elevated in most hemizygous female patients. Thus, reliable biomarkers for Fabry disease are needed, particularly for female patients.

In our study, we used a proteomic approach to identify biomarkers in heterozygous adult female Fabry patients. Capillary electrophoresis coupled to mass spectrometry (CE-MS) is a reliable high-throughput method to simultaneously measure the excretion of hundreds of polypeptides and small proteins in the urine [13]. This technique utilizes capillary electrophoresis (CE) to separate small proteins according to their electrophoretic characteristics, directly followed by mass spectrometric analysis (MS) by electron spray ionization (ESI) and time-of-flight mass spectrometry (TOF-MS). Thus, every detected peptide will be unambiguously characterized by the migration time in CE and the molecular mass determined by MS. CE-MS is characterized by a low amount of sample required, a short analysis time and a high reproducibility owing to the constant buffer composition and flow characteristics of CE that allow stable ESI conditions for coupling to MS throughout the run. Using CE-MS, a total of over 100,000 different peptides have been detected in human urine, and 5,000 of those are detectable in at least 20% of urine samples [14], rendering CE-MS based urine proteomic analysis a powerful tool for the discovery of potential biomarkers. Here, we used CE-MS of urine to identify a proteomic pattern that characterizes female Fabry patients.

Results

Patient characteristics

We examined a total of 52 treatment-naïve and 11 ERT treated adult female Fabry patients from three clinical centers. The untreated patients were randomly divided in a 2:1 ratio into a training cohort and a validation cohort. Clinical characteristics of these two cohorts and the patients under ERT are given in **Table 1**. Patient characteristics did not differ among centers (data not shown). Overall, patients had relatively few symptoms and well preserved renal and cardiac functions. The Mainz Severity Score Index (MSSI) [15] was available for 19 patients of the training cohort (median 9.0, range 0–24) and 8 patients of the validation cohort (median 6.5, range 1–16).

Fabry disease is characterized by a unique urinary biomarker profile

The compiled data of the CE-MS analysis of all urine samples from the 35 untreated female Fabry patients and the 89 age-matched female healthy controls of the training cohort are shown in **Figure 1 a and b**, respectively. The comparison of the abundance of individual urinary peptides between patients and controls resulted in the identification of 152 peptides with significantly altered urinary

Table 1. Clinical characteristics of all studied female Fabry patients.

cohort	training	validation	ERT
N	35	17	11
age (years)	40.9±12.6	35.7±12.8	36.4±16.4
renal manifestations			
GFR (ml/min/1.73 m^2)	87±23	91±13	85±20
urine protein (mg/g crea), median (range)	65 (20–1364)	59 (44–1248)	55 (50–195)
urine albumin (mg/g crea), median (range)	14 (3–864)	10 (5–258)	8 (5–106)
microalbuminuria, N (%)	7 (21%)	4 (24%)	1 (9%)
macroalbuminuria, N (%)	3 (9%)	0 (0%)	0 (0%)
cardiac manifestations			
LVMI (g/m^2)	83±29	81±19	111±77
LVH, N (%)	5 (14%)	1 (6%)	3 (27%)
arrhythmia, N (%)	1 (3%)	0 (0%)	0 (0%)
nervous system involvement			
stroke, N (%)	2 (6%)	0 (0%)	2 (18%)
acroparesthesia, N (%)	13 (41%)	8 (47%)	11 (100%)
other manifestations			
angiokeratoma, N (%)	4 (13%)	2 (12%)	1 (9%)
hypohydrosis, N (%)	6 (19%)	1 (6%)	4 (36%)

ERT, enzyme replacement therapy; GFR, glomerular filtration rate; LVMI, left ventricular mass index; LVH, left ventricular hypertrophy (defined as LVMI≥110 g/m^2). Data are mean ± SD, unless otherwise stated.

excretion (adjusted p-value<0.05). The CE-MS characteristics of these markers and their regulation in Fabry disease are given in **Table S1**. Due to the fact that the number of potential biomarkers exceeded the number of samples studied, we attempted to identify the most consistent markers by randomly excluding 30% of all patients and controls from the analysis. After repeating this analysis 30 times as an iterative algorithm, we chose only those 64 markers that significantly differed between patients and controls in at least 50% of all permutations. Based on these 64 markers (**Figure 1 c and d**) we next created a support-vector-machine (SVM)-based model to distinguish Fabry patients from controls. The SVM-based model combines the amplitude of all 64 markers for a given urine sample into a score, which denotes the distance of that sample in a 64-dimensional space (every dimension representing the amplitude of one marker) from a hyperplane that is designed to separate the cases from controls. This model correctly classifies all cases and

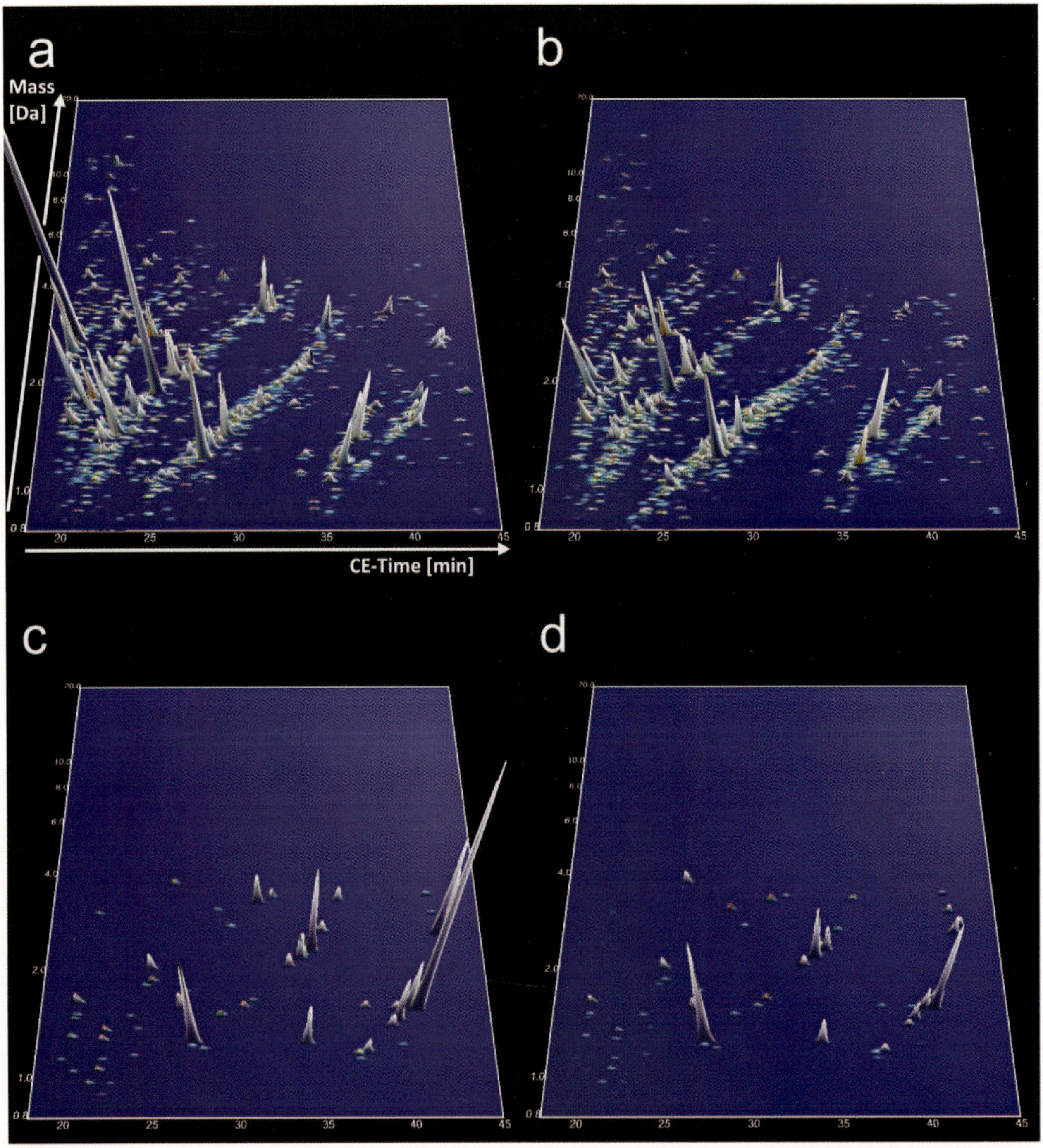

Figure 1. Compiled urinary protein profiles of female Fabry patients (a) and healthy controls (b) included in the training cohort. Normalized MS molecular weight (800–20,000 Da) in logarithmic scale is plotted against normalized CE migration time (18–45 min). The mean signal intensity of polypeptides is given as peak height. 3-D contour plots of the 64 diagnostic markers in the Fabry (c) and healthy control (d) patient cohort with 5× zoom compared to (a) and (b).

controls in the training cohort, corresponding to an area under the receiver-operator-characteristics curve (AUC) of 1. Complete take-one-out crossvalidation in the training cohort yielded an AUC of 0.939 (95% CI 0.882–0.974) (**Figure 2 a**). We then tested the diagnostic model in an independent validation cohort consisting of 17 untreated female Fabry patients and 45 age- and sex-matched healthy controls. Using as a diagnostic cut-off value the mean between the highest and lowest possible cut-off values that would yield 100% sensitivity and 100% specificity in the training cohort, the model achieved a sensitivity of 88.2% and a specificity of 97.8% in the validation cohort (AUC 0.970, 95% CI 0.891–0.996) (**Figure 2 b**) using genetic mutation analysis as a reference. The two Fabry patients from the validation cohort with false-negative proteomic test results did not obviously differ from the remaining patients, in particular they had both GLA mutations which were not unique in the cohort (one missense and one nonsense mutation).

To further evaluate the specificity of the biomarker model for Fabry disease as compared to other disorders, we applied it to a total of 412 previously analyzed urine probes from female patients suffering from a wide variety of renal, metabolic and cardiovascular diseases. The overall specificity of the model applied to these 412 patients was 97%, i.e. the rate of false positive results for Fabry disease among patients with other diseases was very low (**Table 2**).

To gain insight into pathophysiologic mechanisms, we attempted to identify the peptides with altered excretion in Fabry disease. Because the small sample volume used for capillary electrophoresis is not usually sufficient for tandem mass spectrometry based sequencing, we used liquid chromatography-tandem mass spectrometry (LC-MS/MS) for peptide sequencing. We were able to identify the amino acid sequence of 50 out of all 152 differentially excreted peptides, and among the 64 markers used in the diagnostic model, 13 could be identified. The peptide sequences of all identified markers are given along with their CE-MS characteristics in **Table S1**. The majority of identified regulated peptides were collagen fragments with 2/3 of them being up- and 1/3 being downregulated. Interestingly, the C-terminal sequences PPG and PGP were very frequent among the upregulated fragments (6/24 and 11/24, respectively), whereas they were hardly present among the downregulated (0/12 and 1/12, respectively).

Correlation of biomarkers with disease severity and progression

We wondered whether the proteomic changes could reflect disease severity and predict progression in addition to a potential diagnostic use. We therefore correlated the intensity of all 64 diagnostic biomarkers with GFR, albuminuria, and left ventricular mass index (LVMI) in the total treatment-naïve study population consisting of the training and validation cohorts. As a measure of disease progression, we calculated GFR slope by regressing estimated GFR over time for every patient. Follow-up serum creatinine measurements were available for 36 patients. In these 36 patients, an average of 3.6 (range: 2–7) creatinine measurements were available over a mean period of 3.5±1.9 years (1.8±1.7 years before and 1.7±1.4 years after urine sampling for CE-MS analysis). In the unadjusted analysis, several markers showed significant correlations with these clinical measures of disease severity (6 with GFR, 6 with albuminuria, and 11 with LVMI). However, after adjustment for multiple testing, only two correlations remained significant (both with GFR).

Effects of enzyme replacement therapy on the biomarker profile

To analyze the effects of enzyme replacement therapy on the urine proteome in Fabry disease, we analyzed spot urine samples of 11 female Fabry patients that were receiving ERT. The clinical characteristics of these patients are summarized in **Table 1**. Notably, the treated patients did not differ significantly in terms of their clinical parameters from the untreated patients except for a higher rate of reported acroparesthesia ($p<0.001$). In particular, GFR, albuminuria and LVMI were not significantly different. Their median MSSI was 11 (range 5–30) and tended to be higher than in the untreated patients. Details on the type of ERT product, duration and dose, and timing of urine sampling relative to ERT are given in **Table 3**.

The compiled proteomic data of all treated patients are graphically depicted in **Figure 3 a**. Of the 64 biomarkers (**Figure 3 b**) from the diagnostic model, 31 differed significantly between treated and untreated (training and validation cohort) patients in the unadjusted analysis and 16 remained significant after adjustment for multiple testing. The mean levels of all of these biomarkers were changed toward their mean levels in healthy control subjects. Importantly, when applying the diagnostic biomarker model to the treated patients, only three out of 11 scored positive. Thus, ERT seams to have a profound effect on the urinary proteome, changing it toward that of healthy controls. The 3 ERT treated patients who still scored positive for Fabry disease did not significantly differ from the remaining 8 in terms of treatment duration (4.1±2.1 vs. 3.4±2.3 years, $p=0.557$) or time interval between the last ERT infusion and urine sampling for

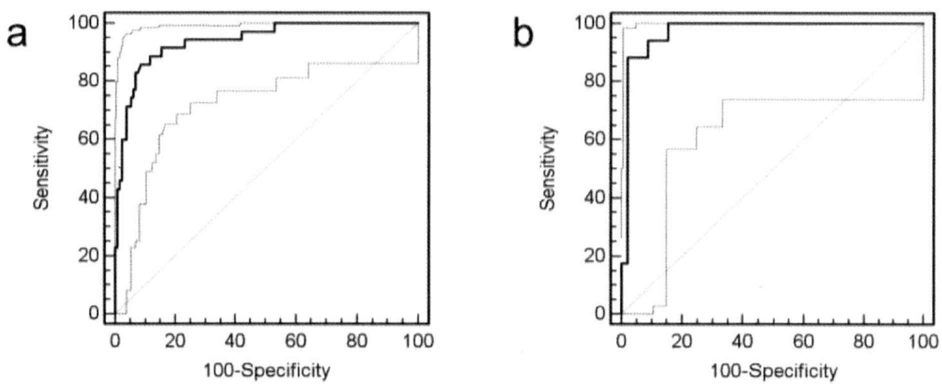

Figure 2. ROC curves for differentiation of Fabry female patients and female healthy controls in the training set upon complete take-one-out crossvalidation (a) and in the independent validation set (b).

Table 2. Specificity of the biomarker model for differentiating Fabry disease from other renal, metabolic and cardiovascular diseases.

Disease	Age	False positive/total N	Specificity (%)
ADPKD	31±8	6/78	92
diabetic nephropathy	58±13	0/47	100
FSGS	42±23	0/27	100
heart failure	68±10	1/9	89
hypertension	66±11	1/17	94
IgA nephropathy	35±13	0/24	100
cardiovascular disease	66±7	3/47	94
minimal change disease	42±10	0/12	100
membranous nephropathy	54±20	0/9	100
kidney stones	56±8	0/8	100
renal cell carcinoma	64±11	0/42	100
bladder cancer	66±11	4/46	91
systemic lupus erythematodes	41±11	0/19	100
ANCA vasculitis	67±6	0/27	100

ADPKD, autosomal dominant polycystic kidney disease; FSGS, focal segmental glomerulosclerosis; ANCA, anti-neutrophil cytoplasmic antibodies. Data are mean ± SD, unless otherwise stated.

proteomic analysis (7.0±4.4 vs. 10.0±8.3 days, $p = 0.364$), although one of them received only a reduced dose of ERT.

Discussion

We have identified and validated a distinct peptide profile in the urine that characterizes adult female Fabry patients. This pattern distinguishes female Fabry patients from healthy controls and from patients with various other forms of kidney or systemic diseases and responds to ERT.

Until now, no study demonstrated the usefulness of a biomarker in adult female Fabry patients as diagnostic marker or as a surrogate marker for disease severity and ERT response. Proteomic techniques offer an unbiased approach to discover unanticipated biomarkers. In addition, the simultaneous detection of hundreds of polypeptides allows for the definition of proteomic biomarker patterns (proteomic profiling), rather than single biomarkers. We used urine rather than serum or plasma for proteomic analysis due to several advantages of urine as sample source that have been discussed in detail elsewhere [16,17]: First, blood contains a high dynamic range between low-level and highly abundant proteins. Removal of highly abundant proteins, such as albumin, which would otherwise obscure the detection of low-level proteins, leads to a concommitant loss of other proteins due to their binding to albumin or unspecific interaction with the affinity column. Second, urine is relatively stable in its composition if handled properly, which may be in part explained by the completion of endogenous proteolysis at the time of urine voidance. Blood, in contrast, contains high level of endogenous protease activity. Third, urine normally does not contain relevant amounts of cellular elements, obviating the need for preanalytical separation. Finally, urine is enriched in low-molecular-weight proteins and peptides, which can be transferred without an initial protease digestion step directly to protein mass spectrometry (top-down MS). Compared to other methods of proteomic analysis, such as 2-dimensional gel electrophoresis (2DGE) or liquid chromatography (LC) followed by mass spectrometry, CE-MS has the advantage of robustness, high reproducibility, low sample volume required, and short analysis time, which make it particularly suitable for clinical proteomic profiling.

Two studies have been previously published that used a proteomic approach to biomarker discovery in Fabry disease. Moore et al. [18] compared serum samples of 12 male and 1 female pediatric Fabry patients before and after 6 months of ERT by LC-MS/MS and found 5 of 50 identified proteins to be significantly altered under therapy. Vojtova et al. [19] compared 11 male and 9 female Fabry patients with or without ERT to 10 healthy controls using 2DGE followed by MALDI-TOF/TOF and identified 5 differentially expressed proteins. However, none of the above mentioned studies validated their results in an independent cohort. Given the large number of peptides being simultaneously detected using proteomic techniques, vigorous adjustment for multiple testing and validation of the results in an

Table 3. Duration, dose and timing of ERT in the analyzed treated patients.

age (years)	body weight (kg)	ERT product and dose/2 weeks	interval from last ERT dose to urine sampling (days)	treatment duration (years)	biomarker score
62	72	agalsidase alfa 0.22 mg/kg	13	0.6	−1.999 (neg)
28	60	agalsidase alfa 0.18 mg/kg	1	3.6	−1.436 (neg)
25	49	agalsidase alfa 0.21 mg/kg	7	3.8	−1.129 (neg)
17	51	agalsidase alfa 0.20 mg/kg	13	2.4	−0.601 (neg)
43	51	agalsidase alfa 0.28 mg/kg	5	1.1	−0.563 (neg)
59	52	agalsidase alfa 0.20 mg/kg	2	5.6	−0.313 (neg)
22	59	agalsidase alfa 0.20 mg/kg	7	5.6	−0.245 (neg)
34	63	agalsidase alfa 0.22 mg/kg	6	0.1	0.060 (neg)
33	55	agalsidase beta 1.27 mg/kg	13	6.4	0.241 (pos)
20	45	agalsidase alfa 0.20 mg/kg	1	5.9	0.316 (pos)
57	58	agalsidase alfa 0.12 mg/kg	17	2.3	0.455 (pos)

ERT, enzyme replacement therapy. The diagnostic cut off value for the biomarker score is 0.1.

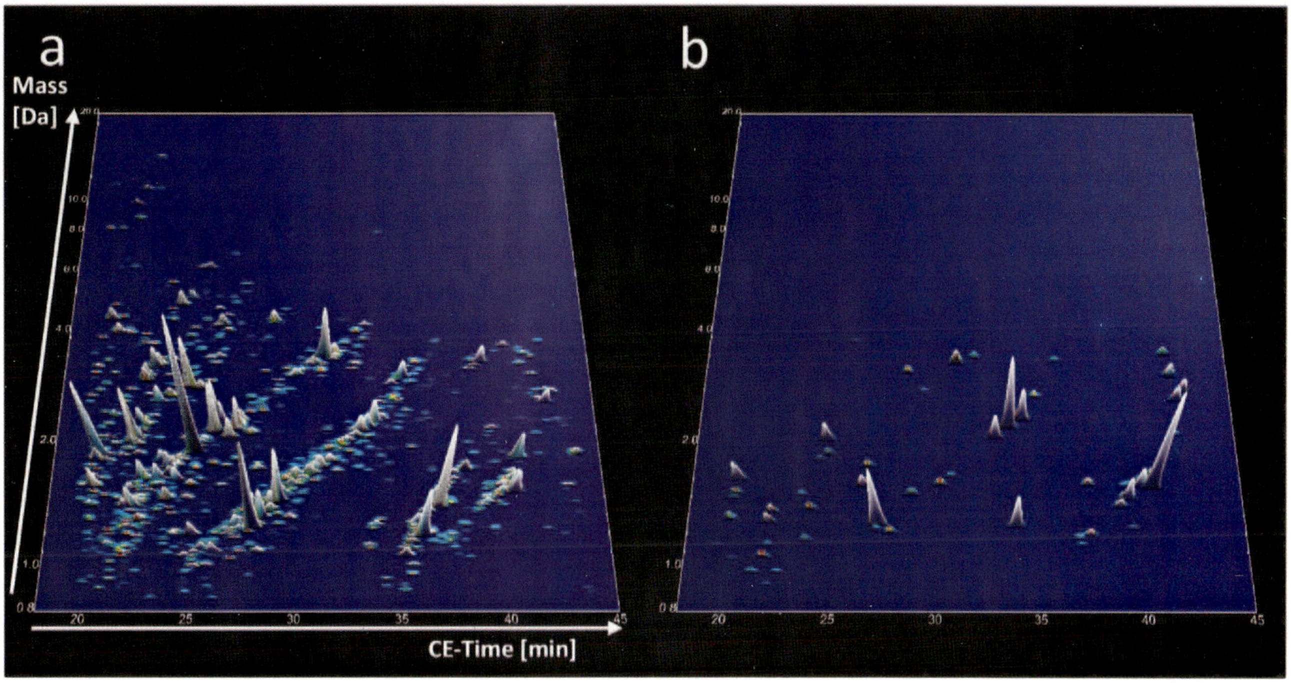

Figure 3. Compiled urinary protein profiles of ERT treated female Fabry patients (a). Normalized MS molecular weight (800–20,000 Da) in logarithmic scale is plotted against normalized CE migration time (18–45 min). The mean signal intensity of polypeptides is given as peak height. (b) 3-D contour plots of the 64 specific markers in the treated Fabry cohort with 5× zoom compared to (a). Note that the proteomic pattern resembles more that of healthy controls (Figure 1b and d) than that of untreated female Fabry patients (Figure 1a and c).

independent cohort are of particular importance [20]. Our study is, to our knowledge, the first proteomic study in Fabry disease, which compares both, treatment-naïve and ERT treated patients to healthy controls and validated the results in an independent cohort.

The biomarker model that we describe distinguishes adult untreated female Fabry patients not only from age-matched healthy controls but also from a large number of different renal diseases with a high degree of specificity. This makes CE-MS particularly useful as a noninvasive diagnostic screening test in unexplained renal, cardiac or cerebrovascular disease. Several recent studies have shown a high prevalence of Fabry disease in populations with unexplained renal failure [21,22,23,24], stroke [25,26,27] or hypertrophic cardiomyopathy [28,29,30]. However, screening these populations for Fabry disease is hampered by the low sensitivity of GLA activity measurement in female patients (50% [31]–67% [32]) whereas diagnostic sequencing of the GLA gene is not feasible given the high cost (currently ca. 2,000–3,000 USD). CE-MS is available for clinical use and considerably cheaper than genetic testing (currently ca. 500 USD, i.e. similar to the price of GLA activity assays). In terms of diagnostic accuracy, CE-MS also favourably compares to urinary Gb_3, for which an AUC of 0.876 has been reported [33] (vs. 0.970 for CE-MS in our study), although lyso-Gb_3 seems to perform better than total Gb_3 [34]. In addition, because similarly accurate CE-MS based diagnostic models have been developed for a variety of other renal and cardiovascular diseases [13,35,36,37,38,39], CE-MS may give hints to an alternative diagnosis in Fabry negative patients, i.e. this approach may offer an efficient diagnostic method, which can detect a variety of diseases using a single diagnostic test. With 97.8%, specificity was high, thus reducing the false positive rate if screening preselected patients. Certainly, the specificity is not ideal, and as a consequence, to avoid high false positive rates, CE-MS is not suitable for screening women at very low risk for Fabry disease, e.g. the general population. Also, mutation analysis will be required for diagnostic confirmation, in particular before initiating a costly therapy. In summary, CE-MS as a diagnostic tool for Fabry disease in females may be clinically useful primarily in the evaluation of patients with unexplained renal disease, hypertrophic cardiomyopathy or cerebrovascular disease, followed by mutation analysis for patients scoring positive in CE-MS.

Importantly, most ERT treated female Fabry patients scored negative in the diagnostic model. Thus, ERT seems to reduce the Fabry-specific alterations in the urinary polypeptide pattern to a level below the diagnostic threshold in most patients receiving ERT. Hence, CE-MS could be useful for monitoring response to treatment, i.e. lack of the urine proteome to normalize may be an indicator of insufficient dosing of ERT. This finding is noteworthy, as ERT dosing recommendations are largely arbitrary to date. Further studies are needed to determine whether the response of the urine proteomic profile to ERT is of prognostic value and whether it is dose-dependent. Given that treated and untreated patients were similar with respect to their end-organ manifestations, reversibility of proteomic alterations under therapy indicates that these alterations probably reflect ongoing pathophysiological processes rather than established organ damage. Thus, it is likely that the changes in the urine proteome that we identified are both dose-dependent and may be of prognostic value as they mirror disease activity.

We found correlations with disease severity for only a minority of the diagnostic biomarkers, which may be explained by a number of reasons: *First*, the diagnostic markers were selected with the aim to achieve a high sensitivity and specificity. Thus, only robust markers that were altered in most patients have been included in the model and these markers may not be the most useful for a severity score. *Second*, most included patients had few manifestations of Fabry disease and the study cohort did not cover the whole spectrum of disease severity. *Third*, most variables used to assess disease severity may be affected by factors other than Fabry disease and show a considerable variation even in healthy subjects. *Fourth*, clinical measures of disease severity mostly reflect irreversible organ damage, whereas many diagnostic pattern biomarkers, as stated above, responded to treatment and thus did not reflect irreversible organ damage. Further studies using larger patient cohorts, including a broader spectrum of disease severity as well as longer follow up time, will be needed to define prognostic markers and to generate a prognostic biomarker model.

Sequencing of naturally occurring peptides by MS/MS still represents a challenge [17]. We were able to identify nearly one third of differentially excreted peptides. Similar to other diseases that have been studied using CE-MS [35,36,38,39,40], most diagnostic biomarkers identified represent collagen fragments. Indeed, collagen fragments appear to be the major constituents of urinary peptides identified to date [39]. The predominance of collagen fragments among identified urinary peptides may be somewhat biased due to the fact that they are more easily fragmented and detected by MS/MS owing to their high content in proline residues. Nevertheless, urinary collagen fragments likely reflect a high normal physiological turnover of the extracellular matrix that may be altered in disease. Of note, most collagen fragments upregulated in female Fabry disease exhibited one of two characteristic C-terminal motivs, PPG or PGP. This particular pattern seems relatively specific for Fabry disease. Further study is needed to test whether these fragments arise from cleavage by a particular type of protease. It is tempting to speculate that lysosomal proteases, such as cathepsins, are released in Fabry disease due to lysosomal accumulation of Gb_3 and lead to cleavage of collagen. Among the other identified peptides, 6 were uromodulin fragments, all of which were upregulated. Interestingly, these were all C-terminal fragments. It has previously been shown that Fabry patients excrete reduced amounts of full-length uromodulin but abnormally processed uromodulin lacking the C-terminus [41]. Efforts to sequence the remaining urinary polypeptides are ongoing and may in the future provide additional pathopysiological insights.

We have limited the analysis to adult female Fabry patients, because we felt that biomarkers to guide diagnosis and treatment decisions are particularly needed for in this patient subgroup. Furthermore, we focused on Fabry patients with relatively few manifestations, aiming to identify markers of early disease progression. Future work will address the use of urine proteomics in both, adult male Fabry patients and in children.

In summary, we defined a urinary biomarker model that allows diagnostic evaluation of female patients for Fabry disease with high accuracy and might be used to monitor response to ERT. Further study is needed to identify prognostic markers and to establish a dose-response relationship between ERT and urinary peptide changes.

Methods

Ethics Statement

Collection of patient data and collection, storage and analysis of urine samples have been approved by the local ethics committees of the three participating centers (Kantonale Ethikkommission Zürich, Ethik-Kommission bei der Medizinischen Fakultät der Universität Würzburg, and Royal free Hospital and Medical School research ethics committee, respectively). All participating subjects gave written informed consent. This study was performed in accordance with the Helsinki Declaration.

Patients and Procedures

52 treatment-naïve and 11 ERT-treated female Fabry patients from three clinical centers were studied. The diagnosis of Fabry disease was confirmed by mutation analysis in all patients. Control urine samples were taken from healthy volunteers and patients with a variety of other renal, metabolic and cardiovascular diseases. These samples have been previously collected as part of several clinical studies (refs [13,35,36,37,38,39] and as yet unpublished studies). All samples were collected in the morning from midstream urine, frozen at −20°C without prior centrifugation and without addition of protease inhibitors, as suggested in recently published recommendations [42].

Sample preparation and CE-MS analysis

All urine samples for CE-MS analyses were stored in accordance with current recommendations of EuroKUP and HUPO/HKUPP (http://www.eurokup.org/sites/default/files/StandardProtocolforUrine Collection.pdf) at −20°C until analysis and underwent a maximum of 2 freeze/thaw cycles. A 0.7 mL aliquot was thawed immediately before use, diluted with 0.7 mL of 2 M urea, 10 mM NH_4OH and 0.02% SDS, filtered using Centrisart ultracentrifugation filter devices (20 kDa MWCO; Sartorius, Goettingen, Germany) at 3,000 g until 1.1 ml of filtrate was obtained and desalted on a PD-10 desalting column (Amersham Bioscience, Uppsala, Sweden) equilibrated in 0.01% NH_4OH in HPLC-grade H_2O. Finally, all samples were lyophilized, stored at 4°C, and resuspended in HPLC-grade H_2O shortly before CE-MS analysis.

CE-MS analysis was performed as described previously [13,43] using a P/ACE MDQ capillary electrophoresis system (Beckman Coulter, Fullerton, USA) on-line coupled to a Micro-TOF MS (Bruker Daltonic, Bremen, Germany). The ESI sprayer (Agilent Technologies, Palo Alto, CA, USA) was grounded, and the ion spray interface potential was set between −4 and −4.5 kV. Data acquisition and MS acquisition methods were automatically controlled by the CE *via* contact-close-relays. Spectra were accumulated every 3 s, over a range of m/z 350 to 3000. Accuracy, precision, selectivity, sensitivity, reproducibility, and stability of the analytical platform were demonstrated and described in great detail elsewhere [13].

Data processing, cluster analysis and statistical methods

Mass spectral ion peaks representing identical molecules at different charge states were deconvoluted into single masses using MosaiquesVisu software [44]. Migration time and ion signal intensity (amplitude) were normalized using internal polypeptide standards [45,46]. For the identification of potential biomarkers, the reported p-values were calculated using the Wilcoxon Rank-Sum test followed by adjustment for multiple testing using the method described by Benjamini and Hochberg [47]. Disease-specific polypeptide patterns were generated using SVM based MosaCluster software [48]. Sensitivity and specificity were calculated based on tabulating the number of correctly classified samples. Confidence intervals (95% CI) based on exact binomial calculations were carried out in MedCalc version 8.1.1.0 (MedCalc Software, Mariakerke, Belgium, http://www.medcalc.be). The Receiver Operating Characteristic (ROC) plot was obtained by plotting all sensitivity values on the y-axis against their equivalent 1-specificity values on the x-axis for all available thresholds (MedCalc Software). The AUC was evaluated, as it provides a single measure of overall accuracy that is not dependent upon a particular threshold [49]. To correlate individual biomarkers with measures of disease severity or with response to treatment, Kendall Tau and Mann-Whiney U-test were used, respectively, and adjustment for multiple testing was done using the Bonferroni correction.

Sequencing of polypeptides

Some of the candidate biomarkers have been previously sequenced using liquid chromatography coupled to tandem mass spectrometry (LC-MS/MS) analysis as recently described in detail [50]. We further tried to identify as yet unidentified urinary peptides that were regulated in Fabry disease. ESI LTQ-OT MS using HCD (higher collisional dissociation) was performed on a LTQ Orbitrap XL equipped with a NanoAcquity system from Waters. Peptides were trapped on a home-made 5 µm 200 Å Magic C18 AQ (Michrom) 0.1×20 mm pre-column and separated on a home-made 5 µm 100 Å Magic C18 AQ (Michrom) 0.75×150 mm column with a gravity-pulled emitter. The analytical separation was run for 65 min using a gradient of H2O/FA 99.9%/0.1% (solvent A) and CH3CN/FA 99.9%/0.1% (solvent B) as follows: 0–1 min 95% A and 5% B, then to 65% A and 35% B at 55 min, and 20% A and 80% B at 65 min at a flow rate of 220 nL/min. For MS survey scans, the OT resolution was set to 60000 and the ion population was set to 5E5 with an m/z window from 400 to 2000. Three precursor ions were selected for collision-induced dissociation in the supplementary hexapole prior to Orbitrap analysis. For this, the ion population was set to 2E5, with an isolation width of 2.5 *m/z* units. The normalized collision energies were set to 40%. Spectral data was converted into .dta files (RAW files generated by ion traps from Thermo Fisher Scientific) and searched against human entries in the Swiss-Prot database (Swiss-Prot Number 2010.06) using the Open Mass Spectrometry Search Algorithm (OMSSA; free from NCBI, http://pubchem.ncbi.nlm.nih.gov/omssa/); e-value cut-off was 0.01. All matched sequences were manually validated.

Acknowledgments

We thank Ruth Russi and Markus Blum for technical assistance and Atul Mehta for collaboration with the care of London patients.

Author Contributions

Conceived and designed the experiments: ADK DGW HM RPW ALS. Performed the experiments: JS AS WM. Analyzed the data: ADK JS HM. Contributed reagents/materials/analysis tools: ADK FB PJ CW DAH RPW ALS. Wrote the paper: ADK ALS.

References

1. Wilcox WR, Oliveira JP, Hopkin RJ, Ortiz A, Banikazemi M, et al. (2008) Females with Fabry disease frequently have major organ involvement: lessons from the Fabry Registry. Mol Genet Metab 93: 112–128.
2. Dobyns WB, Filauro A, Tomson BN, Chan AS, Ho AW, et al. (2004) Inheritance of most X-linked traits is not dominant or recessive, just X-linked. Am J Med Genet A 129A: 136–143.
3. Guffon N (2003) Clinical presentation in female patients with Fabry disease. J Med Genet 40: e38.
4. Desnick RJ, Brady R, Barranger J, Collins AJ, Germain DP, et al. (2003) Fabry disease, an under-recognized multisystemic disorder: expert recommendations for diagnosis, management, and enzyme replacement therapy. Ann Intern Med 138: 338–346.
5. Andrade J, Waters PJ, Singh RS, Levin A, Toh BC, et al. (2008) Screening for Fabry disease in patients with chronic kidney disease: limitations of plasma alpha-galactosidase assay as a screening test. Clin J Am Soc Nephrol 3: 139–145.
6. Eng CM, Guffon N, Wilcox WR, Germain DP, Lee P, et al. (2001) Safety and efficacy of recombinant human alpha-galactosidase A–replacement therapy in Fabry's disease. N Engl J Med 345: 9–16.
7. Schiffmann R, Kopp JB, Austin HA, 3rd, Sabnis S, Moore DF, et al. (2001) Enzyme replacement therapy in Fabry disease: a randomized controlled trial. Jama 285: 2743–2749.
8. El Dib RP, Pastores GM (2010) Enzyme replacement therapy for Anderson-Fabry disease. Cochrane Database Syst Rev 5: CD006663.
9. Kitagawa T, Ishige N, Suzuki K, Owada M, Ohashi T, et al. (2005) Non-invasive screening method for Fabry disease by measuring globotriaosylceramide in whole urine samples using tandem mass spectrometry. Mol Genet Metab 85: 196–202.
10. Rozenfeld PA, De Francesco NP, Borrajo GJ, Ceci R, Fossati CA (2009) An easy and sensitive method for determination of globotriaosylceramide (Gb3) from urinary sediment: utility for Fabry disease diagnosis and treatment monitoring. Clin Chim Acta 403: 194–197.
11. Whitfield PD, Calvin J, Hogg S, O'Driscoll E, Halsall D, et al. (2005) Monitoring enzyme replacement therapy in Fabry disease–role of urine globotriaosylceramide. J Inherit Metab Dis 28: 21–33.
12. Young E, Mills K, Morris P, Vellodi A, Lee P, et al. (2005) Is globotriaosylceramide a useful biomarker in Fabry disease? Acta Paediatr Suppl 94: 51–54; discussion 37–58.
13. Theodorescu D, Wittke S, Ross MM, Walden M, Conaway M, et al. (2006) Discovery and validation of new protein biomarkers for urothelial cancer: a prospective analysis. Lancet Oncol 7: 230–240.
14. Coon JJ, Zurbig P, Dakna M, Dominiczak AF, Decramer S, et al. (2008) CE-MS analysis of the human urinary proteome for biomarker discovery and disease diagnostics. Proteomics Clin Appl 2: 964.
15. Whybra C, Kampmann C, Krummenauer F, Ries M, Mengel E, et al. (2004) The Mainz Severity Score Index: a new instrument for quantifying the Anderson-Fabry disease phenotype, and the response of patients to enzyme replacement therapy. Clin Genet 65: 299–307.
16. Metzger J, Luppa PB, Good DM, Mischak H (2009) Adapting mass spectrometry-based platforms for clinical proteomics applications: The capillary electrophoresis coupled mass spectrometry paradigm. Crit Rev Clin Lab Sci 46: 129–152.
17. Mischak H, Coon JJ, Novak J, Weissinger EM, Schanstra JP, et al. (2009) Capillary electrophoresis-mass spectrometry as a powerful tool in biomarker discovery and clinical diagnosis: an update of recent developments. Mass Spectrom Rev 28: 703–724.
18. Moore DF, Krokhin OV, Beavis RC, Ries M, Robinson C, et al. (2007) Proteomics of specific treatment-related alterations in Fabry disease: a strategy to identify biological abnormalities. Proc Natl Acad Sci U S A 104: 2873–2878.
19. Vojtova L, Zima T, Tesar V, Michalova J, Prikryl P, et al. (2010) Study of urinary proteomes in Anderson-Fabry disease. Ren Fail 32: 1202–1209.
20. Mischak H, Apweiler R, Banks R, Conaway M, Coon J, et al. (2007) Clinical Proteomics: a need to define the field and to begin to set adequate standards. Proteomics Clin Appl 1: 148–156.
21. Kotanko P, Kramar R, Devrnja D, Paschke E, Voigtlander T, et al. (2004) Results of a nationwide screening for Anderson-Fabry disease among dialysis patients. J Am Soc Nephrol 15: 1323–1329.
22. Tanaka M, Ohashi T, Kobayashi M, Eto Y, Miyamura N, et al. (2005) Identification of Fabry's disease by the screening of alpha-galactosidase A activity in male and female hemodialysis patients. Clin Nephrol 64: 281–287.
23. Merta M, Reiterova J, Ledvinova J, Poupetova H, Dobrovolny R, et al. (2007) A nationwide blood spot screening study for Fabry disease in the Czech Republic haemodialysis patient population. Nephrol Dial Transplant 22: 179–186.
24. Gaspar P, Herrera J, Rodrigues D, Cerezo S, Delgado R, et al. (2010) Frequency of Fabry disease in male and female haemodialysis patients in Spain. BMC Med Genet 11: 19.
25. Rolfs A, Bottcher T, Zschiesche M, Morris P, Winchester B, et al. (2005) Prevalence of Fabry disease in patients with cryptogenic stroke: a prospective study. Lancet 366: 1794–1796.
26. Baptista MV, Ferreira S, Pinho EMT, Carvalho M, Cruz VT, et al. (2010) Mutations of the GLA gene in young patients with stroke: the PORTY-STROKE study–screening genetic conditions in Portuguese young stroke patients. Stroke 41: 431–436.
27. Brouns R, Thijs V, Eyskens F, Van den Broeck M, Belachew S, et al. (2010) Belgian Fabry study: prevalence of Fabry disease in a cohort of 1000 young patients with cerebrovascular disease. Stroke 41: 863–868.

28. Nakao S, Takenaka T, Maeda M, Kodama C, Tanaka A, et al. (1995) An atypical variant of Fabry's disease in men with left ventricular hypertrophy. N Engl J Med 333: 288–293.
29. Sachdev B, Takenaka T, Teraguchi H, Tei C, Lee P, et al. (2002) Prevalence of Anderson-Fabry disease in male patients with late onset hypertrophic cardiomyopathy. Circulation 105: 1407–1411.
30. Chimenti C, Pieroni M, Morgante E, Antuzzi D, Russo A, et al. (2004) Prevalence of Fabry disease in female patients with late-onset hypertrophic cardiomyopathy. Circulation 110: 1047–1053.
31. Mehta A, Ricci R, Widmer U, Dehout F, Garcia de Lorenzo A, et al. (2004) Fabry disease defined: baseline clinical manifestations of 366 patients in the Fabry Outcome Survey. Eur J Clin Invest 34: 236–242.
32. Linthorst GE, Vedder AC, Aerts JM, Hollak CE (2005) Screening for Fabry disease using whole blood spots fails to identify one-third of female carriers. Clin Chim Acta 353: 201–203.
33. Paschke E, Fauler G, Winkler H, Schlagenhauf A, Plecko B, et al. (2010) Urinary Total Globotriaosylceramide and Isoforms to Identify Women With Fabry Disease: A Diagnostic Test Study. Am J Kidney Dis.
34. Auray-Blais C, Ntwari A, Clarke JT, Warnock DG, Oliveira JP, et al. (2010) How well does urinary lyso-Gb3 function as a biomarker in Fabry disease? Clin Chim Acta 411: 1906–1914.
35. Delles C, Schiffer E, von Zur Muhlen C, Peter K, Rossing P, et al. (2010) Urinary proteomic diagnosis of coronary artery disease: identification and clinical validation in 623 individuals. J Hypertens 28: 2316–2322.
36. Kistler AD, Mischak H, Poster D, Dakna M, Wuthrich RP, et al. (2009) Identification of a unique urinary biomarker profile in patients with autosomal dominant polycystic kidney disease. Kidney Int 76: 89–96.
37. Haubitz M, Good DM, Woywodt A, Haller H, Rupprecht H, et al. (2009) Identification and validation of urinary biomarkers for differential diagnosis and evaluation of therapeutic intervention in anti-neutrophil cytoplasmic antibody-associated vasculitis. Mol Cell Proteomics 8: 2296–2307.
38. Schiffer E, Vlahou A, Petrolekas A, Stravodimos K, Tauber R, et al. (2009) Prediction of muscle-invasive bladder cancer using urinary proteomics. Clin Cancer Res 15: 4935–4943.
39. Good DM, Zurbig P, Argiles A, Bauer HW, Behrens G, et al. (2010) Naturally occurring human urinary peptides for use in diagnosis of chronic kidney disease. Mol Cell Proteomics 9: 2424–2437.
40. Rossing K, Mischak H, Dakna M, Zurbig P, Novak J, et al. (2008) Urinary proteomics in diabetes and CKD. J Am Soc Nephrol 19: 1283–1290.
41. Vylet'al P, Hulkova H, Zivna M, Berna L, Novak P, et al. (2008) Abnormal expression and processing of uromodulin in Fabry disease reflects tubular cell storage alteration and is reversible by enzyme replacement therapy. J Inherit Metab Dis 31: 508–517.
42. Thongboonkerd V (2007) Practical points in urinary proteomics. J Proteome Res 6: 3881–3890.
43. Wittke S, Mischak H, Walden M, Kolch W, Radler T, et al. (2005) Discovery of biomarkers in human urine and cerebrospinal fluid by capillary electrophoresis coupled to mass spectrometry: towards new diagnostic and therapeutic approaches. Electrophoresis 26: 1476–1487.
44. Neuhoff N, Kaiser T, Wittke S, Krebs R, Pitt A, et al. (2004) Mass spectrometry for the detection of differentially expressed proteins: a comparison of surface-enhanced laser desorption/ionization and capillary electrophoresis/mass spectrometry. Rapid Commun Mass Spectrom 18: 149–156.
45. Theodorescu D, Fliser D, Wittke S, Mischak H, Krebs R, et al. (2005) Pilot study of capillary electrophoresis coupled to mass spectrometry as a tool to define potential prostate cancer biomarkers in urine. Electrophoresis 26: 2797–2808.
46. Jantos-Siwy J, Schiffer E, Brand K, Schumann G, Rossing K, et al. (2009) Quantitative urinary proteome analysis for biomarker evaluation in chronic kidney disease. J Proteome Res 8: 268–281.
47. Reiner A, Yekutieli D, Benjamini Y (2003) Identifying differentially expressed genes using false discovery rate controlling procedures. Bioinformatics 19: 368–375.
48. Decramer S, Wittke S, Mischak H, Zurbig P, Walden M, et al. (2006) Predicting the clinical outcome of congenital unilateral ureteropelvic junction obstruction in newborn by urinary proteome analysis. Nat Med 12: 398–400.
49. DeLeo J Receiver operating characteristic laboratory (ROCLAB): Software fordeveloping decision strategies that account for uncertainty; 1993 Apr 25, 318–325.
50. Zurbig P, Renfrow MB, Schiffer E, Novak J, Walden M, et al. (2006) Biomarker discovery by CE-MS enables sequence analysis via MS/MS with platform-independent separation. Electrophoresis 27: 2111–2125.

14

Gene Therapy in a Humanized Mouse Model of Familial Hypercholesterolemia Leads to Marked Regression of Atherosclerosis

Sadik H. Kassim[1], Hui Li[2], Luk H. Vandenberghe[1], Christian Hinderer[1], Peter Bell[1], Dawn Marchadier[2], Aisha Wilson[2], Debra Cromley[2], Valeska Redon[2], Hongwei Yu[1], James M. Wilson[1], Daniel J. Rader[2]*

1 Gene Therapy Program, Department of Pathology and Laboratory Medicine, University of Pennsylvania, Philadelphia, Pennsylvania, United States of America, **2** Institute for Translational Medicine and Therapeutics, University of Pennsylvania, Philadelphia, Pennsylvania, United States of America

Abstract

Background: Familial hypercholesterolemia (FH) is an autosomal codominant disorder caused by mutations in the low-density lipoprotein receptor (*LDLR*) gene. Homozygous FH patients (hoFH) have severe hypercholesterolemia leading to life threatening atherosclerosis in childhood and adolescence. Mice with germ line interruptions in the *Ldlr and Apobec1* genes (*Ldlr*$^{-/-}$*Apobec1*$^{-/-}$) simulate metabolic and clinical aspects of hoFH, including atherogenesis on a chow diet.

Methods/Principal Findings: In this study, vectors based on adeno-associated virus 8 (AAV8) were used to deliver the gene for mouse *Ldlr* (*mLDLR*) to the livers of *Ldlr*$^{-/-}$*Apobec1*$^{-/-}$ mice. A single intravenous injection of AAV8.*mLDLR* was found to significantly reduce plasma cholesterol and non-HDL cholesterol levels in chow-fed animals at doses as low as 3×10^9 genome copies/mouse. Whereas *Ldlr*$^{-/-}$*Apobec1*$^{-/-}$ mice fed a western-type diet and injected with a control AAV8.null vector experienced a further 65% progression in atherosclerosis over 2 months compared with baseline mice, *Ldlr*$^{-/-}$ *Apobec1*$^{-/-}$ mice treated with AAV8.*mLDLR* realized an 87% regression of atherosclerotic lesions after 3 months compared to baseline mice. Immunohistochemical analyses revealed a substantial remodeling of atherosclerotic lesions.

Conclusions/Significance: Collectively, the results presented herein suggest that AAV8-based gene therapy for FH may be feasible and support further development of this approach. The pre-clinical data from these studies will enable for the effective translation of gene therapy into the clinic for treatment of FH.

Editor: Harald H. H. W. Schmidt, Maastricht University, Netherlands

Funding: National Heart Lung and Blood Institute P01-HL059407 (JMW) and National Institute of Diabetes and Digestive and Kidney Diseases P30-DK047757 (JMW). The funders had no role in study design, data collection and analysis, decision to publish, or preparation of the manuscript.

Competing Interests: J.M.W. is a consultant to ReGenX Holdings, and is a founder of, holds equity in, and receives a grant from affiliates of ReGenX Holdings; in addition, he is an inventor on patents licensed to various biopharmaceutical companies, including affiliates of ReGenX Holdings. This does not alter the authors' adherence to all the PLoS ONE policies on sharing data and materials, as detailed online in the guide for authors.

* E-mail: rader@mail.med.upenn.edu

Introduction

Familial hypercholesterolemia (FH) is a life-threatening genetic disease caused by mutations in the LDL receptor (*LDLR*) gene [1]. Patients with loss-of-function mutations in both *LDLR* alleles (homozygous FH – hoFH) develop atherosclerosis before age 20 and, if not treated, rarely survive past age 30. Patients with hoFH are minimally responsive to conventional LDL-lowering pharmacologic therapy. Orthotopic liver transplantation has been demonstrated to substantially reduce LDL-cholesterol (LDL-C) in hoFH patients, but obvious disadvantages and risks are associated with this approach [2,3]. The current standard of care in hoFH is LDL apheresis, a physical method of purging the plasma of LDL-C which can transiently reduce LDL-C by more than 50% [4,5,6]. However, there is re-accumulation of LDL-C in plasma [7], and therefore apheresis has to be repeated every one to two weeks. Anecdotal evidence suggests that this procedure may delay the onset of atherosclerosis [8]; nonetheless it is laborious, expensive, and not readily available. Furthermore, although the procedure is generally well tolerated, the fact that it needs frequent repetition and IV access can be challenging for many patients and associated with morbidity. Therefore, there is a tremendous unmet medical need for new therapies for hoFH.

Liver-directed gene therapy has been tested as a possible alternative therapy for liver metabolic diseases such as hoFH. Initial attempts to treat FH with gene therapy utilized an *ex vivo* approach wherein autologous hepatocytes transduced with retroviruses containing *LDLR* cDNA were transplanted into homozygous FH patients [9]. Although this approach was well-tolerated by patients, the impact on cholesterol metabolism was modest and variable due in part to the limited amount of gene transfer achievable [9,10]. More recently, attention has focused on the potential of liver directed *in vivo* gene therapy for hoFH.

Nearly all *in vivo* gene therapy based attempts to correct FH have used first generation adenoviral (Ad) vectors or helper-dependent adenoviral vector systems [11,12,13,14]. While these vectors have proven to be quite efficient, they are associated with substantial toxicity due in part to capsid mediated activation of innate immunity and local and systemic inflammation [15,16]. Compared to adenoviral constructs, vectors based on adeno-associated virus (AAV) demonstrate the attractive property of long-term expression without evidence of inflammation [15,16,17]. Initial AAV studies used AAV serotype 2 (AAV2) to express *LDLR* [17]. This approach led to a transient drop in the cholesterol of fat-fed *Ldlr*$^{-/-}$ mice but also triggered a transgene-specific immune response and loss of liver-associated vector DNA; furthermore transduction efficiency was low and efficacy was incomplete. AAVs based on novel capsids have recently been identified [18]; these vector candidates have shown impressive pre-clinical data. One particular vector -AAV8- has shown great promise in mouse and monkey models of liver directed gene transfer, including higher transduction efficiency, less pre-existing humoral immunity in humans, and diminished T cell responses to the capsid [19,20,21]. AAV mediated gene transfer with these new vectors showed long-term correction of the metabolic defect in fat-fed *Ldlr*$^{-/-}$ mice [22] and prevention of atherosclerosis in apoliporotein E deficient (*ApoE*$^{-/-}$) mice [19] and fat-fed *Ldlr*$^{-/-}$ mice [22].

Intrinsic differences in the lipoprotein metabolism of FH animal models used in gene therapy studies and humans, however, limit the relevance of previous preclinical studies to the potential for human application. In humans, the liver synthesizes solely the full-length form of apolioprotein B (APOB), called APOB100, which contains in its carboxy terminal region the motif mediating binding to LDLR. However, mice express in liver high levels of the APOB mRNA editing catalytic polypeptide-1 (APOBEC1), which results in editing of the *ApoB* RNA transcript and the production of a truncated form of the APOB protein called APOB48, which does not bind to LDLR. Mice deleted in the *Apobec1* gene synthesize only APOB100 protein in the liver and thus more closely resemble human physiology. *Ldlr*$^{-/-}$*Apobec1*$^{-/-}$ mice much more closely simulate the metabolic and clinical aspects of FH than do *Ldlr*$^{-/-}$ mice [23]. On a chow diet, these mice develop spontaneous and substantial hypercholesterolemia with a lipoprotein profile similar to that of human hoFH patients. Furthermore, in contrast to *Ldlr*$^{-/-}$ mice which require a high-fat diet to develop atherosclerosis and develop relatively simple macrophage-rich atherosclerotic lesions, *Ldlr*$^{-/-}$*Apobec1*$^{-/-}$ mice fed a chow diet develop extensive atherosclerosis throughout the aorta, including most of the branch points; these lesions range in morphology from simple lesions of macrophage foam cells to more complex lesions containing smooth muscle cells and extracellular matrix [24]. Feeding a high-fat diet to *Ldlr*$^{-/-}$*Apobec1*$^{-/-}$ mice further enhances the rate of progression of atherosclerosis [23]. To date, no gene therapy studies have evaluated FH correction in this mouse model.

For *in vivo* gene therapy of FH to become a clinical reality, pre-clinical studies need to be conducted using the proper combination of vector, transgene, and animal model that accurately reflects FH pathophysiology. The advent of AAV8 and the availability of *Ldlr*$^{-/-}$*Apobec1*$^{-/-}$ mice provide an opportunity to critically evaluate the potential of gene therapy for hoFH using current models and gene transfer technology.

Materials and Methods

Animals

Male C57BL/6 *Ldlr*$^{-/-}$*Apobec1*$^{-/-}$ mice were bred in house and have been described elsewhere [23]. For expression and efficacy studies, mice were given unrestricted access to water and were fed a standard chow diet. The vector was injected via an intravenous tail-vein injection with specified genome copies (gc)/mouse. Animals were sacrificed 35 days after gene transfer. For all studies, blood was obtained at least one times before and at designated time-points after gene transfer. For atherosclerosis regression studies, three groups of male mice (n = 10 per group) were given unrestricted access to water and were fed a high-fat western diet (0.15% cholesterol, 21% butterfat; DYETS, PA, USA) starting 8 weeks prior to vector injection and maintained on this diet throughout the experiment. After 8 weeks on the high-fat diet, prior to vector injection, one group of mice (baseline) was sacrificed for various analyses. The second and third groups were injected with 1×10^{11} GC of AAV8.TBG.*mLDLR* or AAV8.TBG.*nLacZ* vector, respectively. Eight weeks after vector treatment, mice were sacrificed for the indicated analyses. *Ldlr*$^{-/-}$*Apobec1*$^{-/-}$*ApoB*$^{+/+}$ mice were generated by crossing *Ldlr*$^{-/-}$*Apobec1*$^{-/-}$ [23] with human *ApoB* transgenic mice [25]. *Ldlr*$^{-/-}$*Apobec1*$^{-/-}$*ApoB*$^{+/+}$ mice are viable, fertile, and do not display any gross physical or behavioral abnormalities. These animals were bred in house and maintained on a chow diet. All study protocols were approved by the Institutional Animal Care and Use Committee at The University of Pennsylvania (Protocol Approval #800791).

Cloning and AAV Production

The mouse *Vldlr* and *Ldlr* AAV constructs were cloned in an AAV ITR flanked construct named pENN AAV TBG PI construct which drives expression from a thyroxine-binding globulin (TBG) hepatocyte specific promoter with a chimeric intron from Promega Corporation (Madison, Wisconsin) encoding the 5′-donor site from the first intron of the human b-globin and the branch and 3′-acceptor site from the intron located between the leader and body of an immunoglobulin gene heavy chain variable region. The cDNA sequences were amplified from PCR from constructs acquired from openbiosystems.com (*Ldlr*: genbank accession number BC019207; *Vldlr*: BC013622) with primers:

MLU-mLDLR F (gtaagcACGCGTaagctaaggatgagcaccgcgga-tctgat),

MLU-mLDLR R (TTGAttcACGCGTtcatgccacatcgtcctccagg-ctgaccatc),

MLU-mVLDLR F (gtaagcACGCGTgcgggcagcatgggcacgtccg-cgcgctgg),

SAL-mVLDLR R (ggaatcGTCGACtcaagccagatcatcatctgtgctta-caac).

The *Vldlr* construct was generated by MluI-SalI insertion of the cDNA insert into pENN AAV TBG PI construct. *Ldlr* was cloned by MluI insertion of the cDNA amplicon into the same AAV construct. AAV vector was generated by triple transfection of the AAV ITR flanked construct with the packaging plasmid pAAV2/8 and the helper plasmid pdF6 as previously described [20,21]. AAV vector particles were purified by double CsCl gradient banding as described in Wang et al [21].

En Face Quantification of Atherosclerotic Lesions in the Aorta

Mice were anesthetized, the aorta was gently perfused with saline via the left ventricle, and the heart was cut off at the base and embedded in OCT. The rest of the aorta was removed and fixed in 10% formalin/PBS for at least 3 days. Aortic arch lesion area was quantitated using a method similar to that previously described [26,27]. After the adventitial and adipose tissue was removed, the aortic arches were stained with oil red O solution (1.8% oil red O, wt/vol, in 60% isopropanol, filtered twice through a 0.2-μm filter) for 15 minutes and destained with 60% isopropanol for 5 minutes to eliminate background staining. The outer curvature of the arch was cut longitudinally, and the arch was laid open on a glass slide and mounted in Supermount (BioGenex). The image was captured with the use of a Leica MZIZ microscope and digitized, and the oil red O–stained lesion area was quantitated using the Image J image analysis system. All data capture and quantitation were performed in a blinded fashion.

Immunohistochemistry and Quantification of Atherosclerosis Lesions in the Aortic Root

LDLR expression in liver was detected on frozen sections that were fixed in acetone (−20C) for 5 min, air dried, blocked with 1% goat serum in PBS for 20 min, and incubated for 1 h with a rabbit serum against LDLR (a gift from Dr. William Lagor and Dr. Gene C. Ness) diluted 1:200 in blocking buffer [28]. After washing in PBS, the sections were treated for 30 min with FITC-labeled secondary antibodies against rabbit IgG diluted in blocking buffer (Vector Laboratories, 1:200) and mounted with Vectashield containing DAPI (Vector). Fresh-frozen OCT-embedded hearts were used for Immunohistochemistry of lesions in the aortic root. Serial sections of the aortic root were mounted on masked slides. Sections were fixed in acetone, air-dried, and rehydrated in PBS containing 0.02% NaN_3 and blocked with 1% BSA in PBS/NaN_3 and 1% goat serum. For lesion analysis, sections were stained with oil-red-o or hematoxylin and eosin. Images were captured digitally with a video camera connected to a Leica microscope. The digitized images were analyzed with Image J image analysis software. Total lesion area was quantified by manual tracing of entire intimal lesion in 10 equally spaced aortic root sections per mouse. The acquisition of images and analysis of lesions were performed in a blinded fashion. For detection of macrophages, or VCAM-1, sections were reacted with rat antibodies against CD68 (clone FA-11, Serotec) and VCAM-1 (clone 429, BD Pharmingen) diluted 1:200 and 1:25 in blocking buffer, respectively. A Vectastain Elite ABC kit (Vector) was used according to the manufacturer's protocol to visualize bound rat antibodies. Collagen was detected by trichrome staining using a staining kit from Sigma following the manufacturer's protocol.

Analytical Methods

The plasma total cholesterol levels were measured in individual mice at each time point with an enzymatic assay on a Cobas Fara II (Roche Diagnostic Systems Inc) with the use of Sigma reagents (Sigma Chemical Co). Plasma samples from groups of 5 mice were pooled at each time point and subjected to fast protein liquid chromatography (FPLC) gel filtration (Pharmacia LKB Biotechnology) on two Superose 6 columns. Cholesterol concentrations in the fractions were determined with an enzymatic assay (Wako Pure Chemical Industries, Ltd). For hepatic cholesterol and triglyceride analysis, liver was homogenized in a saline solution (~250 mg liver/ml saline). Cholesterol and triglyceride were measured as described [29] after solubilization of lipid by deoxycholate using cholesterol reagent or triglyceride reagent and lipid lintrol standards.

Statistical Analyses

Atherosclerotic lesion area data were subjected to a 1-way ANOVA. Experimental groups were compared with the baseline group by using the Dunnett test. Repeated-measures ANOVA was used to compare cholesterol levels among different groups of mice

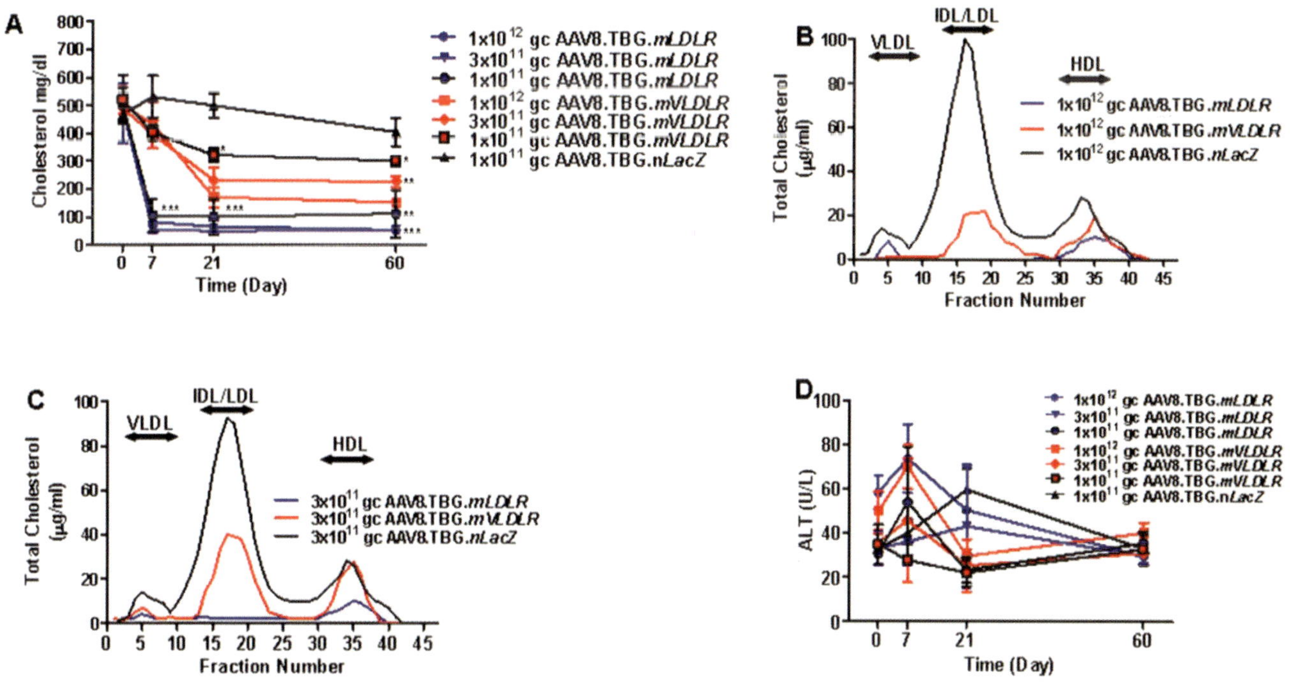

Figure 1. Evaluation of AAV8 encoding mouse *Vldlr* or mouse *Ldlr* in Ldlr-/-Apobec1-/- Mice. (A) Plasma cholesterol levels in *Ldlr-/-Apobec1-/-* mice after treatment with AAV8.TBG.*mVLDLR* or AAV8.TBG.*mLDLR* (n = 5 animals per dose group). Each point represents mean ± s.d. *P<0.05, **P<0.01, ***P<0.001 (B and C) Pooled mouse plasma from AAV-injected *Ldlr-/-Apobec1-/-* (n = 5) were analyzed by FPLC fractionation and the cholesterol content of each fraction was determined. (B) Lipoprotein profile of animals injected with 1×10^12 GC of vector 28 days after treatment. (C) Lipoprotein profile of animals injected with 3×10^11 GC of vector 28 days after treatment. (D) Plasma ALT levels in *Ldlr-/-Apobec1-/-* mice after treatment with AAV8.TBG.*mVLDLR* or AAV.TBG.*mLDLR* (n = 5 animals per dose group). Each point represents mean ± s.d. At all time points and doses examined, no significant differences in ALT were detected between AAV8.TBG.*mLDLR* and AAV8.TBG.*mVLDLR*.

over time after gene transfer. Statistical significance for all comparisons was assigned at P<0.05. Graphs represent mean± SD values.

Results

mLDLR is more effective than *mVLDLR* in correcting hypercholesterolemia

Although *LDLR* is the logical transgene to use for gene therapy of FH, we and others have considered an alternative approach using the gene encoding the very-low-density lipoprotein receptor (*VLDLR*) which is a member of the *LDLR* super family that binds with high affinity to APOE containing lipoproteins such as VLDL [14,17]. While this gene is not expressed in liver, vector mediated gene transfer of *VLDLR* to liver does partially ameliorate hypercholesterolemia in rabbits [13] and mice deficient in *Ldlr* [12,13,17]. One advantage of VLDLR is that it should be viewed as a self protein in hoFH patients and therefore should not elicit adaptive immune responses [12,17].

A proximal step in the development of a clinical trial of gene therapy for hoFH is the selection of the transgene which, in the case of hoFH, could be *LDLR* or *VLDLR*. We performed a direct comparison of AAV8 mediated gene transfer of the murine versions of both genes at three doses (1×10^{12}, 3×10^{11} and 1×10^{11} GC/mouse) in chow-fed *Ldlr*$^{-/-}$*Apobec1*$^{-/-}$ mice using a liver specific promoter, thyroxine binding globulin (TBG). Within seven days of vector administration, a marked reduction in plasma cholesterol was realized in *Ldlr*$^{-/-}$*Apobec1*$^{-/-}$ mice injected with AAV8.TBG.*mLDLR* at all doses compared to control AAV8.TBG.*nLacZ* treated animals, in which serum lipids were maintained at the high baseline levels throughout the study (Fig. 1A). In the low-dose (1×10^{11} GC/mouse) group, for example, plasma cholesterol levels significantly fell from a baseline level of 505±59 mg/dl to 112±34 mg/dl. AAV8.TBG.*mVLDLR* treated animals realized much less significant decreases in levels of total plasma cholesterol (Fig. 1A). We also examined FPLC fraction cholesterol levels 28 days after treatment with the high and (Fig. 1B) and intermediate-dose of vector (Fig. 1C). AAV8.TBG.*mLDLR* at both doses was considerably more effective than AAV8.TBG.*mVLDLR* in reducing levels of VLDL and IDL/LDL in *Ldlr*$^{-/-}$*Apobec1*$^{-/-}$ mice; in contrast, a prominent IDL/LDL peak was detected at both doses of AAV8.TBG.*mVLDLR*

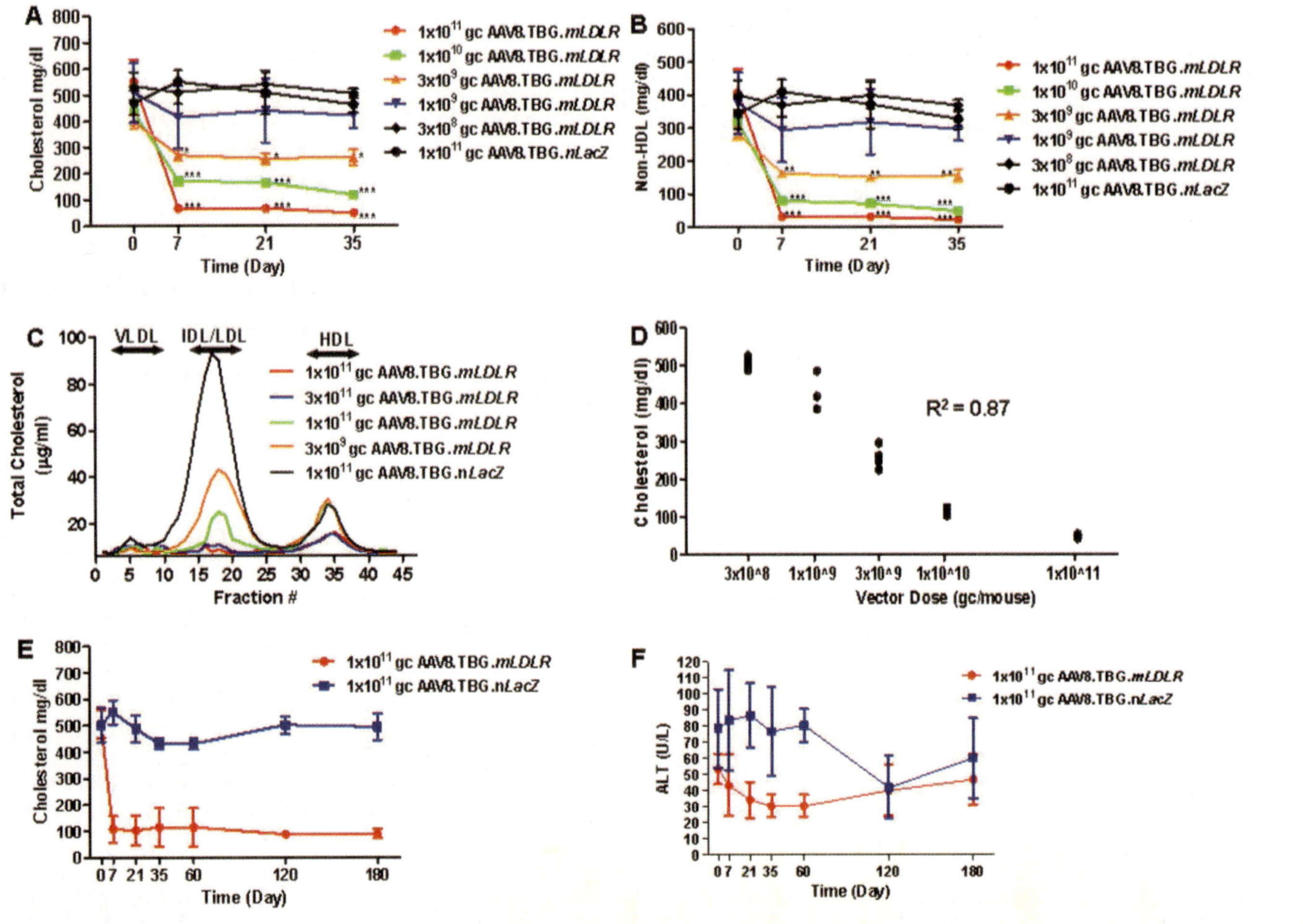

Figure 2. Evaluation of the minimum effective dose of AAV.TBG.*mLDLR* vector in *Ldlr-/-Apobec1-/-* Mice. Amounts of (A) Plasma cholesterol and (B) non-HDL cholesterol were evaluated in *Ldlr-/-Apobec1-/-* mice up to day 35 after treatment with different doses of AAV8.mLDLR (n = 9 animals per dose group). Each point represents mean ± s.d. *P<0.05, **P<0.01, ***P<0.001. (C) Pooled mouse plasma from AAV-injected *Ldlr-/-Apobec1-/-* (n = 5, per dose group) were analyzed by FPLC fractionation and the cholesterol content of each fraction was determined. (D) Dose response analysis of Day 60 samples examining cholesterol levels as a function of vector dose. (E) Plasma cholesterol and (F) Alanine transaminase were evaluated in *Ldlr-/-Apobec1-/-* mice up to day 180 days after treatment with 1×10^11 GC of AAV8.TBG.*mLDLR* (n = 10) or 1×10^11 GC of AAV8.TBG.*nLacZ* (n = 9). Each point represents mean ± s.d.

treatment. No elevation of transaminases was detected in any group (Fig. 1D). Given these results, the remaining experiments focused exclusively on characterizing AAV8.TBG.*mLDLR* function *in vivo*.

AAV8 mediated gene transfer of mLDLR is effective at low doses of vector

Critical to the success of gene therapy is the demonstration of efficacy at doses of vector that are safe and can be easily manufactured. Formal regulatory review of a proposed human study requires an assessment of the minimal dose that shows some metabolic/clinical effect [30]. Chow-fed male *Ldlr*$^{-/-}$*Apobec1*$^{-/-}$ mice were treated with a single intravenous injection of AAV8.TBG.mLDLR; doses ranged from 1×10^{12} genome copies/mouse to 3×10^{8} genome copies (GC)/mouse. Thirty-five days after vector injection, mice were necropsied and livers were harvested and processed for presence and abundance of vector genomes and LDLR protein [21].

Correction of hypercholesterolemia was found to be dose dependent. With respect to total cholesterol (Fig. 2A) and non-HDL cholesterol (Fig. 2B), reduction was realized within seven days of vector treatment. The most significant decreases were observed at the highest treatment doses. Surprisingly, reduction was observed with doses as low as 3×10^{9} GC/mouse with total cholesterol levels dropping 35% from 397±26 mg/dl at baseline to 256±29 mg/dl on day 35 and non-HDL cholesterol levels decreasing by 45% from 284±19 mg/dl at baseline to 154±17 mg/dl (Fig. 2B) on day 35. This magnitude of correction is comparable to that seen in *Ldlr*$^{-/-}$*Apobec1*$^{-/-}$ mice treated with 1×10^{11} GC/mouse of AAV8.TBG.*mVLDLR* (Fig. 1A), suggesting that AAV8.TBG.*mLDLR* is at least 30 fold more effective than AAV8.TBG.*mVLDLR*. With respect to FPLC fraction cholesterol levels, all doses of AAV8.TBG.*mLDLR*, except 3×10^{8} GC, led to substantial reductions in the IDL/LDL peak compared to AAV8.TBG.*nLacZ* treated *Ldlr*$^{-/-}$*Apobec1*$^{-/-}$ mice. Only the higher doses of 1×10^{11} GC/mouse and 1×10^{10} GC/mouse also reduced the HDL-C levels compared to control *Ldlr*$^{-/-}$*Apobec1*$^{-/}$

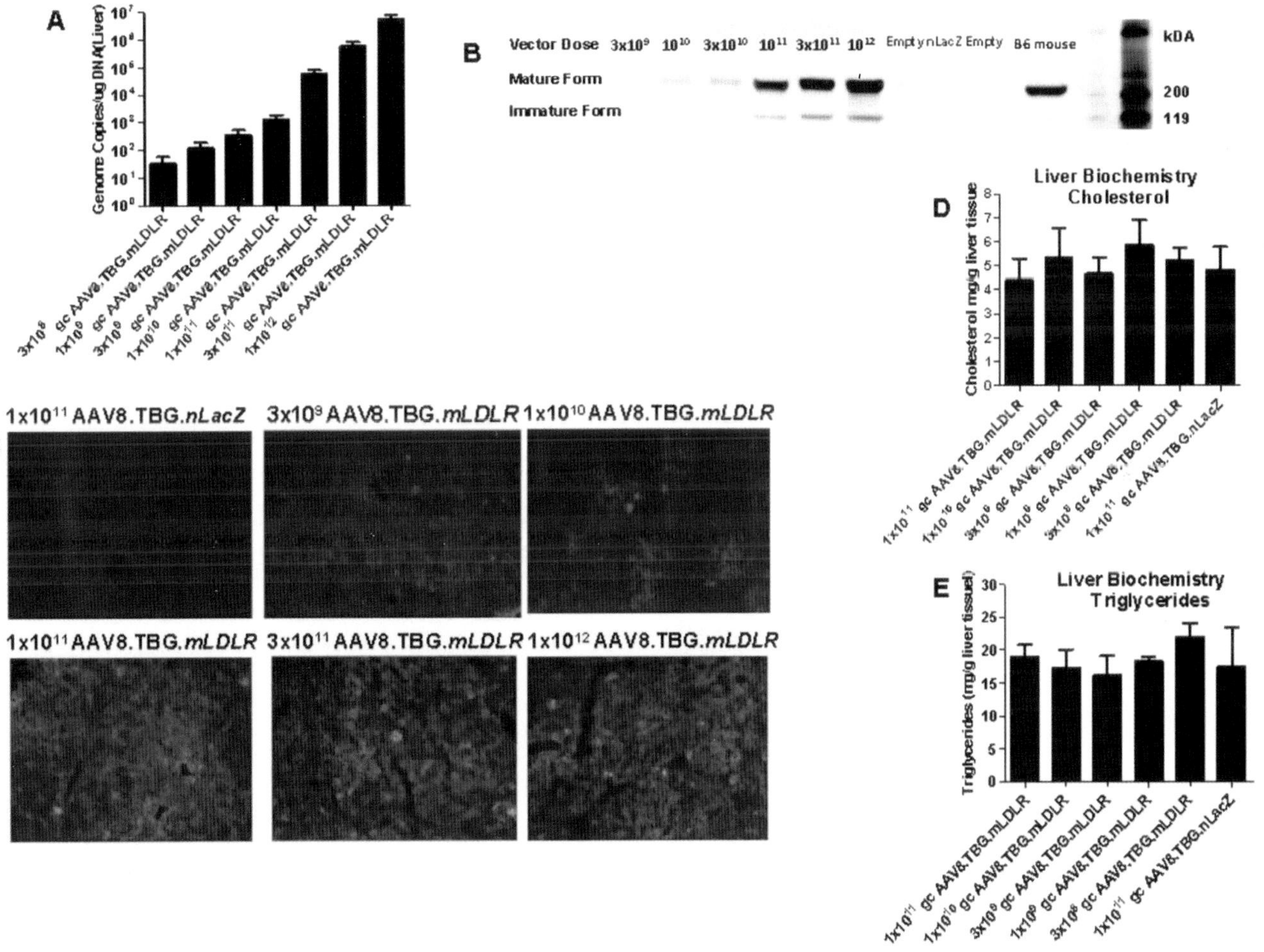

Figure 3. Efficacy of vector mediated transgene expression in liver. (A) Vector DNA expression in the liver. The amount of vector genomes in the liver *Ldlr-/-Apobec1-/-* mice (n = 9 mice per group) was assessed by Taqman analysis of total genomic DNA harvested at day 35 after vector administration. The limit of detection is 10 genome copies/μg DNA. (B) Membrane fraction of liver extract at day 35 was prepared from AAV-treated *Ldlr-/-Apobec1-/-* mice and subjected to Western blot analysis for the detection of transgene expression using LDLR specific antiserum. Positive control is liver extracts from B6 mice. Negative control is liver extracts from AAV8.TBG.*nLacZ* treated *Ldlr-/-Apobec1-/-* mice. (C) Histological analysis of mouse liver. Immunofluorescence staining was performed on mouse liver sections for detection of LDLR expression in *Ldlr-/-Apobec1-/-* mouse at day 35 after vector administration. Cryo-preserved liver section were prepared and probed with rabbit serum against LDLR followed by FITC labeled secondary antibody. Total levels of cholesterol (D) and (E) triglycerides were measured in the livers of *Ldlr-/-Apobec1-/-* mice at day 35. No significant differences were detected between any of the treatment groups (n = 5 mice per treatment group).

$^{-}$ mice (Fig. 2C). Regression analysis of the day 35 post-injection data revealed a clear dose-dependent response with regard to reduction of total cholesterol levels (Fig. 2D). Long-term studies revealed that treatment of *Ldlr*$^{-/-}$*Apobec1*$^{-/-}$ mice with 1×10^{11} GC AAV8.TBG.*mLDLR* resulted in significant correction of cholesterol (Fig. 2E) in the absence of ALT elevation for up to 6 months after injection of vector (Fig. 2F). Collectively, these data reveal that 1×10^{10} GC/mouse is the minimum effective dose required for complete correction; furthermore, partial correction can be attained with as little as 3×10^{9} GC/mouse. Importantly, this correction was maintained for up to 6 months after treatment with no detectable inflammation.

Taqman analysis revealed a dose dependent recovery of vector genomes from the liver (Fig. 3A). Using Western blot analysis, we detected LDLR immunoreactive protein in the liver of AAV8.TBG.mLDLR treated mice with vector doses equal to or greater than 1×10^{10} GC (Fig. 3B). At 1×10^{10} GC/mouse, only the mature form of the LDLR protein (160 kDa band) was detected, whereas in the higher dose groups, both the mature and immature incompletely glycosylated forms (120 kDa band) were present [31]. Immunofluroesence analysis revealed dose dependent expression of immunoreactive LDLR in liver (Fig. 3C); specifically, within 35 days of vector treatment, 60 to 70% of hepatocytes expressed immunoreactive LDLR following injection with 1×10^{12} GC/mouse whereas between 5 to 10% of hepatocytes expressed detectable LDLR at the lowest dose showing some metabolic improvement (i.e., 3×10^{9} GC/mouse). As expected, no LDLR protein was observed in the livers of AAV8.TBG.*nLacZ* treated *Ldlr*$^{-/-}$*Apobec1*$^{-/-}$mice (Fig. 3B and 3C). Importantly, over-expression of *mLDLR* did not result in the pathologic accumulation of hepatic cholesterol (Fig. 3D) or hepatic triglycerides (Fig. 3E) at any of the doses examined.

AAV8.mLDLR Induces marked regression of atherosclerosis

Given that AAV8.TBG.*mLDLR* markedly lowered total cholesterol and non-HDL cholesterol, we next examined whether AAV8.TBG.*mLDLR* had any effect on the progression or even the regression of atherosclerotic lesions. Three groups of male *Ldlr*$^{-/-}$*Apobec1*$^{-/-}$ mice were fed a high-fat western-type diet to hasten the progression of atherosclerosis. After two months of the atherogenic diet, one group of mice received a single intravenous injection of 1×10^{11} GC/mouse of control AAV8.TBG.*nLacZ* vector, one group received 1×10^{11} GC/mouse of AAV8.TBG.*mLDLR* vector, while a third baseline group of animals was necropsied for atherosclerosis lesion quantification. The mice who received vectors were maintained on the high-fat diet for an additional 60 days at which time they were necropsied. Animals that received the AAV8.TBG.*mLDLR* vector realized a rapid drop in total cholesterol from 1555 ± 343 mg/dl at baseline to 266 ± 78 at day 7 and to 67 ± 13 by day 60 after treatment (Fig. 4A). By contrast, the plasma cholesterol levels of AAV8.TBG.*nLacZ* treated mice remained virtually unchanged from 1566 ± 276 at baseline to 1527 ± 67 when measured 60 days after vector (Fig. 4A). The same trend was observed with respect to non-HDL cholesterol (Fig. 4B). All animals developed slight increases in serum transaminanses following the 2 months on the high fat diet, which remained elevated following treatment with the AAV8.TBG.*nLacZ* vector but diminished three-fold to normal levels after treatment with the AAV8.TBG.*mLDLR* vector (Fig. 4C).

Evolution of pre-existing atherosclerotic lesions was assessed by two independent methods. In the first method the aortas were opened from the arch to the iliac bifurication and stained with Oil Red O (Fig. 5A); morphometric analyses quantified the percent of aorta

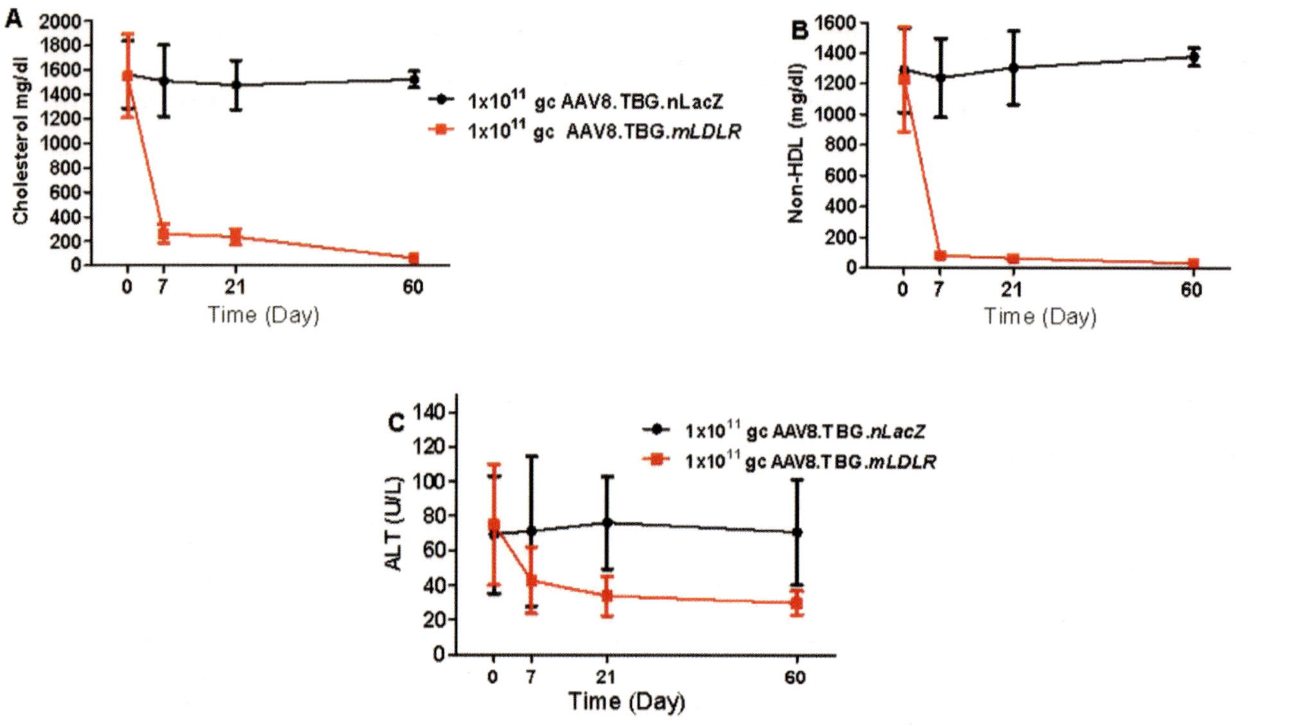

Figure 4. Evaluation of AAV8.TBG.*mLDLR* vector in high fat fed *Ldlr-/-Apobec1-/-* mice. Amounts of (A) Plasma cholesterol (B) non-HDL cholesterol, and (C) Alanine transaminase were evaluated in *Ldlr-/-Apobec1-/-* mice up to day 60 after treatment with 1x10^11 GC of AAV8.TBG.*mLDLR* (n = 10) or 1×1011 GC of AAV8.TBG.*nLacZ* (n = 9). Each point represents mean ± s.d. *P<0.05, ‡ P<0.001.

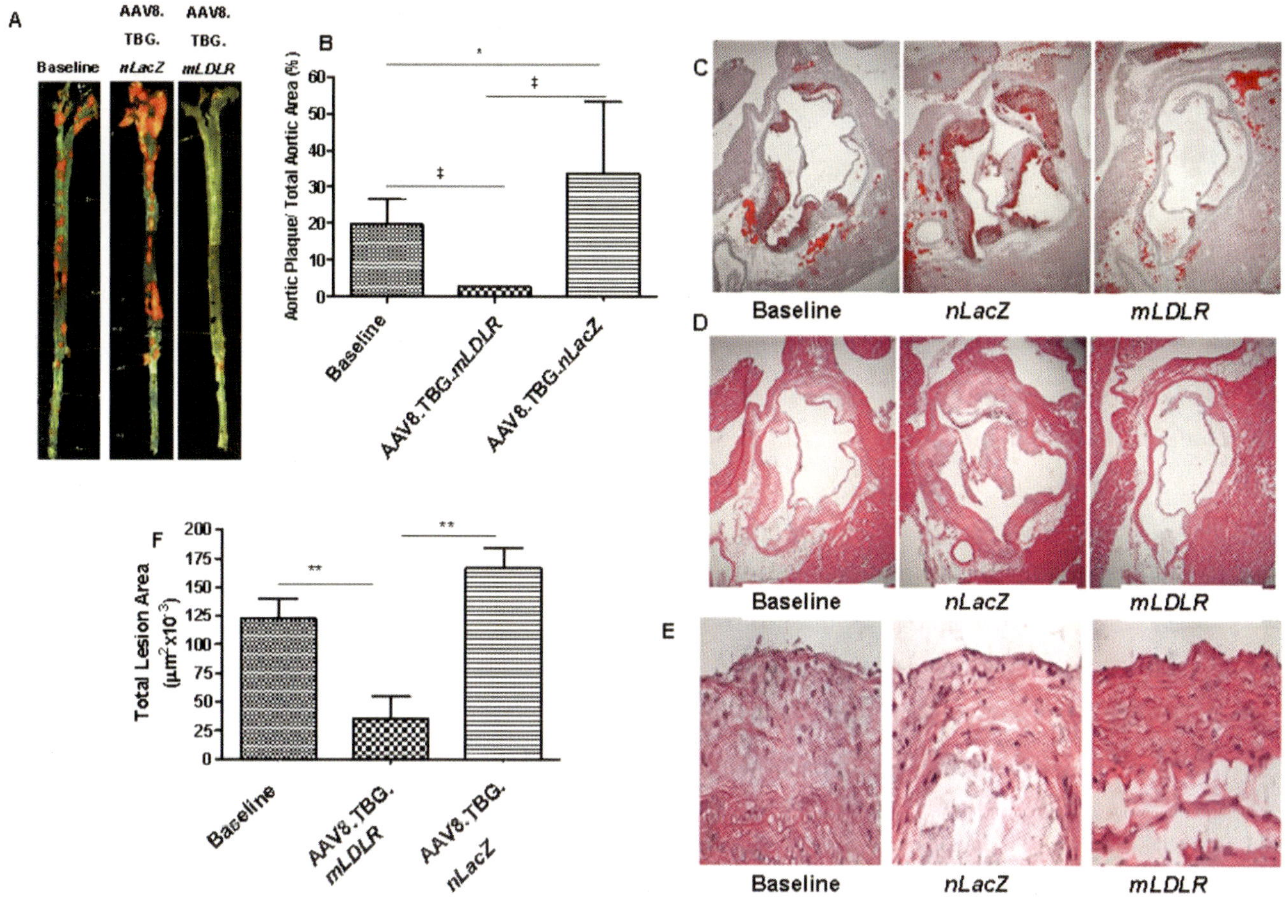

Figure 5. AAV8.TBG.*mLDLR* mediated regression of atherosclerotic lesions in high-fat fed *Ldlr-/-Apobec1-/-*mice. (A) En face Sudan IV staining. Mouse aortas were pinned and stained with Sudan IV, which stains neutral lipids. Representative aortas from animals treated with 1×10^11 of AAV8.TBG.*nLacZ,* 1×10^11 of AAV8.TBG.*mLDLR* at day 60 after vector administration (day 120 on high-fat diet), or at baseline (day 60 on high-fat diet) are shown. (B) The percent Sudan IV staining of the total aortic surface In baseline (n = 10), AAV.TBG.*nLacZ* (n = 9) and AAV8.TBG.*mLDLR* (n = 10) was determined as described under Materials and Methods. Aortic roots from these mice were stained with oil red o (C) or hematoxylin and eosin (H&E) (D) 10× magnification. Quantification was conducted on oil red o lesions (E) as described in the materials and methods. Each column represents mean ± s.d. $^*P<0.05$, $^{**}P<0.01$, $^{***}P<0.001$, ‡ $P<0.001$. (F) H&E stained aortic roots at 40× magnification show a thin fibrous cap and expanded necrotic core in lesions of baseline and AAV8.nLacZ treated mice compared to AAV8.mLDLR injected animals.

stained with Oil Red O along the entire length of the aorta (Fig. 5B). Two months of high fat diet resulted in extensive atherosclerosis covering 20% of the aorta reflecting the baseline disease at the time of vector; this increased to 33% over an additional two month period following treatment with the AAV8.TBG.*nLacZ* vector, representing a 65% further progression in atherosclerosis. In contrast, treatment with the AAV8.TBG.*mLDLR* vector led to a regression of atherosclerosis by 87% over two months, from 20% of the aorta covered by atherosclerosis at baseline to only 2.6% of the aorta covered by atherosclerosis 60 days after vector administration.

In the second method, total lesion area was quantified in the aortic root (Fig. 5C–5F). This analysis revealed the same overall trends, with AAV8.TBG.*nLacZ* injected mice showing a 44% progression over 2 months compared to baseline mice, while AAV8.TBG.*mLDLR* injected mice demonstrating a 64% regression in lesion compared with baseline mice. In summary, expression of LDLR via injection of AAV8.TBG.*mLDLR* induced marked reduction in cholesterol and substantial regression of atherosclerosis over 2 months as assessed by 2 independent methods of quantification at 2 different sites within the aorta.

For further assessment of lesion remodeling, immunostaining was performed on fresh-frozen sections of the aortic root. Samples were examined for CD68, a foam cell marker (Fig. 6A), VCAM-1, an adhesion molecule that plays a role in atherosclerotic lesion formation (Fig. 6B), and collagen, a molecule that determines the mechanical stability of atherosclerotic plaques (Fig. 6C). Lesions in baseline treated groups were advanced, with many necrotic centers, CD68+ macrophages and macrophage-derived foam cells, and extensive VCAM-1 and collagen in the expanded neointima (Fig. 5F and 6A–6C) These results demonstrate the complexity of the lesions in the pre-injected aorta (i.e., that they had progressed past the early macrophage foam cell stage). AAV8.TBG.*nLacZ* treated animals displayed similar advanced pathology. In contrast, AAV8.TBG.*mLDLR* treated mice had much smaller lesions with decreased areas of CD68, VCAM-1, and collagen immunostaining in the intima and media. These results indicate a change in smooth muscle cell phenotype that is part of the wide-scale remodeling process that occurred during the 2 months in which systemic lipid levels where normalized.

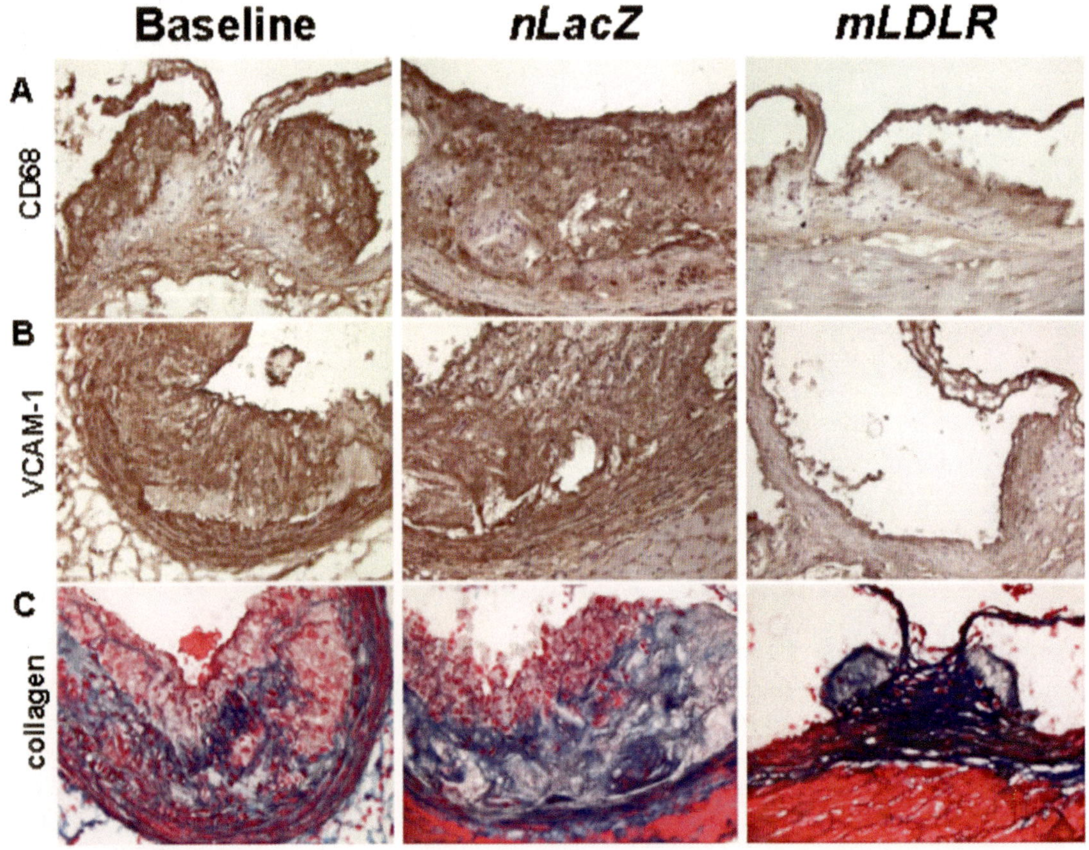

Figure 6. Immunohistochemical analysis of mouse atherosclerotic lesions. Representative aortic root sections immunostained for the foam cell marker CD68 (A), VCAM-1 (B), or Masson trichrome blue stain for collagen content (C). Original magnification, 40×. Note abundant immunostaining for foam cell marker, CD68 (brown), VCAM-1 adhesion molecules (also brown), and presence of collagen αblue) within lesion in baseline and AAV.TBG.*nLacZ* injected *Ldlr-/-Apobec1-/-*animals.

Discussion

Homozygous FH emerged as a model for liver-directed gene therapy in the 1980s with the demonstration of metabolic correction in patients following liver transplantation and genetic correction of deficient hepatocytes *ex vivo* with retroviruses[9,10]. The optimal approach is *in vivo* targeting of hepatocytes following systemic delivery of vector, which is facilitated by the presence of fenestrae in liver capillaries[32]. Genotype/phenotype studies in patients with hoFH indicated the potential for efficacy in those with complete deficiency of *LDLR* following less than complete genetic reconstitution from gene therapy [9,10,33]. Finally, a simple measurement of serum lipids provides a specific, sensitive and relevant read out of gene transfer and clinical efficacy.

One of the biggest challenges in evaluating a novel gene therapy approach for the clinic is the identification of an authentic animal model for assessing efficacy and safety. This is particularly important when the underlying pathology of the disease may impact on vector performance as may be the case for the steatosis of liver in hoFH [34]. Animal models of hoFH have been described in rabbits and monkeys although they suffer from some significant limitations in terms of biology, genetics, available reagents and accessibility [35,36,37]. The mouse provides some substantial advantages especially as it relates to germ line engineering to render animal more "human like" as was the case with the mouse models used in this study.

Studies with AAV8 expressing *mLDLR* in the $Ldlr^{-/-}Apobec1^{-/-}$ mouse showed impressive efficacy. Reductions in serum cholesterol of 35%, which according to human phenotype/genotype studies should be beneficial [33], were achieved with 3×10^{9} GC/mouse. This dose translates to 3×10^{12} GC for a 20 kg adolescent and 1×10^{13} GC for a 70 kg adult which is well within the reach of current manufacturing protocols [38]. Most importantly, we show that complete amelioration of hypercholesterolemia led to marked regression of atherosclerosis over two months despite continuation of the western-type diet. This result represents the fastest and most substantial regression of atherosclerosis seen in a murine model after reduction in plasma cholesterol.

A formal evaluation of safety awaits GLP toxicology studies, although our data to date demonstrated no toxicity up to 10^{12} GC. In fact, normalization of cholesterol following gene therapy actually improved the hepatotoxicity associated with steatosis that occurred when the animals were on a high fat diet (Fig. 4C). Recent reports suggest that the constitutive over-expression of *LDLR* may lead to pathological accumulation of lipids and cholesterol in hepatocytes and that the use of physiologically controlled expression elements is required for the design of FH gene therapy [39,40]. This effect has been seen *in vitro* and *in vivo* following delivery of *LDLR* expression plasmids under the control of strong viral promoters [39,40]. No such pathologies (Fig. 3D–3E) were observed in our studies highlighting the importance of selecting the proper transgene/promoter/vector combination in designing gene therapy strategies.

Several additional aspects of AAV biology should be considered in possible clinical trials. We have shown that even low levels of pre-existing neutralizing antibodies (NAB) due to natural AAV infections will diminish gene transfer and potentially change vector bio-distribution[41]. AAV8 was isolated from a rhesus macaque and NABs to it are lower in humans than what is present to presumably human derived AAVs like AAV2 [18,42]. However, some humans do show low levels of NAB to AAV8 [43]. Mouse studies like the ones described in this paper demonstrate the remarkable result of tolerance to antigenic transgenes [44] although our primate [45] and canine studies [20,46] indicate that the threshold for T cell tolerance is lower in larger animals and presumably humans. Based on these findings we suggest that initial clinical trials be restricted to hoFH subjects who 1) are AAV8 NAB negative and 2) have at least one allele that expresses LDLR protein that spans most of its open reading frame to promote deletion of T cells to wild type LDLR. A final concern relates to the activation of T cells to capsids and killing of transduced hepatocytes which is a hypothesis that emerged from an AAV2 clinical trial in hemophilia [47,48]. It seems prudent to consider a similar biology may occur with other AAV serotypes although our studies indicate this is unlikely to happen with AAV8 as it lacks the necessary dendritic cell interactions to effect cross presentation of capsids [49,50].

In summary, our results suggest that the intravenous injection in mice of a low dose of an AAV8-based vector encoding the *LDLR* cDNA generates sustained expression of the LDLR protein in the liver without evidence of hepatic inflammation or toxicity and is highly effective in markedly reducing plasma cholesterol levels and regressing atherosclerosis in a "humanized" murine model of hoFH. These results suggest that AAV8-based gene therapy for hoFH may be feasible and support further development of this approach.

Acknowledgments

We thank Julie Johnston, Martin Lock, and Arbans Sandhu (Penn Vector Core) for supplying vectors. Also, we are grateful to Dr. William Lagor (University of Pennsylvania School of Medicine) and Dr. Gene Ness (College of Medicine, University of South Florida) for donation of LDLR anti-serum. Finally, we would like to thank Deirdre McMenamin, Regina Munden, Natalie Ridge, Edwige Edouard, Dr. Mao-Sen Sun, and Dr. Jeffrey Billheimer for excellent technical support.

Author Contributions

Conceived and designed the experiments: SHK HL JMW DJR. Performed the experiments: SHK CH PB AW DC VR HY. Analyzed the data: SHK LHV CH PB DM JMW DJR. Contributed reagents/materials/analysis tools: SHK HL LHV DM DJR. Wrote the paper: SHK JMW DJR. Primary Investigator: DJB. Provided extensive technical and experimental support: LHV CH PB AW DC HY. Co-Investigator: JMW. Senior Author: JMW.

References

1. Rader DJ, Cohen J, Hobbs HH (2003) Monogenic hypercholesterolemia: New insights in pathogenesis and treatment. Journal of Clinical Investigation 111: 1795–1803.
2. Deckelbaum RJ, Lees RS, Small DM (1977) Failure of complete bile diversion and oral bile acid therapy in the treatment of homozygous familial hypercholesterolemia. New England Journal of Medicine 296: 465–470.
3. Bilheimer DW, Goldstein JL, Grundy SM (1984) Liver transplantation to provide low-density-lipoprotein receptors and lower plasma cholesterol in a child with homozygous familial hypercholesterolemia. New England Journal of Medicine 311: 1658–1664.
4. Rela M, Muiesan P, Heaton ND, Corbally M, Hajj H, et al. (1995) Orthotopic liver transplantation for hepatic-based metabolic disorders. Transplant International 8: 41–44.
5. Beigel R, Beigel Y (2009) Homozygous familial hypercholesterolemia: Long term clinical course and plasma exchange therapy for two individual patients and review of the literature. Journal of Clinical Apheresis 24: 219–224.
6. Borberg H (2009) 26 Years of LDL - Apheresis: A review of experience. Transfusion and Apheresis Science 41: 49–59.
7. Thompson GR (2003) LDL apheresis. Atherosclerosis 167: 1–13.
8. Thompson GR, Maher VMG, Matthews S, Kitano Y, Neuwirth C, et al. (1995) Familial Hypercholesterolaemia Regression Study: A randomised trial of low-density-lipoprotein apheresis. Lancet 345: 811–816+807–808.
9. Grossman M, Raper SE, Kozarsky K, Stein EA, Engelhardt JF, et al. (1994) Successful ex vivo gene therapy directed to liver in a patient with familial hypercholesterolaemia. Nature Genetics 6: 335–341.
10. Grossman M, Rader DJ, Muller DWM, Kolansky DM, Kozarsky I, et al. (1995) A pilot study of ex vivo gene therapy for homozygous familial hypercholesterolaemia. Nature Medicine 1: 1148–1154.
11. Vaessen SFC, Twisk J, Kastelein JJP, Kuivenhoven JA (2007) Gene therapy in disorders of lipoprotein metabolism. Current Gene Therapy 7: 35–47.
12. Kozarsky KF, Jooss K, Donahee M, Strauss IiiJF, Wilson JM (1996) Effective treatment of familial hypercholesterolaemia in the mouse model using adenovirus-mediated transfer of the VLDL receptor gene. Nature Genetics 13: 54–62.
13. Kozarsky KF, McKinley DR, Austin LL, Raper SE, Stratford-Perricaudet LD, et al. (1994) In vivo correction of low density lipoprotein receptor deficiency in the Watanabe heritable hyperlipidemic rabbit with recombinant adenoviruses. Journal of Biological Chemistry 269: 13695–13702.
14. Nomura S, Merched A, Nour E, Dieker C, Oka K, et al. (2004) Low-density lipoprotein receptor gene therapy using helper-dependent adenovirus produces long-term protection against atherosclerosis in a mouse model of familial hypercholesterolemia. Gene Therapy 11: 1540–1548.
15. McCaffrey AP, Fawcett P, Nakai H, McCaffrey RL, Ehrhardt A, et al. (2008) The host response to adenovirus, helper-dependent adenovirus, and adeno-associated virus in mouse liver. Molecular Therapy 16: 931–941.
16. Wu Z, Asokan A, Samulski RJ (2006) Adeno-associated Virus Serotypes: Vector Toolkit for Human Gene Therapy. Molecular Therapy 14: 316–327.
17. Chen SJ, Rader DJ, Tazelaar J, Kawashiri MA, Gao GP, et al. (2000) Prolonged correction of hyperlipidemia in mice with familial hypercholesterolemia using an adeno-associated viral vector expressing very-low-density lipoprotein receptor. Molecular Therapy 2: 256–261.
18. Gao GP, Alvira MR, Wang L, Calcedo R, Johnston J, et al. (2002) Novel adeno-associated viruses from rhesus monkeys as vectors for human gene therapy. Proceedings of the National Academy of Sciences of the United States of America 99: 11854–11859.
19. Kitajima K, Marchadier DHL, Miller GC, Gao GP, Wilson JM, et al. (2006) Complete prevention of atherosclerosis in ApoE-deficient mice by hepatic human ApoE gene transfer with adeno-associated virus serotypes 7 and 8. Arteriosclerosis, Thrombosis, and Vascular Biology 26: 1852–1857.
20. Wang L, Calcedo R, Nichols TC, Bellinger DA, Dillow A, et al. (2005) Sustained correction of disease in naive and AAV2-pretreated hemophilia B dogs: AAV2/8-mediated, liver-directed gene therapy. Blood 105: 3079–3086.
21. Wang L, Wang H, Bell P, McCarter RJ, He J, et al. (2009) Systematic Evaluation of AAV Vectors for Liver directed Gene Transfer in Murine Models. Molecular Therapy.
22. Lebherz C, Gao G, Louboutin JP, Millar J, Rader D, et al. (2004) Gene therapy with novel adeno-associated virus vectors substantially diminishes atherosclerosis in a murine model of familial hypercholesterolemia. Journal of Gene Medicine 6: 663–672.
23. Powell-Braxton L, VÃ©niant M, Latvala RD, Hirano KI, Won WB, et al. (1998) A mouse model of human familial hypercholesterolemia: Markedly elevated low density lipoprotein cholesterol levels and severe atherosclerosis on a low-fat chow diet. Nature Medicine 4: 934–938.
24. Daugherty A (2002) Mouse models of atherosclerosis. American Journal of the Medical Sciences 323: 3–10.
25. Sanan DA, Newland DL, Tao R, Marcovina S, Wang J, et al. (1998) Low density lipoprotein receptor-negative mice expressing human apolipoprotein B-100 develop complex atherosclerotic lesions on a chow diet: No accentuation by apolipoprotein(a). Proceedings of the National Academy of Sciences of the United States of America 95: 4544–4549.
26. Tangirala RK, PraticÃ3 D, FitzGerald GA, Chun S, Tsukamoto K, et al. (2001) Reduction of isoprostanes and regression of advanced atherosclerosis by apolipoprotein E. Journal of Biological Chemistry 276: 261–266.
27. Tangirala RK, Tsukamoto K, Chun SH, Usher D, Puré E, et al. (1999) Regression of atherosclerosis induced by liver-directed gene transfer of apolipoprotein A-I in mice. Circulation 100: 1816–1822.
28. Ness GC, Zhao Z (1994) Thyroid hormone rapidly induces hepatic LDL receptor mRNA levels in hypophysectomized rats. Archives of Biochemistry and Biophysics 315: 199–202.
29. Tsukamoto K, Tangirala RK, Chun S, Usher D, Pure E, et al. (2000) Hepatic Expression of Apolipoprotein E Inhibits Progression of Atherosclerosis without

Reducing Cholesterol Levels in LDL Receptor-Deficient Mice. Molecular Therapy 1: 189–194.
30. Schale S, Renner M, Longhurst S, Narayanan G (2009) Regulatory requirements for clinical trial and marketing authorisation application for gene therapy medicinal products. Bundesgesundheitsblatt - Gesundheitsforschung - Gesundheitsschutz. pp 1–8.
31. Goldstein JL, Brown MS, Anderson RG, Russell DW, Schneider WJ (1985) Receptor-mediated endocytosis: concepts emerging from the LDL receptor system. Annual review of cell biology 1: 1–39.
32. Jacobs F, Wisse E, De Geest B () The Role of Liver Sinusoidal Cells in Hepatocyte-Directed Gene Transfer. Am J Pathol 176: 14–21.
33. Soutar AK, Naoumova RP (2007) Mechanisms of Disease: genetic causes of familial hypercholesterolemia. Nat Clin Pract Cardiovasc Med 4: 214–225.
34. Garg A, Misra A (2002) Hepatic Steatosis, Insulin Resistance, and Adipose Tissue Disorders. J Clin Endocrinol Metab 87: 3019–3022.
35. Russell JC, Proctor SD () Small animal models of cardiovascular disease: tools for the study of the roles of metabolic syndrome, dyslipidemia, and atherosclerosis. Cardiovascular Pathology 15: 318–330.
36. Moghadasian MH, Frohlich JJ, McManus BM () Advances in Experimental Dyslipidemia and Atherosclerosis. Lab Invest 81: 1173–1183.
37. Scanu A, Khalil A, Neven L, Tidore M, Dawson G, et al. (1988) Genetically determined hypercholesterolemia in a rhesus monkey family due to a deficiency of the LDL receptor. J Lipid Res 29: 1671–1681.
38. Wright JF (2008) Manufacturing and characterizing AAV-based vectors for use in clinical studies. Gene Therapy 15: 840–848.
39. Cichon G, Willnow T, Herwig S, Uckert W, Löser P, et al. (2004) Non-physiological overexpression of the *low density lipoprotein receptor* (LDLr) gene in the liver induces pathological intracellular lipid and cholesterol storage. The Journal of Gene Medicine 6: 166–175.
40. Hibbitt OC, McNeil E, Lufino MMP, Seymour L, Channon K, et al. (2009) Long-term Physiologically Regulated Expression of the Low-density Lipoprotein Receptor In Vivo Using Genomic DNA Mini-gene Constructs. Mol Ther.
41. Wang L, Calcedo R, Wang H, Bell P, Grant R, et al. (2009) The Pleiotropic Effects of Natural AAV Infections on Liver-directed Gene Transfer in Macaques. Mol Ther 18: 126–134.
42. Gao G, Vandenberghe LH, Alvira MR, Lu Y, Calcedo R, et al. (2004) Clades of Adeno-Associated Viruses Are Widely Disseminated in Human Tissues. J Virol 78: 6381–6388.
43. Calcedo R, Vandenberghe LukÂ H, Gao G, Lin J, Wilson JamesÂ M (2009) Worldwide Epidemiology of Neutralizing Antibodies to Adeno Associated Viruses. The Journal of Infectious Diseases 199: 381–390.
44. Breous E, Somanathan S, Vandenberghe LH, Wilson JM (2009) Hepatic regulatory T cells and Kupffer cells are crucial mediators of systemic T cell tolerance to antigens targeting murine liver. Hepatology 50: 612–621.
45. Gao G, Wang Q, Calcedo R, Mays L, Bell P, et al. (2009) Adeno-associated virus-mediated gene transfer to nonhuman primate liver can elicit destructive transgene-specific T cell responses. Human Gene Therapy 20: 930–942.
46. Sarkar R, Tetreault R, Gao G, Wang L, Bell P, et al. (2004) Total correction of hemophilia A mice with canine FVIII using an AAV 8 serotype. Blood 103: 1253–1260.
47. Manno CS, Arruda VR, Pierce GF, Glader B, Ragni M, et al. (2006) Successful transduction of liver in hemophilia by AAV-Factor IX and limitations imposed by the host immune response. Nature Medicine 12: 342–347.
48. Hasbrouck NC, High KA (2008) AAV-mediated gene transfer for the treatment of hemophilia B: problems and prospects. Gene Ther 15: 870–875.
49. Vandenberghe LH, Wang L, Somanathan S, Zhi Y, Figueredo J, et al. (2006) Heparin binding directs activation of T cells against adeno-associated virus serotype 2 capsid. Nat Med 12: 967–971.
50. Mays LE, Vandenberghe LH, Xiao R, Bell P, Nam H-J, et al. (2009) Adeno-Associated Virus Capsid Structure Drives CD4-Dependent CD8+ T Cell Response to Vector Encoded Proteins. J Immunol 182: 6051–6060.

15

Female Mucopolysaccharidosis IIIA Mice Exhibit Hyperactivity and a Reduced Sense of Danger in the Open Field Test

Alex Langford-Smith[1], Kia J. Langford-Smith[1], Simon A. Jones[2], Robert F. Wynn[3], J. E. Wraith[2], Fiona L. Wilkinson[1], Brian W. Bigger[1]*

1 Stem Cell and Neurotherapies, School of Biomedicine, Faculty of Medical and Human Sciences, University of Manchester, Manchester, United Kingdom, **2** Genetic Medicine, St. Mary's Hospital, Manchester, United Kingdom, **3** Blood and Marrow Transplant Unit, Royal Manchester Children's Hospital, Manchester, United Kingdom

Abstract

Reliable behavioural tests in animal models of neurodegenerative diseases allow us to study the natural history of disease and evaluate the efficacy of novel therapies. Mucopolysaccharidosis IIIA (MPS IIIA or Sanfilippo A), is a severe, neurodegenerative lysosomal storage disorder caused by a deficiency in the heparan sulphate catabolising enzyme, sulfamidase. Undegraded heparan sulphate accumulates, resulting in lysosomal enlargement and cellular dysfunction. Patients suffer a progressive loss of motor and cognitive function with severe behavioural manifestations and premature death. There is currently no treatment. A spontaneously occurring mouse model of the disease has been described, that has approximately 3% of normal enzyme activity levels. Behavioural phenotyping of the MPS IIIA mouse has been previously reported, but the results are conflicting and variable, even after full backcrossing to the C57BL/6 background. Therefore we have independently backcrossed the MPS IIIA model onto the C57BL/6J background and evaluated the behaviour of male and female MPS IIIA mice at 4, 6 and 8 months of age using the open field test, elevated plus maze, inverted screen and horizontal bar crossing at the same circadian time point. Using a 60 minute open field, we have demonstrated that female MPS IIIA mice are hyperactive, have a longer path length, display rapid exploratory behaviour and spend less time immobile than WT mice. Female MPS IIIA mice also display a reduced sense of danger and spend more time in the centre of the open field. There were no significant differences found between male WT and MPS IIIA mice and no differences in neuromuscular strength were seen with either sex. The altered natural history of behaviour that we observe in the MPS IIIA mouse will allow more accurate evaluation of novel therapeutics for MPS IIIA and potentially other neurodegenerative disorders.

Editor: Stephen D. Ginsberg, Nathan Kline Institute and New York University School of Medicine, United States of America

Funding: This work was funded by the UK Society for Mucopolysaccharide Diseases, The Irish Society for Mucopolysaccharide Diseases, The Sanfilippo Children's Research Foundation, and the Biotechnology and Biological Sciences Research Council. The funders had no role in study design, data collection and analysis, decision to publish, or preparation of the manuscript.

Competing Interests: The authors have declared that no competing interests exist.

* E-mail: Brian.Bigger@Manchester.ac.uk

Introduction

Mucopolysaccharidosis IIIA (MPS IIIA, OMIM #252900), or Sanfilippo Type A, is an autosomal recessive lysosomal storage disorder that affects 0.82 in 100,000 live births in the United Kingdom [1]. The disease is characterised by severe and progressive loss of cognitive and motor functions, behavioural difficulties and eventually death in the second decade of life, although the severity and progression of the disease varies widely [1,2,3]. MPS IIIA is caused by mutations in the *SGSH* gene that result in deficiency of the N-sulfoglucosamine sulfohydrolase enzyme (sulfamidase, EC 3.10.1.1) and subsequent accumulation of undegraded heparan sulphate, lysosomal enlargement and cellular and organ dysfunction [4,5,6,7]. Patients exhibit progressive neurodegeneration and behavioural problems including hyperactivity, a reduced sense of danger, aggression and sleep disturbances [7,8,9,10,11,12].

Although there are no current therapies, several strategies are in development for MPS IIIA or the phenotypically indistinguishable MPS IIIB disease, including substrate reduction therapy [13,14,15], intrathecal enzyme replacement therapy [16,17,18,19,20] and gene therapy with lentiviral [21], adenoviral [22] or adeno-associated-viral [23] vectors. Most strategies make use of the ability of exogenous enzyme to complement affected cells, however the presence of the blood brain barrier limits efficient enzyme distribution. Biomarkers for MPS IIIA or related diseases are still in development [24,25], thus the accurate evaluation of neurodegeneration using behavioural phenotyping in the mouse model of disease is paramount. A spontaneously occurring mouse model of MPS IIIA on a mixed 129SvJ, C57BL/6, SJL, and CD1 background has been previously described with around 3% of normal enzyme activity and exhibiting many of the features observed in patients [26]. The MPS IIIA mice exhibit severe neuropathology characterised by enlarged lysosomes, primary storage of HS, secondary storage of GM2 and GM3 gangliosides and cholesterol and chronic neuroinflammation [19,23,26,27,28]. The MPS IIIA mice are euthanized between 9 and 12 months of age due to urine retention, a phenotype not seen in the patients but also seen in MPS IIIB mice [29]. The MPS IIIA mouse model has been backcrossed to the C57BL/6 background by Professor John Hopwood's Lysosomal Diseases Research Unit [30] and to the C57BL/6J background by Jackson laboratories [31].

Although the behaviour of the MPS IIIA mouse model has been evaluated in the open field test at several ages, using different sexes, by several groups and on different strain backgrounds, there is a remarkable amount of variability in the outcome of the test as outlined in Table 1.

Using the mixed background mouse, at many of the time points measured, no differences are observed between either male or female WT and MPS IIIA mice, with initial findings of hyperactivity and later hypoactivity in males [18,32]. After back crossing the MPS IIIA mice on to a C57BL/6 background, the behaviour was extensively studied by Crawley *et al.* at different time points. Hyperactivity in males was observed at 12 weeks of age, and females at 22 and 32 weeks of age, although these mice were not naively tested [30]. At most time points, no differences were seen. However male, but not female, MPS IIIA mice were shown to be hypoactive at some time points in the work of Lau *et al* [33] and male MPS IIIA mice were hypoactive at 15 weeks of age in a more recent paper by Lau *et al.* [34]. Hypoactivity in male mice was also observed at some time points in McIntyre *et al.* [21]. In columns 7, 8, 9 and 10 of Table 1 (marked as bold) we have also presented markedly variable outcomes of observations of locomotor behaviour of MPS IIIA and WT mice that received control intracranial injections [18,21,23,35].

Patients with MPS IIIA are believed to have a reduced sense of danger, which can be inferred in mice by the amount of time spent in the centre of the open field test or by use of the elevated plus maze test, both of which can be used to measure their tendency to avoid open spaces and remain close to cover (thigmotaxis). No difference in the time in centre of the open field was detected by Lau *et al.* [33], however this could be due to the small size of the open field used. In the elevated plus maze, male MPS IIIA mice were reported to display reduced anxiety with a greater proportion of their path length (distance travelled) spent in the open arms at some time points but not others [33,34].

Overall, there are discrepancies in behaviour of this mouse model that could be due to gender differences, the age of testing and the methodology used to perform the tests. Therefore we have attempted to perform a standardised analysis of MPS IIIA mice by first backcrossing them to the C57BL/6J background for over 10 generations and subsequently testing a cohort of MPS IIIA and WT mice at the same circadian time point at 4, 6 and 8 months (16, 24 and 32 weeks) of age in the 60 minute open field test, the elevated plus maze, as well as several other neuromuscular evaluations that we have previously shown to be effective for phenotyping MPS IIIB mice [36]. The female MPS IIIA mice were hyperactivity, had a recued sense of danger and no neuromuscular differences. The open field test performed at the same point in the circadian rhythm was a consistent, sensitive and reliable behavioural test for the evaluation of novel therapeutic strategies in MPS IIIA mice.

Methods

Mouse maintenance

The MPS IIIA mouse colony was maintained through heterozygous breeding at the University of Manchester, all procedures were ethically approved by the University of Manchester Ethical Review Process Committee and in accordance with the UK Home Office regulations under project licence PPL 40/3117. Mice were housed in individually ventilated cages, had access *ad libitum* to food and water and were in a 12 hour light and dark cycle. Male mice were singly housed at 14 weeks of age due to aggressive tendencies but female mice remained housed in groups of 4–6. The MPS IIIA mice (B6.Cg-Sgsh^{mps3a}) have been backcrossed from the original mixed 129SvJ, C57BL/6, SJL, and CD1 background [26] onto the C57BL/6J background by more than 10 generations of backcrossing with C57BL/6J mice (Harlan, UK) and were maintained by heterozygous breeding. WT and MPS IIIA littermates have been used in all behavioural experiments.

Genotyping MPS IIIA mice

MPS IIIA mice have a G to A mutation in the *SGSH* gene which removes a *Msp*1I restriction enzyme digestion site. Genotyping is performed by PCR amplification of DNA followed by *Msp*1I digestion and observation of the size of DNA fragments produced. Genomic DNA was extracted from ear punches using the GenElute Mammalian Genomic DNA Miniprep Kit (Sigma Aldrich) following the manufacturer's instructions and *SGSH* was amplified by PCR using the forward primer 5′ GTGTTCCCTGCCTGCTCAC 3′ and reverse primer 5′ CCAGTCCCCTCATCCCACTA 3′. The DNA was digested with *Msp*1I (New England Biolabs, UK) and the DNA fragments were separated by 2% agarose gel electrophoresis. The genotype was determined from the pattern of DNA fragments; wild type (WT) reveals 199 bp, 118 bp and 78 bp fragments, mutant (MUT) 317 bp and 78 bp fragments and heterozygous (HET) 317 bp, 199 bp, 118 bp and 78 bp.

Behavioural testing

At 4, 6 and 8 months (16, 24 and 32 weeks) of age, the same cohorts of 10 male WT and 10 male MPS IIIA mice and 10 female WT and 11 MPS IIIA mice were analysed with the following behavioural tests. 1.5 hours into the 12 hour light phase the mice were dropped into the centre of an open field arena (width 450 mm, depth 450 mm, height 500 mm) made of matt white acrylic. The behaviour was recorded for 60 minutes using a digital camcorder (Sony) and analysed using Top Scan software (Clever Sys. Inc., USA). The path length, frequency (number of times) and duration of rapid exploratory behaviour (speed >100 mm/s), frequency and duration of immobility (speed <5 mm/s) and frequency of entering the centre and duration in the centre (75 mm from each edge) was analysed. Rearing in the open field was analysed by counting the number of unsupported rears (front paws off the floor) and supported rears (front paws on the wall) in the first 10 minutes. The same researcher performed all experiments and was blinded to genotype.

After a 30 minute rest, the mice were placed onto the end of an open arm of an elevated plus maze. The maze was constructed of matt white acrylic, comprised of four 500 mm long by 100 mm wide arms, two of which were enclosed by 500 mm high walls, and was raised on a stand 500 mm off the floor. Mice were placed so they faced towards the centre of the maze and were given 10 minutes to explore the maze before returning to a cage. The maze was cleaned using 70% ethanol. 30 minutes later the mice were tested for a second time, in the same manner. The results were analysed using Top Scan software (Clever Sys) to examine the amount of time spent on the open arm, the percentage of path length in the open arm, and the percentage of open arm entries.

30 minutes later the inverted screen test was performed, as described previously [36]. In brief, at 4, 6 and 8 months of age the mouse was placed on a 470 mm square with a 13 mm square wire mesh. The screen was then rotated through 180° over 1–2 seconds. The mouse was then suspended upside down over a

Table 1. Summary of the significant differences in the open field activity of MPS IIIA mice in the literature.

Paper		Hemsley *et al.*		Hemsley *et al.*	Lau *et al.*		Lau *et al.*	McIntyre *et al.*	Crawley *et al.*		** Hemsley et al.*	** Hemsley et al.*	** McIntyre et al.*	** Fraldi et al.*	This Study	
Year		2005		2007	2008		2010	2010	2006		*2007*	*2009*	*2010*	*2007*		
Background		Mixed		Mixed	C57BL/6		C57BL/6	C57BL/6	C57BL/6		*Mixed*	*C57BL/6*	*C57BL/6*	*C57BL/6*	C57BL/6J	
Measure		Line Crossing		Line Crossing	Zone Entries		Path Length	Line crossing	Line Crossing		*Line Crossing*	*Path Length*	*Line crossing*	*Path Length*	Path Length	
Sex		Male	Female	Male	Male	Female	Male	Male	Male	Female	*Male*	*Male*	*Male*	*Male*	Male	Female
Age (Weeks)	**3**	Hyper	Hyper		NS	NS										
	4								NS	Hypo						
	5				NS	NS										
	6	Hypo	NS	Hypo					NS	NS						
	8								NS	NS	*NS* +Hypo**					
	10	NS	NS		Hypo	NS			NS	NS				*NS**		
	12								Hyper	NS	*NS* +Hypo**	*Hypo**				
	15	Hypo	NS		NS	NS	Hypo		NS	NS				*NS**		
	16														NS	Hyper
	18				Hypo	NS			NS	NS	*Hypo**			*NS**		
	20	NS	NS					Hypo					*NS**			
	21													*Hyper**		
	22				Hypo	NS			NS	Hyper						
	24							NS					*NS**		NS	Hyper
	25								NS	NS						
	28							NS					*NS**			
	32								NS	Hyper					NS	Some Hyper
	40	NS	NS						NS	NS						

Hyper indicates significant hyperactive behaviour and hypo indicates significant hypoactive behaviour in the open field test. NS indicates no significant difference and * indicates mice that have recieved intracranial injections. Control injections contained: 2.5 µl of 50 mM sodium acetate, 100 mM sodium chloride at pH 5.0 in Hemsley *et al* 2007, 4 µl 10 mM sodium phosphate, 140 mM sodium chloride pH 7.0 in Hemsley *et al.* 2009, 5 µl 0.9% (w/v) sodium chloride in McIntyre *et al.* 2010 and 1 µl GFP adeno-associated viral vector in Fraldi *et al.* 2007. The work of Hemsley et *al.* 2007 contained multiple control treated groups and where there were differences between groups, both have been shown. Where female mice are not mentioned or cells are blank no testing was performed.

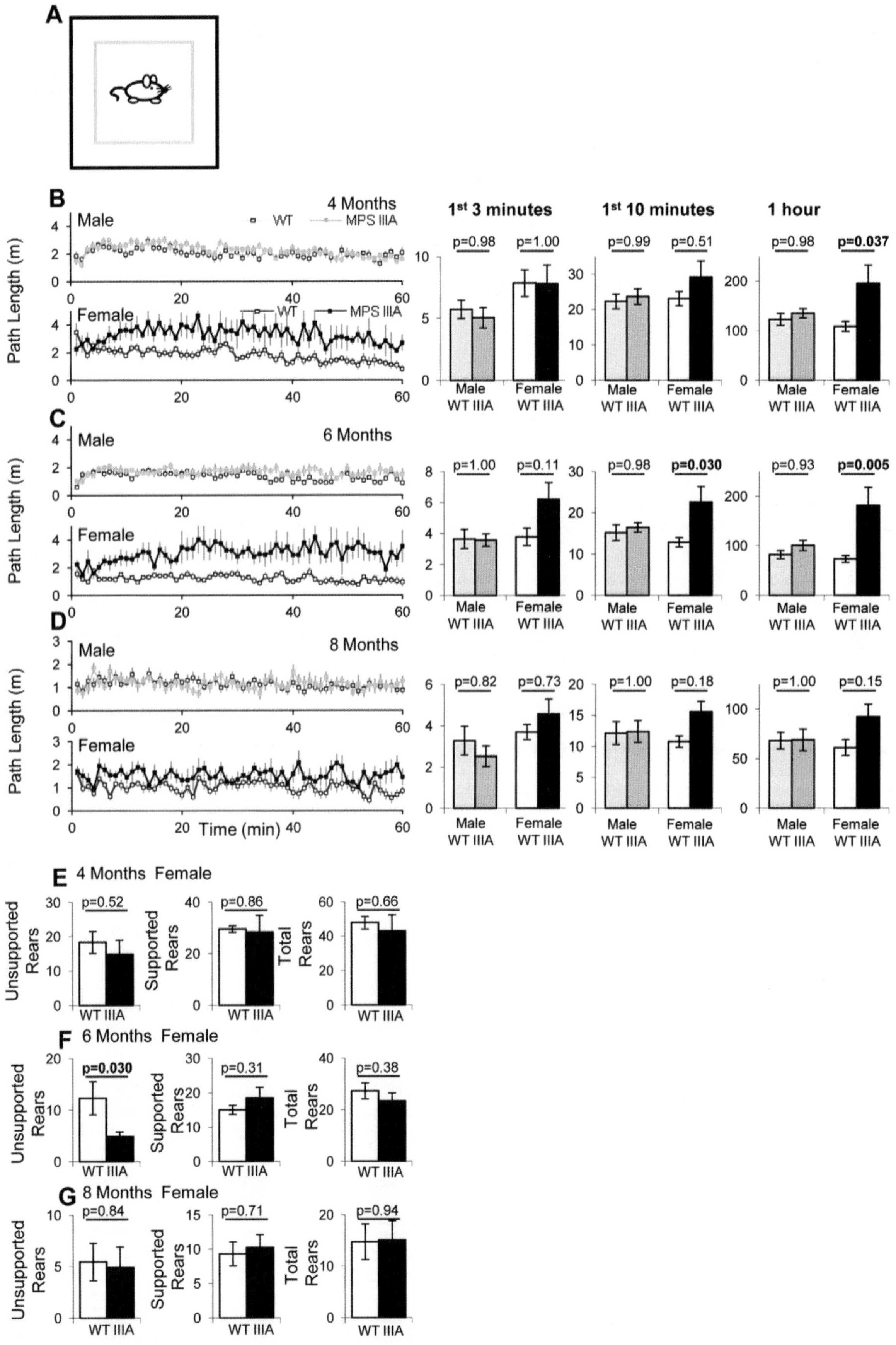
A
B
4 Months
Male
WT
MPS IIIA
Female
Path Length (m)
1st 3 minutes
1st 10 minutes
1 hour
p=0.98
p=1.00
p=0.99
p=0.51
p=0.98
p=0.037
Male
Female
WT IIIA
C
6 Months
p=1.00
p=0.11
p=0.98
p=0.030
p=0.93
p=0.005
D
8 Months
p=0.82
p=0.73
p=1.00
p=0.18
p=1.00
p=0.15
Time (min)
E
4 Months Female
Unsupported Rears
Supported Rears
Total Rears
p=0.52
p=0.86
p=0.66
F
6 Months Female
p=0.030
p=0.31
p=0.38
G
8 Months Female
p=0.84
p=0.71
p=0.94

Figure 1. Open field path length and rearing. At 4, 6 and 8 months (16, 24 and 32 weeks) of age, 10 WT male (light grey squares), 10 MPS IIIA male (dark grey squares), 10 WT female (white squares) and 11 MPS IIIA female (black squares) were placed in the open field and the behaviour was recorded for 60 minutes (A). The results of the open field behaviour are presented as a 60 minute period with the average of every minute presented and as a bar chart of the first 3 minutes, first 10 minutes and the whole hour. Error bars represent the standard error of the mean (SEM). p values were calculated by 2 Way ANOVA. The mean average path length in Metres at 4 (B), 6 (C) and 8 (D) months have been presented. The number of unsupported, supported and total rears in the first 10 minutes at 4 (E), 6 (F) and 8 (G) months of age have also been presented.

padded surface; the rear leg moves were counted and the duration suspended was recorded up to 2 minutes.

One hour later the horizontal bar test was performed as described previously [14,36]. In brief, a 2 mm diameter, 300 mm long metal wire was secured between 2 posts, 320 mm above a padded surface. The mouse was allowed to grip the centre of the wire and the time taken to fall or to reach the side was recorded up to 2 minutes. The test was repeated three times as a training run followed by a 10 minute rest before three test runs. The results were scored as follows: crossing the bar in x seconds was scored as 240-x, remaining on the bar was scored as 120 and falling off the bar after y seconds was recorded as y.

Urine retention

Upon sacrifice 9 male WT, 8 male MPS IIIA, 7 female WT and 8 female MPS IIIA mice at 8 months (32 weeks) of age were dissected and the urine was removed from the bladder and volume measured using an insulin syringe (BD).

Statistical analysis

Statistical analysis was performed using JMP software (SAS Institute Inc, Cary, NC, USA) and analysed by MANOVA with repeated measures for overall significances and by one or two way ANOVA, as appropriate, with Tukey post hoc tests at individual time points. Significance was set at $p \leq 0.05$. For the MANOVA analysis the Genotype significance determines if there is a difference between WT and MPS IIIA mice irrespective of the age of the mice, the Time significance determines if there is a change in the behaviour of the mice at different ages irrespective of the genotype and the Genotype*Time significance determines if MPS IIIA mouse behaviour changes over time in a different manner to WT mice.

Results

Cohorts of male and female, WT and MPS IIIA mice (n = 10–11 per group) were monitored in a 60 minute open field test as outlined in Figure 1A. The path length minute by minute over 60 minutes is shown at 4 months (16 weeks) in Figure 1B, 6 months (24 weeks) in Figure 1C and at 8 months (32 weeks) in Figure 1D. The behaviour in the first 3 minutes, 10 minutes and 60 minutes is presented to allow comparison against published data and to identify the minimum amount of time required for statistically significant analyses. At 4 months of age, female MPS IIIA mice were significantly hyperactive and travel almost twice as far as the WT mice over 60 minutes ($p = 0.037$; Figure 1B). Examining the behaviour over the first 3 minutes showed no difference and no trend in female behaviour, but over 10 minutes there was a non-significant trend towards hyperactivity. No difference was found in the path length of male WT or MPS IIIA mice at 4 months.

At 6 months of age the same female MPS IIIA mice demonstrated increased path length with significant differences after 10 minutes ($p = 0.030$) and greater differences after 60 minutes ($p = 0.005$; Figure 1C). No difference was detected between male WT and MPS IIIA mice (Figure 1C).

At 8 months of age there was a trend for the female mice to be hyperactive but no significant differences were found after 3 ($p = 0.73$), 10 ($p = 0.15$) or 60 minutes ($p = 0.18$; Figure 1D). Similarly, no significant differences were found with male mice after 3, 10 or 60 minutes. Overall, using MANOVA repeated measure analysis, a significant genotype difference ($p = 0.011$), time difference ($p = 1.2 \times 10^{-7}$) and a time*genotype difference ($p = 0.021$) were found. This indicates that overall, MPS IIIA mice are significantly more hyperactive than WT mice, that this changes with time and that MPS IIIA and WT mice change their behaviour in a different manner over time.

The number of unsupported rears (front paws off the floor), supported rears (front paws on a wall) and total rears were counted manually in the first 10 minutes of the open field test. The only significant change observed was a decrease in the number of unsupported rears by female MPS IIIA mice at 6 months of age (Figure 1F). However, given that there were no other significant genotype effects, this may be just a chance occurrence (Figure 1E and G). MANOVA repeated measure analysis of the data showed no significant genotype effect in the three rearing measures, but there was a significant decline in all measures with time (unsupported, $p = 0.004$, supported and total $p = 0.00003$) irrespective of genotype.

Rapid exploratory motion was analysed by measuring the frequency and duration of speed over 100 mm/s (Figure 2A–F). At 4 months of age, female MPS IIIA mice show significant increases in both the frequency ($p = 0.048$; Figure 2A) and duration ($p = 0.05$; Figure 2D) of rapid exploration over 60 minutes. However, no significant differences were observed after 3 or 10 minutes, although a trend was detected after 10 minutes (Figure 2A). No significant differences were found between male MPS IIIA or WT mice at 4 months of age.

At 6 months of age, there was a trend towards increased frequency (Figure 2B) and duration (Figure 2E) of rapid exploratory motion after 3 minutes in the female MPS IIIA mice ($p = 0.23$, $p = 0.10$). After 10 ($p = 0.021$, $p = 0.034$) and 60 minutes ($p = 0.0003$, $p = 0.0057$), female MPS IIIA mice had significantly increased frequency (Figure 2B) and duration (Figure 2E) of rapid exploratory motion over 100 mm/s. No significant differences were observed between male WT and MPS IIIA mice. This rapid exploratory behaviour is visible in Video S1 which shows the median female WT and MPS IIIA mouse at 6 months of age at 4 times normal speed.

At 8 months of age, female MPS IIIA mice show a trend towards increased frequency of rapid exploratory motion over 60 minutes ($p = 0.18$) (Figure 2C), with a trend to increase in duration after 10 minutes ($p = 0.083$) and a significant increase after 60 minutes ($p = 0.02$) (Figure 2F). Male MPS IIIA and WT mice were indistinguishable. Using MANOVA repeated measure analysis, there was a significant difference between WT and MPS IIIA mice over all three time points for frequency (Genotype; $p = 0.004$) and duration (Genotype; $p = 0.013$) of rapid exploratory motion. There was a significant decline in frequency (Time; $p = 9.7 \times 10^{-15}$) and duration (Time, $p = 4.5 \times 10^{-8}$) of rapid exploratory motion with time and also between genotypes over

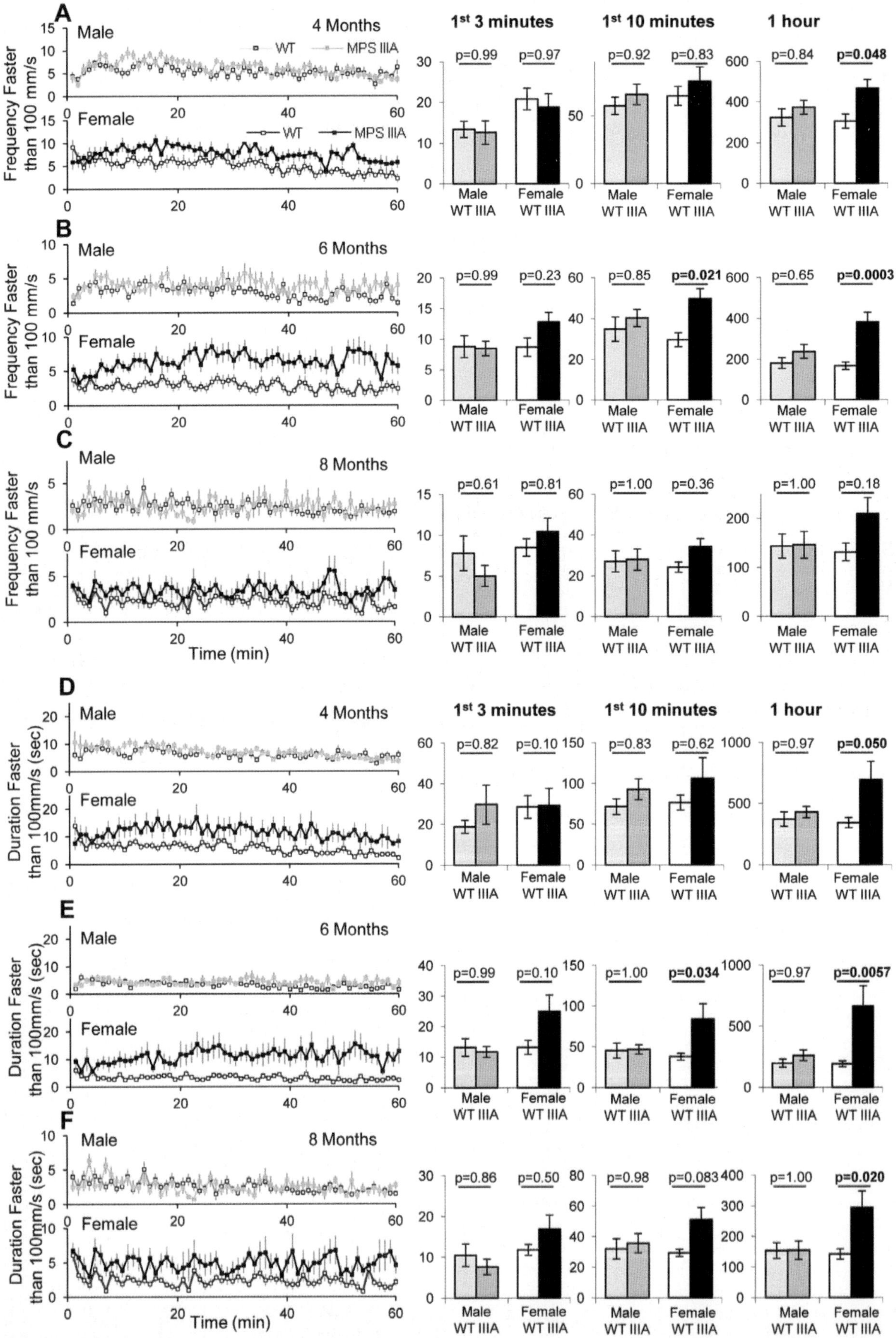
A
Male
4 Months
WT
MPS IIIA
Female
Frequency Faster than 100 mm/s
1st 3 minutes
1st 10 minutes
1 hour
p=0.99
p=0.97
p=0.92
p=0.83
p=0.84
p=0.048
Male WT IIIA
Female WT IIIA
B
Male
6 Months
Female
Frequency Faster than 100 mm/s
p=0.99
p=0.23
p=0.85
p=0.021
p=0.65
p=0.0003
C
Male
8 Months
Female
Frequency Faster than 100 mm/s
Time (min)
p=0.61
p=0.81
p=1.00
p=0.36
p=1.00
p=0.18
D
Male
4 Months
Female
Duration Faster than 100mm/s (sec)
1st 3 minutes
1st 10 minutes
1 hour
p=0.82
p=0.10
p=0.83
p=0.62
p=0.97
p=0.050
E
Male
6 Months
Female
Duration Faster than 100mm/s (sec)
p=0.99
p=0.10
p=1.00
p=0.034
p=0.97
p=0.0057
F
Male
8 Months
Female
Duration Faster than 100mm/s (sec)
Time (min)
p=0.86
p=0.50
p=0.98
p=0.083
p=1.00
p=0.020

Figure 2. Open field rapid exploratory behaviour. At 4, 6 and 8 months of age 10 WT male (light grey squares), 10 MPS IIIA male (dark grey squares), 10 WT female (white squares) and 11 MPS IIIA female (black squares) were placed in the open field and the behaviour was recorded for 60 minutes. The results of this test are presented as a 60 minute period with the average of every minute presented and as a bar chart of the first 3 minutes, first 10 minutes and the whole hour. Error bars represent the SEM. p values were calculated by 2 Way ANOVA. The frequency of moving faster than 100 mm/s at 4 (A), 6 (B) and 8 (C) months and the duration spent moving faster than 100 mm/s at 4 (D), 6 (E) and 8 (F) months of age have been presented.

time for frequency (Time*Genotype $p = 0.00005$) and duration (Time*Genotype, $p = 0.036$).

The frequency and duration the mice spent immobile was also recorded (Figure 3A–F). There were no significant differences in frequency of immobility between either male or female MPS IIIA and WT mice at any time point. However, female WT mice had significantly increased duration of immobility over 60 minutes at 4 ($p = 0.005$) and 6 months ($p = 0.004$) but not at 8 months ($p = 0.70$). Male MPS IIIA or WT mice had indistinguishable duration of immobility at all time points measured. Using MANOVA repeated measures there was an overall increase in the frequency of WT immobility over MPS IIIA mice over the three time points (Genotype; $p = 0.027$), but no change with time (Time; $p = 0.543$), or genotype with time interaction (Genotype*-Time; $p = 0.636$). MANOVA repeated measures analysis of duration of immobility demonstrated a significant genotype effect over the three time points (Genotype; $p = 0.05$), that changes significantly with time (Time; $p = 1.5 \times 10^{-9}$) and changes differently with time between the two genotypes (Genotype*Time; $p = 0.030$).

Mice being a prey species tend to display thigmotaxis, remaining close to the sides of an open field arena. Increased frequency and duration of time spent in the centre of the open field test therefore demonstrates reduced thigmotaxis and this is commonly considered to be a measure of reduced anxiety or reduced sense of danger that the animal experiences [37]. Male MPS IIIA and WT mice showed no significant differences in frequency of centre entries at any age (Figure 4A, B and C). At 4 months of age, female MPS IIIA mice showed significantly increased centre entries at 60 minutes ($p = 0.0045$). At 6 months female MPS IIIA mice entered the centre significantly more at 3, 10 and 60 minutes ($p = 0.057$, $p = 0.023$, $p = 0.0005$; Figure 4B). At 8 months of age female MPS IIIA showed no significant increases in centre entries ($p = 0.37$)(Figure 4C). Using MANOVA MPS IIIA mice showed significantly increased centre entries (Genotype; $p = 0.003$), which changed significantly over time (Time; $p = 2.3 \times 10^{-11}$) and between genotypes over time (Genotype*Time; $p = 0.0013$).

The duration spent in the centre has also been analysed. At 4 months of age, female MPS IIIA mice spent significantly more time in the centre than WT, after 60 minutes ($p = 0.012$; Figure 4D). Males were not significantly different. At 6 months of age female MPS IIIA mice had increase duration in the centre after 60 minutes ($p = 0.012$) and showed an almost significant trend in male mice ($p = 0.055$; Figure 4E). At 8 months of age there are no significant differences between genotypes (Figure 4F). By MANOVA repeated measure analysis MPS IIIA mice spend significantly increased duration in the centre area (Genotype; $p = 0.001$), this changes significantly over time (Time; $p = 2.5 \times 10^{-6}$) and between genotypes over time (Time*Genotype; $p = 0.005$).

Thirty minutes after behavioural analysis in the open field, the same cohort of mice were tested on an elevated plus maze (Figure 5A) for ten minutes, followed by a 30 minute rest and another 10 minute trial. Several parameters were measured (frequency of entering open arm, percentage of entries into the open arm, path length in open arm, percentage of path length in open arm and time in open arm) but none reached significance. Here we have presented the percentage of entries to the open arms, percentage of path length in the open arms and duration in the open arms as measure of anxiety (Figure 5B, C, D), which is representative of many of the other measures. At 4, 6 and 8 months of age there was no significant difference in male or female WT or MPS IIIA open arm entries (Figure 5B, C, D). At 4, 6 and 8 months there was no difference between WT and MPS IIIA mice in the repeat elevated plus maze and no difference between first and second elevated plus maze tests except that in the second test, all the mice performed fewer entries and had a shorter path length (Figure S1A–C). Statistical analysis by MANOVA showed no significant difference in genotype, or time but there was a significant difference in how the genotypes behaved over time in the percentage of path length in the open arm ($p = 0.019$) as the MPS IIIA mouse path length decreased at 8 months but the WT increased.

The inverted screen test (Figure 6A) and horizontal bar crossing test (Figure 6B) were also performed. The inverted screen test measures neuromuscular strength and the bar crossing test measures both neuromuscular strength and motor coordination. The bar crossing test showed no significant differences between WT and MPS IIIA of either sex at 4, 6 or 8 months of age (Figure 6C–E). Over time, there was a significant decrease in the number of moves and time spent on the inverted screen ($p = 1.7 \times 10^{-6}$, $p = 1.2 \times 10^{-5}$), and a significant sex difference in the number of moves with females moving more ($p = 0.004$). Bar crossing showed no genotype effect and no time effect but there was a significant Time*Sex effect ($p = 0.044$), as the female score decreased over time but the male score increased at 6 months and then decreased at 8 months.

Discussion

We have backcrossed the mixed background MPS IIIA mouse model onto the C57BL/6J background and characterised a behavioural phenotype that can be used to accurately distinguish female MPS IIIA mice from WT littermates. Our findings clearly show that male mice show no significant difference to WT littermates in the open field test or elevated plus maze, whilst female MPS IIIA mice demonstrate characteristic hyperactive behaviour initially at 4 months (16 weeks) and more strongly at 6 months (24 weeks), which declines again at 8 months (32 weeks) of age. We also show that these mice have a reduced thigmotaxis at 4 and 6 months of age which would indicate a reduced sense of danger. Hyperactivity and a reduced sense of danger are observed in the behavioural phenotype of the MPS IIIA patients [1,7,10,11].

In this study we observed no significant behavioural differences between WT and MPS IIIA male mice. This is in contrast to Hemsley *et al.* 2005 where hyperactivity was initially observed at 3 weeks, hypoactivity at 6 and 15 weeks and no changes at 10, 20 and 40 weeks in male mixed background mice [32]. Lau *et al.* 2008 used male MPS IIIA mice that had been back crossed onto the C57BL/6 background and observed no differences at 3, 5 and 15

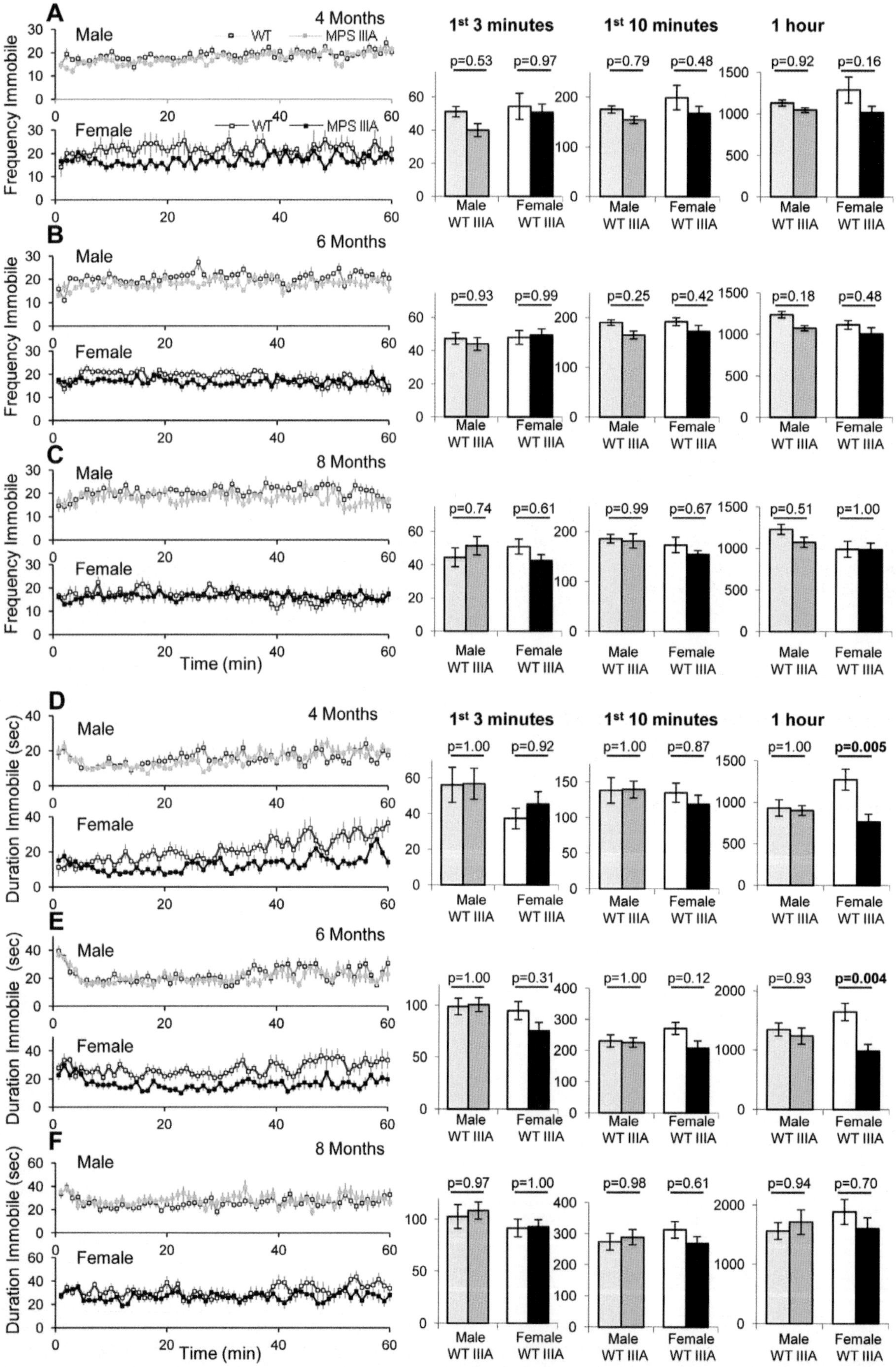
A
4 Months
B
6 Months
C
8 Months
D
4 Months
E
6 Months
F
8 Months
Male
Female
WT
MPS IIIA
Frequency Immobile
Duration Immobile (sec)
Time (min)
1st 3 minutes
1st 10 minutes
1 hour
WT IIIA
p=0.005
p=0.004

Figure 3. Open field immobile behaviour. At 4, 6 and 8 months of age 10 WT male (light grey squares), 10 MPS IIIA male (dark grey squares), 10 WT female (white squares) and 11 MPS IIIA female (black squares) were placed in the open field and the behaviour was recorded for 60 minutes. The results of this test are presented as a 60 minute period with the average of every minute presented and as a bar chart of the first 3 minutes, first 10 minutes and the whole hour. Error bars represent the SEM. p values were calculated by 2 Way ANOVA. The frequency of not moving at 4 (A), 6 (B) and 8 (C) months and the duration spent not moving at 4 (D), 6 (E) and 8 (F) months of age have been presented.

weeks, with significant hypoactivity at 10, 18 and 22 weeks [33] but subsequently observed hypoactivity in 15 week old male mice [22]. Crawley *et al.*, using male MPS IIIA mice on the same C57BL/6 background, found no changes at 4, 6, 8, 10, 15, 18, 22, 25, 32 and 40 weeks and only observed hyperactivity at 12 weeks [30]. Finally, using male mice independently crossed onto the C57BL/6J background by Jackson laboratories, hypoactivity was observed in MPS IIIA mice at 20 weeks of age by McIntyre *et al.* but no difference was found at 24 or 32 weeks [38]. Clearly, it is hard to obtain consistent behavioural readouts from male mice in this context and it is always difficult to know if hypoactivity could be confounded by any parameter affecting the mouse's physical ability to move. We find male MPS IIIA mice to be very aggressive and are unable to keep them group housed, which is likely to change their behaviour. Singly housing male C57BL/6 mice has been shown to increase locomotor activity and reduce anxiety [39] or alternatively in other researchers hands to have no effect [40]. At the very least, it certainly leads to weight gains, which will restrict movement, and this may confound reliable open field measures. Additionally we find that all MPS IIIA mice retain urine over time, with male mice retaining significantly more urine at 8 months of age and urine retention is the humane endpoint (Figure S2). Clearly urinary retention could be restricting movement which would confound behavioural measures. Lastly, it is worth pointing out that many male mouse studies are on mixed, C57BL/6 or C57BL/6J backgrounds, some of which have been performed in different laboratories, which could lead to inconsistencies in outcomes. Overall, we would argue that comparisons of male MPS IIIA mice with WT are not appropriate (or easy to perform) for determination of treatment responses.

Several studies analysed behaviour of male MPS IIIA mice following control intracranial injections. Fraldi *et al.* tested male mice and found that the MPS IIIA mice were hyperactive at 21 weeks of age but not prior to this, but these mice had received intracranial injections and this may have adversely affected the mouse's behaviour [23]. Other studies where intracranial injections have been given to MPS IIIA mice all used male mice and generally observed either no changes or hypoactivity [18,21,35]. It is worth considering that intracranial injections could have altered the natural behaviour of the mouse and this may be why hypoactivity is observed.

We found female MPS IIIA mice to be hyperactive, having a significantly increased path length, frequency and duration of rapid exploratory behaviour and reduced duration of immobility at 4 and 6 months of age, (16 and 24 weeks) whilst duration of rapid exploratory behaviour was significantly increased at 8 months (32 weeks). At 4 months of age differences are only significant after 60 minutes, but at 6 months they are all significant after both 10 and 60 minutes. This indicates that the 60 minute test is a more sensitive test to identify hyperactivity than the 10 or 3 minutes tests. No significant differences were observed over the first 3 minutes at any time point, thus we would suggest that studies such as that of Crawley *et al.* 2006 where this short test has been used are not likely to yield significant differences [30].

Our hyperactivity findings in females are supported by Crawley *et al*, where hyperactivity was observed at 22 and 32 weeks of age in a 3 minute test with female MPS IIIA C57BL/6 mice, however no difference was observed at any point prior to 18 weeks or at 25 or 40 weeks of age [30]. They also observed hypoactivity in females at 4 weeks of age but we do not have comparative data to comment on this. The longer testing time utilised in our study may have meant that we were better able to detect behavioural changes in the mice that were not detectable with the 3 minute test.

On the mixed background, female MPS IIIA mice were hyperactive at 3 weeks of age but at subsequent ages no differences were observed at 6, 10, 15, 20, 30 or 40 weeks of age [32]. In the work of Lau *et al.*, using the C57BL/6 backcross, no differences were observed between female WT and MPS IIIA C57BL/6 mice between 3–22 weeks of age [33].

MPS IIIB is a phenotypically indistinguishable disease to MPS IIIA. In the mouse model of MPS IIIB, hyperactivity has been observed in a 10 minute open field test [41] but hypoactivity in an 8 minute open field test performed half in the light half in the dark [42]. A 60 minute open field test did not report differences in path length in male or female mice [43], but a 60 minute open field test that we performed on female mice at the same circadian time as this study observed hyperactivity at 8 months of age [36], which is consistent with our findings here. We also observed significant increases in hyperactivity in male MPS IIIB mice at 8 months of age, although they were less significant differences than those observed in females [14]. The MPS IIIB mouse is a complete knockout and thus may be slightly more severe than the MPS IIIA mouse with ~3% residual enzyme activity. This may explain why we were able to detect significant genotype differences at 8 months of age in MPS IIIB in all parameters but only some in MPS IIIA. We believe that the 60 minute open field test is still measuring habituation behaviour due to the profiles of activity observed in both MPSIIIA mice in this paper and in MPSIIIB mice [36] over time. We found that differences in behaviour between MPS IIIB and WT mice [36] and MPS IIIA and WT mice (Figure 1B and C) became more pronounced from 3 to 10 to 60 minutes and diverged in the first few minutes from a similar initial response. When we compared MPS IIIB and WT mice over a 24 hour period following 24 hours of habituation [36] the differences were significantly muted and over 14 days there was no significant difference [44]. This suggests that a 60 minute open field test does not reflect home cage behaviour but instead probably measures extended habituation to a novel environment.

A significant decrease in the number of unsupported rears by female MPS IIIA mice was observed at 6 months of age, however, there was no difference in the overall number of rears, or supported rears, at this or any other time point. No consistent trend in the number of rears with female mice is apparent in the literature, Crawley *et al.* reported that female MPS IIIA mice reared less at 15 and 25 weeks of age but there were no significant differences at 9 other time points [30]. No significant differences in rearing were observed in Lau *et al.* who also used backcrossed mice [33], or Hemsley *et al* who used mixed background mice [32]. A more consistent trend is observed in male mice with MPS IIIA rearing less [18,30,32,33,35], but increased rearing has been observed at 3 weeks [32]. However, at most time points no significant difference is observed. Manual measurement of rears

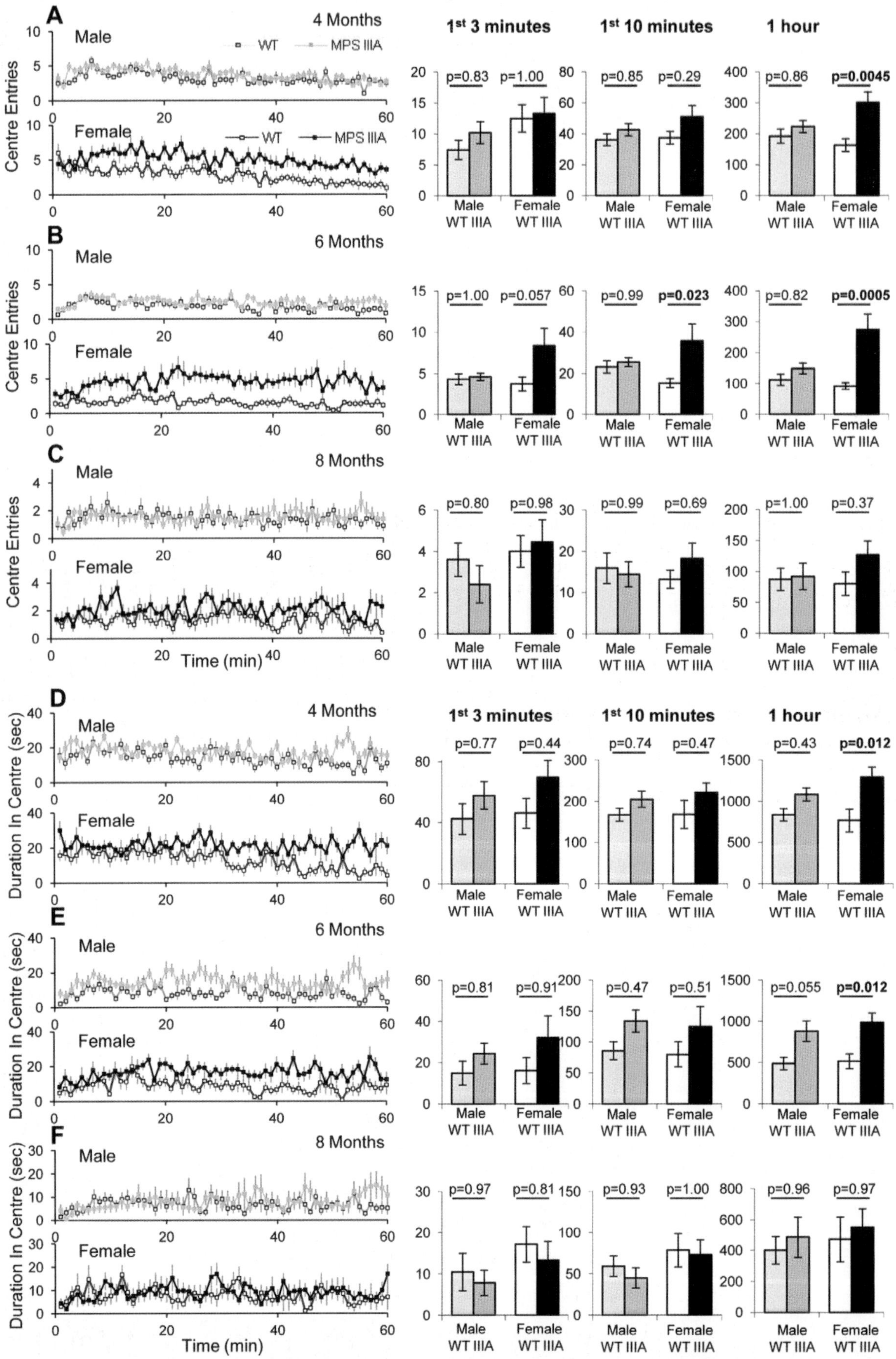
A
4 Months
Male
WT
MPS IIIA
Female
Centre Entries
1st 3 minutes
1st 10 minutes
1 hour
p=0.83
p=1.00
p=0.85
p=0.29
p=0.86
p=0.0045
Male WT IIIA
Female WT IIIA
B
6 Months
p=1.00
p=0.057
p=0.99
p=0.023
p=0.82
p=0.0005
C
8 Months
p=0.80
p=0.98
p=0.99
p=0.69
p=1.00
p=0.37
Time (min)
D
Duration In Centre (sec)
p=0.77
p=0.44
p=0.74
p=0.47
p=0.43
p=0.012
E
p=0.81
p=0.91
p=0.47
p=0.51
p=0.055
p=0.012
F
p=0.97
p=0.81
p=0.93
p=1.00
p=0.96
p=0.97

Figure 4. Open field sense of danger behaviour. At 4, 6 and 8 months of age 10 WT male (light grey squares), 10 MPS IIIA male (dark grey squares), 10 WT female (white squares) and 11 MPS IIIA female (black squares) were placed in the open field and the behaviour was recorded for 60 minutes. The results of this test are presented as a 60 minute period with the average of every minute presented and as a bar chart of the first 3 minutes, first 10 minutes and the whole hour. Error bars represent the SEM. p values were calculated by 2 Way ANOVA. The frequency of entering the centre at 4 (A), 6 (B) and 8 (C) months and the duration spent in the centre at 4 (D), 6 (E) and 8 (F) months of age have been presented.

can be subjective and there may be variations in the rearing behaviour, such as amount of time per rear that cannot be measured by simply counting the number of rears. This is why we examined the number of supported and unsupported rears [36,45]. In the MPS IIIB mouse model, no difference in rearing was observed in the first 10 minutes of an open field test with female mice at 8 months of age [36] and no difference in the first 30 minutes but a significant decrease in the number of rears by 4.5–5 month old male MPS IIIB mice in the second 30 minutes of a 60 minute open field test [43]. Our conclusion is that rearing is too variable an outcome in MPS IIIA and IIIB mice and is therefore not a valuable informative test.

At 4 and 6 months of age the MPS IIIA female mice had a reduced sense of danger and spent a greater proportion of time in

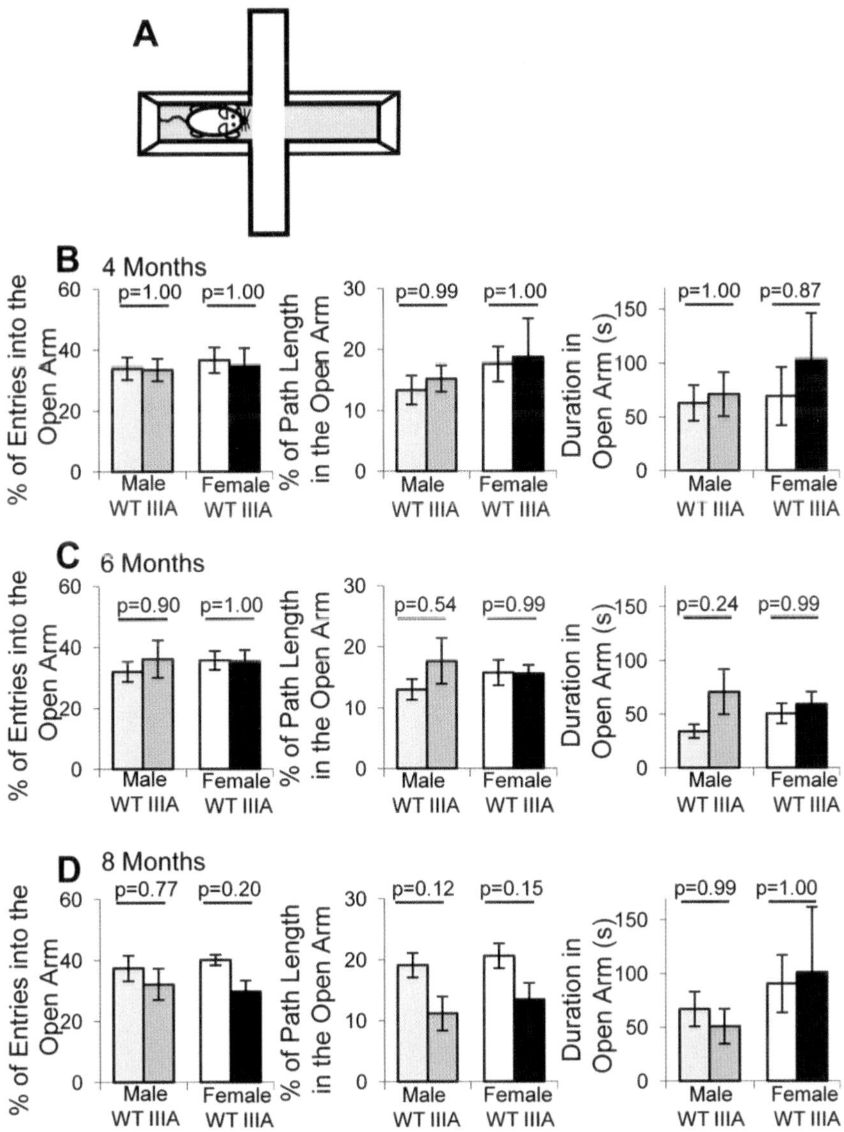

Figure 5. Elevated plus maze behaviour. At 4, 6 and 8 months of age 7–11 WT male (light grey bars), MPS IIIA male (dark grey bars), WT female (white bars) and MPS IIIA female (black bars) were placed on the elevated plus maze (A) and the behaviour was recorded for 10 minutes. After a 30 minute rest, the test was repeated. The results of the first test are presented as the mean of each measure with error bars representing the SEM. p values were calculated by 2 Way ANOVA. The following measures have been presented; the percentage of total entries that were into the open arm, the percentage of the path length in the open arm and the duration spent on the open arm at 4 (B), 6 (C) and 8 (D) months of age.

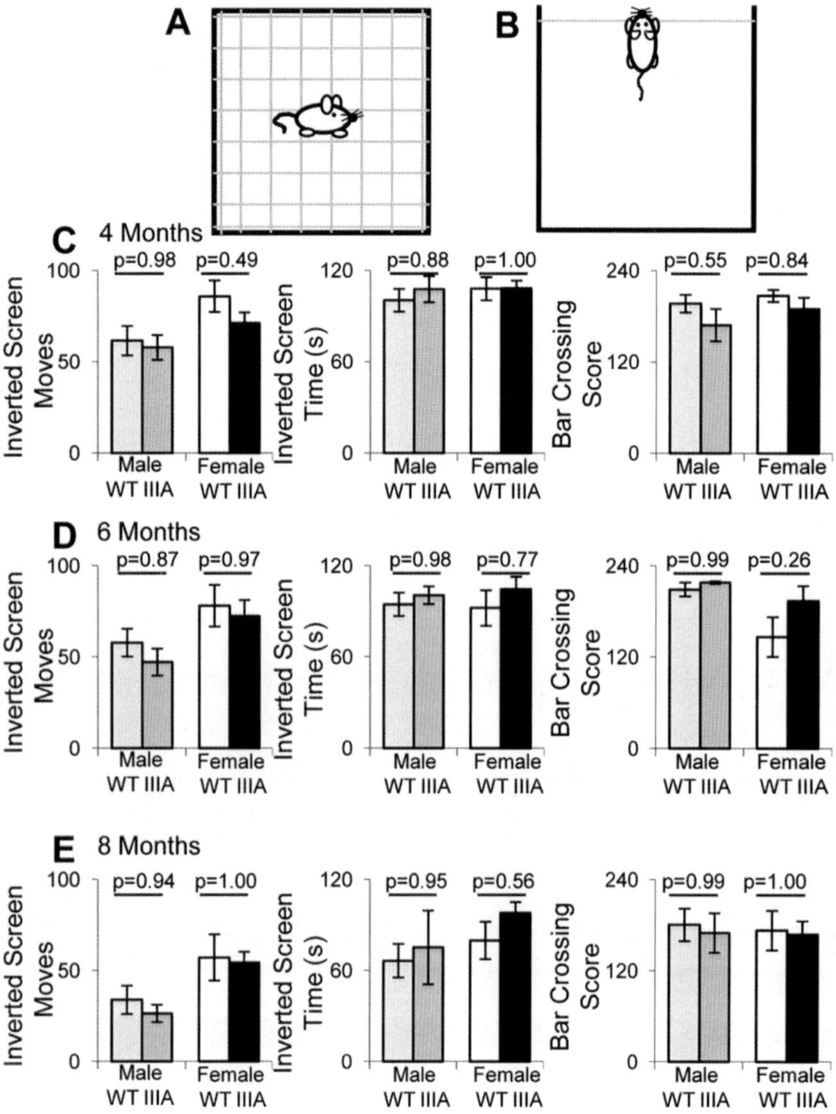

Figure 6. Neuromuscular behaviour. At 4, 6 and 8 months of age 8–11 WT male (light grey bars), MPS IIIA male (dark grey bars), WT female (white bars) and MPS IIIA female (black bars) were placed on the inverted screen test (A) and horizontal bar crossing test (B). The number of rear leg moves, the time spent on the inverted screen and the bar crossing score are presented at 4 (C), 6 (D) and 8 (E) moths of age. Error bars represent the SEM and p values were calculated by 2 Way ANOVA.

the centre of the open field, this measure was significant after 60 minutes but not after 3 or 10 minutes. This is supported by the patients with MPS IIIA which are believed to have a reduced sense of danger [1]. No difference in the time in centre was detected by Lau *et al.* in both male and female mice [33], however this could be because the open field was larger in our study and therefore more sensitive to thigmotaxis [45,46]. In the MPS IIIB mouse model no differences were observed in the duration spent in the centre of the open field [36] but the open field used in that study was also smaller than the one used in this study.

The elevated plus maze did not demonstrate a decrease in anxiety or sense of danger in the MPS IIIA mice. There were also no differences between repeat tests, and both WT and MPS IIIA mice appeared to habituate equally. Lau *et al.* 2010, observed no significant differences with male mice at 6.5 months (26 weeks) of age with a 5 minute elevated plus maze test, but there was a trend towards reduced anxiety [34]. However in Lau *et al.* 2008 a significant increase in the time the male MPS IIIA mice spent in the open arms at 18 weeks of age, the percentage of the path length on the open arms at 15 and 18 weeks and the percentage of entries into the open arms at 20 weeks was observed [33]. Additionally they observed significant differences between repeats of the elevated plus maze, male MPS IIIA mice had a significantly longer path length in the repeat elevated plus maze test while WT mice remained unchanged [33]. We did not observe decreased anxiety or a change in behaviour between repeat elevated plus maze tests. The width of the arms could be affecting this test as this study used 10 cm wide arms and Lau *et al.*, used 7 cm wide arms. It has been demonstrated that when using 5, 7 or 9 cm wide arms, NMRI mice spent more time in the wider open arms compared to C57BL/10J mice that showed no difference [47]. Ten minutes on the elevated plus maze may also be too short a time to detect the sense of danger differences in the MPS IIIA mice as the only centre measure on open field that is significant after 10 minutes is the number of centre entries in female mice at 6 months of age ($p = 0.023$). A lack of difference in the elevated plus maze performed in daylight is supported by MPS IIIB mice which showed no difference in the light but were less anxious in the dark [41]. The increased number of centre entries and duration in the open field could perhaps reflect increased but undirected anxiety whereby mice are actually more agitated but have lost the ability to determine what is dangerous. A more pragmatic explanation could be due to the mice not being naively tested as they only received a 30 minute break after the open field test before starting the elevated plus maze test. Prior behavioural tests can affect the result of elevated plus maze tests with C57BL/6J mice that have previously been tested in an open field test [48].

No significant differences were observed in the inverted screen or bar crossing tests which is consistent with the work of Crawley *et al.* who observed no difference in neuromuscular strength with back crossed MPS IIIA mice [30]. However on the mixed background strain, there was a significant decrease in neuromuscular strength with MPS IIIA mice being unable to grip the inverted screen for as long as the WT mice from 20 weeks of age [32]. The work in our study is supported by work with the MPS IIIB mouse model that does not show a decline in motor function at 5 months of age by accelerating rotarod [43,49] but does by a rocking rotarod test from 9 months onwards [50,51]. The decline in motor function could relate to the presence of increasing urine retention in the MPS IIIA and B mouse models [14,26,29]. Our own tests in the MPS IIIB mouse model found that neuromuscular decline only occurred at 10 months of age (40 weeks) [14,36]. Given that the MPS IIIA mouse has residual enzyme activity, it is possible that progression of MPS IIIA disease is slightly less rapid than in MPS IIIB which would explain why we did not see a trend to changes in motor function at 8 months in MPS IIIA mice.

Standardisation of tests is a very important aspect of behavioural test design that may have affected comparison of our tests to those of other laboratories. In this study the size of the open field was larger than that described in many studies and the behaviour was observed for much longer (60 minutes compared to 3 minutes). The increased size and time of the test allows better spatial and temporal resolution of the mouse behaviour and so makes the test more sensitive [45]. Video analysis software was used which has been shown to be more sensitive than line crossing determined by an observer or beam breaks [52]. In this study, the mouse was placed in the centre of the open field rather than in the corner and the test was carried out at the same time point of circadian rhythm for all mice as there is a known peak in activity in the similar MPS IIIB mouse model [44]. The mice in this study were also housed differently; females were group housed and male mice were singly housed from 14 weeks of age. The background of the mice can affect the behavioural phenotype, therefore we backcrossed the MPS IIIA mice in this study onto the C57BL/6J background for more than 10 generations. Other groups have used MPS IIIA mice on a mixed background [18,32], or on a C57BL/6 [23,30,33,34] or C57BL/6J [21] background. Strain specific differences can also significantly affect behavioural outcomes [53].

Conclusion

We have demonstrated that we can reliably detect differences in the behaviour of female but not male MPS IIIA mice at 4 and 6 months (16 and 24 weeks) of age and these differences match the patient phenotype. Male mice were singly housed due to their aggression which may change comparative behavioural responses. Female MPS IIIA mice are hyperactive, with a longer path length, increased frequency and duration of rapid exploratory behaviour, and spend less time immobile. They also show a trend to this behaviour at 8 months of age with significantly increased duration of rapid exploratory behaviour. Female MPS IIIA mice demonstrate a reduced sense of danger with a greater proportion of the time spent in the centre of the open field with a greater number of centre entries. These two time points and multiple measures are ideal to evaluate novel therapies for MPS IIIA as the effect of a therapy can be sensitively determined using multiple measures. This behavioural phenotype is supported by both the phenotype of the patients and our recent similar observations in the MPS IIIB mouse model [14,36]. The increased size of the open field, the increased length of the test, the use of video analysis software and performing the test at consistent point in the circadian rhythm have produced a sensitive and robust test to evaluate the effect of therapies on female MPS IIIA mice.

Supporting Information

Figure S1 Repeat elevated plus maze behaviour. At 4, 6 and 8 months of age 7–11 WT male (light grey bars), MPS IIIA male (dark grey bars), WT female (white bars) and MPS IIIA female (black bars) were placed on the elevated plus maze (A) and the behaviour was recorded for 10 minutes. After a 30 minute rest, the test was repeated. The results of the repeat test are presented as the mean of each measure with error bars representing the SEM. p values were calculated by 2 Way ANOVA. The following measures have been presented; the percentage of total entries that were into the open arm, the percentage of the path length in the open arm and the duration spent on the open arm at 4 (A), 6 (B) and 8 (C) months of age.

Figure S2 Urine retention at 8 months. At 8 months of age 9 WT male (light grey bars), 8 MPS IIIA male (dark grey bars), 7 WT female (white bars) and 8 MPS IIIA female (black bars) were sacrificed and the urine volume in the bladder measured. The results are presented as the mean with error bars representing the SEM. p values were calculated by 2 Way ANOVA.

Video S1 Open field behaviour video. A video running at 4 times the normal speed showing the median female WT and MPS IIIA mouse at 6 months of age. The MPS IIIA mouse is on the left and the WT mouse is on the right.

Acknowledgments

The authors gratefully acknowledge the help and assistance of the staff of the Manchester BSU, Dr Richard Preziosi for statistical advice and the Manchester Biomedical Research Centre.

Author Contributions

Conceived and designed the experiments: AL-S KJL-S FLW BWB. Performed the experiments: AL-S KJL-S. Analyzed the data: AL-S KJL-S FLW BWB. Wrote the paper: AL-S KJL-S SAJ RFW JEW FLW BWB.

References

1. Heron B, Mikaeloff Y, Froissart R, Caridade G, Maire I, et al. (2011) Incidence and natural history of mucopolysaccharidosis type III in France and comparison with United Kingdom and Greece. American journal of medical genetics Part A 155A: 58–68.

2. Meyer A, Kossow K, Gal A, Muhlhausen C, Ullrich K, et al. (2007) Scoring evaluation of the natural course of mucopolysaccharidosis type IIIA (Sanfilippo syndrome type A). Pediatrics 120: e1255–1261.
3. Valstar MJ, Neijs S, Bruggenwirth HT, Olmer R, Ruijter GJG, et al. (2010) Mucopolysaccharidosis type IIIA: Clinical spectrum and genotype-phenotype correlations. Annals of Neurology 68: 876–887.
4. Kresse H (1973) Mucopolysaccharidosis 3 A (Sanfilippo A disease): deficiency of a heparin sulfamidase in skin fibroblasts and leucocytes. Biochem Biophys Res Commun 54: 1111–1118.
5. Kresse H, Neufeld EF (1972) The Sanfilippo A corrective factor. Purification and mode of action. J Biol Chem 247: 2164–2170.
6. Scott HS, Blanch L, Guo XH, Freeman C, Orsborn A, et al. (1995) Cloning of the sulphamidase gene and identification of mutations in Sanfilippo A syndrome. Nat Genet 11: 465–467.
7. Valstar M, Ruijter G, van Diggelen O, Poorthuis B, Wijburg F (2008) Sanfilippo syndrome: A mini-review. Journal of Inherited Metabolic Disease 31: 240–252.
8. Malm G, Månsson JE (2010) Mucopolysaccharidosis type III (Sanfilippo disease) in Sweden: clinical presentation of 22 children diagnosed during a 30-year period. Acta Pædiatrica 99: 1253–1257.
9. Fraser J, Wraith JE, Delatycki MB (2002) Sleep disturbance in mucopolysaccharidosis type III (Sanfilippo syndrome): a survey of managing clinicians. Clin Genet 62: 418–421.
10. Bax MC, Colville GA (1995) Behaviour in mucopolysaccharide disorders. Arch Dis Child 73: 77–81.
11. Cleary MA, Wraith JE (1993) Management of mucopolysaccharidosis type III. Arch Dis Child 69: 403–406.
12. Fraser J, Gason AA, Wraith JE, Delatycki MB (2005) Sleep disturbance in Sanfilippo syndrome: a parental questionnaire study. Arch Dis Child 90: 1239–1242.
13. Roberts AL, Rees MH, Klebe S, Fletcher JM, Byers S (2007) Improvement in behaviour after substrate deprivation therapy with rhodamine B in a mouse model of MPS IIIA. Mol Genet Metab 92: 115–121.
14. Malinowska M, Wilkinson FL, Langford-Smith KJ, Langford-Smith A, Brown JR, et al. (2010) Genistein improves neuropathology and corrects behaviour in a mouse model of neurodegenerative metabolic disease. PLoS ONE 5: e14192.
15. Malinowska M, Wilkinson FL, Bennett W, Langford-Smith KJ, O'Leary HA, et al. (2009) Genistein reduces lysosomal storage in peripheral tissues of mucopolysaccharide IIIB mice. Molecular Genetics and Metabolism 98: 235–242.
16. Hemsley KM, Norman EJ, Crawley AC, Auclair D, King B, et al. (2009) Effect of cisternal sulfamidase delivery in MPS IIIA Huntaway dogs–a proof of principle study. Mol Genet Metab 98: 383–392.
17. Hemsley KM, Beard H, King BM, Hopwood JJ (2008) Effect of high dose, repeated intra-cerebrospinal fluid injection of sulphamidase on neuropathology in mucopolysaccharidosis type IIIA mice. Genes, Brain and Behavior 7: 740–753.
18. Hemsley KM, King B, Hopwood JJ (2007) Injection of recombinant human sulfamidase into the CSF via the cerebellomedullary cistern in MPS IIIA mice. Mol Genet Metab 90: 313–328.
19. Savas PS, Hemsley KM, Hopwood JJ (2004) Intracerebral injection of sulfamidase delays neuropathology in murine MPS-IIIA. Mol Genet Metab 82: 273–285.
20. Gliddon BL, Hopwood JJ (2004) Enzyme-replacement therapy from birth delays the development of behavior and learning problems in mucopolysaccharidosis type IIIA mice. Pediatr Res 56: 65–72.
21. McIntyre C, Byers S, Anson DS (2010) Correction of mucopolysaccharidosis type IIIA somatic and central nervous system pathology by lentiviral-mediated gene transfer. The journal of gene medicine 12: 717–728.
22. Lau AA, Hopwood JJ, Kremer EJ, Hemsley KM (2010) SGSH gene transfer in mucopolysaccharidosis type IIIA mice using canine adenovirus vectors. Mol Genet Metab 100: 168–175.
23. Fraldi A, Hemsley K, Crawley A, Lombardi A, Lau A, et al. (2007) Functional correction of CNS lesions in an MPS-IIIA mouse model by intracerebral AAV-mediated delivery of sulfamidase and SUMF1 genes. Hum Mol Genet 16: 2693–2702.
24. Langford-Smith KJ, Mercer J, Petty J, Tylee K, Church H, et al. (2011) Heparin cofactor II-thrombin complex and dermatan sulphate:chondroitin sulphate ratio are biomarkers of short- and long-term treatment effects in mucopolysaccharide diseases. Journal of inherited metabolic disease 34: 499–508.
25. Langford-Smith K, Arasaradnam M, Wraith JE, Wynn R, Bigger BW (2010) Evaluation of heparin cofactor II-thrombin complex as a biomarker on blood spots from mucopolysaccharidosis I, IIIA and IIIB mice. Molecular Genetics and Metabolism 99: 269–274.
26. Bhaumik M, Muller VJ, Rozaklis T, Johnson L, Dobrenis K, et al. (1999) A mouse model for mucopolysaccharidosis type III A (Sanfilippo syndrome). Glycobiology 9: 1389–1396.
27. McGlynn R, Dobrenis K, Walkley SU (2004) Differential subcellular localization of cholesterol, gangliosides, and glycosaminoglycans in murine models of mucopolysaccharide storage disorders. J Comp Neurol 480: 415–426.
28. Arfi A, Richard M, Gandolphe C, Bonnefont-Rousselot D, Therond P, et al. (2011) Neuroinflammatory and oxidative stress phenomena in MPS IIIA mouse model: the positive effect of long-term aspirin treatment. Molecular genetics and metabolism 103: 18–25.
29. Gografe SI, Sanberg PR, Chamizo W, Monforte H, Garbuzova-Davis S (2009) Novel pathologic findings associated with urinary retention in a mouse model of mucopolysaccharidosis type IIIB. Comparative medicine 59: 139–146.
30. Crawley AC, Gliddon BL, Auclair D, Brodie SL, Hirte C, et al. (2006) Characterization of a C57BL/6 congenic mouse strain of mucopolysaccharidosis type IIIA. Brain Res 1104: 1–17.
31. The Jackson Laboratory Website Available: http://jaxmice.jax.org/strain/003780.html. Accessed 2011 Sep 12.
32. Hemsley KM, Hopwood JJ (2005) Development of motor deficits in a murine model of mucopolysaccharidosis type IIIA (MPS-IIIA). Behav Brain Res 158: 191–199.
33. Lau AA, Crawley AC, Hopwood JJ, Hemsley KM (2008) Open field locomotor activity and anxiety-related behaviors in mucopolysaccharidosis type IIIA mice. Behav Brain Res 191: 130–136.
34. Lau AA, Hannouche H, Rozaklis T, Hassiotis S, Hopwood JJ, et al. (2010) Allogeneic stem cell transplantation does not improve neurological deficits in mucopolysaccharidosis type IIIA mice. Experimental neurology 225: 445–454.
35. Hemsley KM, Luck AJ, Crawley AC, Hassiotis S, Beard H, et al. (2009) Examination of intravenous and intra-CSF protein delivery for treatment of neurological disease. The European journal of neuroscience 29: 1197–1214.
36. Langford-Smith A, Malinowska M, Langford-Smith KJ, Wegrzyn G, Jones S, et al. (2011) Hyperactive behaviour in the mouse model of mucopolysaccharidosis IIIB in the open field and home cage environments. Genes, Brain and Behavior 10: 673–682.
37. Simon P, Dupuis R, Costentin J (1994) Thigmotaxis as an index of anxiety in mice. Influence of dopaminergic transmissions. Behav Brain Res 61: 59–64.
38. McIntyre C, Derrick Roberts AL, Ranieri E, Clements PR, Byers S, et al. (2008) Lentiviral-mediated gene therapy for murine mucopolysaccharidosis type IIIA. Mol Genet Metab 93: 411–418.
39. Voikar V, Polus A, Vasar E, Rauvala H (2005) Long-term individual housing in C57BL/6J and DBA/2 mice: assessment of behavioral consequences. Genes, brain, and behavior 4: 240–252.
40. Arndt SS, Laarakker MC, van Lith HA, van der Staay FJ, Gieling E, et al. (2009) Individual housing of mice–impact on behaviour and stress responses. Physiology & behavior 97: 385–393.
41. Cressant A, Desmaris N, Verot L, Brejot T, Froissart R, et al. (2004) Improved behavior and neuropathology in the mouse model of Sanfilippo type IIIB disease after adeno-associated virus-mediated gene transfer in the striatum. J Neurosci 24: 10229–10239.
42. Li HH, Yu WH, Rozengurt N, Zhao HZ, Lyons KM, et al. (1999) Mouse model of Sanfilippo syndrome type B produced by targeted disruption of the gene encoding alpha-N-acetylglucosaminidase. Proc Natl Acad Sci U S A 96: 14505–14510.
43. Fu H, Kang L, Jennings JS, Moy SS, Perez A, et al. (2007) Significantly increased lifespan and improved behavioral performances by rAAV gene delivery in adult mucopolysaccharidosis IIIB mice. Gene Ther 14: 1065–1077.
44. Canal MM, Wilkinson FL, Cooper JD, Ed Wraith J, Wynn R, et al. (2010) Circadian rhythm and suprachiasmatic nucleus alterations in the mouse model of mucopolysaccharidosis IIIB. Behav Brain Res 209: 212–220.
45. Benjamini Y, Lipkind D, Horev G, Fonio E, Kafkafi N, et al. (2010) Ten ways to improve the quality of descriptions of whole-animal movement. Neuroscience and biobehavioral reviews 34: 1351–1365.
46. Crawley JN (2007) What's wrong with my mouse? : behavioral phenotyping of transgenic and knockout mice. Hoboken, NJ: John Wiley. xvi, 523 p.
47. Lamberty Y, Gower AJ (1996) Arm width and brightness modulation of spontaneous behaviour of two strains of mice tested in the elevated plus-maze. Physiology & behavior 59: 439–444.
48. Voikar V, Vasar E, Rauvala H (2004) Behavioral alterations induced by repeated testing in C57BL/6J and 129S2/Sv mice: implications for phenotyping screens. Genes, brain, and behavior 3: 27–38.
49. Fu H, DiRosario J, Kang L, Muenzer J, McCarty DM (2010) Restoration of central nervous system alpha-N-acetylglucosaminidase activity and therapeutic benefits in mucopolysaccharidosis IIIB mice by a single intracisternal recombinant adeno-associated viral type 2 vector delivery. The journal of gene medicine 12: 624–633.
50. Heldermon CD, Hennig AK, Ohlemiller KK, Ogilvie JM, Herzog ED, et al. (2007) Development of sensory, motor and behavioral deficits in the murine model of Sanfilippo syndrome type B. PLoS ONE 2: e772.
51. Heldermon CD, Ohlemiller KK, Herzog ED, Vogler C, Qin E, et al. (2010) Therapeutic efficacy of bone marrow transplant, intracranial AAV-mediated gene therapy, or both in the mouse model of MPS IIIB. Mol Ther 18: 873–880.
52. Kafkafi N, Lipkind D, Benjamini Y, Mayo CL, Elmer GI, et al. (2003) SEE locomotor behavior test discriminates C57BL/6J and DBA/2J mouse inbred strains across laboratories and protocol conditions. Behavioral neuroscience 117: 464–477.
53. Gerlai R (1996) Gene-targeting studies of mammalian behavior: is it the mutation or the background genotype? Trends in neurosciences 19: 177–181.

Substrate Reduction Augments the Efficacy of Enzyme Therapy in a Mouse Model of Fabry Disease

John Marshall[1]*, Karen M. Ashe[1], Dinesh Bangari[1], KerryAnne McEachern[1], Wei-Lien Chuang[1], Joshua Pacheco[1], Diane P. Copeland[1], Robert J. Desnick[2], James A. Shayman[3], Ronald K. Scheule[1], Seng H. Cheng[1]

1 Applied Discovery Research, Genzyme Corporation, Framingham, Massachusetts, United States of America, **2** Genetics and Genomic Sciences, Mount Sinai School of Medicine, New York, New York, United States of America, **3** Internal Medicine – Nephrology, Genzyme Corporation, University of Michigan, Ann Arbor, Michigan, United States of America

Abstract

Fabry disease is an X-linked glycosphingolipid storage disorder caused by a deficiency in the activity of the lysosomal hydrolase α-galactosidase A (α-gal). This deficiency results in accumulation of the glycosphingolipid globotriaosylceramide (GL-3) in lysosomes. Endothelial cell storage of GL-3 frequently leads to kidney dysfunction, cardiac and cerebrovascular disease. The current treatment for Fabry disease is through infusions of recombinant α-gal (enzyme-replacement therapy; ERT). Although ERT can markedly reduce the lysosomal burden of GL-3 in endothelial cells, variability is seen in the clearance from several other cell types. This suggests that alternative and adjuvant therapies may be desirable. Use of glucosylceramide synthase inhibitors to abate the biosynthesis of glycosphingolipids (substrate reduction therapy, SRT) has been shown to be effective at reducing substrate levels in the related glycosphingolipidosis, Gaucher disease. Here, we show that such an inhibitor (eliglustat tartrate, Genz-112638) was effective at lowering GL-3 accumulation in a mouse model of Fabry disease. Relative efficacy of SRT and ERT at reducing GL-3 levels in Fabry mouse tissues differed with SRT being more effective in the kidney, and ERT more efficacious in the heart and liver. Combination therapy with ERT and SRT provided the most complete clearance of GL-3 from all the tissues. Furthermore, treatment normalized urine volume and uromodulin levels and significantly delayed the loss of a nociceptive response. The differential efficacies of SRT and ERT in the different tissues indicate that the combination approach is both additive and complementary suggesting the possibility of an improved therapeutic paradigm in the management of Fabry disease.

Editor: Raphael Schiffmann, National Institutes of Health, United States of America

Funding: All support for these studies was provided by Genzyme Corporation, the employer of all the authors except RJD and JAS. The described studies were part of the drug development program at Genzyme Corporation. The internal publication review committee approved the manuscript for publication.

Competing Interests: The authors have read the journal's policy and have the following conflicts: John Marshall, Karen Ashe, Dinesh Bangari, Kerry Anne McEachern, Wei-Lien Chuang, Joshua Pacheco, Diane Copeland, Ronald Scheule, and Seng Cheng are all employees of and shareholders in Genzyme Corporation. James Shayman is an employee of the University of Michigan and co-inventor of Genz-112638 which is licensed to Genzyme by the University of Michigan. Genzyme funded all the studies and is developing Eliglustat tartrate for treatment of type 1 Gaucher disease. Patents regarding this approach have been filed. This does not alter the authors' adherence to all the PLoS ONE policies on sharing data and materials.

* E-mail: john.marshall@genzyme.com

Introduction

The lysosomal storage disorder (LSD) Fabry disease is caused by mutations in the gene encoding the lysosomal hydrolase α-galactosidase A (α-gal) [1]. Deficiency in α-gal activity results in the abnormal accumulation of neutral glycosphingolipids, in particular globotriaosylceramide (GL-3) in many cell types. Vascular endothelium accumulation plays a major role, leading to kidney dysfunction, cardiac and cerebrovascular disease [2]. The current standard of care for Fabry patients is enzyme-replacement therapy (ERT) through periodic infusions of recombinant human α-gal (agalsidase beta or agalsidase alpha). This treatment has been shown to be effective at slowing the loss of renal function [3,4] and at reducing the cardiac disease [5]. However, its ability to abate disease progression particularly in patients with more advanced manifestations is more modest [6,7]. Also, the degree of accumulated GL-3 clearance varies depending upon the cell-type [8]. Hence, alternative or adjuvant therapies may provide an improvement over the existing treatment paradigm.

Several alternative therapeutic options have been evaluated for LSDs [9], with substrate reduction therapy (SRT) being the most promising based on its demonstrated efficacy in Gaucher disease and oral availability [10,11]. SRT works on the principle of limiting the production of the pathologic substrate, which in the case of Fabry disease is primarily GL-3. This can be achieved by inhibiting the enzyme glucosylceramide synthase which catalyzes the first step in the synthesis of glycosphingolipids (GL-1) and therefore subsequent molecules including GL-3. The premise of SRT for Fabry disease using inhibitors of glucosylceramide synthase has been evaluated in mouse models [12–14] and shown to be of some benefit in lessening the burden of glycolipid accumulation. A candidate inhibitor, miglustat, is approved for treatment of type 1 Gaucher disease (in patients for whom ERT is not a therapeutic option). It is however associated with adverse side effects [15,16] that may compound reported Fabry disease symptoms (*e.g.* diarrhea, peripheral neuropathy) and is not approved for this indication [17]. It is desirable to have alternative small molecule drugs with the appropriate safety profile for SRT of Fabry disease. However, it should be noted that because the majority of Fabry patients are null for α-gal activity, SRT as a monotherapy is unlikely to be as effective as it has been shown for type 1 Gaucher patients, whom invariably retain some residual glucocerebrosidase activity. This distinction suggests that a combination of ERT and SRT may be a more beneficial approach to managing Fabry disease.

To evaluate the relative merits of a combined SRT and ERT approach for Fabry disease, we utilized a drug already shown to be active in SRT for Gaucher disease [11], namely eliglustat tartrate (Genz-112638). As an inhibitor of glucosylceramide synthase, eliglustat tartrate has been shown to be effective as both a monotherapy and in combination with ERT in a mouse model of Gaucher disease [18,19]. In the current studies, we evaluated this molecule in an α-galactosidase A knockout mouse [20] that exhibits many similarities with the human disease. Although the disease manifestations are less severe than noted in human, the mouse models of Fabry disease [20,21] nevertheless can provide valuable information on the merits of various therapeutic interventions [22]. Evaluations of potential therapies in these mice have focused mainly on tissue levels of GL-3, but other disease relevant symptoms could also be measured, such as heat-sensitivity as a marker of peripheral neuropathy [23,24]. Here, we describe our evaluation of SRT (using eliglustat tartrate) as a monotherapy as well as SRT in combination with ERT (using recombinant human α-galactosidase A) in a Fabry mouse model. We demonstrate that the therapeutic benefit of the combined therapy approach is both additive and complementary for treating this disease.

Results

The majority of our studies with SRT using eliglustat tartrate were performed using immunocompetent Fabry mice. However, because infusions of α-gal elicited the production of antibodies against the recombinant human enzyme (that may complicate interpretation of the results), studies that involved the use of ERT were performed using the Fabry-Rag mouse model, which does not generate a humoral response to recombinant human α-gal (data not shown). Although multiple symptoms are apparent in patients, Fabry mouse models are relatively normal except for modest accumulation of GL-3. We have noted previously [23] that the Fabry mouse also displays a progressive functional deficit in heat sensitivity as well as pathology in the dorsal root ganglia. In addition to monitoring this sensory readout, we also measured renal parameters to monitor the potential impact of treatment on kidney function.

SRT reduces the rate of GL-3 accumulation in visceral tissues

One-month old Fabry mice were either untreated or dosed with eliglustat tartrate (in food) and sacrificed over time to quantify tissue GL-3 levels. **Figure 1** shows that in untreated mice, all the visceral tissues evaluated (liver, kidney, heart and spleen) as well as whole blood, accumulated GL-3 over the 11 month course of the study to levels at least 100-fold higher than wild-type control GL-3 levels. Treated Fabry mice also continued to accumulate GL-3 throughout the course of the study, but did so at a reduced rate, generally resulting in significant net GL-3 reductions of 40–50% by the end of the study. One exception was the brain, where no difference was seen between treated and untreated mice, though the increase of GL-3 in both treated and untreated Fabry mice was significant ($p<0.0001$) relative to the wild-type control. This lack of treatment efficacy in the CNS was expected, because eliglustat tartrate is a substrate for P-glycoprotein [11] and as such fails to distribute to the brain parenchyma effectively. Overall, these results are consistent with an ability of eliglustat tartrate to inhibit (to some degree) the synthesis of glycosphingolipids such as GL-3, but because this inhibition is not complete and given the total absence of α-gal in the model, these glycosphingolipids continue to accumulate in most tissues albeit at a significantly reduced rate.

SRT normalizes urine volume and decreases urine GL-3 levels

In untreated Fabry patients, GL-3 deposition in the kidney leads to proteinuria and progressively decreasing glomerular filtration rates. Later stage renal dysfunction then leads to uremia and is a common cause of death [2]. Initial renal symptoms, however, may include polyuria due to a concentration defect [25]. Enzyme replacement therapy can successfully ameliorate these symptoms, especially in patients with early-stage renal insufficiency [26]. As a model, the Fabry mouse appears to recapitulate early, rather than later effects of the disease process. Thus, for example, there was no evidence of renal failure in 80-week old mice in one Fabry mouse model [27]. Consistent with this view, a screening of renal parameters in our mouse model revealed increases in urine volume and urine GL-3 that could be used as biomarkers related to the disease process. **Figure 2A** shows that the volume of urine produced by the cohort of untreated Fabry mice trended toward a higher level relative to that produced by wild-type mice; SRT normalized urine volume to wild-type levels. **Figure 2B** shows that there was an ~20-fold increase in urine GL-3 levels in the untreated Fabry mice relative to that of age-matched wild-type controls. Treating Fabry mice with eliglustat tartrate (SRT) reduced the urine GL-3 concentration to about 50% that of the untreated mice, mirroring the benefit observed in the visceral tissues (Figure 1). It should be noted that the carbon chain length and form of the urine GL-3 acyl groups more closely matched those detected in the mouse kidney profile and differed significantly from that of the blood (data not shown). This suggests that the source of the urine GL-3 is not a representative blood filtrate but more likely derived from the kidney. **Figure 2C** depicts the total GL-3 excreted over 24 h, showing that although SRT significantly decreased urine GL-3 (~2.5-fold relative to untreated Fabry mice), it remained ~10-fold higher than wild-type levels. Together with the data in Figure 1 showing GL-3 deposition in the kidney over time, these results demonstrate renal involvement in the Fabry mouse with physiologic consequences that may mirror the early stages of kidney pathophysiology in Fabry patients. They also suggest that SRT may provide benefit in terms of delaying the loss of renal function.

SRT delays the onset of heat-insensitivity in Fabry mice

Fabry disease is characterized by small fiber dysfunction in both male and female patients that results in increased thresholds for both heat and cold stimuli [28–31]. Consistent with this small fiber neuropathy, Fabry mice also develop a demonstrable deficit in their ability to respond to a heat stimulus [22,23]. Potential therapeutics can be evaluated in this model for their effects on a nociceptive response to a heat stimulus by measuring the time taken by the mouse to react (latency) after being placed on a 55°C hot-plate. **Figure 3** shows that there was no difference in latency between treated and untreated Fabry mice at 3 months of age, although both groups reacted more slowly to heat than the wild-type mice at this initial time point. Wild-type mice showed no change in latency throughout the study. However, consistent with our earlier report [23], untreated Fabry mice developed a progressive thermal

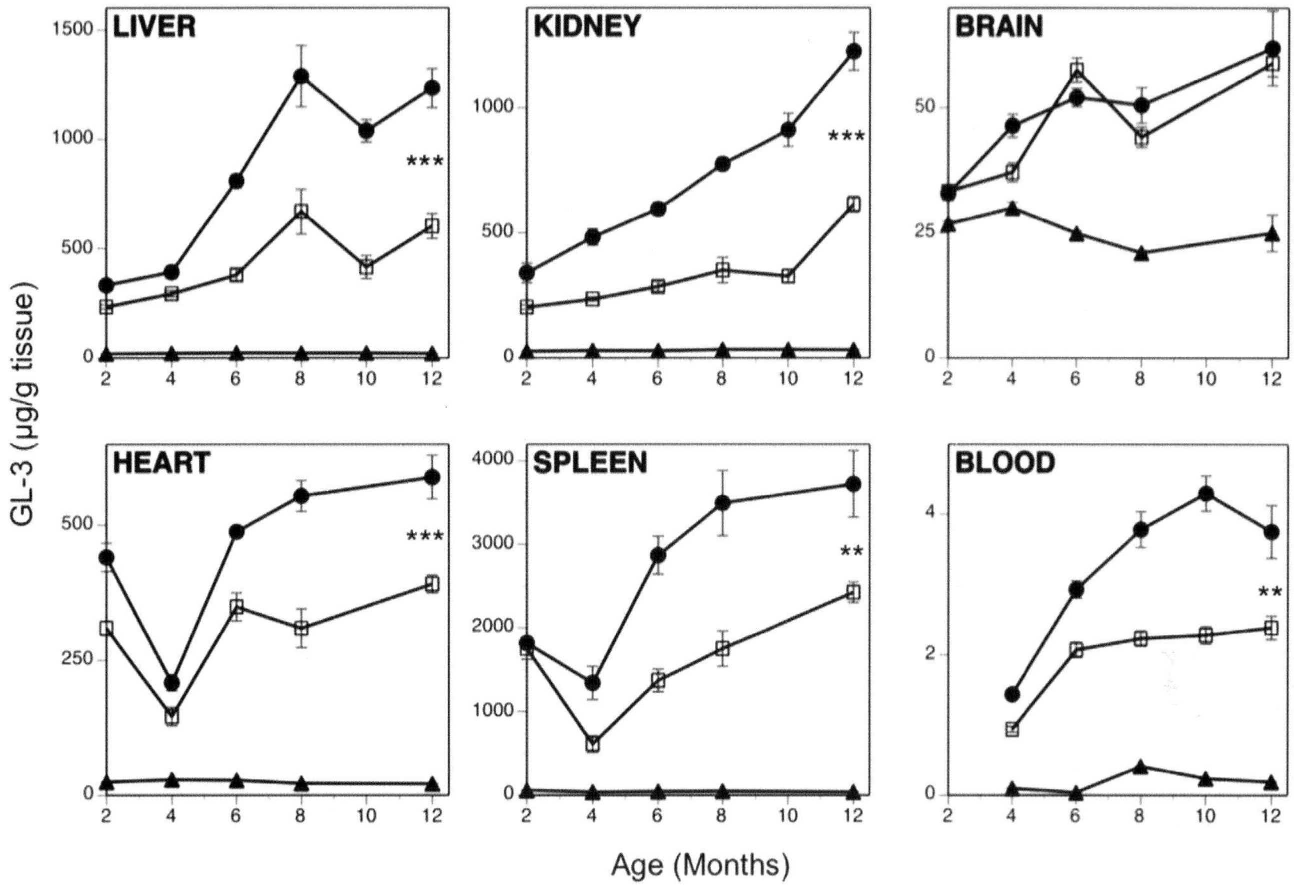

Figure 1. Substrate reduction therapy delays the accumulation of GL-3 in visceral tissues of Fabry mice. Treated Fabry mice received eliglustat tartrate as a component of their food beginning at 5 weeks of age. The GL-3 levels in various tissues of untreated control Fabry (●), eliglustat tartrate-treated Fabry (□) and wild-type mice (▲) were determined using a mass spectrometry assay and are presented as µg GL-3/g wet tissue. Data are shown as mean ± SEM (n = 5 mice/time point). Statistics were performed using the Graphpad Prism software t test (** = $p<0.01$; *** = $p<0.001$).

hypoalgesia beginning at 5 months of age. An equivalent deficit was not observed in the eliglustat tartrate-treated Fabry mice until 7 months of age. This two-month delay in the progression of loss of heat-sensitivity between the treated and untreated Fabry mice was consistent and significant throughout the course of the study. Collectively, these results in the Fabry mouse suggest that SRT with eliglustat tartrate can provide benefit by delaying GL-3 accumulation and its attendant (renal and neurologic) symptoms. Because the Fabry mouse is null for α-gal, we reasoned that stabilization or actual reduction of the GL-3 burden would be more likely if recombinant α-gal were included in the treatment regime. To evaluate this possibility, we chose to use the Fabry-Rag model (these mice do not develop mature B or T cells), thereby eliminating any humoral immune response to α-gal epitopes that might complicate interpretation of the experimental results.

Combined ERT and SRT is most effective at reducing GL-3 levels in tissues of the Fabry-Rag mouse

The combination of ERT and SRT was evaluated in 3-month old Fabry-Rag mice, an age at which significant GL-3 has accumulated; absolute GL-3 levels were comparable between Fabry and Fabry-Rag mice (data not shown). Fabry mice were treated either by ERT or SRT alone or by combination SRT and ERT. For the monotherapy studies, Fabry mice were administered either 300 mg/kg/day eliglustat tartrate in the food throughout the course of the study (SRT) or α-gal (1 mg/kg) every 2 months (ERT2). For the combination studies, animals received 300 mg/kg/day eliglustat tartrate and α-gal (1 mg/kg) dosed IV every 2 months (ERT2+SRT) or 4 months (ERT4+SRT). The latter was designed to determine whether the frequency of enzyme treatments could be reduced when combined with SRT. Mice were killed beginning at 3-months of age, and tissue GL-3 levels determined. Visceral tissues (liver, kidney, heart and spleen), whole blood and urine all demonstrated elevated levels of GL-3 in the Fabry-Rag mouse relative to the wild-type controls at all time points (data not shown).

Figure 4A shows that although all treatment paradigms reduced GL-3, the greatest and most consistent reductions regardless of tissue were obtained using infusions of α-gal every two months plus eliglustat tartrate. **Figure 4B** shows the results for liver, kidney, heart and urine at the end of the study (11 months of age). In the liver and heart, ERT was the more effective monotherapy strategy, with additional benefit realized in the liver when SRT was deployed in combination. In the kidney, ERT and SRT alone were equally effective, but their combination was significantly more effective. Urine GL-3 was effectively reduced by SRT, with some added benefit by ERT. The kidney and urine both showed highly significant improvements in GL-3 levels with either regimen of combination therapy (ERT2 or ERT4) when compared to the ERT alone group. This observation suggests that a combination of ERT and SRT may benefit those Fabry patients whose renal function continues to decline even when on ERT

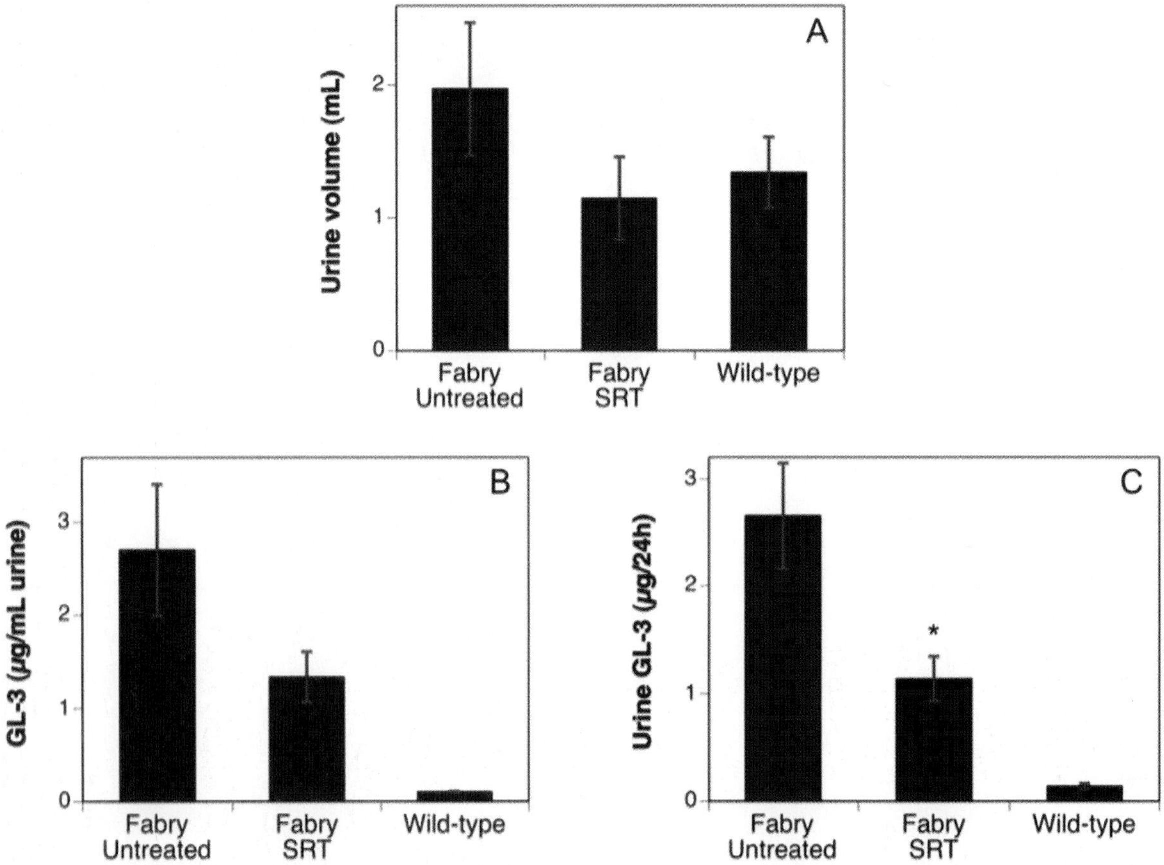

Figure 2. Substrate reduction therapy normalizes urine volume and decreases urine GL-3 levels. Treated Fabry mice received eliglustat tartrate as a component of their food beginning at 5 weeks of age. Urine was collected from eliglustat tartrate (SRT)-treated or untreated Fabry mice and also from age-matched wild-type mice (11-months of age) housed in metabolic cages for 24 h. (**A**) Total urine volume. (**B**) Concentration of GL-3 in the urine. (**C**) Total GL-3 excreted in urine over 24 h. Data are shown as mean ± SEM (n = 15 mice/group). Statistics were determined using the Graphpad Prism software t test (* = p<0.05 compared to Fabry untreated).

[26]. Taken together, these results suggest that in all the tissues tested, maximum GL-3 reduction can be obtained using a combination of ERT plus SRT, and that within this context, more frequent dosing with enzyme appears to be more effective.

Combined ERT and SRT is most effective at reducing uromodulin levels in the urine of Fabry-Rag mice

Uromodulin (Tamm-Horsfall glycoprotein) is the most abundant protein in normal mammalian urine. It resides as a glycophosphatidylinositol-anchored protein on the tubular epithelial cells of the ascending loop of Henle from where it is proteolytically cleaved and excreted. Uromodulin expression and processing appears to be abnormal in Fabry patients [32]. Characterization of the Fabry-Rag mouse showed that urine uromodulin levels were significantly elevated. **Figure 5** shows that although monotherapy by SRT and ERT had some ability to decrease urine uromodulin concentrations (20–25% reduction compared to untreated), combining ERT and SRT appeared to result in an additive effect, reducing uromodulin concentrations by at least 50%. Taking into account the effects of combination ERT and SRT on urine volume (data not shown; see Figure 2), total uromodulin amounts excreted over a 24 h period were most effectively reduced by the combined ERT and SRT approaches (~75% compared to untreated; data not shown).

In untreated Fabry patients, uromodulin excretion has been reported as being reduced [32], while we found an increase in the untreated Fabry-Rag mouse model. In addition to possible differences in the extent of kidney pathology between the mouse model and patients, it is worth noting that differences in ELISA capture antibodies together with post-translational processing of uromodulin [32] may help account for these apparent discrepancies. In any case, excreted uromodulin may be reflecting GL-3 buildup in the distal tubules, and these changes can be normalized most effectively in the mouse model by a combined ERT plus SRT approach.

SRT is most effective at delaying the onset of heat-insensitivity in Fabry-Rag mice

The effects of the different therapeutic regimes on thermal sensitivity in Fabry-Rag mice were also evaluated using the hot-plate assay (Figure 3). **Figure 6** shows that the latency of Fabry-Rag mice at 3 months of age (start of study) to react upon being placed on a hot-plate was already significantly increased relative to that of wild-type mice that were 11 months of age (end of study). Left untreated, the latency of Fabry-Rag mice to react to the hot-plate essentially doubled over the eight months of the experiment. Although this progressive increase in latency in the Fabry-Rag was qualitatively similar to that observed in the Fabry model (Figure 3), it was not as dramatic, and did not approach the latency (60 sec) seen in the immunocompetent Fabry mouse. Consistent with the wild-type result shown in Figure 3, latency in the wild-type mouse cohort was unchanged over this same time frame (data not shown).

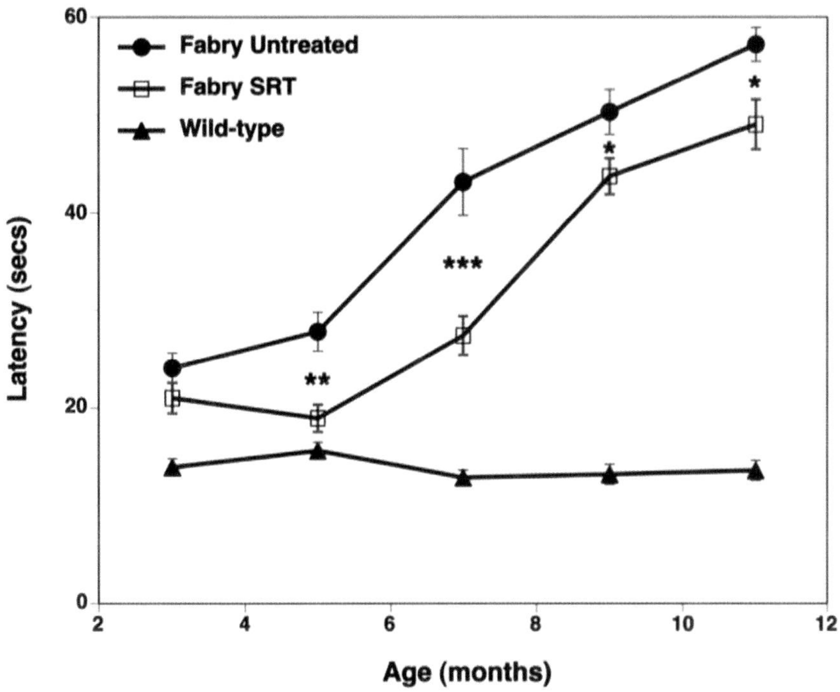

Figure 3. Substrate reduction therapy delays the onset of heat-insensitivity in Fabry mice. Treated Fabry mice received eliglustat tartrate as a component of their food beginning at 5 weeks of age. Mice were placed on a 55°C hot-plate and the time for them to respond (latency) recorded. Latency was measured every two months from 3-months of age for untreated control Fabry (●), eliglustat tartrate treated Fabry (□), and wild-type mice (▲). Statistics compare the treated to the untreated Fabry mice. Data are shown as mean ± SEM (n = 15 mice/time point). Statistics were determined using the Graphpad Prism software t test (* = $p<0.05$; ** = $p<0.01$; *** = $p<0.001$).

Fabry-Rag mice treated with ERT alone showed no improvement in response time compared to untreated controls. Mice that received SRT alone or SRT combined with ERT showed similarly reduced response times and were all significantly more sensitive to the heat stimulus than untreated Fabry-Rag controls. Taken together, these data suggest that SRT is more effective than ERT at delaying the loss of heat sensitivity in the Fabry-Rag mouse and may therefore provide benefit in treating the peripheral nervous system related symptoms of Fabry patients.

Combined ERT and SRT is most effective at reducing the number of vacuolated neurons in the dorsal root ganglia of Fabry-Rag mice

Cell bodies of primary sensory neurons are located in the dorsal root ganglia (DRG); their afferent axons project into the spinal column. The neuropathic pain characteristic of Fabry disease may have its origin in the accumulation of GL-3 in DRG neurons and their subsequent destruction [33]. We had previously shown that at nine months of age, the DRG cell bodies of Fabry mice appear vacuolated and distended, and that this vacuolation could be partially prevented by providing exogenous α-gal from a gene therapy vector [23]. We therefore monitored the DRG morphology to assess the relative efficacies of SRT and ERT in the Fabry-Rag model. Vacuolated DRG neurons were quantified after 8 months of treatment. Spinal cords were processed for H&E staining to reveal the presence of vacuolated cells in the dorsal root ganglia. **Figure 7** (left panel) shows qualitatively that the untreated Fabry-Rag DRGs had the most severe vacuolation (lighter shaded cell bodies), consistent with our previous findings in the immunocompetent Fabry model. Treatment with ERT alone appeared to decrease vacuolation. Combination ERT and SRT decreased vacuolation to a greater extent, but still did not normalize morphology to that seen in age-matched wild-type mice. **Figure 7** (right panel) compares the quantitative analysis of DRG vacuolation resulting from the different treatment regimes. In untreated animals, the degree of DRG vacuolation approached 75%, *i.e.* three of every four DRG neurons were vacuolated. Although both ERT and SRT monotherapies decreased DRG vacuolation relative to that seen in untreated mice, the combination of ERT and SRT produced the largest beneficial effect, decreasing vacuolation by ~50%. The reductions in all treatment groups were significant relative to the untreated Fabry-Rag control. Comparison of the ERT only treated group with the combination bi-monthly ERT with SRT (ERT2+SRT) showed significant benefit of the combined therapy approach. There was no significant difference between the ERT alone and the ERT every 4 months plus SRT (ERT4+SRT) indicating that for DRG vacuolation these treatments are equally effective. Collectively, these results imply that any aspect of Fabry peripheral neuropathy that may have been derived from DRG pathology (*e.g.* acroparesthesias, neuropathic pain) might be mitigated by a combined ERT plus SRT approach.

Discussion

Clinical experience with ERT using recombinant human α-galactosidase A has shown it to be an effective therapy for many Fabry patients. Treatment results in positive effects on the heart, kidneys, peripheral nervous system and quality of life [34]. There is, however, evidence that ERT could be improved upon. For example, enzyme replacement with α-gal is unable to remove GL-3 from all tissues to the same degree. Endothelial cell clearance is much better than clearance from kidney podocytes, other

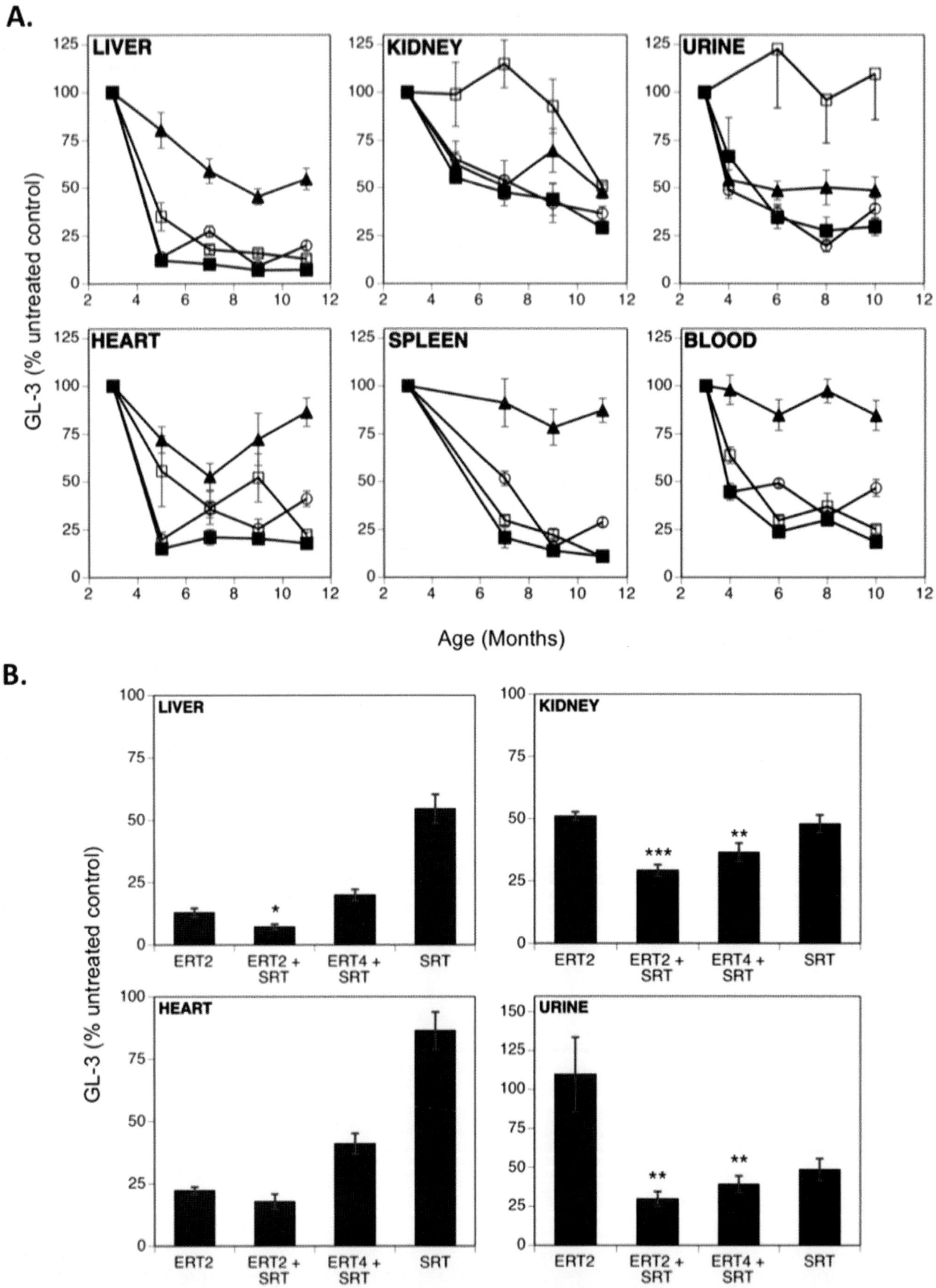
A.
LIVER
KIDNEY
URINE
HEART
SPLEEN
BLOOD
GL-3 (% untreated control)
Age (Months)
B.
LIVER
KIDNEY
HEART
URINE
GL-3 (% untreated control)
ERT2
ERT2 + SRT
ERT4 + SRT
SRT

Figure 4. Combined enzyme-replacement therapy and substrate reduction therapy is most effective at reducing GL-3 levels in visceral tissues and fluids of the Fabry-Rag mouse. Untreated age-matched Fabry-Rag mice were used to standardize the GL-3 levels. (**A**) GL-3 levels over time for groups treated with ERT every two months (□),ERT every two months+eliglustat tartrate (■), ERT every four months+eliglustat tartrate (○) and eliglustat tartrate alone (▲). (**B**) GL-3 levels at the end of the study in liver, kidney, heart (all 11-months old) and urine (10-months old) for groups treated with ERT every two months (ERT2), ERT every two months+eliglustat tartrate (ERT2+SRT), ERT every four months+eliglustat tartrate (ERT4+SRT) and eliglustat tartrate alone (SRT). Statistical comparisons are to the ERT2 treatment group. Data are shown as mean ± SEM (n = 5 mice/time point except 11-month tissue and all blood and urine samples where n = 10 mice/time point). Statistics were determined using the Graphpad Prism software t test (* = p<0.05; ** = p<0.01; *** = p<0.001).

epithelial cells, smooth muscle cells and cardiac myocytes [8,35]. This is possibly due to restricted accessibility of the protein to these cell types. Given these considerations, alternative or additional therapeutic options could prove beneficial for Fabry patients.

A SRT approach has proven effective for Gaucher disease [11]. Because the pharmacodynamics and biodistribution of a small-molecule drug might differ from that of an enzyme, a SRT approach might provide benefit in tissues less accessible to ERT. The different functional modality of these two approaches was demonstrated by their differential effects on the lipid composition of the caveolae of vascular endothelium from Fabry mice [36]. However, as most male Fabry patients have essentially no α-gal enzyme activity, a SRT approach is unlikely to be effective as a monotherapy. This point was demonstrated in our studies evaluating SRT monotherapy using eliglustat tartrate in the Fabry mouse, in which a reduction in the rate of accumulation was achieved, but the GL-3 substrate continued to increase over time (Figure 1). This is in contrast to observations using SRT for type 1 Gaucher disease in which there are significant levels of residual enzyme activity and a monotherapy could successfully prevent or reverse disease progression [11,19]. We went on to demonstrate that the most effective treatment at reducing the levels of GL-3 was by combining ERT every two months with SRT. This yielded the

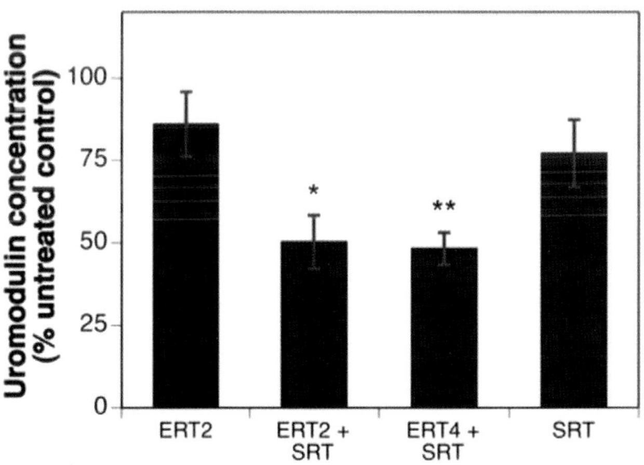

Figure 5. Combined enzyme-replacement therapy and substrate reduction therapy is most effective at reducing uromodulin levels in the urine of Fabry-Rag mouse. Urine was collected from 10-month old Fabry-Rag mice. Mice receiving no treatment were used to standardize urine volume and uromodulin levels for those treated with ERT every two months (ERT2), ERT every two months+eliglustat tartrate (ERT2+SRT), ERT every four months+eliglustat tartrate (ERT4+SRT) and eliglustat tartrate alone (SRT). Relative urine uromodulin levels from the Fabry-Rag mice were determined using a sandwich ELISA. Data are presented as % of uromodulin concentration relative to an age-matched untreated control Fabry-Rag mouse. Data are shown as mean ± SEM (n = 10 mice/time point). Statistical comparisons are to the ERT2 treatment group and were determined using the Graphpad Prism software t test (* = p<0.05; ** = p<0.01; *** = p<0.001).

best efficacy at every time point in all tissues tested (Figure 4A) and was significantly better than ERT alone in the liver, kidney and urine. When comparing ERT alone to the ERT every two months plus SRT, significant improvements were also observed in urine uromodulin levels (Figure 5), loss of heat-sensitivity (Figure 6) and prevention of DRG cell vacuolation (Figure 7). These therapeutic improvements in divergent systems suggest that the combination therapy may be both additive and complementary.

As well as just adding SRT to the existing ERT, we evaluated the potential for a reduced frequency of ERT in combination with SRT (ERT4+SRT) as being another treatment option. In some assays, notably kidney and urine GL-3 levels (Figure 4), urine uromodulin level (Figure 5), heat-sensitivity (Figure 6) and degree of DRG vacuolation (Figure 7), this therapeutic option was as, or more effective than, ERT every two months alone. These results suggest that by using SRT the frequency of ERT infusions could be reduced, improving quality of life while maintaining therapeutic efficacy.

Although Fabry disease is caused by an X-linked mutation and therefore is often considered a predominantly male disorder, through lyonization there are many female Fabry heterozygotes that are also symptomatic [2,37,38]. Although the degree of disease severity tends to be milder and onset of disease symptoms delayed relative to males, there are female patients who are severely affected. These patients, who are already on ERT, would likely also benefit from the combination enzyme replacement and substrate reduction therapy. However, there is a subset of female Fabry patients whose disease symptoms are relatively mild or more slowly progressing who currently do not receive ERT. The option of a SRT alone may provide a realistic treatment alternative for these mildly affected patients. The SRT monotherapy studies in Fabry mice reported here provide evidence that therapeutic benefit might be attained through this approach. Similar effects were achieved in the preventative study (starting at one month of age) and the treatment study (starting at 3 months of age) with SRT alone, thus suggesting potential benefits for symptomatic patients. Furthermore, as mildly affected female Fabry patients express α-gal in a proportion of their cells, this might allow for some degree of enzyme cross-correction and render them amenable to an SRT monotherapy approach, *i.e.* similar to a type 1 Gaucher patient.

Conceptually, some symptoms of Fabry disease are unlikely to be treated effectively with ERT due to limited access of the protein therapeutic. These could include disease manifestations that may be related to the peripheral or central nervous systems, such as acroparesthesia, gastrointestinal distress, and psychological aspects [39] as well as hearing deficiencies and corneal opacity. A small molecule SRT-based treatment option may provide more benefit for such manifestations, as evidenced by the delayed loss of heat-sensitivity of Fabry-Rag mice treated with SRT (Figure 6). A second-generation molecule with properties similar to those of eliglustat tartrate, but able to cross the blood-brain barrier, may prove efficacious for treating eye, ear and CNS deficiencies.

In summary, our preclinical results in mouse models of Fabry disease suggest that for α-galactosidase A null Fabry patients, SRT as a monotherapy is unlikely to correct disease symptoms effectively. If this approach is combined with ERT, two new

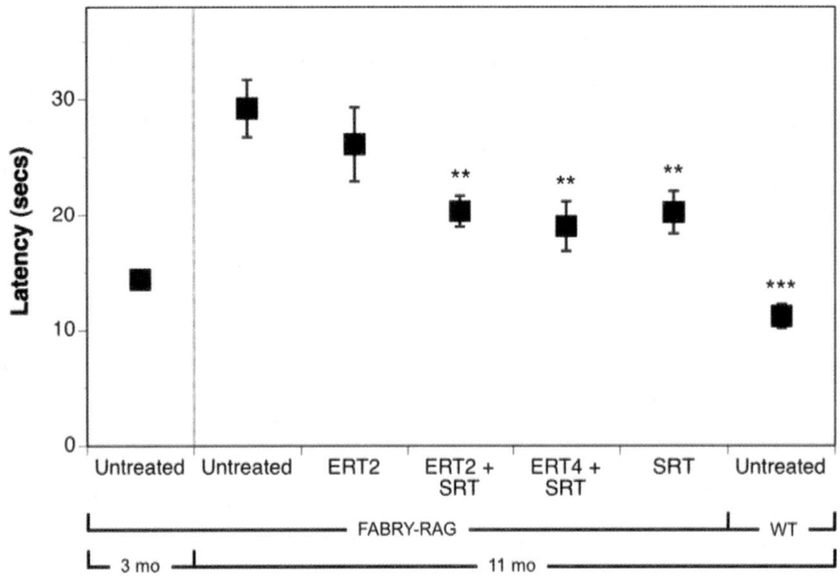

Figure 6. Substrate reduction therapy is most effective at delaying the onset of heat-insensitivity in Fabry-Rag mice. Treatments were begun at 3 months of age. Latency in treated Fabry-Rag mice and in an age-matched wild-type control group was measured at 11 months of age; a 3-month old untreated Fabry-Rag cohort was included for comparison. Mice were placed on a 55°C hot-plate and the time for them to respond (latency) recorded. Latency is shown for wild-type mice, Fabry-Rag mice treated with ERT every two months (ERT2), ERT every two months+eliglustat tartrate (ERT2+SRT), ERT every four months+eliglustat tartrate (ERT4+SRT), eliglustat tartrate alone (SRT) and an untreated Fabry-Rag cohort. Data are shown as mean ± SEM (n = 10 mice/time point). Statistical comparisons are to the untreated Fabry-Rag mice at 11 months of age, and were determined using the Graphpad Prism software t test (* = $p<0.05$; ** = $p<0.01$; *** = $p<0.001$).

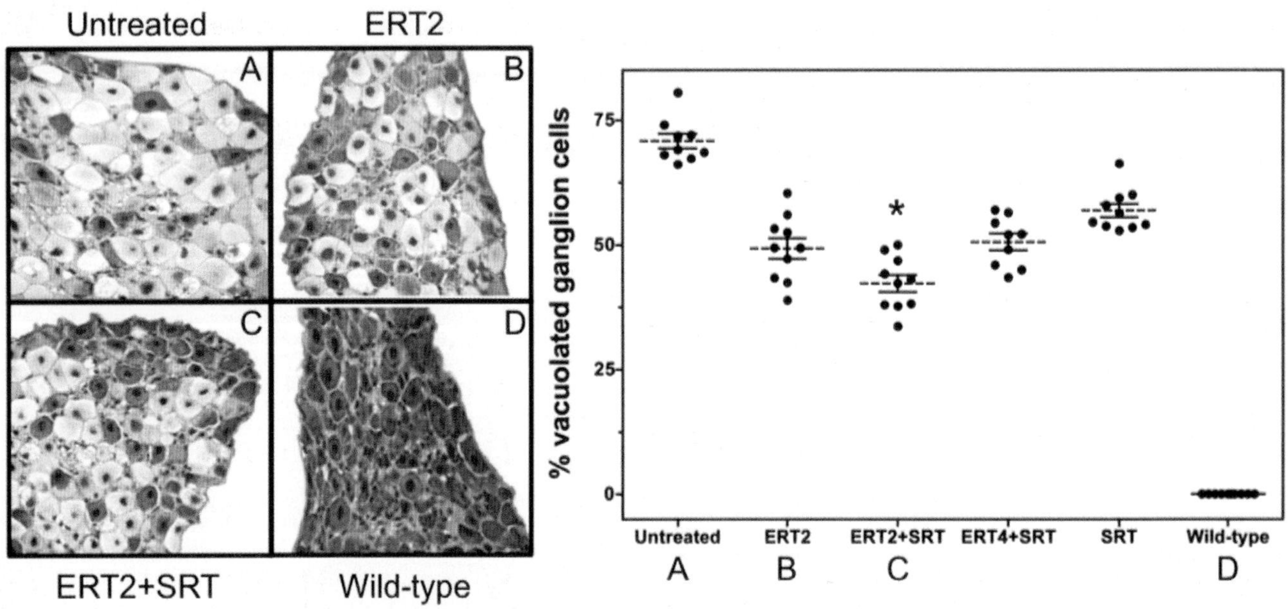

Figure 7. Combined enzyme-replacement therapy and substrate reduction therapy is most effective at reducing the number of vacuolated ganglion cells in DRGs of the Fabry-Rag mouse. Spinal cords from 11-month old mice were processed for hematoxylin and eosin staining. Photomicrographs (400×) of the dorsal root ganglia were taken to highlight the degree of vacuolation in the ganglion cells of the thoracic section. (**Left Panel**) Representative images are shown for (**A**) untreated Fabry-Rag mice, (**B**) Fabry-Rag mice treated with ERT every two months only (ERT2), (**C**) Fabry-Rag mice treated with ERT every two months and SRT (ERT2+SRT), and (**D**) wild-type controls. (**Right Panel**) Multiple sections were examined microscopically and the percent vacuolated DRG cells in each section determined. Groups of Fabry-Rag mice were treated with ERT every two months (ERT2), ERT every two months+eliglustat tartrate (ERT2+SRT), ERT every four months+eliglustat tartrate (ERT4+SRT), eliglustat tartrate alone (SRT). Age-matched untreated Fabry-Rag and wild-type mice were included as controls. Data are shown as individual scores (•), mean (dashed line) ± SEM (n = 10 mice/time point). Statistics were determined using the Graphpad Prism software t test (* = $p<0.05$ compared to ERT2 treated).

viable treatment options become possible. One allows for a reduced frequency of ERT while on SRT maintenance therapy, improving quality of life through a reduced dependency on enzyme infusions. The second approach adds SRT to the existing ERT, perhaps resulting in a treatment modality that is both additive and complementary with a more beneficial outcome than either treatment alone. For the currently under-treated mildly-affected female population, SRT alone may provide therapeutic benefit, as has been demonstrated for type 1 Gaucher patients. With carefully designed treatment regimens, adding SRT to the medical options for all Fabry patients could provide significant therapeutic and quality-of-life benefits.

Materials and Methods

Animal Studies

Ethics Statement. Procedures involving mice were reviewed and approved by the Genzyme Corporation Institutional Animal Care and Use Committee (Protocol 07-1115-2-BC) following guidelines established by the Association for Assessment of Accreditation of Laboratory Animal Care (AAALAC).

Wild-type 129/Sv mice were obtained from Taconic Laboratories (Germantown, NY). Fabry mice (α-galactosidase A knock-out) [21] were contract bred at Charles River Labs (Bedford, MA). Fabry-Rag mice are a stable cross of a Fabry mouse and a Rag-1 mouse [40] to generate an immune-deficient strain of mouse that accumulates GL-3 and can receive repeat doses of recombinant human α-galactosidase without developing a humoral immune response. Pathological and glycosphingolipid characterization revealed no discernible differences to the parental Fabry mouse line (data not shown), though differences in the rate of loss of heat-sensitivity (measured in the hot-plate assay – see below) were observed.

Urine was collected every two months. Mice were housed individually in metabolic cages for 24 h with unrestricted access to food and water. Blood samples were collected from the orbital venous plexus under anesthesia (2–3% isoflurane) into EDTA microhematocrit capillary tubes. Animals were killed by carbon dioxide inhalation, their tissues harvested immediately and snap frozen on dry ice. Spinal columns were taken whole and fixed in 10% neutral buffered formalin before processing for histological analysis.

Treatment regimens

Animals in SRT treatment groups received eliglustat tartrate (Genz-112638; (1*R*,2*R*)-octanoic acid [2-(2,3-dihydro-benzo[1,4] dioxin- 6-yl)-2-hydroxy-1-pyrrolidin-1-ylmethyl -ethyl]-amide-L-tartaric acid salt) as a component of the pellet food diet. Drug was formulated at 0.15% w/w in standard mouse chow (TestDiet, Richmond, IN) and provided *ad libitum*. This formulation provided 300 mg/kg of eliglustat tartrate per day for a 25 g mouse eating 5 g of food per day. This dose of eliglustat tartrate was selected based on earlier pilot tolerability and efficacy studies (data not shown). Mice receiving recombinant human α-galactosidase A (1 mg/kg) were dosed by tail-vein injection. Mice dosed with α-gal every 2 months received injections at 3-, 5-, 7- and 9-months of age; the cohort receiving α-gal every 4 months was dosed at 3- and 7-months of age. Samples were collected prior to dosing.

Measurement of peripheral sensory function using the hot-plate test

A nociceptive response to a heat stimulus was measured as described previously [23]. Mice were individually placed on a 55°C surface (Analgesia meter, Columbus Instruments, Columbus, OH) and the time taken to respond with a characteristic hind paw shake was recorded as the latency. If no response was evident by 60 sec the mouse was removed to prevent injury. The assay was performed every two months to minimize any potential learning effect.

Quantitation of globotriaosylceramide (GL-3) levels

Tissue. On the day of extraction, tissues were removed from the −80°C freezer and placed on dry ice. Pieces of tissue were cut and placed into 20 mL glass vials and 1 mL of extraction solvent (80% methanol, 15% acetonitrile, 4% 10mM ammonium acetate solution, 1% formic acid) was added per 2.5 mg of tissue. Tissues were then homogenized (TissueTearor, BioSpec Products, Inc., Bartlesville, OK) and sonicated for 10 min at room temperature in a sonicating water bath. The resulting suspension was transferred to a 15 mL conical tube and the debris pelleted by centrifugation at 1500g for 5 min. A 4 mL aliquot of the supernatant was then transferred to an autosampler vial containing dried internal standard (N-heptadecanoyl ceramide trihexoside). The resulting solutions were vortexed for 5 min to ensure dissolution prior to analysis.

Urine. On the day of extraction, urine samples were removed from the −80°C freezer and allowed to thaw. An internal standard (N-heptadecanoyl ceramide trihexoside) was added to microcentrifuge tubes and dried under nitrogen gas. Urine (20 µl) was placed into the tubes, and vortexed 30 sec to solubilize the internal standard. Protein was precipitated from the sample by adding 100µl extraction solvent followed by sonication (sonicating waterbath for 10 min) and centrifugation (16,200g for 5 min) and an aliquot of the supernatant was then transferred to an autosampler vial for analysis.

Dried-Blood Spots. On the day of extraction, samples were removed from a −20°C freezer and allowed to come to room temperature. An internal standard (N-heptadecanoyl ceramide trihexoside) was added to microcentrifuge tubes and dried under nitrogen gas. A single 3.2 mm spot was punched from each card into a tube containing the dried internal standard. Protein was precipitated from the sample by adding 200µl extraction solvent followed by sonication (sonicating waterbath for 10 min) and centrifugation (16,200g for 5 min). An aliquot of the supernatant was then transferred to an autosampler vial for analysis.

LC/MS/MS. Samples were analyzed on a system consisting of an HTC PAL autosampler, Agilent 1200 HPLC, and API-5000 and 4000 Qtrap mass spectrometer. During analysis, samples were stored at 9°C in the autosampler cool stack. The HPLC was run in isocratic mode with a normal-phase silica column, and MS/MS was performed in MRM mode. Matrix based calibration curves were prepared to quantify GL-3 concentrations in urine, DBS and tissue.

Quantitation of urine uromodulin

A sandwich ELISA was developed using commercially available reagents to quantitate uromodulin levels in the urine. The capture antibody was a goat polyclonal against an internal region of mouse Tamm-Horsfall protein (G-20; Santa Cruz Biotechnology, Inc., Santa Cruz, CA) and the detection antibody was the biotinylated sheep polyclonal anti-mouse uromodulin antibody (Cat# BAF5175, R&D Systems, Inc., Minneapolis, MN). Following incubation with streptavidin-HRP (Cat# 21127, Thermo Scientific, Rockland, IL) signal was detected using TMB HRP substrate (BioFX Laboratories, Inc., Owings Mills, MD).

Histopathology

At the termination of the study, mice were killed by carbon dioxide asphyxiation. Whole spinal columns were fixed in 10% neutral buffered formalin and subsequently decalcified using buffered formic acid for 5–7 days. Decalcified spinal columns containing the spinal cord and DRGs were embedded in paraffin and 5–6 micron thick cross sections were stained with hematoxylin and eosin (H&E). A board-certified veterinary pathologist who was blinded to the study design examined multiple sections of spinal column including spinal cord and DRGs microscopically. For each section, the total number of normal or enlarged/vacuolated DRG cells was manually counted in a representative microscopic field at ×400 magnification. For quantitative assessment, the percent vacuolated DRG cells in each section were calculated by dividing the number of vacuolated DRG cells by the total number of DRG cells.

Acknowledgments

The authors thank Leah Curtin, Terry Hartnett, Amy Sullivan and members of the Department of Comparative Medicine at Genzyme for animal husbandry and assistance with the animal studies, Craig Siegel for chemistry support, Scott Bercury and Nathan Gumlaw for invaluable technical assistance, and members of the Histology and Pathology Department for their expertise in processing tissues.

Author Contributions

Conceived and designed the experiments: JM KMA DB KM DPC JAS RKS SHC. Performed the experiments: JM KMA DB KM WC JP. Analyzed the data: JM KMA DB WC JP DPC RJD JAS RKS SHC. Contributed reagents/materials/analysis tools: JM DB WC DPC RJD JAS. Wrote the paper: JM RKS SHC.

References

1. Desnick R, Ioannou Y, Eng C (2001) α-Galactosidase A deficiency: Fabry disease. In Scriver C, Beaudet A, Sly W, Valle D, eds. The Metabolic and Molecular Basis of Inherited Disease (8th ed.), McGraw-Hill, New York. pp 3733–3774.
2. Waldek S, Patel MR, Banikazemi M, Lemay R, Lee P (2009) Life expectancy and cause of death in males and females with Fabry disease: Findings from the Fabry Registry. Genet Med 11: 790–796.
3. Schiffman R, Ries M, Timmons M, Flaherty JT, Brady RO (2006) Long-term therapy with agalsidase alfa for Fabry disease: safety effects on renal function in a home infusion setting. Nephrol Dial Transplant 21: 345–354.
4. Germain DP, Waldek S, Banikazemi M, Bushinsky DA, Charrow J, et al. (2007) Sustained, long-term renal stabilization after 54 months of agalsidase beta therapy in patients with Fabry disease. J Am Soc Nephrol 18: 1547–1557.
5. Banikazemi M, Bultas J, Waldek S, Wilcox WR, Whitley CB, et al. (2007) Agalsidase-beta therapy for advanced Fabry disease: a randomized trial. Ann Intern Med 146: 77–86.
6. Wilcox WR, Banikazemi M, Guffon N, Waldek S, Lee P, et al. (2004) Long-term safety and efficacy of enzyme replacement therapy for Fabry disease. Am J Hum Genet 75: 65–74.
7. Vedder AC, Linthorst GE, Houge G, Groener JE, Ormel EE, et al. (2007) Treatment of Fabry disease: outcome of a comparative trial with agalsidase alfa or beta at a dose of 0.2mg/kg. PLoS ONE 2: e598.
8. Thurberg BL, Rennke H, Colvin RB, Dikman S, Gordon RE, et al. (2002) Globotriaosylceramide accumulation in the Fabry kidney is cleared from multiple cell types after enzyme replacement therapy. Kidney Int 62: 1933–1946.
9. Platt FM, Lachmann RH (2009) Treating lysosomal storage disorders: Current practice and future prospects. Biochim Biophys Acta 1793: 737–745.
10. Cox TM, Aerts JM, Andria G, Beck M, Belmatoug N, et al. (2003) The role of the iminosugar N-butyldeoxynojirimycin (miglustat) in the management of type 1 (non-neuropathic) Gaucher disease: a position statement. J Inherit Metab Dis 26: 513–526.
11. Lukina E, Watman N, Arreguin EA, Banikazemi M, Dragosky M, et al. (2010) A Phase 2 study of eliglustat tartrate (Genz-112638), an oral substrate reduction therapy for Gaucher disease type 1. Blood 116: 893–899.
12. Abe A, Gregory S, Lee L, Killem PD, Brady RO, et al. (2000) Reduction of globotriaosylceramide in Fabry disease mice by substrate deprivation. J Clin Invest 105: 1563–1571.
13. Shu L, Murphy HS, Cooling L, Shayman JA (2005) An in Vitro Model of Fabry Disease. J Am Soc Nephrol 16: 2636–2645.
14. Heare T, Alp NJ, Priestman DA, Kulkarni AB, Qasba P, et al. (2007) Severe endothelial dysfunction in the aorta of a mouse model of Fabry disease; partial prevention by N-butyldeoxynojirimycin treatment. J Inherit Metab Dis 30: 79–87.
15. Pastores GM, Barnett NL, Kolodny EH (2005) An open-label, noncomparative study of miglustat in type 1 Gaucher disease: efficacy and tolerability over 24 months of treatment. Clin Ther 27: 1215–1227.
16. Hollak CE, Hughes D, van Schaik IN, Schwierin N, Bembi B (2009) Miglustat (Zavesca®) in type 1 Gaucher disease: 5-year results of a post-authorisation safety surveillance programme. Pharmacoepidemiol Drug Saf 18: 770–777.
17. Hoffman B, Schwarz M, Mehta A, Keshav S (2007) Gastrointestinal symptoms in 342 Patients with Fabry Disease: Prevalence and response to enzyme replacement therapy. Clin Gastroent Hepat 12(5): 1447–1453.
18. McEachern K, Fung J, Komarnitsky S, Siegel CS, Chuang W-L, et al. (2007) A specific and potent inhibitor of glucosylceramide synthase for substrate inhibition therapy of Gaucher disease. Molec Genet Metab 91: 259–267.
19. Marshall J, McEachern KA, Chuang W-L, Hutto E, Siegel CS, et al. (2010) Improved management of lysosomal glucosylceramide levels in a mouse model of type 1 Gaucher disease using enzyme and substrate reduction therapy. J Inherit Metab Dis 33: 281–289.
20. Wang AM, Ioannou YA, Zeidner KM, Gotleb RW, Dikman S, et al. (1996) Generation of a mouse model with α-galactosidase A deficiency. Am J Hum Genet 59: A208.
21. Ohshima T, Murray GJ, Swaim WD, Longenecker G, Quirk JM, et al. (1997) Alpha-galactosidase A deficient mice: a model of Fabry disease. Proc Natl Acad Sci USA 94: 2540–2544.
22. Moore DF, Gelderman MP, Fuhrmann SR, Schiffmann R, Brady RO, et al. (2006) Fabry disease and vascular risk factors: future strategies for patient-based studies and the knockout murine model. Acta Paediatrica S451: 69–71.
23. Ziegler RJ, Cherry M, Barbon CM, Li C, Bercury SD, et al. (2007) Correction of the biochemical and functional deficits in Fabry mice following AAV8-mediated hepatic expression of α-galactosidase A. Molec Ther 15: 492–500.
24. Rodrigues LG, Ferraz MJ, Rodrigues D, Pais-Vieira M, Lima D, et al. (2009) Neurophysiological, behavioral and morphological abnormalities in the Fabry knockout mice. Neurobiol Dis 33: 48–56.
25. Sessa A, Meroni M, Battini G, Righetti A, Maglio A, et al. (2003) Renal involvement in Anderson-Fabry disease. J Nephrol 16: 310–313.
26. Schiffmann R, Askari H, Timmons M, Robinson C, Benko W, et al. (2007) Weekly enzyme replacement therapy may slow decline of renal function in patients with Fabry disease who are on long-term biweekly dosing. J Am Soc Nephrol 18: 1576–1583.
27. Ohshima T, Schiffmann R, Murray GJ, Kopp J, Quirk JM, et al. (1999) Aging accentuates and bone marrow transplantation ameliorates metabolic defects in Fabry disease mice. Proc Natl Acad Sci USA 96: 6423–6427.
28. Dutsch M, Marthol H, Stemper B, Brys M, Haendl T, et al. (2002) Small fiber dysfunction predominates in Fabry neuropathy. J Clin Neurophys 19: 575–586.
29. Torvin Moller A, Winther Bach F, Feldt-Rasmusen U, Rasmussen A, Hasholt L, et al. (2009) Functional and structural nerve fiber findings in heterozygote patients with Fabry disease. Pain 145: 237–245.
30. Luciano CA, Russell JW, Banerjee TK, Quirk JM, Scott LJC, et al. (2002) Physiological characterization of neuropathy in Fabry's disease. Muscle & Nerve 26: 622–629.
31. Schiffmann R, Scott LJC (2002) Pathophysiology and assessment of neuropathic pain in Fabry disease, Acta Paediatrica. International Journal of Paediatrics Supplement 91(439): 48–52.
32. Vylet'al P, Hulkova H, Zivna M, Berna L, Novak P, et al. (2008) Abnormal expression and processing of uromodulin in Fabry disease reflects tubular cell storage alteration and is reversible by enzyme replacement therapy. J Inherit Metab Dis 31: 508–517.
33. Gadoth N, Sandbank U (1983) Involvement of dorsal root ganglia in Fabry's disease. J Mol Genet 20: 309–313.
34. Lidove O, Joly D, Barbey F, Bekri S, Alexandra J-F, et al. (2007) Clinical results of enzyme replacement therapy in Fabry disease: a comprehensive review of literature. Int J Clin Pract 61: 293–302.
35. Thurberg BL, Fallon JT, Mitchell R, Aretz T, Gordon RE, et al. (2009) Cardiac microvascular pathology in Fabry disease: evaluation of endomyocardial biopsies before and after enzyme replacement therapy. Circulation 119: 2561–2567.
36. Shu L, Shayman JA (2007) Caveolin-associated accumulation of globotriaosylceramide in the vascular endothelium of α-galactosidase A null mice. J Biol Chem 282: 20960–20967.
37. Wilcox WR, Oliveira JP, Hopkin RJ, Ortiz A, Banikazemi M, et al. (2008) Females with Fabry disease frequently have major organ involvement: Lessons from the Fabry Registry. Molec Genet Metab 93: 112–128.
38. Kobayashi M, Ohashi T, Sakuma M, Ida H, Eto Y (2008) Clinical manifestations and natural history of Japanese heterozygous females with Fabry disease. J Inherit Metab Dis Online Report #003 DOI 10.1007/s10545-007-0740-6.
39. Wilson Crosbie T, Packman W, Packman S (2009) Psychological aspects of patients with Fabry disease. J Inherit Metab Dis 32: 745–753.
40. Mombaerts P, Iacomini J, Johnson RS, Herrup K, Tonegawa S, et al. (1992) RAG-1-Deficient mice have no mature B and T lymphocytes. Cell 68: 869–877.

Can Multiple Lifestyle Behaviours Be Improved in People with Familial Hypercholesterolemia? Results of a Parallel Randomised Controlled Trial

Karen Broekhuizen[1], Mireille N. M. van Poppel[1]*, Lando L. Koppes[2], Iris Kindt[3], Johannes Brug[4], Willem van Mechelen[1]

1 Department of Public and Occupational Health, EMGO+ Institute for Health and Care Research, VU University Medical Centre, Amsterdam, The Netherlands, **2** Division of Work and Employment, TNO, Hoofddorp, The Netherlands, **3** Foundation for the Identification of Persons with Inherited Hypercholesterolemia, Amsterdam, The Netherlands, **4** EMGO+ Institute for Health and Care Research, VU University Medical Centre, Amsterdam, The Netherlands

Abstract

Objective: To evaluate the efficacy of an individualised tailored lifestyle intervention on physical activity, dietary intake, smoking and compliance to statin therapy in people with Familial Hypercholesterolemia (FH).

Methods: Adults with FH (n = 340) were randomly assigned to a usual care control group or an intervention group. The intervention consisted of web-based tailored lifestyle advice and face-to-face counselling. Physical activity, fat, fruit and vegetable intake, smoking and compliance to statin therapy were self-reported at baseline and after 12 months. Regression analyses were conducted to examine between-group differences. Intervention reach, dose and fidelity were assessed.

Results: In both groups, non-significant improvements in all lifestyle behaviours were found. Post-hoc analyses showed a significant decrease in saturated fat intake among women in the intervention group ($\beta = -1.03$; CI $-1.98/-0.03$). In the intervention group, 95% received a log on account, of which 49% logged on and completed one module. Nearly all participants received face-to-face counselling and on average, 4.2 telephone booster calls. Intervention fidelity was low.

Conclusions: Individually tailored feedback is not superior to no intervention regarding changes in multiple lifestyle behaviours in people with FH. A higher received dose of computer-tailored interventions should be achieved by uplifting the website and reducing the burden of screening questionnaires. Counsellor training should be more extensive.

Trial Registration: Dutch Trial Register NTR1899

Editor: D. William Cameron, University of Ottawa, Canada

Funding: This project was financed by ZonMw (Netherlands Organisation for Health, Research and Development). The publication of the manuscript was funded by The Netherlands Organization of Scientific Research. The funders had no role in study design, data collection and analysis, decision to publish, or preparation of the manuscript.

Competing Interests: The authors have declared that no competing interests exist.

* E-mail: mnm.vanpoppel@vumc.nl

Introduction

Familial hypercholesterolemia (FH) is an autosomal dominant disorder of the lipoprotein metabolism. Due to a defect of the low density lipoprotein (LDL) receptor gene, plasma concentrations of LDL cholesterol (LDL-C) are elevated [1]. In most Western countries, approximately one in 500 people is affected with FH [2]. Elevated serum LDL-C and therefore FH is associated with an elevated risk of premature cardiovascular disease (CVD) [3], which is the disease with the highest burden in disability adjusted life years in the Netherlands [4]. If elevated LDL-C is not diagnosed and treated, the cumulative risk of developing coronary artery disease by the age of 60 years is over 60% for men, and over 30% for women [5].

Yet, research has mainly been focused on the effectiveness of pharmaceutical therapy, whereas achieving (additional) improvement by lifestyle change has hardly been investigated in people with FH. Large primary and secondary prevention trials with statins have clearly demonstrated the benefit of reducing LDL-C in subjects with high LDL-C [6,7]. Also, Versmissen and colleagues showed an overall risk reduction in a large cohort (n = 2146) of people with FH that used statins [8]. However, lifestyle factors also appear to play an important role in moderating the course of FH [9,10]. The EUROASPIRE III survey, conducted in 2006–2007 in 22 European countries, showed a high prevalence of unhealthy lifestyles among CVD patients treated by cardiologists, and moreover, use of medication was often inadequate to achieve treatment goals [11]. Overall, two main strategies are of importance to optimally reduce CVD risk among people with FH: 1) Improvement of compliance to statin therapy, and 2) Improvement of CVD-risk-related lifestyle.

A healthy lifestyle is mentioned as an aspect of the treatment of FH with many benefits beyond LDL-C-lowering drugs [12]. In the most recent European guidelines on cardiovascular disease prevention [13], lifestyle modification is recommended for individuals at high risk for CVD. Results of primary prevention trials in high-risk persons and secondary prevention trials in CVD patients both show that substantial reductions in the CVD risk can be obtained through lifestyle changes [14–15]. For example, the INTERHEART study showed that eating fruit and vegetables daily, being physically active regularly and avoiding smoking were effective in reducing the risk of a myocardial infarction by 80% [16]. Particularly, interpersonal and tailored interventions matching an individual's specific needs and preferences have shown promising results within a range of lifestyle behaviours [17,18].

There is a lack of evidence-based interventions that incorporate a comprehensive approach to optimise treatment goals of people with FH in the Netherlands, as well as elsewhere. We assume that lifestyle improvements can positively change biological CVD risk indicators, and that this would eventually lead to a reduction of the CVD risk. In the PRO-FIT project, we developed an individually tailored lifestyle intervention aimed at a CVD risk reduction in individuals with FH. At first, we investigated the efficacy of the intervention on biological CVD risk indicators: lipids (LDL-C, HDL-C, TC and triglycerides), systolic blood pressure, glucose, body mass index (BMI) and waist circumference [19]. In this paper, we report the efficacy on smoking, physical activity, dietary intake and compliance to statin therapy.

Materials and Methods

Design and participants

The protocol for this trial and supporting CONSORT checklist are available as supporting information; see Checklist S1 and Protocol S1. A parallel randomised controlled trial was conducted with measurements at baseline and at 12 months post-baseline. Participants diagnosed with FH through DNA analyses from January 1st 2007 to April 15th 2009, aged from 18 to 70 years and with a LDL-level>75th percentile (age and gender specific) were recruited from the national cascade screening program of the Foundation for the Identification of Persons with Inherited Hypercholesterolemia (StOEH) [20]. Access to internet, sufficient fluency in Dutch and residency <150 km radius from Amsterdam were additional eligibility criteria. Invitation brochures were send by a research assistant to 986 people during six months (from February 1st 2009 until August 1st 2009) and resulted in 340 participants (34%), of whom 336 (99%) completed the baseline questionnaire, and 318 (94%) completed the baseline and follow-up questionnaire. The follow-up period of 12 months lasted until August 2010. Details on recruitment and participant flow can be found in figure S1. Details on power calculation can be found elsewhere [21].

The content of this paper was guided by the recommendations for reporting randomised controlled trials of the CONSORT (Consolidated Standards of Reporting Trials) statement [22]. The PRO-FIT project was approved by the Medical Ethics Committee of the VU University Medical Centre (under registration number: NL23932.029.08) and all participants gave written informed consent. The trial is registered at the Dutch Trial Register (under registration number: NTR1899).

Procedure

After the participant had confirmed to participate and had signed the informed consent form, the baseline questionnaire was sent out. Thereafter, the concealed randomisation procedure was carried out by an independent researcher. Participants were randomly assigned to either the usual care control group (n = 159) or the intervention group (n = 181) through a stratified computerised randomisation procedure using Microsoft© Office Access 2003 software. At first, participants were stratified according to cholesterol lowering medication use, assuming that medication use implicates treatment by a general practitioner and/or medical specialist, who could have already given lifestyle advice. In addition, we expected that a decrease in LDL-C – the primary outcome of this project - because of the intervention is smaller if a participant already uses medication. Family members of the same household were clustered and subsequently randomised as a cluster to prevent contamination of the intervention effect due to spill over of communication about the intervention among participants. For this reason, the allocation ratio was 1:1.1.

Theoretical framework

The intervention of the PRO-FIT project was developed according to the integrated model for exploring motivational and behavioural change, the I-Change model (2.0) [21,23]. Briefly, it assumes that the behavioural change process can be distinguished in three phases: awareness, motivation and action/behaviour. Hypothetically, due to gained knowledge and awareness of one's CVD risk, a participant will become motivated to change lifestyle behaviour(s), and subsequently, implementation intentions and action plans will be formed to actually achieve (maintenance of) behavioural change. In addition, it is assumed that this will eventually lead to a reduction in CVD risk (see figure S2).

Intervention

The intervention consisted of a combination of tailored web-based advice (*PRO-FIT*advice*) and face-to-face counselling complemented with telephone booster sessions (*PRO-FIT*coach*). The goal was to: 1) improve awareness of the cardiovascular disease risk through an increase of specific knowledge, cues to action and change in risk perception, 2) improve motivation with respect to healthy behaviour through an increase of specific knowledge and a change in attitude, self-efficacy and social influences, 3) adopt and maintain a healthier lifestyle, with regard to physical activity, saturated fat intake, fruit and vegetables intake, smoking and compliance to statin therapy, and 4) lower the level of LDL-C and other biological CVD risk indicators and thereby reducing the CVD risk.

The intervention has been described in detail elsewhere [22]. Briefly, participants were encouraged to visit a weblink referring to the project website, where generic CVD risk information was presented, containing feedback on CVD risk behaviours, their contribution to overall CVD risk, and cues on how to change behaviours. Thereafter, participants could log on to a personal account, consisting of six tailored advice modules on smoking, physical activity, saturated fat intake, fruit intake, vegetables intake and compliance to statin therapy. The module on compliance to statin therapy was developed at the Rijksuniversiteit Groningen, the Netherlands. The other modules were based on existing tailored information modules of the 'Healthy Life Check' (in Dutch: 'Gezondlevencheck') of the Netherlands Heart Foundation [24]. The modules on fruit and vegetables were mainly based on existing modules of the Live Healthy Coach (in Dutch: Leefgezondcoach) of the Dutch Diabetes Federation, developed at the Erasmus University Medical Centre in Rotterdam, the Netherlands.

On-screen personalised feedback was tailored to personal performance level (current lifestyle behaviour), awareness of one's own performance, as well as personal motivation to change, outcome expectations, attitude and self-efficacy. Personalised feedback to compliance to statin therapy was tailored on knowledge and personal beliefs about (the effect of) statin therapy, potential side effects of the prescribed drug and current compliance.

Subsequently, the participant and the personal coach further established the level of the participant's knowledge/awareness about FH and CVD risk factors. Furthermore, the assessment(s) and advice(s) within the participant's personal *PRO-FIT*advice* account were discussed and ambivalence and barriers related to the recommended behaviour changes were explored based on Motivational Interviewing (MI) techniques [25]. Further, an additional one to five counsellor-initiated booster telephone sessions were performed to further encourage the participant's behavioural changes. The two personal coaches had lifestyle coaching and nursing/teaching backgrounds and had received an additional 3-day MI workshop, incorporating both introductive lessons and practical training sessions with professional actors. Both participant and personal coach were not blinded for group assignment and intervention implementation.

The control group received care as usual.

Measurements

Lifestyle related outcomes. The level of physical activity in minutes of moderate to vigorous physical activity performed per week, as well as whether participants either did meet or did not meet the physical activity guideline of 30 minutes of moderate- to vigorous physical activity on at least 5 days a week [26], was measured by the Short QUestionnaire to ASsess Health-enhancing physical activity (SQUASH), which has been found to be fairly reliable and reasonably valid [27].

Saturated fat, fruit and vegetables intake were measured by the short Dutch questionnaire on total and saturated fat intake and on fruit and vegetable intake, that have been validated as related to seven day dietary records [28,29]. For the fruit and vegetable questionnaire also biomarker validity has been established [30]. From this questionnaire, a score for saturated fat intake, ranging from 0 (lowest) to 80 (highest) fat points was computed, as well as servings of fruit and grams of vegetables per day. One fat point equals 2 gram of saturated fat. Subsequently, it was assessed whether a participant met the Dutch recommendations for daily saturated fat intake, being ≤28 gram/day for men and ≤22 gram/day for women, as well as for daily fruit intake (2 servings/day) and daily vegetable intake (200 gram/day) [31]. Smoking behaviour was assessed by a self-reported measure, asking participants if they were a current smoker, an ex-smoker, or a never smoker. Consequently, they were categorized as either smoker (if currently smoking) or non-smoker (if ex-smoker or never smoker) [32].

The five-item Medication Adherence Report Scale (MARS-5) was used to measure self-reported compliance to statin therapy, which was found to have good reliability and validity [33]. Scores on five items were combined to a total score ranging from 5 (lowest) to 25 (highest). The items referred to whether participants always (1)/never (5) forget or stop their medication, decide to miss out a dose, take less than instructed or alter the dose of their medication without consulting a medical doctor and/or pharmacist. Based on former research, low compliance is suggested if one or more doses are missing, thereby assuming an overestimation of the actual compliance [34,35]. As a consequence, participants with a score of 25 were categorised as compliant to statin therapy, others (score<25) as non-compliant.

Other outcomes. Intention to change was assessed with a self-report measure, asking participants whether they plan to change behaviour X on a 5-point Likert scale (certainly yes (1) to certainly no (5)) and how sure they are of this (absolutely sure (1) to absolutely not sure(5)). Both scores were averaged and participants were categorised into motivated (average score≤2) or unmotivated (average score>2) to change behaviour for each specific behaviour [36].

Both height (in cm) and body weight (in kg) were measured twice on calibrated scales. Body Mass Index (BMI) was calculated from the average scores. LDL-C was measured with fasting finger stick samples analysed on a Cholestech LDX desktop analyser (Cholestech, Hayward, USA). The reproducibility and precision of lipids measurement by the LDX analyser are within the guidelines of the NCEP [37,38]. The Cholestech LDX analyser has been validated for point-of-care lipid measurements in clinical practice [39].

A process evaluation was carried out, taking into account the process elements reach, dose (delivered and received) and fidelity. The research methods of this evaluation, as well as the results and discussion are extensively described elsewhere [40]. In short, reach (the number of people with FH that took part in the project, as well as how representative the participants in the intervention group were for the study population and non-participants) was assessed by consulting the StOEH client database, as well as the PRO-FIT client database. The dose of all delivered elements of the intervention was assessed by logs that were kept by the coaches and the project database. Dose received, i.e. the way participants used PRO-FIT*advice (% of participants that logged on, number of modules finished), was assessed by means of log on rates and website use data. Whether face-to-face counselling sessions were implemented as planned according to MI guidelines (i.e. MI fidelity) was assessed by two MI experts, following the Motivational Interviewing Treatment Integrity code (MITI 3.1.1.) [41].

Self-reported measures were collected through digital questionnaires that were sent by email. Body height, weight and lipid measurements were conducted at the participants' homes by a research assistant.

Statistical analyses

Potential baseline differences were checked between intervention and control group with linear and logistic regression analyses, including group allocation as an independent variable, and the following dependent variables: gender, age, education, BMI, medication use, LDL-C and whether participants met the recommendations on the different lifestyle behaviours at baseline. In addition, differences between dropouts and non-dropouts regarding the above-mentioned baseline characteristics were tested with linear and logistic regression analyses as well. If baseline differences were found, the variable concerned was included in further analyses. Effect modification of the above-mentioned variables and intention to change was checked and confirmed if the p-value of the interaction term was <0.05. Only in case of significant effect modification, outcomes were presented per category of the effect modifier (e.g. for women and men separately) as well.

Primary, a complete case analysis was conducted at the participant level, restricted to those who filled in questionnaires at both baseline and follow-up. These numbers vary for different outcome measures. Subsequently, an intention-to-treat analysis was conducted, involving all participants who were randomly assigned ($n = 340$). Missing data on physical activity, dietary saturated fat, fruit and vegetable intake, smoking and compliance to statin therapy were imputed using multiple imputations. Five different datasets were created in SPSS (version 18.0) using Fully Conditional Specification and Predictive Mean Matching procedures. All available data on the above-mentioned lifestyle outcomes, as well as on group allocation, gender, age, education,

BMI, medication use and LDL-C were included in the imputation model. Thereafter the multiple datasets were analysed as described below, using SPSS (version 18.0). Pooled estimates were computed following the rules as described by Rubin [42]. As no major differences were found, only the results of the complete case analysis are presented.

In order to investigate whether the PRO-FIT intervention had had an effect on physical activity, dietary saturated fat, fruit and vegetable intake, smoking and compliance to statin therapy, regression analyses were conducted. Linear regression analyses were conducted, including group allocation as an independent variable and the following continuous outcome measures as dependent variables: saturated fat intake, fruit and vegetables intake, physical activity, compliance to statin therapy). Because data on physical activity were skewed, we log-transformed them and conducted log-linear regression analyses. Binary logistic regression analyses were conducted, including group allocation as an independent variable and smoking as a dependent variable. The post-test scores were regressed on study group and baseline measure of the outcome variable.

Results

Baseline characteristics of participants

In Figure S1 the recruitment, participant and retention flow is presented. As can be seen from Table 1, the participants were equally distributed with regard to gender. Overall, a mainly middle-aged, medium to highly educated, fairly overweight sample participated in the project. The majority had an elevated LDL-C and used cholesterol-lowering medication. Baseline differences between control and intervention group were found for BMI ($\beta = -1.10$; CI $-2.17- -0.04$). As a consequence, this variable was included in the regression analyses. No differences were found between dropouts and participants regarding the baseline characteristics.

Effects on physical activity

No significant between-group differences were found regarding physical activity. As can be seen from Table 2, after 12 months, the control and intervention group performed more minutes of moderate to vigorous physical activity per week. The majority of both groups was compliant to the Dutch guideline of physical activity at baseline (both 78%) and after 12 months (both 80%).

Table 1. Baseline characteristics of the control and intervention group.

	Control group	Intervention group
Gender (% female; N)	56.3; N = 159	57.1; N = 181
Age (years, mean ± SD; N)	45.9 (13.0); N = 159	44.7 (12.9); N = 181
Education[1] (%; N)		
low	3.6	3.1
medium	62.8	58.2
high	33.6; N = 137	38.7; n = 163
BMI (kg/m^2, mean ± SD; N)	**27.1 (5.3); N = 159**	**26.0 (4.7); N = 181**
Medication use (% yes; N)	69.6; N = 159	68.8; N = 181
LDL-C (mmol/l, mean ± SD; N)	3.7 (1.2); N = 130	3.7 (1.3); N = 146

[1]Classification according to National Monitor Public Health: www.monitorgezondheid.nl.
N = sample size; SD = standard deviation; BMI = body mass index; Significant differences between control and intervention group (P<0.05) are printed in bold font.

Effects on saturated fat and fruit and vegetable intake

After 12 months, the control and intervention group consumed less fat points compared to baseline values. No significant between-group effect was found. Gender appeared to be a significant effect modifier ($p = 0.03$). Post-hoc analysis showed a significant decreased fat consumption specifically among women in the intervention group compared to the control group after 12 months (see Table 2). In general, after 12 months, 13% more participants in the intervention group met the recommendations for fat intake, compared to 1% more in the control group.

No significant between-group differences were found regarding fruit intake. A minimal change was seen in the amount of servings of fruit per day consumed by both control and intervention group after 12 months (see Table 2). In both control and intervention group, the percentage of participants meeting the recommendations for fruit intake slightly increased (+2% and 7%).

No significant between-group differences were found regarding vegetables intake. More grams of vegetables per day were consumed in both control and intervention group after 12 months (see Table 2). After 12 months, 12% more participants in the control group met the recommendations for vegetable intake, as opposed to 4% more participants in the intervention group.

Effects on smoking behaviour

No significant between-group effect was found on smoking behaviour. A decrease in the overall percentage of smokers was seen in both control and intervention group after 12 months (see Table 2). Changes in smoking behaviour were similar in both groups. The majority (control group: 80%; intervention group: 85%) continued not-smoking, and 13% (control group) and 10% (intervention group) continued to be a smoker. Respectively 7% (control group) and 5% (intervention group) quitted smoking in the past year, and 1% in both groups started smoking.

Effects on compliance to statin therapy

No significant between-group effect was found on compliance to statin therapy. Of the participants who used cholesterol lowering medication at baseline, 44% of the participants in the control group was categorised as compliant at baseline, associated with a score of 25 on the MARS-5 questionnaire, compared to 38% in the intervention group. After 12 months, an increase in compliance was seen in both the control group and the intervention group.

Process

A 34% ($n = 181$) representative proportion of the intended intervention group was reached during the recruitment phase; participants did not differ from non-participants ($n = 623$) on age, gender and LDL-C levels. Of the participants, 95% received a PRO-FIT*advice log on account, of which 49% actually logged on and completed at least one advice module. Nearly all participants received a face-to-face counselling session and on average, 4.2 telephone booster calls were delivered. None of the face-to-face sessions were implemented according to MI guidelines.

Discussion

In this paper, we aimed to investigate the efficacy of an individualised lifestyle intervention on physical activity, dietary intake, smoking and compliance to statin therapy among people with FH. After 12 months, improvements were seen in both

Table 2. Lifestyle behaviours at baseline and follow-up and intervention effects from linear or logistic regression analyses.[1]

	Control group	Intervention group		
	Mean (SD);N	Mean (SD);N	β	95% CI
MVPA[2] (min/wk)				
Baseline	363.1 (3.5); N = 146	422.0 (3.1); N = 171		
12 months	428.0 (3.7); N = 146	501.0 (3.3); N = 171		
Difference	+64.9	+79.0	1.11[3]	−0.12–0.33
Saturated fat intake (fat points/day)				
Baseline	14.3 (4.9) N = 146	15.4 (4.8) N = 171		
12 months	13.7 (4.6) N = 146	14.0 (5.0) N = 171		
Difference	−0.6	−1.4	−0.61	−1.35–0.14
Fruit intake (servings/day)				
Baseline	1.4 (1.1); N = 145	1.5 (1.3); N = 169		
12 months	1.4 (1.1); N = 145	1.6 (1.1); N = 169		
Difference	+0.0	+0.1	0.05	−0.12–0.22
Vegetables intake (grams/day)				
Baseline	151.2 (77.8); N = 144	162.1 (75.8); N = 169		
12 months	163.4 (77.2); N = 146	171.5 (76.6); N = 169		
Difference	+12.2	+9.4	3.26	−9.78–16.29
Smokers (%)				
Baseline	15.2; N = 145	18.3; N = 171		
12 months	10.2; N = 146	13.5; N-171		
Difference	−5	−4.8	OR = 1.15	0.39–3.33
Compliant to statin therapy (%)[4]				
Baseline	44.4; N = 99	38.1; N = 118		
12 months	51.4; N = 105	44.5; N = 119		
Difference	+7.0	+6.4	OR = 0.99	0.51–1.94
Post-hoc analyses				
Saturated fat intake (fat points/day) **in men**				
Baseline	16.3 (5.3); N = 63	16.7 (4.9); N = 73		
12 months	15.2 (4.5); N = 63	15.5 (5.2); N = 73		
Difference	−1.1	−1.2	−0.06	−1.30–1.16
Saturated fat intake (fat points/day) **in women**				
Baseline	12.8 (3.9); N = 82	14.4 (4.5); N = 98		
12 months	12.6 (4.4); N = 83	12.8 (4.6); N = 98		
Difference	−0.2	−1.6	**−1.03**	**−1.98–−0.08**

[1]Differences between control and intervention group after 12 months are tested through linear of logistic regression analyses, controlled for baseline values and baseline BMI. N = sample size; SD = standard deviation; β/OR = beta or Odds ratio as effect indicators from linear or logistic regression analyses; 95% CI = 95% confidence interval as effect indicator from linear or logistic regression analyses; Significant differences between control and intervention group ($P<0.05$) printed in bold font.
[2]MVPA = Physical activity with moderate to vigorous intensity; means are geometric means;
[3]Log-linear regression was conducted;
[4]Assessed with the MARS-5 questionnaire, a score = 25 is defined as compliant, <= 24 is defined as noncompliant.
Since no major differences were found between intention-to-treat analysis and complete case analysis, only the results of the complete case analysis are presented.

control and intervention group in physical activity, saturated fat intake, fruit and vegetable intake, smoking and compliance to statin therapy. Although most changes were more pronounced among participants in the intervention group, the between-group differences were small and not significant. Post-hoc analyses showed a significant decrease in the intervention group in saturated fat intake among women.

This lack of effects is in contrast with the latest evidence in the field of computer-tailored promotion of healthy lifestyle behaviours; recent reviews and meta-analyses indicate that such tailored interventions are likely to be effective [18,25,43–47] [48–50]. However, evidence on the effects of such and other lifestyle interventions in a FH population is scarce. In a review on dietary interventions in a FH population, Shafiq and colleagues emphasise the need for large, parallel randomised controlled trials, since no reliable conclusions could be drawn from the included studies [51]. Until now, no indisputable effects have been published so far.

It may be that the intervention reach and true exposure (dose received) was insufficient to initiate behaviour changes. The content of the intervention was largely based on earlier tailored interventions, that were effective on behaviour changes, and our process evaluation indicates that participants were sufficiently exposed to the intervention. However, the results also indicate that only half of the participants logged on at the *PRO-FIT*advice* website and completed at least one of the advice modules, and that face-to-face counselling sessions were delivered with low MI fidelity. Mixed evidence has been published on computer-tailored interventions addressing more than one lifestyle behaviour. In their latest review, Sweet and colleagues concluded that single health behaviour interventions are more effective at changing specific health behaviours than multiple-behaviour interventions [52]. Further, it appears from literature that multiple-behaviour interventions may be burdensome for some individuals, and advices may be too long [53–55]. Regarding the low MI fidelity, it has often been reported that skills required for effective MI may take longer to develop than the 3-day MI workshop in our project [56,57]. Probably, the provided MI workshop was not sufficient and more thorough monitoring and supervision of counselling skills during the intervention should have been built in.

The lack of large improvements in both control and intervention group, might be caused by the relatively healthy lifestyle of our population. Results showed that the majority of the people with FH in this project already met the recommendations on physical activity and smoking behaviour at baseline (physical activity: 78%; non-smokers: 81–85%). However, this was the case for both control and intervention group. On this point, the FH population obviously differed from the general Dutch population, as survey data show that only 53% of the Dutch general population is sufficiently physically active and 73% of all Dutch adults are non-smokers [58] [26]. Though, there was much room for improvement with regard to saturated fat and fruit and vegetable consumption. Only 49–57% of our study population met the Dutch recommendations on saturated fat consumption, and only one third on fruit and vegetable consumption.

The baseline self-reported compliance to statin therapy in our project (38–44%) is comparable to those reported in the literature. Our results showed no significant intervention effect. According to recent reviews, the effects of compliance-improving interventions are generally small [34,59]. About 50% of the interventions proved to be efficacious, and effects on treatment outcomes (p.e. LDL-C) were often absent. So far, little is known about the determinants of compliance [34]. Julius and colleagues recommended assessing patients' motivation to take prescribed medications, and to identify and address potential barriers to compliance [60].

To our knowledge, the PRO-FIT intervention is the first to evaluate the effects of an innovative lifestyle intervention on multiple lifestyle behaviours among people with FH. The RCT was conducted in a sample representative for the general FH population with a small drop-out rate. The intervention is innovative in combining three communication channels: the individualised web-based approach added by the social interaction of the face-to-face and telephone coaching sessions. So far, few studies have evaluated the effects of an intervention that had combined web-based computer-tailored lifestyle education *and* motivational interviewing techniques on multiple lifestyles [61–63]. Thereby, the step-wise approach of raising awareness first, then giving tailored feedback and thereafter motivating people towards behavioural change, is thoroughly described and based on a firm theoretical framework [22,23]. Moreover, from the process measures reach and dose it can be said that the implementation of the intervention was feasible. Confidence in the validity of our findings is increased by the parallel randomised study design and absence of differential attrition.

This project also had limitations. Behaviour is multi-dimensional and complex to measure by self-report. The use of inappropriate or crude measures has serious implications and could likely have led to misleading results, for instance an underestimation of effect sizes. Although fairly reliable and valid questionnaires were used, the choice of a (self-report) measure often remains a compromise between the research aim, accuracy level and feasibility [64].

Despite randomization of 4 clusters of family members living in the same household, communication among family members of control and intervention group was unavoidable. The Dutch screening program works cascade-wise; once a person is diagnosed (the index patient), pedigrees are consulted to trace other potentially FH positive family members. In a relative small country such as the Netherlands, families appeared to be wide-spread and overlapping each other, making it rather challenging to prevent communication, which therefore should be taken into account when interpreting the results.

Conclusions

In conclusion, this project suggests that in general individually tailored feedback is not superior to generic feedback regarding changes in multiple lifestyle behaviours in people with FH. Women aged 18–40 years in the intervention group consumed significantly less saturated fats, and compliance to statin therapy significantly improved among unmotivated medication users in the intervention group. These results should be carefully interpreted, due to post-hoc analyses of relatively small subgroups. Research is needed to gain more insight in the characteristics of this specific high-risk population, for instance risk perceptions and determinants of behaviour, such as self-efficacy, attitude, motivation and social influence. The effects of the small lifestyle changes on CVD risk remains (and is due) to be investigated.

In practice, it is crucial to achieve an optimal received dose of a computer-tailored intervention, by e.g. reducing the burden of filling in (screening) questionnaires to a minimum in order to keep participants motivated, e.g. by creating a joint questionnaire, for both evaluative and tailoring purposes. Thereby, it is known that incorporating iterative feedback and interactive website components are positively associated with exposure to web-based interventions [65]. Further, MI training of counsellors should be more extensive, incorporating more thorough monitoring and supervision of counselling skills.

Supporting Information

Figure S1 Recruitment, participant and retention flow. People diagnosed with FH from January 1st 2007 to April 15th 2009, aged from 18 to 70 years, with a LDL-C level>75th percentile (age and gender specific), with access to internet, sufficient fluency in Dutch and residency <150 km radius from Amsterdam were considered as eligible for participation and recruited from the national cascade screening programme of the Foundation for the Identification of Persons with Inherited Hypercholesterolemia (StOEH). Invitation brochures were send to 986 people. The recruitment period lasted 6 months and resulted in 340 participants. Three hundred and eighteen participants (94%) completed the baseline and follow-up questionnaires. Missing data on physical activity, saturated fat intake, fruit and vegetables intake, smoking and compliance to statin therapy were imputed using multiple imputations, allowing an intention-to-treat analysis based on 340 participants.

Figure S2 The I-Change model 2.0. The I-Change model assumes that the behavioural change process can be distinguished in three phases: 1) Awareness, 2) Motivation and 3) Action. Hypothetically, due to gained knowledge and awareness of one's CVD risk, a participant will become motivated to change lifestyle behaviour(s), and subsequently, implementation intentions and action plans will be formed to actually achieve (maintenance of) behavioural change. In addition, it is assumed that this will eventually lead to a reduction in CVD risk.

Protocol S1 Trial protocol.

Checklist S1 CONSORT checklist.

Acknowledgments

We would like to acknowledge the patient organization for people with (inherited) CVD (in Dutch: Hart & Vaatgroep/Stichting Bloedlink) for initiating this project, and the Cascade screening program of the Dutch Foundation for the Identification of Persons with Inherited Hypercholesterolemia (in Dutch: StOEH) for their support regarding the recruitment of participants. We are grateful to dr. A. Oenema of the Erasmus University Medical Centre in Rotterdam, the Netherlands and prof. dr. A. Dijkstra of the Rijksuniversiteit Groningen, the Netherlands, for sharing their computer-tailored advice modules.

Author Contributions

Conceived and designed the experiments: KB. Performed the experiments: KB. Analyzed the data: KB. Contributed reagents/materials/analysis tools: MNMvP. Wrote the paper: KB. Assisted in designing the experiments and writing the manuscript: MNMvP LLK IK WvM JB.

References

1. Kasper DL, Braunwald E, Fauci AS, Hauser SL, Longo DL, et al. (2008) Harrison's principles of internal medicine New York: McGraw-Hill Medical Publishing Division.
2. Goldstein J, Hobbs H, Brown M (2001) Familial Hypercholesterolemia. In: edited by C . Scriver, et al. The Metabolic and Molecular Bases of Inherited Disease. New York:McGraw-Hill. pp. 2863–2913.
3. Yuan G, Wang J, Hegele RA (2006) Heterozygous familial hypercholesterolemia: an underrecognized cause of early cardiovascular disease. CMAJ 174:1124–1129.
4. Treurniet HF, Hoeymans N, Gijsen R, Poos MJ, van Oers JA, et al. (2005) Health status and the challenges for prevention in The Netherlands. Public Health 119:159–166.
5. Betteridge DJ (1991) Risk of fatal coronary heart disease in familial hypercholesterolaemia. Scientific Steering Committee on behalf of the Simon Broome Register Group. Br Med J 303: 893–6.
6. Baigent C, Keech A, Kearney PM, Blackwell L, Buck G, et al. (2005) Efficacy and safety of cholesterol-lowering treatment: prospective meta-analysis of data from 90,056 participants in 14 randomised trials of statins Lancet 366:1267–1278.
7. Kearney PM, Blackwell L, Collins R, Keech A, Simes J, et al. (2008) Efficacy of cholesterol-lowering therapy in 18,686 people with diabetes in 14 randomised trials of statins: a meta-analysis. Lancet 371:117–125.
8. Versmissen J, Oosterveer DM, Yazdanpanah M, Defesche JC, Basart DC, et al. (2008) Efficacy of statins in familial hypercholesterolaemia: a long term cohort study. BMJ 337:a2423
9. Hegele RA (2002) Environmental modulation of atherosclerosis end points in familial hypercholesterolemia. Atheroscler Suppl 2:5–7.
10. Austin MA, Hutter CM, Zimmern RL, Humphries SE (2004) Familial hypercholesterolemia and coronary heart disease: a HuGE association review. Am J Epidemiol 160:421–429.
11. Kotseva K, Wood D, Backer GD, Bacquer DD, Pyorala K, et al. (2009) EUROASPIRE III: a survey on the lifestyle, risk factors and use of cardioprotective drug therapies in coronary patients from 22 European countries. Journal of Cardiovascular Risk 16:121–137.
12. Civeira F (2004) Guidelines for the diagnosis and management of heterozygous familial hypercholesterolemia. Atherosclerosis 173:55–68.
13. Graham I, Atar D, Borch-Johnsen K, Boysen G, Burell G, et al (2007) European guidelines on cardiovascular disease prevention in clinical practice: executive summary. European Heart Journal 28:2375–2414.
14. Kromhout D, Menotti A, Kesteloot H, Sans S (2002) Prevention of coronary heart disease by diet and lifestyle: evidence from prospective cross-cultural, cohort, and intervention studies. Circulation 105:893–898.
15. Blokstra A, van DI, Verschuren WM (2012) Efficacy of multifactorial lifestyle interventions in patients with established cardiovascular diseases and high risk groups. Eur J Cardiovasc Nurs 11:97–104.
16. Yusuf S, Hawken S, Ounpuu S, Dans T, Avezum A, et al. (2004) Effect of potentially modifiable risk factors associated with myocardial infarction in 52 countries (the INTERHEART study): case-control study. Lancet 364:937–952.
17. Hettema J, Steele J, Miller WR (2005) Motivational interviewing. Annu Rev Clin Psychol 1:91–111.
18. Noar SM, Benac CN, Harris MS (2007) Does tailoring matter? Meta-analytic review of tailored print health behavior change interventions. Psychol Bull 133:673–693.
19. Broekhuizen K, van Poppel MNM, Koppes LL, Kindt I, Brug J, et al. (2012) No significant improvement of cardiovascular disease risk indicators by a lifestyle intervention in people with Familial Hypercholesterolemia compared to usual care: results of a randomised controlled trial. BMC Res Notes 5:181
20. Foundation for the Identification of Persons with Inherited Hypercholesterolemia (2010) Annual Report 2009. Amsterdam: Foundation for the Identification of Persons with Inherited Hypercholesterolemia. 15p.
21. Broekhuizen K, van Poppel MNM, Koppes LL, Brug J, van Mechelen W (2010) A tailored lifestyle intervention to reduce the cardiovascular disease risk of individuals with Familial Hypercholesterolemia (FH): design of the PRO-FIT randomised controlled trial. BMC Public Health 10:69
22. Schulz KF, Altman DG, Moher D (2010) CONSORT 2010 Statement: Updated guidelines for reporting parallel group randomised trials. J Clin Epidemiol 63:834–840.
23. de Vries H, Mesters I, van 't Riet J, Willems K, Reubsaet A (2006) Motives of Belgian adolescents for using sunscreen: the role of action plans. Cancer Epidemiol Biomarkers Prev 15:1360–1366.
24. Oenema A, Brug J, Dijkstra A, de Weerdt I, de Vries H (2008) Efficacy and use of an internet-delivered computer-tailored lifestyle intervention, targeting saturated fat intake, physical activity and smoking cessation: a randomized controlled trial. Ann Behav Med 35:125–135.
25. Rubak S, Sandbaek A, Lauritzen T, Christensen B (2005) Motivational interviewing: a systematic review and meta-analysis. Br J Gen Pract 55:305–312.
26. Kostalova B, Frenken F, Storm I (2011) Norm gezond bewegen 2001–2004. Bilthoven:RIVM.
27. Wendel-Vos GC, Schuit AJ, Saris WH, Kromhout D (2003) Reproducibility and relative validity of the short questionnaire to assess health-enhancing physical activity. J Clin Epidemiol 56:1163–1169.
28. van Assema P, Brug J, Ronda G, Steenhuis I (2001) The relative validity of a short Dutch questionnaire as a means to categorize adults and adolescents to total and saturated fat intake. J Hum Nutr Diet 14:377–390.
29. van Assema P, Brug J, Ronda G, Steenhuis I, Oenema A (2002) A short dutch questionnaire to measure fruit and vegetable intake: relative validity among adults and adolescents. Nutr Health 16:85–106.
30. Bogers RP, van Assema P, Kester AD, Westerterp KR, Dagnelie PC (2004) Reproducibility, validity, and responsiveness to change of a short questionnaire for measuring fruit and vegetable intake. Am J Epidemiol 159:900–909.
31. Voedingscentrum (2011) Richtlijnen Voedselkeuze. Den Haag: Voedingscentrum.
32. Mudde AN, Willemsen MC, Kremers S, de Vries H (2000) Meetinstrumenten voor onderzoek naar roken en stoppen met roken. Den Haag:STIVORO.
33. Horne R, Weinman J (1999) Patients' beliefs about prescribed medicines and their role in adherence to treatment in chronic physical illness. J Psychosom Res 47:555–567.
34. Haynes RB, Ackloo E, Sahota N, McDonald HP, Yao X (2008) Interventions for enhancing medication adherence. Cochrane Database Syst Rev CD000011.
35. Stephenson BJ, Rowe BH, Haynes RB, Macharia WM, Leon G (1993) The rational clinical examination. Is this patient taking the treatment as prescribed? JAMA 269:2779–2781.
36. De Vet E, de Nooijer J, de Vries NK, Brug J (2006) The Transtheoretical model for fruit, vegetable and fish consumption: associations between intakes, stages of change and stage transition determinants. Int J Behav Nutr Phys Act 3:13
37. Panz VR, Raal FJ, Paiker J, Immelman R, Miles H (2005) Performance of the CardioChek PA and Cholestech LDX point of care analysers compared to clinical diagnostic laboratory methods for the measurement of lipids. Cardiovasc J S Afr 16:112–117.

38. Issa JS, Strunz C, Giannini SD, Forti N, Diament J (1996) Precision and accuracy of blood lipid analyses by a portable device (Cholestech-LDX). Arq Bras Cardiol 66:339–342.
39. Carey M, Markham C, Gaffney P, Boran C, Maher V (2006) Validation of a point of care lipid analyser using a hospital based reference laboratory. Ir J Med Sci 175:30–35.
40. Broekhuizen K, Jelsma JG, van Poppel MNM, Koppes LL, Brug J, et al. (2012) Is the process of delivery of an individually tailored lifestyle intervention associated with improvements in LDL cholesterol and multiple lifestyle behaviours in people with Familial Hypercholesterolemia? BMC Public Health 12:348
41. Moyers TB, Martin T, Manual JK, Miller WR, Ernst D (2007): Revised Global Scales: Motivational Interviewing Treatment Integrity 3.0 (MITI 3.0) casaa.unm.edu/download/MITI3_1.pdf. University of New Mexico, Center on Alcohol Substance Abuse and Addictions.
42. Rubin DB (1987) Multiple Imputation for Nonresponse in Surveys. New York;J Wiley & Sons.
43. Krebs P, Prochaska JO, Rossi JS (2010) A meta-analysis of computer-tailored interventions for health behavior change. Prev Med 51:214–221.
44. Kroeze W, Werkman A, Brug J (2006) A systematic review of randomized trials on the effectiveness of computer-tailored education on physical activity and dietary behaviors. Ann Behav Med 31:205–223.
45. Neville LM, O'Hara B, Milat A (2009) Computer-tailored physical activity behavior change interventions targeting adults: a systematic review. Int J Behav Nutr Phys Act 6:30
46. Neville LM, Milat AJ, O'Hara B (2009) Computer-tailored weight reduction interventions targeting adults: a narrative systematic review. Health Promot J Austr 20:48–57.
47. Lustria M, Cortese J, Noar S, Glueckauf R (2009) Computer-tailored health interventions delivered over the Web: review and analysis of key components. Patient Educ Couns 74:156–173.
48. Civljak M, Sheikh A, Stead LF, Car J (2010) Internet-based interventions for smoking cessation. Cochrane Database Syst Rev CD007078
49. Shahab L, McEwen A (2009) Online support for smoking cessation: a systematic review of the literature. Addiction 104:1792–1804.
50. Heckman CJ, Egleston BL, Hofmann MT (2010) Efficacy of motivational interviewing for smoking cessation: a systematic review and meta-analysis. Tob Control 19:410–416.
51. Shafiq N, Singh M, Kaur S, Khosla P, Malhotra S (2010) Dietary treatment for familial hypercholesterolaemia. Cochrane Database Syst Rev CD001918.
52. Sweet SN, Fortier MS (2010) Improving physical activity and dietary behaviours with single or multiple health behaviour interventions? A synthesis of meta-analyses and reviews Int J Environ Res Public Health 7:1720–1743.
53. Nigg CR, Allegrante JP, Ory M (2002) Theory-comparison and multiple-behavior research: common themes advancing health behavior research. Health Educ Res 17:670–679.
54. Prochaska JJ, Spring B, Nigg CR (2008) Multiple health behavior change research: an introduction and overview. Prev Med 46:181–188.
55. Prochaska JJ, Sallis JF (2004) A randomized controlled trial of single versus multiple health behavior change: promoting physical activity and nutrition among adolescents. Health Psychol 23:314–318.
56. Britt E, Hudson SM, Blampied NM (2004) Motivational interviewing in health settings: a review. Patient Educ Couns 53:147–155.
57. Levensky ER, Forcehimes A, O'Donohue WT, Beitz K (2007) Motivational interviewing: an evidence-based approach to counseling helps patients follow treatment recommendations. Am J Nurs 107:50–58.
58. Zantinge E (2009) Roken samengevat. In: Volksgezondheid Toekomst Verkenning, Nationaal Kompas Volksgezondheid. Bilthoven:RIVM.
59. Kripalani S, Yao X, Haynes RB (2007) Interventions to enhance medication adherence in chronic medical conditions: a systematic review. Arch Intern Med 167:540–550.
60. Julius RJ, Novitsky MA Jr, Dubin WR (2009) Medication adherence: a review of the literature and implications for clinical practice. J Psychiatr Pract 15:34–44.
61. van Keulen H, Mesters I, Ausems M, van Breukelen G, Campbell M, et al. (2011) Tailored print communication and telephone motivational interviewing are equally successful in improving multiple lifestyle behaviors in a randomized controlled trial. Ann Behav Med 41:104–118.
62. Campbell MK, Carr C, Devellis B, Switzer B, Biddle A, et al. (2009) A randomized trial of tailoring and motivational interviewing to promote fruit and vegetable consumption for cancer prevention and control. Ann Behav Med 38:71–85.
63. Prochaska JO, Butterworth S, Redding CA, Burden V, Perrin N, et al. (2008) Initial efficacy of MI, TTM tailoring and HRI's with multiple behaviors for employee health promotion. Prev Med 46:226–231.
64. Warren JM, Ekelund U, Besson H, Mezzani A, Geladas N, et al. (2010) Assessment of physical activity - a review of methodologies with reference to epidemiological research: a report of the exercise physiology section of the European Association of Cardiovascular Prevention and Rehabilitation. Eur J Cardiovasc Prev Rehabil 17:127–139.
65. Brouwer W, Kroeze W, Crutzen R, de Nooijer J, de Vries NK, et al. (2011) Which intervention characteristics are related to more exposure to internet-delivered healthy lifestyle promotion interventions? A systematic review. J Med Internet Res 13:e2.

18

Reproducibility and Absolute Quantification of Muscle Glycogen in Patients with Glycogen Storage Disease by ^{13}C NMR Spectroscopy at 7 Tesla

Katja Heinicke[1,2*¶], Ivan E. Dimitrov[3,4¶], Nadine Romain[1], Sergey Cheshkov[3], Jimin Ren[3], Craig R. Malloy[3], Ronald G. Haller[1,2,5]

1 Neuromuscular Center, Institute for Exercise and Environmental Medicine, Texas Health Presbyterian Hospital, Dallas, Texas, United States of America, **2** Department of Neurology and Neurotherapeutics, University of Texas Southwestern Medical Center, Dallas, Texas, United States of America, **3** Advanced Imaging Research Center, University of Texas Southwestern Medical Center, Dallas, Texas, United States of America, **4** Philips Medical Systems, Cleveland, Ohio, United States of America, **5** Department of Neurology, North Texas VA Medical Center, Dallas, Texas, United States of America

Abstract

Carbon-13 magnetic resonance spectroscopy (^{13}C MRS) offers a noninvasive method to assess glycogen levels in skeletal muscle and to identify excess glycogen accumulation in patients with glycogen storage disease (GSD). Despite the clinical potential of the method, it is currently not widely used for diagnosis or for follow-up of treatment. While it is possible to perform acceptable ^{13}C MRS at lower fields, the low natural abundance of ^{13}C and the inherently low signal-to-noise ratio of ^{13}C MRS makes it desirable to utilize the advantage of increased signal strength offered by ultra-high fields for more accurate measurements. Concomitant with this advantage, however, ultra-high fields present unique technical challenges that need to be addressed when studying glycogen. In particular, the question of measurement reproducibility needs to be answered so as to give investigators insight into meaningful inter-subject glycogen differences. We measured muscle glycogen levels *in vivo* in the calf muscle in three patients with McArdle disease (MD), one patient with phosphofructokinase deficiency (PFKD) and four healthy controls by performing ^{13}C MRS at 7T. Absolute quantification of the MRS signal was achieved by using a reference phantom with known concentration of metabolites. Muscle glycogen concentration was increased in GSD patients (31.5±2.9 g/kg w. w.) compared with controls (12.4±2.2 g/kg w. w.). In three GSD patients glycogen was also determined biochemically in muscle homogenates from needle biopsies and showed a similar 2.5-fold increase in muscle glycogen concentration in GSD patients compared with controls. Repeated inter-subject glycogen measurements yield a coefficient of variability of 5.18%, while repeated phantom measurements yield a lower 3.2% system variability. We conclude that noninvasive ultra-high field ^{13}C MRS provides a valuable, highly reproducible tool for quantitative assessment of glycogen levels in health and disease.

Editor: Gisela Nogales-Gadea, Institut de Recerca de la Santa Creu i Sant Pau, Spain

Funding: This project was supported by the Muscular Dystrophy Association, the Giant Tiger Foundation, Texas Health Presbyterian Hospital Dallas, National Center for Research Resources, and the National Institute of Biomedical Imaging and Bioengineering of the National Institutes of Health through Grant Number DK058398 and EB015908. The funders had no role in study design, data collection and analysis, decision to publish, or preparation of the manuscript.

Competing Interests: The authors have read the journal's policy and the authors of this manuscript have the following competing interests: the author Ivan E. Dimitrov is employed by Philips Medical Systems, Cleveland. This does not alter the authors' adherence to PLOS ONE policies on sharing data and materials.

* Email: katjaheinicke@hotmail.com

¶ These authors contributed equally to this work.

Introduction

Glycogen is a critical energy source in human skeletal muscle that is needed to support normal exercise capacity. Blocked glycogen breakdown in muscle glycogen storage diseases (GSD) causes severe exercise intolerance marked by premature fatigue with muscle contractures and rhabdomyolysis triggered by more vigorous exercise [1,2]. In McArdle disease (MD, GSD type V) muscle glycogen breakdown is blocked due to muscle phosphorylase deficiency and in muscle phosphofructokinase deficiency (PFKD, GSD type VII) the utilization of muscle glycogen and blood glucose is prevented, which in both cases severely restricts oxidative and anaerobic metabolism [3,4]. While the diagnosis in GSD V and VII may be achieved by genetic testing or enzymatic analysis of muscle tissue, potential limitations in these methods exist [5,6]. In MD more than 100 mutations in the PGYM gene are known, and molecular screening may fail to identify less common pathogenic mutations or may identify genetic variations of uncertain significance. False positives in the diagnosis of PFKD are common due to the fact that phosphofructokinase is highly labile and enzymatic activity is easily lost by incorrect sample handling. Excess muscle glycogen is a hallmark of these disorders that is usually not recognized unless and until a muscle biopsy is performed. A sensitive means of assessing muscle glycogen noninvasively could facilitate diagnosis and could be used to monitor possible changes in glycogen concentrations with disease progression or in response to therapy. Carbon-13 magnetic resonance spectroscopy (^{13}C MRS) has been reported as a noninvasive method for monitoring *in vivo* metabolites in skeletal muscle without the need for invasive tissue biopsies. Currently, however, the use of glycogen ^{13}C MRS for diagnosis or monitoring therapy in metabolic myopathies has not achieved widespread research or clinical use, partly due to several technical limitations inherent to ^{13}C MRS.

Notably, ^{13}C MRS detects the concentration of glycogen directly by the natural abundance ^{13}C C_1 of glycogen. The low natural abundance of 1.1% of all carbons and low relative sensitivity of the ^{13}C nucleus results in poor signal-to-noise ratio (SNR), [7], therefore, it is appealing to perform ^{13}C MRS in ultra-high fields with the two major advantages of improved SNR and spectral resolution [8]. Concomitant with these advantages, ultra-high fields present unique technical challenges that need to be addressed when studying glycogen. In particular, it is unknown if the expected shorter T2 transverse relaxation time of glycogen at these high fields will result in fast signal decay and poor overall SNR. *In vivo* specific absorption rates (SAR) are also increased at ultra-high fields thus making the application of proton decoupling challenging. Furthermore, there are no studies to investigate the *in vivo* reproducibility of ^{13}C MRS for glycogen detection, thus making quantitative results difficult to interpret. Finally, it is unknown if absolute quantification is feasible given that the radio frequency (RF) transmit field B_1 coil profiles are more inhomogeneous at higher fields and the fact that the excitation and detection sensitivity may be effected by the variability of the subject-specific subcutaneous layer thickness.

In this study we evaluated the *in vivo* skeletal muscle glycogen content of healthy subjects and in patients with glycogen storage disease by performing noninvasive ^{13}C MRS in a 7 Tesla magnet and investigated the feasibility of implementing this technology in the clinical evaluation of metabolic myopathies.

Methods

Subjects & Protocol

The study was approved by the Institutional Review Boards of the University of Texas Southwestern Medical Center and Texas Health Presbyterian Hospital, Dallas. Written informed consent was obtained from all subjects.

Muscle glycogen concentrations were determined by natural abundance ^{13}C MRS in the calf muscle in three MD patients (1 female and 2 males, age 22±4 yrs, mean ± SD), one PFKD patient (male, 42 yrs) and 4 healthy control subjects (1 female and 3 males, age 42±3 yrs). There were no special dietary preparations but a minimum of 12 h rest prior to the measurements was required. In addition to these scans, in order to test reproducibility, one normal subject was scanned on three consecutive days, keeping the time of the day and the time period after a regular meal the same. Glycogen was also determined by diagnostic needle biopsy of the vastus lateralis muscle performed on eight MD patients (6 females and 2 males), one PFKD patient (male) and 4 healthy control subjects (1 female and 3 males). In two MD patients and one PFKD patient, muscle glycogen was measured by both MRS and biopsy.

Due to funding limitations, only local patients previously diagnosed by muscle needle biopsy, a standard method to establish the diagnosis of MD and related disorders, could be studied using MRS at 7T. These biopsies typically are performed on vastus lateralis muscle, whereas the 7T magnet in this study is optimized for the evaluation of calf muscles.

Procedures & Measurements

^{13}C MRS. Spectra were acquired on a whole-body 7T scanner (Achieva, Philips Medical Systems, Cleveland, OH, USA) using a partial volume human calf coil, covering the main part of the gastrocnemius and soleus muscles, operating in quadrature for both proton (^{1}H) and ^{13}C. The ^{1}H portion of the coil consisted of two overlapped rectangular loops, each loop having an 8.6 cm side length. These loops were curved and mounted on a half-cylinder former with a diameter of approximately 16 cm. The ^{13}C portion of the coil consisted of a 9 cm side rectangular curved center loop and an overlapping 10.6 cm butterfly loop. Coupling between ^{1}H and ^{13}C coils was reduced by adding proton traps in the ^{13}C coils. A segmented RF-shield surrounded the bottom and the sides of the coil. The ^{13}C coil was closer than the ^{1}H coil to the surface of the calf, and there was a 10 mm separation between the ^{13}C and ^{1}H coils. The final, usable external diameter of the coil was 14 cm. The coil had a small 10 ml vial of enriched 1,2-^{13}C acetate fixed inside to serve as an external reference for absolute quantification. ^{13}C spectra were acquired by averaging 1024 non-selective free-induction decays (FIDs) with a repetition time (TR) of 800 ms for a total scan time of 14 min. While the relatively long TR was mainly required in order to stay under the FDA-approved specific absorption rate (SAR) limits, it also helped with reducing a potential T1 longitudinal relaxation time bias in the evaluation of the glycogen/total creatine ratio. The excitation was centered at 110 ppm, some 10 ppm away from the glycogen signal, using a broad band (BW = 7812 Hz; 104 ppm) block pulse of duration 128 μs and RF-transmit field (B_1) strength 186 μs. WALTZ-16 decoupling with a 12 μT B_1 pulse centered at 4.1 ppm was used to simplify the spectra and enhance SNR. To avoid power limitations while preserving spectral resolution, the decoupling was performed only during the first 20% of the 256 ms acquisition time. In effect, the decoupling period aimed to cover the acquisition period during which the carbon signal was not completely decayed. No nuclear Overhauser effect (NOE) was applied. The potential NOE effects of the decoupling itself were negligible given that decoupling was performed only for about 50 ms out of a TR of 800 ms. Scans were acquired with BW 16 kHz and 4k points. Total scan time, including patient positioning, surveys and ^{13}C MRS acquisition was about one hour. All subjects tolerated the scan well. Absolute quantification was achieved using the substitution method with a calibration phantom [9]. A 1-L cylindrical bottle was prepared with 100 mM oyster glycogen (molecular weight 180 g/mol), and 40 mM creatine (molecular weight 131.14 g/mol) dissolved in phosphate buffered saline (PBS) at a pH of 7.2. The phantom was scanned immediately after the subject, keeping all power calibration constant and with the same protocol as *in vivo*. No T1 correction was performed on the *in vivo* and phantom signals based on the assumption that glycogen T1 does not differ significantly *in vivo* and *in vitro* [10]. The issue of potential differences in the coil coverage between the *in vivo* and phantom cases was assessed by investigating if the coil sensitivity exceeded the volume of the single cylindrical 1-L volume phantom. First, the dimension along the main static magnetic field (B_0) was checked; this was achieved by scanning two cylindrical phantoms placed with their long symmetry axis collinear. This dual phantom greatly exceeded the physical dimensions of the coil along the B_0 field. It was noted that the signal was only 1% larger in the case of the dual-phantom as compared to a single-phantom. This potential difference in coil sensitivity coverage along the long axis was corrected for by multiplying the measured phantom signal intensities by 1.01. Second, calibration of the coil sensitivity along the short axis

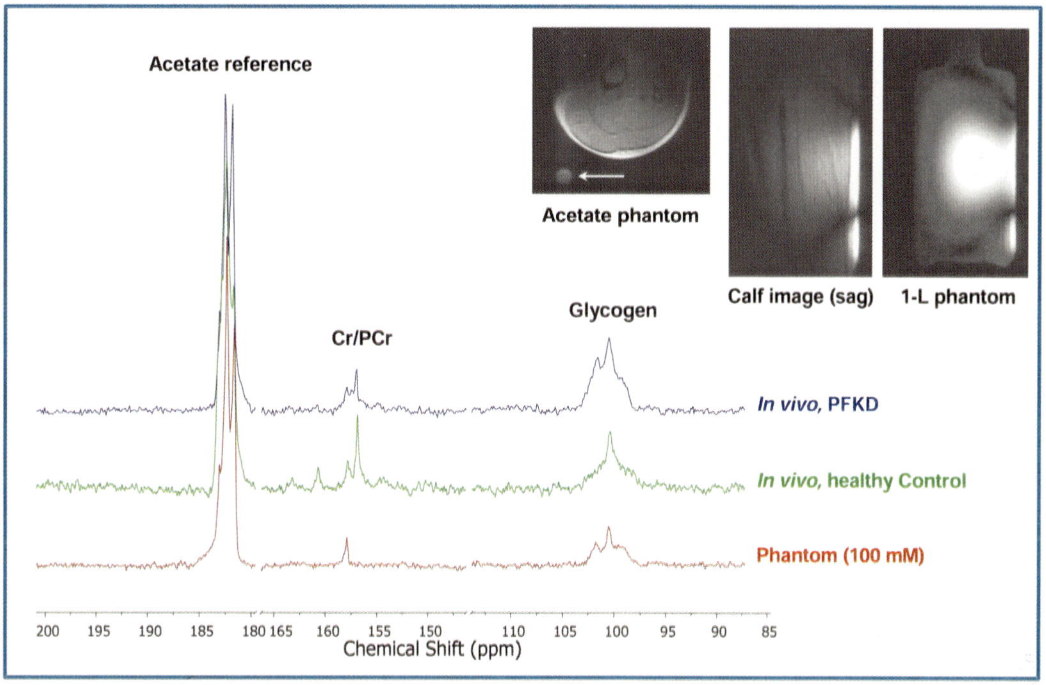

Figure 1. ^{13}C MRS spectra of glycogen and creatine (Cr)/phosphocreatine (PCr) in calf muscle showing glycogen accumulation in a patient with muscle phosphofructokinase deficiency (PFKD) compared with a healthy control subject and the reference quantification phantom at 7T. The observed doublet for the acetate reference is due to the C1-C2 coupling. An axial image of the calf showing the internal acetate phantom (white arrow). Sagittal images of the calf and the 1-L external calibration phantom show the similar approximate sensitivity of the coil.

(anterior-posterior) and the closely related issue of the effects of varying subcutaneous fat thickness on the quantification of glycogen was addressed by performing a set of phantom measurements where the 1-L phantom was placed on fat-pads of different thicknesses and noting the change in the signal. The fat pads were made of small flexible bags filled with olive oil. Care was taken to make sure that the bags had uniform thickness along the phantom body without any noticeable folds or oil voids. Image scouts from the volunteers were used to measure the thickness of the subcutaneous layer and the data was corrected using the interpolated calibration sensitivity curve obtained from the phantom study. System stability and reproducibility of the measurements was established by a) preparing the calibration phantom two different times in order to judge reproducibility in having the same absolute concentrations, and b) by measuring glycogen, creatine and acetate signals three consecutive times, while keeping all the acquisition and scanner calibration parameters the same.

Muscle tissue biopsy and biochemical analysis. Muscle needle biopsies were taken from the mid-portion of the vastus lateralis. The 20 to 30 mg muscle samples were flash-frozen and stored in liquid nitrogen until analyzed. Glycogen content was measured in aliquots of 10% homogenates after boiling for 2 minutes followed by digestion with amyloglucosidase (Sigma A9228) for 2 hours at 37°C. After the addition of perchloric acid and centrifugation, glucose content was measured in aliquots of neutralized supernatants by an enzymatic spectrophotometric assay at 37°C as described by DiMauro et al. [11].

Data analysis

MRS data processing was performed with DC correction, two-fold zero filling, exponential line broadening of 2 Hz, manual phasing and baseline correction. Integrals of the glycogen, total creatine and the reference acetate signals were drawn manually, keeping the intervals of integration consistent across all subjects. The glycogen integration was performed over a region of 10 ppm centered at 100.5 ppm in order to account for the broad baseline glycogen signal. Total creatine integration was performed in the region 157.5–159.5 ppm thus covering both creatine and phosphocreatine. For absolute quantification of glycogen and creatine, the phantom substitution method was used [9]. All quantities are reported in millimoles per liter (mM). To compare MRS data to biopsy data, muscle metabolite concentrations (mM) were converted to grams per kilogram wet weight (g/kg w. w.) using the constant of 1.1 kg·L^{-1} of muscle [12] and the molecular weights used for the phantom. Data are expressed as single values and/or mean ± standard deviation (SD).

Results

Typical ^{13}C MRS spectra of muscle glycogen and total creatine in a PFKD patient, control subject and the reference phantom are shown in Fig. 1, along with typical calf muscle and reference phantom coverage images. The axial muscle T1-weighted image also shows (with white arrow) the circular cross section of the internal acetate calibration phantom, positioned inside the coil. As seen, similar sagittal excitation patterns were observed *in vivo* and in the 1-L external reference phantom, thus suggesting similar coil loading and sensitivities. Mean MRS signal intensities for glycogen and total creatine in mM are shown in Table 1. The values presented reflect a correction for the individual subcutaneous fat thickness, taken from interpolating the results from Fig. 2. For the most volunteers, the average subcutaneous fat thickness was in the

Table 1. Skeletal muscle metabolites - ^{13}C NMR spectroscopy.

Subjects	Glycogen (mM)	Total Creatine (mM)	Glycogen/Total Creatine
MD	192.5±15.1	85.6±22.5	2.3±0.6
PFKD	202.1	124.2	1.6
Controls	75.7±13.6	77.1±8.3	1.0±0.3

Values are expressed individually or group means ± SD. MD, McArdle disease; PFKD, phosphofructokinase deficiency; mM, millimoles per liter.

order of 8–10 mm which would result in individual corrections of 4–5%.

The mean muscle glycogen concentration (Fig. 3A) was 2.5-fold higher in GSD patients (31.5±2.9 g/kg w. w.) compared with control subjects (12.4±2.2 g/kg w. w.). There was no difference in muscle total creatine concentration (Fig. 3B) between the GSD patients (11.2±3.3 g/kg w. w.) and control subjects (9.2±1.0 g/kg w. w.). Muscle biopsy data showed a similar 2.5-fold higher muscle glycogen concentration in GSD patients (24.9±3.5 g/kg w. w.) compared with control subjects (10.0±1.7 g/kg w. w.). Similar values were achieved by both methods in the three GSD patients in whom muscle glycogen was assessed by both MRS (32.9±0.9 g/kg w. w.) and biochemistry (28.0±3.1 g/kg w. w.).

In vivo reproducibility and the corresponding intra-subject variability, as measured by the three identical studies on the same normal subject, showed a reported coefficient of variation 5.18% and 5.71% for glycogen and total creatine, respectively. This is about three times lower than the inter-subject coefficient of variation (17.83% for glycogen and 11.08% for total creatine, in normal subjects) thus making it possible to conduct meaningful comparisons of glycogen values among normal subjects, System stability and hardware measurement reproducibility, as assessed by measuring three times the signal from the concentration reference phantom, showed a standard deviation of 3.2%, and 9.0% for glycogen and creatine, respectively. In addition, the error in the absolute quantification of the metabolites introduced due to fluctuations in the preparation of the calibration phantom was assessed by preparing the phantom two separate times. This sample preparation error was measured at 5.5% and 2.45% for glycogen and creatine, respectively. Assuming independence of the errors, the total combined error of the final quantification is thus calculated to be 6.4% for glycogen and 9.3% for creatine. Comparison of the results of these repeated measurements *in vivo* and in phantoms show that, in terms of reproducibility, the hardware instabilities are smaller than the intra-subject variability, thus attesting to the meaningful comparison of *in vivo* data. However, in terms of absolute quantification, these results suggest that the limiting factor is the accuracy on the preparation of the calibration phantom. Greater care in preparing these calibration phantoms could thus decrease the error in the absolute quantification to the error in the hardware performance, which for our system is in the order of 3% for glycogen.

Discussion

The present study is the first investigation utilizing ^{13}C MRS at 7T for absolute quantification of muscle glycogen concentration in patients with GSD. A major focus of the study is to report on the reproducibility of these studies, both in vivo and in phantoms. The main findings are a 2.5-fold increase in muscle glycogen concentration in MD and PFKD patients in agreement with biochemical measured values, and the demonstration of the high reproducibility of *in vivo* ^{13}C MRS at ultra-high fields as a noninvasive method for clinical diagnosis in GSD patients.

It has been shown that ^{13}C MRS is a valuable method for noninvasive assessments of glycogen levels in skeletal muscle in patients with MD and PFKD [13,14,15], and other GSD's [15,16]. However, these studies were performed at lower magnetic fields with semiquantitative assessment of glycogen expressed as the ratio of glycogen to total creatine. In the present study, the semiquantitative values for glycogen/total creatine ratio in patients and controls were in line with the results found at high magnetic fields (4T), [15] but were below the values found at low magnetic fields (2T), [13,14]. There has been controversy about the complete glycogen visibility by ^{13}C MRS [17], and the discrepancy between the studies might be due to different magnetic field strength and the complex structure of glycogen, a branched polymer of glucose that varies in size and displays heterogeneity in localization within skeletal muscle cells and different muscle fiber types [18]. However, detection and reproducibility of glycogen content in skeletal muscle has been demonstrated earlier at high magnetic fields (4.7T), [19], and there was no difference found in glycogen concentration between calf and thigh muscle in healthy controls [15]. Furthermore, ^{13}C MRS was validated in comparison with skeletal muscle biopsies by biochemical analysis in healthy subjects ($R = 0.95$), [20] and found to be at least as accurate as biopsy measurements (coefficients of variation MRS 4.3% vs. biopsy 9.3%). Using increased signal strength at 7T results in improved measurement accuracy [8] and reduced time

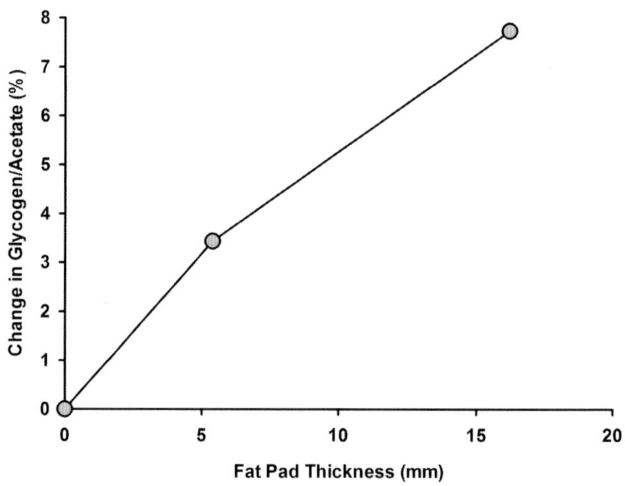

Figure 2. Correction factors for the glycogen/acetate ratio as a function of the thickness of the fat layer underneath the calibration phantom. All *in vivo* data were corrected for the measured thickness of the subcutaneous fat by using interpolated values from this figure. For most subjects this correction was in the order of 4–5%.

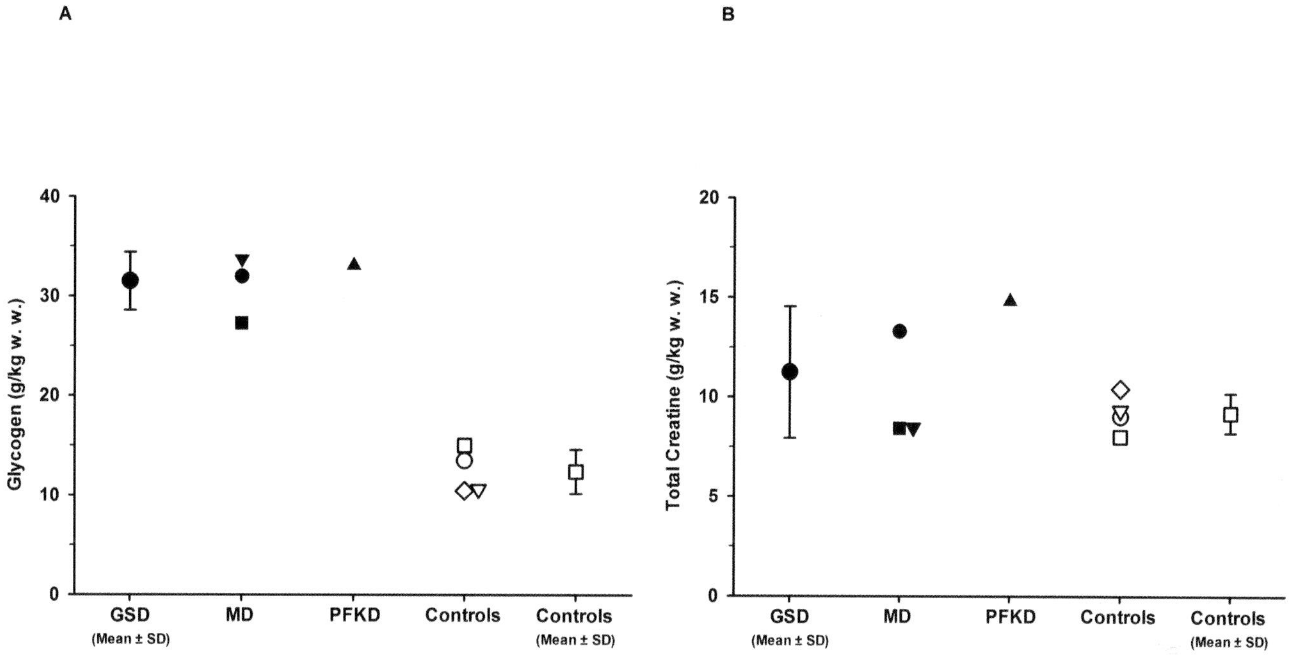

Figure 3. Figure 3A–B. Skeletal muscle glycogen (3A) and total creatine concentrations (3B) measured by ^{13}C MRS. Values are expressed individually or group means ± SD. GSD, glycogen storage diseases; MD, McArdle disease; PFKD, phosphofructokinase deficiency; controls, healthy control subjects; g/kg w. w., grams per kilogram wet weight.

required for glycogen assessment. The SNR for the C_1 peak of glycogen using a phantom was increased by 60% at 7T compared with 3T for the same number of acquisitions. ^{13}C MRS glycogen measurements in our study showed high *in vivo* reproducibility (5.18% for glycogen) with no overlap between the 2.5-fold higher glycogen concentrations in GSD patients compared with control subjects. Glycogen concentrations corresponded closely with the muscle needle biopsy values and absolute glycogen concentrations in control subjects were in agreement with results shown earlier at high magnetic field [20]. Overall, these findings strengthen confidence in the accuracy of our results.

The major advantages of *in vivo* ^{13}C MRS include avoidance of invasive biopsy procedures hence providing the possibility of stress-less and painless assessment of glycogen in a larger muscle volume that would likely be less susceptible to local variations in muscle glycogen concentrations. The accurate quantification of muscle glycogen concentration at ultra-high fields allows assessment of physiological alterations and kinetic changes [9] and also can support the clinical diagnosis in GSD. Little is known regarding possible variations in glycogen storage in MD and PFKD, therefore, it would be beneficial to determine muscle glycogen concentrations in these disorders over time. Monitoring muscle glycogen levels in patients with blocked glycogen breakdown is important in defining the natural history of muscle glycogen levels as well as to determine possible effects of therapy. Both regular aerobic exercise and dietary modifications have been advanced as therapy in GSD V and VII [5,6,21,22]. Fatiguing exercise in healthy humans promotes increased muscle glycogen deposition but the implications for glycogen levels in MD or PFKD are unknown [23]. Blood glucose is a critical alternative fuel in MD and adequate glucose availability as determined by hepatic glycogen stores and dietary carbohydrate, including the ingestion of simple sugars shortly before exercise have been shown to enhance exercise capacity in MD [24,25]. However the implications of dietary carbohydrate for muscle glycogen concentrations are unknown.

In conclusion, muscle glycogen concentrations were 2.5-fold higher in patients with GSD type V and VII, and MRS measurements were consistent with the muscle needle biopsy results. This study clearly demonstrates the feasibility of accurately and reproducibly measuring glycogen in skeletal muscle using *in vivo* ^{13}C MRS at ultra-high fields as a noninvasive method for facilitating clinical diagnosis and monitoring treatment effects in GSD patients.

Acknowledgments

We thank the subjects who participated in the study, P. Wyrick for scientific discussion and J. Davis Baxter and M. Newby for administrative support.

Author Contributions

Conceived and designed the experiments: KH IED CRM RGH. Performed the experiments: KH IED NR SC JR. Analyzed the data: KH IED NR. Contributed reagents/materials/analysis tools: KH IED NR JR RGH SC CRM. Wrote the paper: KH IED NR SC JR CRM RGH.

References

1. DiMauro S (2007) Muscle glycogenoses: an overview. Acta Myol 26: 35–41.
2. Haller RG, Vissing J (2004) Functional evaluation of metabolic myopathies. In: Engel AG, Franzini-Armstrong C, editors. Myology. 3nd ed. New York: McGraw-Hill. pp. 665–679.
3. Haller RG, Vissing J (2002) Spontaneous "second wind" and glucose-induced second "second wind" in McArdle disease: oxidative mechanisms. Arch Neurol 59: 1395–1402.
4. Haller RG, Vissing J (2004) No spontaneous second wind in muscle phosphofructokinase deficiency. Neurology 62: 82–86.

5. Lucia A, Nogales-Gadea G, Perez M, Martin MA, Andreu AL, et al. (2008) McArdle disease: what do neurologists need to know? Nat Clin Pract Neurol 4: 568–577.
6. Sharp LJ, Haller RG (2014) Metabolic and Mitochondrial Myopathies. Neurol Clin 32: 777–799.
7. Boesch C (2007) Musculoskeletal spectroscopy. J Magn Reson Imaging 25: 321–338.
8. Stephenson MC, Gunner F, Napolitano A, Greenhaff PL, Macdonald IA, et al. (2011) Applications of multi-nuclear magnetic resonance spectroscopy at 7T. World J Radiol 3: 105–113.
9. Kreis R (1997) Quantitative localized 1H MR spectroscopy for clinical use. Prog Nucl Magn Reson Spectrosc 31: 155–195.
10. Zang LH, Laughlin MR, Rothman DL, Shulman RG (1990) ^{13}C NMR relaxation times of hepatic glycogen in vitro and in vivo. Biochemistry 29: 6815–6820.
11. DiMauro S, Hartwig GB, Hays A, Eastwood AB, Franco R, et al. (1979) Debrancher deficiency: neuromuscular disorder in 5 adults. Ann Neurol 5: 422–436.
12. Mendez J, Keys A (1960) Density and composition of mammalian muscle. Metabolism 9: 184–188.
13. Jehenson P, Duboc D, Bloch G, Fardeau M, Syrota A (1991) Diagnosis of muscular glycogenosis by in vivo natural abundance 13C NMR spectroscopy. Neuromuscul Disord 1: 99–101.
14. Jehenson P, Duboc D, Labrune P, Fardeau M, Odievre M, et al. (1995) Diagnostic value of the evaluation of glycogen content in muscle diseases by carbon 13 nuclear magnetic resonance. J Chim Phys 92: 1797–1800.
15. Wary C, Laforet P, Eymard B, Fardeau M, Leroy-Willig A, et al. (2003) Evaluation of muscle glycogen content by 13C NMR spectroscopy in adult-onset acid maltase deficiency. Neuromuscul Disord 13: 545–553.
16. Beckmann N, Seelig J, Wick H (1990) Analysis of glycogen storage disease by in vivo 13C NMR: comparison of normal volunteers with a patient. Magn Reson Med 16: 150–160.
17. Murphy E, Hellerstein M (2000) Is in vivo nuclear magnetic resonance spectroscopy currently a quantitative method for whole-body carbohydrate metabolism? Nutr Rev 58: 304–314.
18. Roach PJ, Depaoli-Roach AA, Hurley TD, Tagliabracci VS (2012) Glycogen and its metabolism: some new developments and old themes. Biochem J 441: 763–787.
19. Avison MJ, Rothman DL, Nadel E, Shulman RG (1988) Detection of human muscle glycogen by natural abundance 13C NMR. Proc Natl Acad Sci USA 85: 1634–1636.
20. Taylor R, Price TB, Rothman DL, Shulman RG, Shulman GI (1992) Validation of 13C NMR measurement of human skeletal muscle glycogen by direct biochemical assay of needle biopsy samples. Magn Reson Med 27: 13–20.
21. Haller RG, Wyrick P, Taivassalo T, Vissing J (2006) Aerobic conditioning: an effective therapy in McArdle's disease. Ann Neurol 59: 922–928.
22. Mate-Munoz JL, Moran M, Perez M, Chamorro-Vina C, Gomez-Gallego F, et al. (2007) Favorable responses to acute and chronic exercise in McArdle patients. Clin J Sport Med 17: 297–303.
23. Bergstrom J, Hultman E (1966) Muscle glycogen synthesis after exercise: an enhancing factor localized to the muscle cells in man. Nature 210: 309–310.
24. Andersen ST, Haller RG, Vissing J (2008) Effect of oral sucrose shortly before exercise on work capacity in McArdle disease. Arch Neurol 65: 786–789.
25. Vissing J, Lewis SF, Galbo H, Haller RG (1992) Effect of deficient muscular glycogenolysis on extramuscular fuel production in exercise. J Appl Physiol 72: 1773–1779.

19

Genetic Polymorphisms in *LDLR, APOB, PCSK9* and Other Lipid Related Genes Associated with Familial Hypercholesterolemia in Malaysia

Say-Hean Lye[1], Jagdish Kaur Chahil[1], Pramod Bagali[1], Livy Alex[1]*, Jamunarani Vadivelu[2], Wan Azman Wan Ahmad[2], Siew-Pheng Chan[2], Meow-Keong Thong[2], Shamsul Mohd Zain[3], Rosmawati Mohamed[2]

1 INFOVALLEY® Group of Companies, Jalan Tasik, MINES Resort City, Selangor, Malaysia, **2** Faculty of Medicine, University of Malaya, Kuala Lumpur, Malaysia, **3** The Pharmacogenomics Laboratory, Department of Pharmacology, Faculty of Medicine, University of Malaya, Kuala Lumpur, Malaysia

Abstract

Familial hypercholesterolemia (FH) is an autosomal dominant disorder characterized by elevations in total cholesterol (TC) and low density lipoprotein cholesterol (LDLc). Development of FH can result in the increase of risk for premature cardiovascular diseases (CVD). FH is primarily caused by genetic variations in *Low Density Lipoprotein Receptor* (*LDLR*), *Apolipoprotein B* (*APOB*) or *Proprotein Convertase Subtilisin/Kexin type 9* (*PCSK9*) genes. Although FH has been extensively studied in the Caucasian population, there are limited reports of FH mutations in the Asian population. We investigated the association of previously reported genetic variants that are involved in lipid regulation in our study cohort. A total of 1536 polymorphisms previously implicated in FH were evaluated in 141 consecutive patients with clinical FH (defined by the Dutch Lipid Clinic Network criteria) and 111 unrelated control subjects without FH using high throughput microarray genotyping platform. Fourteen Single Nucleotide Polymorphisms (SNPs) were found to be significantly associated with FH, eleven with increased FH risk and three with decreased FH risk. Of the eleven SNPs associated with an increased risk of FH, only one SNP was found in the *LDLR* gene, seven in the *APOB* gene and three in the *PCSK9* gene. SNP rs12720762 in *APOB* gene is associated with the highest risk of FH (odds ratio 14.78, $p<0.001$). Amongst the FH cases, 108 out of 141 (76.60%) have had at least one significant risk-associated SNP. Our study adds new information and knowledge on the genetic polymorphisms amongst Asians with FH, which may serve as potential markers in risk prediction and disease management.

Editor: Osman El-Maarri, University of Bonn, Institut of Experimental Hematology and Transfusion Medicine, Germany

Funding: The research reported in this research article has been funded by the Ministry of Science, Technology and Innovation (MOSTI), the government of Malaysia (grant number 36-02-03-6058). The funders had no role in study design, data collection and analysis, decision to publish, or preparation of the manuscript.

Competing Interests: Authors LA, JKC, LSH, and PGB are employed by GENERTI (currently renamed as INFOVALLEY LIFE SCIENCES SDN BHD). The other authors named on the manuscript are from University of Malaya. These affliations do not alter the authors' adherence to all the PLOS ONE policies on sharing data and materials,

* E-mail: drlivy@infovalley.net.my

Introduction

Familial hypercholesterolemia (FH) (ICD-10 code E78.0) was the first genetic disease of lipid metabolism to be clinically and molecularly characterized [1]. It is an inherited disorder of lipoprotein metabolism, transmitted in an autosomal dominant manner [2]. FH is characterized by elevated levels of low density lipoprotein cholesterol (LDLc) and total cholesterol (TC) in the circulation, deposits of cholesterol in peripheral tissues, presence of tendon xanthomas and accelerated atherosclerosis, leading to premature cardiovascular events [1,3,4,5,6].

Heterozygous FH is one of the most frequent Mendelian disorders with a frequency of 1 in 500 but has a much higher incidence in certain populations, such as the Afrikaners, Christian Lebanese, Finns, and French-Canadians [7]. The frequency of homozygous FH is 1 in a million, with symptoms appearing in childhood [8].

FH can result primarily from mutations in either *Low Density Lipoprotein-Receptor* gene *(LDLR)*, *Apolipoprotein B-100* gene (*APOB*), *or Proprotein Convertase Subtilisin/Kexin type 9* gene (*PCSK9*), singly or in combination [1]. Genetic variations in the *LDLR* gene are commonly loss-of-function mutations, which result in increased plasma LDLc levels [9]. Genetic variations in the *APOB gene*, and the *PCSK9* gene give rise to the same lipid homeostasis functional defects [1]. To date, genetic variants in an excess of over 1000 have been identified in the *LDLR, APOB & PCSK9* gene as reported by British Heart Foundation (BHF) and other public databases. In addition, other genes associated with lipid control and regulatory regions such as *Upstream Transcription Factor 1* gene (*USF1*), Apolipoprotein *E* gene (*APOE*), *Lipoprotein Lipase* gene (*LPL*), *Fibrinogen Beta Chain* gene (*FGB*), and *Hepatic Lipase* gene (*LIPC*) can manifest as hypercholesterolemia and have been shown to predispose to premature cardiovascular diseases [10,11,12,13,14]. Results from SNPs study should be interpreted with caution, as SNPs may exert their effects individually, or multiple SNPs can act synergistically to cause a functional difference between haplotypes. Interaction among multiple SNPs may jointly affect a disease's risk. Assessing the independent individual SNP without considering the SNP-SNP interactions forms (even on SNPs that show very weak associations with estimated odds ratios) will fail to discover weak associations [15,16].

Clinical management of FH focuses on early detection and control of hypercholesterolemia to decrease the risk of atherosclerosis and to prevent premature cardiovascular disease [17]. Establishing an accurate diagnosis of FH is often difficult. In spite of its prevalence, and considerable benefit associated with its early detection and treatment, FH is often under-diagnosed in many countries [18,19]. Systematic genetic screening for mutations in those at risk of FH has been found to be cost effective and will help in better prognosis [20]. However, most genetic studies in FH were conducted in non-Asian populations and the allelic variants prevailing here in South East Asia are not known. In South East Asia, specifically in Malaysia, only few studies have been carried out on these genes [21,22,23,24,25,26]. Thus, the aim of this study is to determine the genetic variants in the *LDLR*, *APOB*, *PCSK9* and other lipid related genes in a study cohort with clinical FH.

Materials and Methods

Subject Recruitment

Consecutive 141 patients with high LDLc levels above 4 mmol/L were recruited between January 2007 and September 2009 from the medical out-patient clinics at the University Malaya Medical Centre (UMMC), Kuala Lumpur. The FH-Dutch Lipid Clinic Network (DLCN) criteria [27,28] was adopted as the diagnostic scoring method to clinically diagnose/screen for FH, excluding molecular diagnosis criterion, and stratify subjects into possible FH, probable FH or definite FH. One hundred and one control subjects consisted of those who were genetically unrelated, with normal LDLc levels, absence of family history of FH, hyper/hypothyroidism, chronic kidney disease, diabetes, chronic liver disease and characterized as not FH by DLCN criteria (Table S1). The protocol was approved by the UMMC's Medical Ethics Committee (Ref: 546.16) and written informed consents were obtained from all patients.

Questionnaire and Data Collection

The data included socio-demographic characteristics (age, sex, and occupation), personal and family history of hypertension, hypercholesterolemia, CVD and other lifestyle habits, such as smoking status, and physical activity. Body mass index (BMI), waist circumferences (WC) and blood pressure were also measured.

DNA Isolation

Genomic DNA from all subjects was isolated from whole blood using QIAamp DNA Mini Kit (QIAGEN, USA) in 200 µl of total volume according to user protocol. Qualitative and quantitative estimations were carried out on the DNA samples. All DNA samples were normalized to concentration of 50 ng/µl for genotyping.

Selection of Genes/SNPs and Microarray Probes Synthesis

Genetic variations implicated in FH from three publically available databases, BHF (www.ucl.ac.uk) [29], dbSNP (ncbi.nlm.nih.gov/SNP/) [30] and SNPedia (www.snpedia.com), were selected based on the following attributes: i) conventional SNPs known to cause FH in genes encoding *LDLR*, *APOB* and *PCSK9* ii) SNPs in *USF1*, *APOE*, *LPL*, *FGB* and *LIPC* that were known to have functional effects by in vitro assays or were non-synonymous in lipid regulatory regions. Though our initial research and mining led us to 1850 SNPs, which were sent to Illumina for designing the probes, only 1536 could be of designable standards as per Illumina criteria.

A tool called Assay Design Tool (ADT) of Illumina ranks SNPs based on an in-built algorithm where SNPs scoring below 0.4 have a rank of zero suggesting the probe is not designable by Illumina. SNPs scoring between 0.4 and 0.6 get a rank 0.5 whereas a score above 0.6 is ranked 1. SNPs scoring 0.5 and 1 are technically ranked as SNPs that can be successfully designed as probes by Illumina. The assay has an average 30-fold redundancy for each probe thus making the quality control robust. In all, 231 probes had score of 0.5 and 1305 had a score of 1.0. Only 1536 SNPs were chosen because that was the maximum plexity Illumina platform could accommodate.

Most of the reported studies till date were from Caucasian population, and hence we were keenly interested to re-look at the reported SNPs using a population based approach, and check if the interpretations are extrapolatable to Asian population.

Designability scores were graded and qualified probes were selected and synthesized for the custom GoldenGate™ genotyping assay (GGGT) (www.illumina.com). Of the 1850 SNPs mined, 1536 SNPs were synthesized as probes, comprising of 811 in *LDLR*, 245 in *APOB*, 284 in *PCSK9*, and another 196 lipid-regulatory related SNPs.

Genotyping

Genotyping was performed on Universal BeadChips (Illumina, USA) according to the manufacturer's protocol and was carried out in compliance with MIAME (Minimum Information about a Microarray Experiment) guidelines [31]. All the raw data from our GGGT microarray assays were imported into the GenomeStudio™ software (Illumina, USA) for allelic analysis and deviation from Hardy-Weinberg equilibrium. Average call rate of 70–80% was observed, which is expected of a custom GGGT assay.

Statistical Analysis

Statistical analysis was performed using the SPSS software v16.0 (SPSS Inc., Chicago, Illinois). The test of normality (Kolmogorov-Smirnov) was employed to determine the normality of the variables. Descriptive analysis and statistical significance of the association were assessed by independent t-test. Logistic regression was applied to obtain the Odds Ratio (OR) and the p-values for the tested SNPs (p-values ≤ 0.05 were considered to be significant). An $OR > 1.0$ was used as the cut-off for the baseline of risk-associated SNPs, and the baseline risk-lowering SNPs as $OR < 1.0$. An OR equal to 1 was a neutral value and deemed as normal. Analysis of variance (ANOVA) test was conducted for comparison of means between clinical profiles and three genotype groups. Minor allele frequency (MAF) for this study was calculated. MAF for the most closely related ethnic group to our study were also extracted from public database (NCBI dbSNP Build 137). A Chi-Square Test was performed to determine whether there was a significant difference between our study's MAF and public databases' MAF. Bonferroni correction for multiple comparisons of SNPs on the same gene was performed. Unless otherwise specified, all data were presented as means and standard deviations.

Additional Validation of Genotype Calls by Sequencing

Microarray calls were validated by blindly re-genotyping some SNPs in a number of subjects randomly selected from cases using DNA sequencing. Primers were synthesized for regions encompassing a few significant SNPs and the PCR products amplified from the genomic DNA of FH cases were sent for sequencing (First BASE Laboratories, www.base-asia.com).

Results

Subjects Demographics and Clinical Profiles

Of the 141 FH subjects and 111 control subjects included in the study, 24 were classified as definite FH, 25 as probable FH and 92 as possible FH from cases based on DLCN criteria. There was no significant gender bias observed between FH subjects (73 male: 68 female) and control subjects (46 male: 65 female) that were recruited into the study ($p = 0.104$). The mean age of the FH subjects recruited was 46.84 (SD ±11.2), while control subjects were 40.00 (SD ±9.3) with significant difference ($p<0.001$). The BMI ($p = 0.239$), waist circumference ($p = 0.356$) and HDL cholesterol (HDLc) level ($p = 0.420$) were similar between the two study groups. FH subjects were found to have significantly higher levels of triglycerides (TG) ($p = 0.001$), TC and LDLc ($p<0.001$) as compared to controls (Table 1).

FH Associated SNPs

A total of 14 SNPs were found to be significantly associated with FH. Eleven out of 14 were associated with high risk of FH (OR >1), while the remaining three were protective against FH (OR <1). Of the 11 associated SNPs, one (rs2569556) was found in the *LDLR* gene, seven in the *APOB gene* (rs12720762, rs13306187, rs13306194, rs12714238, rs12720772, rs57825321 and rs41291161) and three (rs12084215, rs565436 and rs28362269) in the *PCKS9* gene. The *APOB* rs12720762 is associated with the highest risk of FH with OR of 14.78. Amongst the FH subjects, 108 (76.60%) subjects have had at least one significant risk-associated SNP.17 out of 24 definite FH subjects (70.83%), 19 out 25 probable FH subjects (76%) and 72 out of 92 possible FH subjects (78.26%) had at least one significant risk-associated SNP (Table 2).

The *APOB* rs57825321 and *USF1* rs3737787 and rs2516839 were found to have a protective effect against FH in this case-control association study (Table 2). No significant associations were found with the other 1522 SNPs (99.09%) genotyped (Statistical data not shown but available upon request).

SNPs Association with Clinical and Demographic Profile

We also investigated the association of significant SNPs with the clinical and demographic profile of FH patients. There was no significant association between most of the SNPs with the clinical and demographic profile. However, the *APOB* rs13306194 and rs57825321 were significantly associated with HDLc level ($p<0.001$). *APOB rs12720772* was associated with TC ($p = 0.0275$) and BMI ($p = 0.0337$) while the *PCSK9* rs12084215 was associated with HDLc level ($p = 0.0090$) and BMI ($p = 0.0228$) (Table 3, 4, 5, and 6). Clinical and demographic profile of control subjects was also examined similarly. No significant association was seen between most of the SNPs with the clinical and demographic profile. However, rs12084215 (*PCSK9*) was significantly associated with TG level ($p = 0.0052$) and waist circumference measurement ($p = 0.0214$) (Table 7).

Table 2. FH associated SNPs, ($p<0.05$).

Gene	rs number	Nucleotide change	p-value	OR (CI)
LDLR	rs2569556	[G>A]	0.0140	1.77 (1.12–2.78)
APOB	rs13306187	[G>A]	<0.0001	6.76 (3.28–13.90)
APOB	rs13306194	[G>A]	0.0154	2.25 (1.17–4.34)
APOB	rs12714238	[G>A]	<0.001	8.04 (3.20–20.20)
APOB	rs12720772	[G>A]	0.0130	2.00 (1.16–3.46)
APOB	rs12720762	[G>C]	<0.001	14.78 (5.03–43.44)
APOB	rs41291161	[T>A]	<0.0001	11.51 (4.32–30.69)
APOB	rs57825321	[A>T]	0.0304	2.02 (1.07–3.83)
APOB	rs12714254	[T>G]	<0.001	0.22 (0.11–0.50)
PCSK9	rs12084215	[C>A]	0.0064	3.87 (1.46–10.23)
PCSK9	rs565436	[A>G]	0.0020	5.00 (1.80–13.89)
PCSK9	rs28362269	[G>A]	<0.001	5.43 (2.76–10.65)
USF1	rs3737787	[G>A]	0.0174	0.55 (0.33–0.90)
USF1	rs2516839	[G>A]	0.0317	0.67 (0.46–0.97)

rs number, NCBI Reference SNP (rs) Number, an identification tag assigned by NCBI to SNPs [30].
CI, Confidence interval.
Odds ratio (OR) between groups was determined by logistic regression.

Table 1. Demographics and clinical profiles of the subjects.

Characteristic	Over all FH cases	Definite FH	Probable FH	Possible FH	Controls	p-value Over all FH cases vs. Controls
Males : Females	73:68	11:13	15:10	47:45	46:65	0.104
Age (years)	46.84 (±11.2)	42.37 (±17.4)	45.60 (±18.6)	48.34 (±8.5)	40.00 (±9.3)	<0.001
BMI (kg/m^2)	26.42 (±5.4)	22.79 (±5.1)	26.49 (±5.2)	27.32 (±5.2)	25.62 (±4.9)	0.239
WC (cm)	86.21 (±17.5)	76.64 (±19.1)	85.37 (±18.6)	88.90 (±16.0)	83.05 (±12.2)	0.356
TG (mmol/L)	1.79 (±1.0)	1.99 (±1.8)	2.00 (±1.0)	1.69 (±0.7)	1.23 (±0.7)	0.001
TC (mmol/L)	8.86 (±5.1)	13.23 (±10.7)	9.51 (±2.4)	7.47 (±1.2)	5.18 (±0.9)	<0.001
HDLc (mmol/L)	1.25 (±0.7)	1.17 (±0.4)	1.53 (±1.5)	1.20 (±0.3)	1.34 (±0.3)	0.420
LDLc (mmol/L)	6.37 (±2.3)	9.23 (±3.4)	6.96 (±2.3)	5.49 (±1.0)	3.28 (±0.7)	<0.001

BMI, Body Mass Index.
WC, Waist circumference.
TG, Triglyceride.
TC, Total Cholesterol.
HDLc, High Density Lipoprotein Cholesterol.
LDLc, Low Density Lipoprotein Cholesterol.
The data are expressed as mean (±SD).
p-values were obtained by comparing the phenotypes between the two groups using Student's t-test.

Table 3. Comparison of clinical profiles between rs13306194 genotypes among FH patients.

Clinical Profiles	GG (% = 88)	GA (% = 12)	AA (% = 0)	p-value
Age	47.11±(10.9)	46.18±(12.3)	–	0.7463
TG	1.83±(1.1)	1.54±(0.7)	–	0.2905
TC	8.89±(5.4)	8.86±(2.7)	–	0.9848
HDLc	1.15±(0.3)	1.94±(1.8)	–	<0.001
LDLc	6.42±(2.4)	6.16±(2.4)	–	0.6622
BMI	26.44±(5.5)	26.29±(5.5)	–	0.9173
WC	86.57±(17.3)	82.38±(19.8)	–	0.3720

Data are presented in mean ± SD.
p-values were obtained by comparing the phenotypes among the genotypes using Analysis of Variance (ANOVA).

Table 4. Comparison of clinical profiles between rs57825321 genotypes among FH patients.

Clinical Profiles	AA (% = 86)	AT (% = 14)	TT (% = 0)	p-value
Age	47.02±(11.2)	45.95±(12.0)	–	0.6965
TG	1.83±(1.1)	1.53±(0.7)	–	0.2456
TC	8.89±(5.5)	8.76±(2.5)	–	0.9169
HDLc	1.15±(0.3)	1.88±(1.6)	–	<0.001
LDLc	6.43±(2.4)	6.13±(2.2)	–	0.5995
BMI	26.51±(5.5)	25.97±(5.1)	–	0.6817
WC	86.79±(17.4)	82.44±(18.6)	–	0.3310

Data are presented in mean ± SD.
p-values were obtained by comparing the phenotypes among the genotypes using Analysis of Variance (ANOVA).

Minor Allele Frequency

Information regarding gene, rs number, SNPs region, chromosome, nucleotide change and allele frequency of the associated SNPs observed from this study was summarized. Although, in our study the minor allele of the significant SNPs matched with the information in public database, six of the SNPs (rs13306187 MAF = 0.111, rs12714238 MAF = 0.072, rs12720772 MAF = 0.301, rs41291161 MAF = 0.077, rs57825321 MAF = 0.403, and rs12714254 MAF = 0.405) differed in frequency ($p<0.05$) (Table 8).

Bonferroni Correction

Five out of the eight significant SNPs of *APOB* gene (rs13306187, rs12714238, rs12720762, rs41291161, rs12714254) and all three *PCSK9* gene SNPs (rs12084215, rs565436 and rs28362269) survived significance after a conservative Bonferroni correction for multiple testing, (0.05/9, $p<0.0056$) and (0.05/4, $p<0.0125$) respectively. However, none of the SNPs of *USF1* gene is significant following Bonferroni correction. These 8 SNPs are thus of sufficient interest to warrant further investigation.

Additional Validation of Genotype Calls by Sequencing

A few samples were sent for sequencing to rule out any genotyping errors and results were concordant with the genotype calls generated from the microarray data (Figure S1).

Discussion

Fourteen out of 1536 SNPs evaluated in this study were significantly associated with FH, with 11 SNPs associated with increasing risk for FH, while the remaining three SNPs associated with decreasing risk for FH. Among the risk-increasing SNPs, allele A of rs2569556 in *LDLR* gene was identified among 55 out of 141 FH cases (39.0%), with 48 heterozygous and seven in homozygous genotypes. SNP rs13306187 in *APOB* gene also demonstrated risk association on allele A among 11 FH cases. Ten of the FH cases were heterozygous and only one of the FH case was observed in homozygous genotype. Other risk associated SNPs on *APOB* gene were only observed to occur in heterozygous genotype and these included 64 cases for rs12720772; six cases for rs41291161; 121 cases for rs57825321; 17 cases for rs13306194, six cases for rs12714238, and four cases for rs12720762. Three *PCSK9* SNPs were observed to be associated with increased risk in a heterozygous manner (six cases for rs565436, six cases for rs12084215, and 15 cases for rs28362269). Only two risk-elevating SNPs (rs2569556 in *LDLR* gene and rs13306187 in *APOB* gene) were observed to be in the homozygous state; while other 9 SNPs presented in a heterozygous manner, which may demonstrate a milder phenotypic effect of FH. In general, 17 definite FH subjects (70.83%), 19 probable FH subjects (76%) and 72 possible FH subjects (78.26%) had at least one SNP out of the risk-increasing SNPs. The remaining 33 FH subjects (23.40%) did not have any risk-increasing SNPs indicating that there are other genetic or environmental factors causing hypercholesterolemia that were undetected by our study and which has the potential for future investigation. Besides the risk-increasing SNPs, there were 3 other SNPs with OR<1 (rs12714254 in *APOB* gene, and rs2516839 and rs3737787 in the *USF1* gene) which confer lower risk against FH. *USF1* gene was studied because *USF1* protein regulates the transcriptional activation of a variety of genes involved in glucose, lipid and apolipoproteins (*APOCIII*, *APOAII* and *APOE*) metabolism in the development of atherosclerosis [32,33,34,35]. Results for SNPs in other candidate genes such as *APOE*, *LPL*, *FGB* and *LIPC* were analysed and found not to be significant in our study ($p>0.05$).

Clinical parameters were compared between the significant genotypes among FH patients (Table 3, 4, 5, and 6). Allele A of *APOB* rs12720772 in heterozygous GA patients is associated with significantly higher level of plasma TC compared to the G allele ($p = 0.0275$), while allele A in *APOB* rs12720772 ($p = 0.0337$) and *PCSK9* rs12084215 ($p = 0.0228$) were associated with higher BMI.

Table 5. Comparison of clinical profiles between rs12720772 genotypes among FH patients.

Clinical Profiles	GG (% = 48)	GA (% = 52)	AA (% = 0)	p-value
Age	46.69±(9.0)	47.39±(12.0)	–	0.7175
TG	1.63±(0.8)	1.80±(0.8)	–	0.2683
TC	7.89±(1.9)	8.88±(2.8)	–	0.0275
HDLc	1.23±(0.5)	1.30±(0.9)	–	0.6228
LDLc	5.89±(1.6)	6.68±(2.8)	–	0.0614
BMI	25.18±(3.5)	27.10±(5.9)	–	0.0337
WC	85.04±(13.5)	86.11±(18.8)	–	0.7290

Data are presented in mean ± SD.
p-values were obtained by comparing the phenotypes among the genotypes using Analysis of Variance (ANOVA).

Table 6. Comparison of clinical profiles between rs12084215 genotypes among FH patients.

Clinical Profiles	CC (% = 91)	CA (% = 9)	AA (% = 0)	p-value
Age	44.39±(11.3)	53.50±(2.6)	-	0.0558
TG	1.72±(0.8)	1.68±(0.9)	-	0.9069
TC	8.35±(3.1)	7.65±(1.4)	-	0.5927
HDLc	1.18±(0.5)	2.32±(2.8)	-	0.0090
LDLc	6.32±(3.0)	4.56±(1.8)	-	0.1602
BMI	25.80±(5.7)	31.57±(5.9)	-	0.0228
WC	84.33±(17.0)	94.58±(6.4)	-	0.1518

Data are presented in mean ± SD.
p-values were obtained by comparing the phenotypes among the genotypes using Analysis of Variance (ANOVA).

Table 7. Comparison of clinical profiles between rs12084215 genotypes among Control subjects.

Clinical Profiles	CC (n = 71%)	AC (n = 26%)	AA (n = 3%)	p-value
Age	38.05±(9.11)	37.67±(5.92)	41.00±(4.24)	0.8686
TG	1.07±(0.57)	2.90±(n/a)	-	0.0052
TC	5.11±(0.93)	6.20±(n/a)	-	0.2659
HDLc	1.42±(0.35)	0.98±(n/a)	-	0.2368
LDLc	3.20±(0.78)	3.90±(n/a)	-	0.3934
BMI	25.55±(4.91)	24.98±(5.08)	25.14±(2.27)	0.9313
WC	78.64±(8.96)	98.50±(14.85)	-	0.0214

Data are presented in mean ± SD.
p-values were obtained by comparing the phenotypes among the genotypes using Analysis of Variance (ANOVA).

Interestingly, we observed that 3 risk alleles have the effect of significantly higher level of plasma HDLc in their heterozygous form in 3 SNPs (GA, rs13306194; AT, rs57825321 of *APOB*; CA, rs12084215 of *PCSK9*). For control subjects, similar approach for clinical and demographic profile was also performed. Only allele A in SNP rs12084215 of *PCSK9* was associated with higher level of TG ($p = 0.0052$) and waist circumference measurement ($p = 0.0214$) with heterozygous AC (Table 7). It is noteworthy that all the parameter-associated SNPs presented with homozygous wild type (+/+) and heterozygous (+/−) but extremely low or no homozygous mutant (−/−). This finding is commonly observed among the heterozygous FH associated SNPs [36] (Table 3, 4, 5, 6, and 7).

MAF from the studied population were calculated and compared with the MAF information on public database. Han Chinese subjects, where available, were selected as the targeted group for comparison as this Asian ethnicity were believed to closely resemble the ethnic groups of our study population. The results demonstrated that six of our SNPs differed in the frequency of MAF in public database [37]. Disparity in frequency could be due to founder-effects, natural selection or multi-ethnic groups in the study population [7,38] (Table 8).

Out of the 1536 SNPs that were studied, 1522 SNPs (99.09%) did not show any significant result or association. This is because besides the SNPs being mono-allelic (non-polymorphic) [37], we also observed an almost equal number of the predicted risk alleles present in both case subjects and control subjects across our 252 samples. Thus analyses of these polymorphisms were not statistically significant and therefore, regarded as having non-pathogenic phenotype. These findings suggest that many SNPs published in public databases might just be non-pathogenic polymorphisms in Malaysia. This will require further validation in a larger population of Asian descent.

For the SNPs association study, we included all significant SNPs, inclusive of SNPs with relatively low odds ratio (*LDLR* rs2569556, OR 1.77), as SNPs usually work with other functionally relevant SNPs additively or synergistically, to manifest a disease condition in certain population [16]. Therefore, including these SNPs with relatively low ORs might aid future research on SNP-SNP interaction and polygenic effect of FH. Furthermore, 12 SNPs that were reported as significant were in the intronic and untranslated region (UTR) of genes. These SNPs could be in linkage disequilibrium with other functional SNPs involved in potential regulatory regions or splice site variants that may be associated with lipid related disorders. Exons 2 to 6 fall in the ligand binding region while exons 7 to 14 coded for epidermal growth factor precursor (EGFP)-like domain in *LDLR* gene. Although SNP rs2569556 is in intron 6, this polymorphism may contribute to the disturbance in ligand binding or the internalization of the receptor into the liver cell [29,39].

SNPs rs2569556, rs12720772, rs57825321 and rs12714254 were found to deviate from HWE during the post-hoc analysis (Table S2). These SNPs were retained because not necessarily all HWE deviations indicate genotyping errors. SNPs deviating from HWE may confound trait-allele association as they are thought to reflect genotyping error [40,41] although the contrary has also been argued [42]. Presence of a common deletion polymorphism, a mutant PCR-primer site or a tendency to miscall heterozygotes as homozygotes could also lead to deviation [43]. Deviation from HWE, assuming sources of error have been eliminated, may indicate the association of a locus with disease. As FH homozygous is so rare (one in a million) and deleterious, low count or complete absence of homozygous allele deviated significantly from HWE.

There are several limitations in the current clinical setup on how a subject is diagnosed as FH based solely on elevated cholesterol levels, physical manifestations and family history. Hypercholesterolemia is a silent disease and the underlying aetiology of FH is not routinely defined. Without proper genetic screening, "over-diagnosis" or misdiagnosis of FH may take place because the condition might overlap with other forms of dyslipidemia, sedentary lifestyle, inappropriate dietary intake or metabolic syndrome, which would contribute to hypercholesterolemia. Similarly, FH subjects with milder phenotypes who maintain a healthy lifestyle may have normal cholesterol levels and the phenomenon of "under-diagnosis" occurs. Furthermore, not all clinically diagnosed patients have a known genetic defect, suggesting that other genes besides *LDLR*, *APOB* and *PCSK9* may play a role in the alteration of lipid metabolism which remains yet to be discovered.

One drawback of our approach is there was a significant difference noted in our subjects' age (patients 46.84 SD ±11.2 vs. control 40.00 SD ±9.3), as FH patients recruited were older. Age is acknowledged as risk factor for age-related dyslipidemia. Reason for age-related disruption of lipid homeostasis include the gradual decline in clearance of LDLc with increasing age, the progressively reduced ability to remove cholesterol through conversion to bile acids, the decreased activity of the rate-limiting enzyme in bile acid biosynthesis [44] and progressive decrease in growth hormone secretion with age also causes critical changes in LDLc metabolism. Growth hormone plays an important role in cholesterol

Table 8. Minor allele frequency of significant SNPs.

Gene	rs no.	Region	Chr	Nucleotide change	MAF (Total)	MAF (Cases)	MAF (Controls)	MAF (PD)	p-value (Total vs. PD)	MAF source
LDLR	rs2569556	Intron 6	19	G>A	0.263	0.316	0.223	0.209	0.3853	HapMap-HCB
APOB	rs13306187	Exon 25	2	G>A	0.111	0.197	0.043	0.035	0.0314	HapMap-HCB
APOB	rs13306194	Exon 12	2	G>A	0.091	0.128	0.061	0.133	0.2784	Pilot 1 CHB+JPT low coverage panel
APOB	rs12714238	Intron 5	2	G>A	0.072	0.136	0.022	0.011	0.0311	Pharmacogenetics Network for Cardiovascular Risk Therapy
APOB	rs12720772	Intron 18	2	G>A	0.301	0.352	0.260	0.000	<0.001	HapMap-CHB
APOB	rs12720762	Intron 1	2	G>C	0.076	0.159	0.014	0.021	0.0741	Pharmacogenetics Network for Cardiovascular Risk Therapy
APOB	rs41291161	Intron 14	2	T>A	0.077	0.149	0.021	0.001	<0.001	ABECASIS CLINICAL PANEL
APOB	rs57825321	Intron 16	2	A>T	0.403	0.429	0.369	0.158	<0.001	Pilot 1 CHB+JPT low coverage panel
APOB	rs12714254	Intron 3	2	T>G	0.405	0.342	0.454	0.100	<0.001	Pilot 1 CHB+JPT low coverage panel
PCSK9	rs12084215	Intron 3	1	C>A	0.102	0.164	0.046	NA	NA	NA
PCSK9	rs565436	Intron 9	1	A>G	0.079	0.145	0.036	0.100	0.6627	Pilot 1 CHB+JPT low coverage panel
PCSK9	rs28362269	Intron 9	1	G>A	0.112	0.188	0.053	0.059	0.1289	Pilot 1 YRI low coverage panel
USF1	rs2516839	5′ UTR	1	G>A	0.408	0.360	0.447	0.366	0.5197	HapMap-CHB
USF1	rs3737787	3′ UTR	1	G>A	0.163	0.117	0.199	0.250	0.1032	HapMap-HCB

rs no, NCBI Reference SNP (rs) Number, an identification tag assigned by NCBI to SNPs.
Chr, Chromosome.
p-value obtained by comparing frequencies using Chi-Square Test.
MAF (Total), minor allele frequency obtained from total sum of case and control subjects in this study.
MAF (PD), minor allele frequency information from public database, NCBI dbSNP Build 137.

homeostasis by either modulating the expression of hepatic *LDLR* [45] or controlling the activity of cholesterol 7alpha-hydroxylase (CYP7A1), a rate-limiting enzyme in the synthesis of bile acid from cholesterol [46]. Presence of FH causal SNPs along with increasing age accelerates the hypercholesterolemia. This bias was beyond our control as our recruitment of subjects was based on volunteered patients who visit UMMC.

Another limitation of our study was that the microarray genotyping platform used in this study only allowed us to study published SNPs. It is possible that rare risk-associated SNPs may be discovered in future using other existing technologies such as sequencing. The authors also recognise that the genotype scores are not true reflection of the biological characteristics of FH as all alleles were given the same statistical weight. Therefore, a model of association of SNPs should be created to calculate the overall genetic risk. These 14 SNPs identified could provide more insights in future studies on screening markers for FH management and warrants further investigation.

Acknowledgments

We greatly appreciate the support of the study subjects and their families who participated in this project. We would also like to thank the staff of UM, UMMC and INFOVALLEY® for their timely help during the subject recruitment and sample collection. Our special gratitude goes to Dr. S. Pavai, Dr. Roma, Dr. Haizal, Dr. Alex Tan, Dr. Haliza, Ms. Rajeswari Karuppiah and Ms. Valli in their assistance during patient recruitment, sample collection and administration processes. We thank Prof. Dr. Karuthan Chinna for his helpful guidance in statistical analysis. In addition, we would like to thank the three reviewers for their insightful comments that have helped to improve this paper.

Author Contributions

Conceived and designed the experiments: SHL JKC PB LA JV WAWA SPC MKT RM. Performed the experiments: SHL JKC LA. Analyzed the data: SHL JKC PB LA JV MKT SMZ RM. Contributed reagents/ materials/analysis tools: SHL JKC LA JV WAWA SPC RM. Wrote the paper: SHL JKC LA JV MKT RM.

References

1. Rader DJ, Cohen J, Hobbs HH (2003) Monogenic hypercholesterolemia: new insights in pathogenesis and treatment. J Clin Invest 111: 1795–1803.
2. Alonso R, Defesche JC, Tejedor D, Castillo S, Stef M, et al. (2009) Genetic diagnosis of familial hypercholesterolemia using a DNA-array based platform. Clin Biochem 42: 899–903.
3. Stamler J, Wentworth D, Neaton JD (1986) Is relationship between serum cholesterol and risk of premature death from coronary heart disease continuous and graded? Findings in 356,222 primary screenees of the Multiple Risk Factor Intervention Trial (MRFIT). JAMA 256: 2823–2828.
4. Wilson PW, Garrison RJ, Castelli WP, Feinleib M, McNamara PM, et al. (1980) Prevalence of coronary heart disease in the Framingham Offspring Study: role of lipoprotein cholesterols. Am J Cardiol 46: 649–654.
5. Castelli WP, Anderson K, Wilson PW, Levy D (1992) Lipids and risk of coronary heart disease. The Framingham Study. Ann Epidemiol 2: 23–28.
6. Steinberg D, Witztum JL (1990) Lipoproteins and atherogenesis. Current concepts. JAMA 264: 3047–3052.
7. Marais AD (2004) Familial hypercholesterolaemia. Clin Biochem Rev 25: 49–68.
8. Soutar AK, Naoumova RP (2007) Mechanisms of disease: genetic causes of familial hypercholesterolemia. Nat Clin Pract Cardiovasc Med 4: 214–225.
9. Anderson RG (2003) Joe Goldstein and Mike Brown: from cholesterol homeostasis to new paradigms in membrane biology. Trends Cell Biol 13: 534–539.
10. Lee JC, Weissglas-Volkov D, Kyttala M, Sinsheimer JS, Jokiaho A, et al. (2007) USF1 contributes to high serum lipid levels in Dutch FCHL families and U.S. whites with coronary artery disease. Arterioscler Thromb Vasc Biol 27: 2222–2227.
11. de Knijff P, Havekes LM (1996) Apolipoprotein E as a risk factor for coronary heart disease: a genetic and molecular biology approach. Curr Opin Lipidol 7: 59–63.
12. Alonso-Orgaz S, Moreno L, Macaya C, Rico L, Mateos-Caceres PJ, et al. (2006) Proteomic study of plasma from moderate hypercholesterolemic patients. J Proteome Res 5: 2301–2308.
13. Ando H, Nishimura Y, Nemoto T, Takamura T, Nagai Y, et al. (2001) Severe hypercholesterolemia in a double heterozygote for lipoprotein lipase deficiency (LPL(Arita)) and apolipoprotein epsilon4: a report of a family with LPL(Arita). Endocr J 48: 113–118.
14. Meng L, Ruixing Y, Yiyang L, Xingjiang L, Kela L, et al. (2010) Association of LIPC −250G>A polymorphism and several environmental factors with serum lipid levels in the Guangxi Bai Ku Yao and Han populations. Lipids Health Dis 9: 28.
15. Dinu I, Mahasirimongkol S, Liu Q, Yanai H, Sharaf Eldin N, et al. (2012) SNP-SNP interactions discovered by logic regression explain Crohn's disease genetics. PLoS One 7: e43035.
16. Onay VU, Briollais L, Knight JA, Shi E, Wang Y, et al. (2006) SNP-SNP interactions in breast cancer susceptibility. BMC Cancer 6: 114.
17. Al-Allaf FA, Coutelle C, Waddington SN, David AL, Harbottle R, et al. (2010) LDLR-Gene therapy for familial hypercholesterolaemia: problems, progress, and perspectives. Int Arch Med 3: 36.
18. Dorsch MF, Lawrance RA, Durham NP, Hall AS (2001) Familial hypercholesterolaemia is underdiagnosed after AMI. BMJ 322: 111.
19. Rees A (2008) Familial hypercholesterolaemia: underdiagnosed and undertreated. Eur Heart J 29: 2583–2584.
20. Jarvik GP, Brunzell JD, Motulsky AG (2008) Frequent detection of familial hypercholesterolemia mutations in familial combined hyperlipidemia. J Am Coll Cardiol 52: 1554–1556.
21. Al-Khateeb A, Zahri MK, Mohamed MS, Sasongko TH, Ibrahim S, et al. (2011) Analysis of sequence variations in low-density lipoprotein receptor gene among Malaysian patients with familial hypercholesterolemia. BMC Med Genet 12: 40.
22. Khoo KL, Tan H, Liew YM (2000) Familial hyperlipidaemia in Malaysian children. Med J Malaysia 55: 249–258.
23. Khoo KL, Van Acker P, Tan H, Deslypere JP (2000) Genetic causes of familial hypercholesterolaemia in a Malaysian population. Med J Malaysia 55: 409–418.
24. Khoo KL, van Acker P, Defesche JC, Tan H, van de Kerkhof L, et al. (2000) Low-density lipoprotein receptor gene mutations in a Southeast Asian population with familial hypercholesterolemia. Clin Genet 58: 98–105.
25. Khoo KL, Tan H, Liew YM, Deslypere JP, Janus E (2003) Lipids and coronary heart disease in Asia. Atherosclerosis 169: 1–10.
26. Azian M, Hapizah MN, Khalid BA, Khalid Y, Rosli A, et al. (2006) Use of the denaturing gradient gel electrophoresis (DGGE) method for mutational screening of patients with familial hypercholesterolaemia (FH) and Familial defective apolipoprotein B100 (FDB). Malays J Pathol 28: 7–15.
27. Fouchier SW, Defesche JC, Umans-Eckenhausen MW, Kastelein JP (2001) The molecular basis of familial hypercholesterolemia in The Netherlands. Hum Genet 109: 602–615.
28. Betteridge J (2000) Lipids and vascular disease : current issues. London: Martin Dunitz.
29. Leigh SE, Foster AH, Whittall RA, Hubbart CS, Humphries SE (2008) Update and analysis of the University College London low density lipoprotein receptor familial hypercholesterolemia database. Ann Hum Genet 72: 485–498.
30. Sherry ST, Ward MH, Kholodov M, Baker J, Phan L, et al. (2001) dbSNP: the NCBI database of genetic variation. Nucleic Acids Res 29: 308–311.
31. Brazma A, Hingamp P, Quackenbush J, Sherlock G, Spellman P, et al. (2001) Minimum information about a microarray experiment (MIAME)-toward standards for microarray data. Nat Genet 29: 365–371.
32. Casado M, Vallet VS, Kahn A, Vaulont S (1999) Essential role in vivo of upstream stimulatory factors for a normal dietary response of the fatty acid synthase gene in the liver. J Biol Chem 274: 2009–2013.
33. Ribeiro A, Pastier D, Kardassis D, Chambaz J, Cardot P (1999) Cooperative binding of upstream stimulatory factor and hepatic nuclear factor 4 drives the transcription of the human apolipoprotein A-II gene. J Biol Chem 274: 1216–1225.

34. Pastier D, Lacorte JM, Chambaz J, Cardot P, Ribeiro A (2002) Two initiator-like elements are required for the combined activation of the human apolipoprotein C-III promoter by upstream stimulatory factor and hepatic nuclear factor-4. J Biol Chem 277: 15199–15206.
35. van der Vleuten GM, Isaacs A, Hijmans A, van Duijn CM, Stalenhoef AF, et al. (2007) The involvement of upstream stimulatory factor 1 in Dutch patients with familial combined hyperlipidemia. J Lipid Res 48: 193–200.
36. Yuan G, Wang J, Hegele RA (2006) Heterozygous familial hypercholesterolemia: an underrecognized cause of early cardiovascular disease. CMAJ 174: 1124–1129.
37. Alex L, Chahil JK, Lye SH, Bagali P, Ler LW (2012) Differences in allele frequencies of autosomal dominant hypercholesterolemia SNPs in the Malaysian population. J Hum Genet 57: 358–362.
38. Austin MA, Hutter CM, Zimmern RL, Humphries SE (2004) Genetic causes of monogenic heterozygous familial hypercholesterolemia: a HuGE prevalence review. Am J Epidemiol 160: 407–420.
39. Lombardi P, Sijbrands EJ, van de Giessen K, Smelt AH, Kastelein JJ, et al. (1995) Mutations in the low density lipoprotein receptor gene of familial hypercholesterolemic patients detected by denaturing gradient gel electrophoresis and direct sequencing. J Lipid Res 36: 860–867.
40. Clayton DG, Walker NM, Smyth DJ, Pask R, Cooper JD, et al. (2005) Population structure, differential bias and genomic control in a large-scale, case-control association study. Nat Genet 37: 1243–1246.
41. Salanti G, Amountza G, Ntzani EE, Ioannidis JP (2005) Hardy-Weinberg equilibrium in genetic association studies: an empirical evaluation of reporting, deviations, and power. Eur J Hum Genet 13: 840–848.
42. Cox DG, Kraft P (2006) Quantification of the power of Hardy-Weinberg equilibrium testing to detect genotyping error. Hum Hered 61: 10–14.
43. Balding DJ (2006) A tutorial on statistical methods for population association studies. Nat Rev Genet 7: 781–791.
44. Trapani L, Pallottini V (2010) Age-Related Hypercholesterolemia and HMG-CoA Reductase Dysregulation: Sex Does Matter (A Gender Perspective). Curr Gerontol Geriatr Res: 420139.
45. Matasconi M, Parini P, Angelin B, Rudling M (2005) Pituitary control of cholesterol metabolism in normal and LDL receptor knock-out mice: effects of hypophysectomy and growth hormone treatment. Biochim Biophys Acta 1736: 221–227.
46. Rudling M, Parini P, Angelin B (1997) Growth hormone and bile acid synthesis. Key role for the activity of hepatic microsomal cholesterol 7alpha-hydroxylase in the rat. J Clin Invest 99: 2239–2245.

Functional Characterization of Two Low-Density Lipoprotein Receptor Gene Mutations in Two Chinese Patients with Familial Hypercholesterolemia

Haihong Wang, Shengyuan Xu, Liyuan Sun, Xiaodong Pan, Shiwei Yang, Luya Wang*

Department of Atherosclerosis, Beijing Institute of Heart Lung and Blood Vessel Disease, Beijing Anzhen Hospital Affiliated with Capital Medical University, Beijing, China

Abstract

Background: Familial hypercholesterolemia (FH) is an autosomal dominant disease that primarily results from mutations in the low-density lipoprotein receptor (*LDLR*) gene. We investigated two unrelated Chinese FH patients using gene screening and functional analysis to reveal the pathogenicity and the mechanism by which these mutations cause FH.

Methods: First, the *LDLR* gene was sequenced in these patients. Then, mutant receptors were transfected into human embryo kidney 293(HEK-293) cells, and a confocal laser-scanning microscope was used to observe the localization of mutant proteins. Further, the expression and the internalization activity were analyzed by flow cytometry. Finally, LDLR protein expression and stability was detected by western blot.

Results: Two different *LDLR* class 2B mutations were detected in two patients. The C201F mutation is a known mutation. However, the G615V mutation is novel. Flow cytometry showed that the expression and internalization activity of the mutant LDLRs were reduced to 73.6% and 82.6% for G615V and 33.2% and 33.5% for C201F, respectively.

Conclusions: This study identified two *LDLR* mutations in Chinese patients with FH and analyzed the relationship between the genotype and phenotype of these patients. We found that these mutant LDLRs were defective in transport, which led to a reduction in cholesterol clearance. These results increase our understanding of the mutational spectrum of FH in the Chinese population.

Editor: Maria Cristina Vinci, Cardiological Center Monzino, Italy

Funding: This study was supported by grants from the National Natural Science Foundation of China (81170810, 81271923) and the Beijing Natural Science Foundation (7112022). The funders had no role in study design, data collection and analysis, decision to publish, or preparation of the manuscript.

Competing Interests: The authors have declared that no competing interests exit.

* E-mail: wangluya@126.com

Introduction

Familial hypercholesterolemia (FH) is an autosomal dominant, inherited disease of lipid metabolism. Clinical manifestations of FH are abnormally high concentrations of plasma low-density lipoprotein cholesterol, tendon xanthomas and premature coronary heart disease. Total plasma cholesterol concentrations in heterozygous FH patients are typically in the range of 7 to 15 mmol/L and in homozygous FH range from 20 to 25 mmol/L. FH heterozygotes present manifestations of CHD at the age of 30–40 years, and homozygous FH present CHD before the age of 20 years [1] [2]. It is largely believed that in the general population, the prevalence of the homozygous FH is 1/1,000,000, while the prevalence of heterozygous FH is 1/500 [3–5]. However, in the Copenhagen General Population study, the prevalence of FH was approximately 1/200 [6]. Based on these estimates of prevalence, there are approximately 14–34 million individuals with FH worldwide [7]. Prevalence of FH might be as high as 1/80 in some populations, especially in French Canadians [8]. FH is commonly caused by mutations in the low-density lipoprotein receptor (*LDLR*), apolipoprotein B (*apoB*), or proprotein convertase subtilisin/kexin type 9 (*PCSK9*) genes. In particular, *LDLR* gene mutations are the most frequent cause of FH [9].

The LDLR is a cell-surface glycoprotein responsible for the uptake and removal of cholesterol-rich lipoproteins particles from the circulation [10]. According to biochemical and functional studies of *LDLR*, *LDLR* mutations can be divided into five classes. Class 1 mutations include null alleles with no detectable LDLR protein. Class 2 mutations encode LDLR proteins with defective transport from the endoplasmic reticulum to the Golgi apparatus that is either completely (class 2A) or partially blocked (class 2B).Class 3 mutations produce LDLR proteins that are defective in binding LDL. Class 4 mutations encode LDLR that fails to internalize LDL. Finally, class 5 mutations produce recycling-defective receptors [11–13]. To date, more than 1,200 *LDLR* mutations have been documented worldwide [14]. However, it has been previously shown that the presence of a mutation in the *LDLR* does not necessarily result in FH occurrence [15,16]. Therefore, there is a need for functional validation of *LDLR* mutations to determine their pathogenicity.

In this study, we investigated two unrelated Chinese FH probands and their first-degree relatives. One novel and one previously reported *LDLR* mutation were found. We further investigated the pathogenicity and the mechanism of these FH-causing mutations using a combination of transfection, confocal laser scanning microscopy, flow cytometry analysis, and western blot.

Materials and Methods

Patients

Two probands were recruited from the Beijing Anzhen Hospital that met the following FH clinical diagnostic criteria: 1) for adults, total cholesterol (TC) >7.8 mmol/L or low-density lipoprotein cholesterol (LDL-C) >4.4 mmol/L; 2) for children younger than 16 years old, TC >6.7 mmol/L; 3) patients or their relatives have tendon xanthomas; 4) patients with xanthomas whose TC is higher than 16 mmol/L are diagnosed as homozygous and the others patients are diagnosed as heterozygous [17].

Ethics Statement

The study was reviewed and approved by the ethical committee of the Beijing Anzhen Hospital, and all participants signed an informed consent form. The written informed consent for the minor enrolled in the study was obtained from his guardian.

Blood Lipid Measurements

Peripheral venous blood samples from the two probands and their first-degree relatives were drawn after a 12-hour fast. TC, LDL-C, triglycerides (TG) and high-density lipoprotein cholesterol (HDL-C) were measured using routine commercial kits (Beckman Coulter, Brea, USA) and an automated biochemistry analyzer (Beckman AU 4500, Brea, USA).

Sequencing of *LDLR*, *APOB* and *PCSK9* Genes

Genomic DNA was extracted using the phenol-chloroform centrifugation method. Then, the coding regions of *LDLR* (containing the promoter and 18 exons with flanking intron sequences), and *PCSK9* (containing the 12 exons with flanking intron sequences) genes as well as part of exon 26 of the APOB gene, associated with the apoB -LDLR interaction were amplified by polymerase chain reaction (PCR). The sequences of oligonucleotide used for the amplification are shown in the Table S1, S2 and S3. Thereafter, the amplification products were purified and then sequenced on ABI Prism 3730×l DNA Analyzer. The results were analyzed by phred/phrap/consed package. Finally, when mutations were detected, another sequencing reaction was performed on both genomic DNA from the relative and on a new PCR product from the proband.

Construction of a *LDLR* Mutant

We cloned the wild-type *LDL-R* gene from the hepatocyte cell line BEL 7402 in the OmicsLink (Guangzhou FulenGen, China) mammal cell expression vector, which has an N-terminal enhanced green fluorescent protein (EGFP) tag. The *LDLR* mutations (G615V and C201F) were generated from OmicsLink-LDLR by oligonucleotide site-directed mutagenesis using a QuikChange XL mutagenesis kit (Stratagene) according to the manufacturer's instructions. The following oligonucleotides were used to generate different plasmids carrying the *LDLR* mutations:

5′-TGCCAACCGCCTCACAG**T**TTCCGATGT-CAACTTGT-3′ (mutated base in bold) was used to change the codon GGT, which encodes glycine (G615), to GTT, which encodes valine (V);

5′-TGGTGGCCCCGACTT**T**CAAGGACAAATCTG-3′ (mutated base in bold) was used to change the codon TGC, which encodes cysteine (C201), to TTC, which encodes phenylalanine (F).

The integrity of all of the constructs was confirmed by direct sequence analysis.

Cell Culture and Transfection

Human embryonic kidney 293 (HEK-293) cells, which do not express LDLR [18], were cultured in Dulbecco's modified Eagle's medium (DMEM) supplemented with 10% fetal bovine serum, 100 U/ml penicillin and 100 μg/ml streptomycin at 37°C in a humidified atmosphere of 5% CO_2. In total, 3×10^5 cells were seeded in 6-well plates for 24 hours and plasmids containing wild-type and mutant *LDLR* were transfected into HEK-293 cells using lipofectamine2000 reagent (Invitrogen) according to the manufacturer's instructions. Transfection efficiency was estimated by counting the EGFP positive cells under a fluorescent microscope. Confocal laser scanning microscope and flow cytometry were used to determine the function of the LDLR following a 48-hour culture.

Confocal Laser Scanning Microscope (CLSM)

To determine the cellular localization of the LDLR-EGFP fusion proteins and to analyze the LDLR activity by measuring internalization of LDL in transfected cells, CLSM (Leica) was used. To obtain the fluorescent images, a 63×oil objective was used.

To observe the cellular localization of the LDLR-EGFP fusion proteins, the cells transfected with wild-type protein, G615V or C201F LDLR were grown on cover slips, fixed and permeabilized with 70% ethanol for 10 minutes. Then, the cells were incubated in PBS containing 1 ml/L Triton X-100 for 15 minutes at room temperature. Afterwards, the cells were washed three times in PBS and incubated with tetramethylrhodamine-conjugated concanavalin A (1:100, Molecular Probes) at room temperature for 1 hour. Next, the cells were washed three times with PBS and fixed with 4% paraformaldehyde for 15 minutes at room temperature. Finally, the intracellular fluorescent dye was observed by CLSM.

To analyze the LDLR activity, the cells transfected with wild-type, G615V or C201F LDLR were grown on cover slips and incubated in serum-free media containing 20 μg/ml fluorescent 1,1′-dioctadecyl-3,3,3′3′-tetramethylindocarbocyanine perchlorate (Dil)-conjugated LDL (Molecular Probes) for 4 hours at 37°C. Following the LDL incubation, the medium was removed, and the cells were washed three times with PBS and fixed with 4% paraformaldehyde for 15 minutes at room temperature. Finally, the intracellular fluorescent dye was observed by CLSM.

Flow Cytometry Analysis

Flow cytometry was used to detect the amount of cell-surface LDLR expression and LDL internalization. The fluorescence of 10,000 events for each sample was acquired for data analysis. Forward scatter versus side scatter gates were set to exclude dead cells and debris. Experiments were repeated at least three times with triplicate samples for each cell line.

To measure the amounts of cell-surface LDLR expression, the cells transfected with wild-type, G615V or C201F LDLR were harvested 48 hours after transfection and resuspended in PBS containing 1% BSA. Then, the cells were washed twice in PBS containing 1% BSA and incubated with phycoerythrin (PE)-conjugated mouse monoclonal anti-human LDLR (1:20, R&D) at room temperature for 30 minutes in the dark. Finally, the cells were washed three times with PBS containing 0.1% BSA and resuspended in PBS. PE fluorescence was quantified using a FACS Calibur (Beckman Coulter).

To measure LDLR internalization activity, the cells transfected with wild-type, G615V or C201F LDLR were incubated in serum-free media containing 20 μg/ml Dil-LDL for 4 hours at 37°C. Following the LDL incubation, the medium was removed, and the cells were detached from the culture dish. Afterwards, the cells were washed twice in PBS and resuspended in PBS. The amount of LDL internalization was detected using a FACS Calibur (Beckman Coulter).

Western Blot

Western blot was used to investigate LDLR protein expression levels and stability. The protein contens were normalized to the level of GADPH.

To measure the LDLR protein expression levels and stability, the cells transfected with wild-type, G615V or C201F LDLR were harvested 48 hours after transfection. Fresh cells were harvested with lysis buffer. Protein samples (30 μg) were separated by 8% SDS-PAGE, transferred onto nitrocellulose membranes for incubated with the primary antibodies anti-LDLR (1:500, Abcam, Cambridge, UK) or anti-GADPH (1:3000 diluted in TBS-T, Kangwei, China) at 4°C overnight, then with IR Dye-conjugated secondary antibodies (1:5000, Rockland Immunochemicals, Gilbertsille, PA) for 1 hour. Images were quantified by use of the Odyssey infrared imaging system (LICOR Biosciences Lincoln, NE, USA). All experiments were repeated at least 3 times.

Results

Clinical Features

The blood lipid concentrations of the two probands and their first-degree relatives are shown in the Table 1. The data was collected for the first time in our experiment. The patients had received some lipid-lowering drugs therapy before our experiment.

Proband 1 presented with multiple xanthomas on the bilateral eyelids, extensor tendon and buttocks when the patient was 8 years old. B-mode Doppler ultrasound revealed increased intima-media thickness and multiple atherosclerotic plaques in the common carotid arteries, the bilateral femoral arteries, and the bilateral external iliac arteries. Transthoracic Doppler echocardiography showed that each cardiac chamber was within the normal range and the thickness and motion of each ventricular wall was normal, but the coronary flow velocity reserve (CFVR) in the distal left anterior descending coronary artery (LAD) was reduced to 1.9 (normal value ≥3).

At the age of four years old, proband 2 had two cutaneous xanthomas on his buttocks that gradually increased. In the following years, multiple cutaneous xanthomas were noticed on the bilateral eyelids, hands, elbows and knees. Tendon xanthomas were also discovered on the extensor tendons over the Achilles and the knees. The interphalangeal joints were widened and deformed, the Achilles tendons were widened, and the cornea arcus was apparent. The electrocardiogram indicated a more than 0.05 mV depression in the ST-segment in I, avL, V5 and V6. Transthoracic Doppler echocardiography showed the following: the aorta wall was thickened and the lumen was narrowed, the whole heart was enlarged, and systolic function of the heart was obviously decreased. Mild mitral regurgitation, hydropericardium, valve thickening, and left and right coronary artery diffuse stenosis were also discovered. The ejection fraction (EF) was decreased to 25.5%, and the CFVR was reduced to 1.16.

Table 1. Clinical features and gene identification results of the probancs and their first relatives.

Pedigree	Patient	Sex	Age	TC (mmol/L)	LDL-C (mmol/L)	TG (mmol/L)	HDL-C (mmol/L)	Nucleic acid change	Mutation
I	Proband1	Female	40	16.87	13.93	2.47	0.73	c.1907G>T	p.G615V
	Aunt	Female	58	4.93	3.10	1.40	1.05	c.1907G>T	p.G615V
	Mother	Female	67	8.29	5.71	1.42	1.41	normal	normal
	Sister	Female	46	8.91	5.39	0.98	1.27	c.1907 G>T	p.G615V
	Son	Male	17	4.62	2.83	1.23	1.95	normal	normal
II	Proband2	Male	13	12.79	10.05	1.50	1.19	c.665G>T	p.C201F
	Father	Male	35	5.71	2.69	3.93	0.97	c.665G>T	p.C201F
	Mother	Female	34	6.37	3.61	1.77	2.16	normal	normal

Identification of Gene Mutations

The *LDLR* mutations found in the two probands and their first-degree relatives are shown in the Table 1. No mutations in *apoB* and *PCSK9* genes were detected in these patients.

For proband 1, a single base substitution (G>T) at position 1907 in the thirteenth exon of the *LDLR* gene was identified, which leads to a change from glycine (GGT) to valine (GTT) in the protein sequenced at position 615 (Figure 1A). We were unable to obtain blood from the proband's father and therefore do not have the gene sequence for the *LDLR* from the proband's father. However, we did sequence the *LDLR* from the proband's paternal aunt. Interestingly, the same heterozygous missense mutation at G615V was detected in the proband's aunt. In addition, the proband's sister was also identified as having the G615V mutation. The *LDLR* locus of the proband's mother and son was normal.

Proband 2 had a single base substitution (G>T) in exon 4 of the *LDLR* gene at nucleotide 665, which changes codon 201 in the mature protein from cysteine (TGC) to phenylalanine (TTC) (Figure 1B). The same heterozygous missense mutation was detected in the proband's father. Proband 2′s mother was not identified as having the C210F mutation.

Confocal Laser Scanning Microscopy Analysis of Wild-type and Mutant LDLR in HEK-293 Cells

The localization of LDLR was investigated using co-localization of LDLR and tetramethylrhodamine-conjugated concanavalin A. Concanavalin A specifically binds to mannose-rich glycans in the endoplasmic reticulum (ER) [19]. The results showed that wild-type LDLR was arranged as a circle and was primarily distributed on the cell surface. However, the LDLR accumulated in the cytoplasm for G615V and C201F (Figure 2). Therefore, these two mutations are classified as class 2 mutations. For simplicity, only a single cell is shown in Figure 2, but this cell is representative of the majority of the cells scanned in each field.

LDLR function was analyzed by evaluating the cells ability to internalize Dil-LDL. The results showed that both G615V and

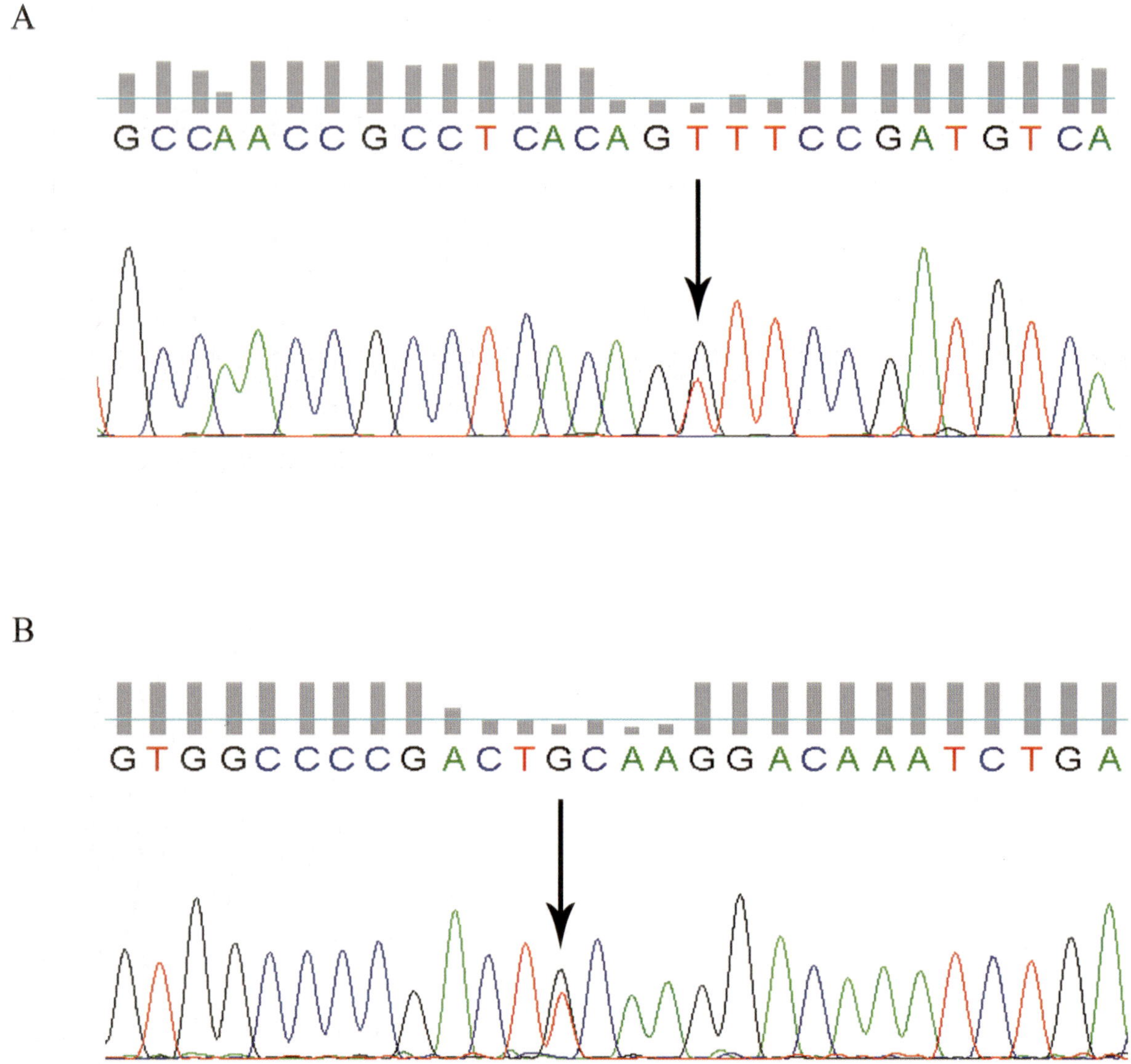

Figure 1. The DNA sequencing results of the two FH probands. (A) The *LDLR* gene of proband 1. The arrow indicates the G>T missense mutation at position 1907 of the thirteenth exon resulting in a glycine to valine substitution; (B) The *LDLR* gene of proband 2. The arrow indicates the G>T missense mutation at position 665 of the fourth exon resulting in a cysteine to phenylalanine substitution.

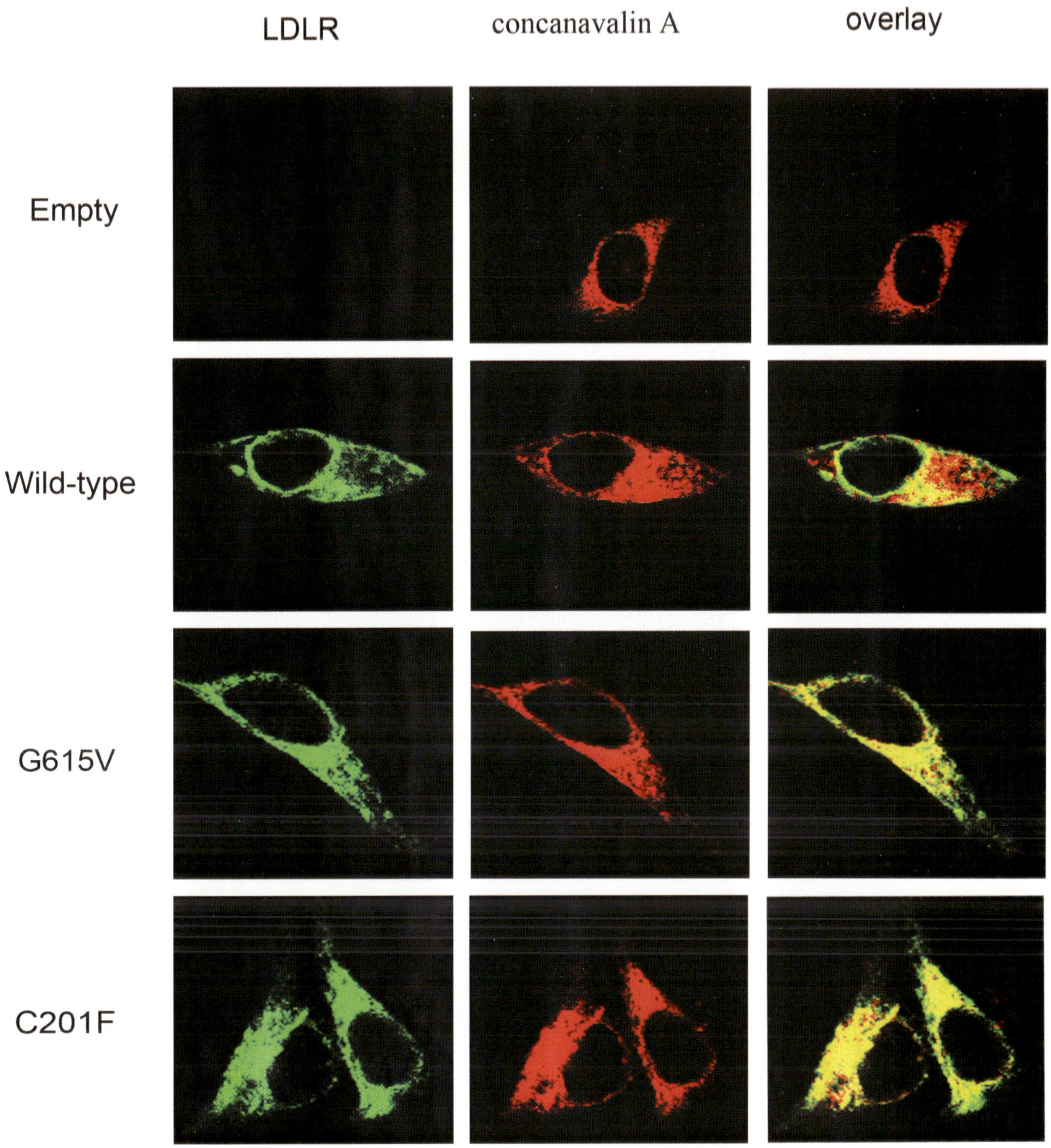

Figure 2. Confocal laser images of wild-type, G615V and C201F LDLR localization in transfected HEK-293 cells. Cells were incubated with tetramethylrhodamine-conjugated concanavalin A at room temperature for 1 hour. Overlays are shown in the right panels with co-localization appearing yellow. Similar results were obtained in 3 separate experiments.

C201F LDLR mutants still retained internalization function (Figure 3). Combined with the above results, we conclude that the two mutations belong to class 2B mutations. Surface expression and activity of the LDLR was further investigated by flow cytometry.

Flow Cytometry Analysis of Cell-surface LDLR Expression and LDL Internalization in HEK-293 Cells

Flow cytometry was used to detect cell-surface LDLR expression and LDL internalization in HEK-293 cells that were transfected with wild-type or mutant LDLR (G615V and C201F). This analysis revealed that the cell-surface expression level of G615V and C201F LDLR were reduced to 73.6% and 33.2%, respectively, when compared with wild-type LDLR (Figure 4). Additionally, it was observed that both mutations

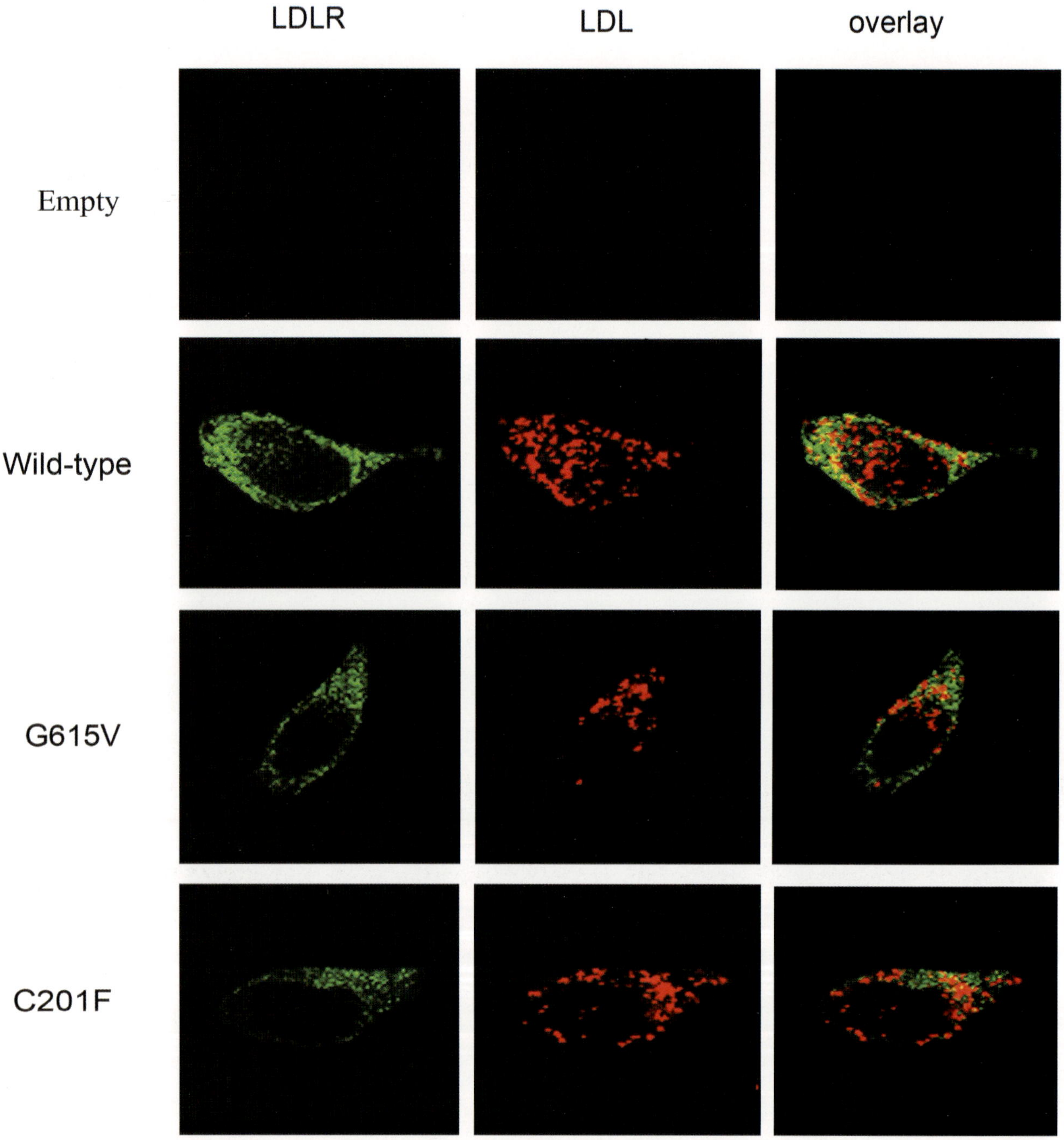

Figure 3. Confocal laser images of wild-type, G615V and C201F LDLR activity in transfected HEK-293 cells. Cells were incubated with 1,1′-dioctadecyl-3,3,3′3′-tetramethylindocarbocyanine perchlorate (DiI)-conjugated LDL for 4 hours at 37°C. Overlays are shown in the right panels with co-localization appearing yellow. Similar results were obtained in 3 separate experiments.

impaired the ability of the LDLR to internalize LDL. Cells expressing G615V and C201F mutant receptors showed 82.6% and 33.5% residual activity, respectively, when compared to cells expressing wild-type LDLR (Figure 5).

Western Blot Analysis of LDLR Protein Expression and Stability in HEK-293 Cells

Western blot was used to detect LDLR protein expression and stability in HEK-293 cells that were transfected with wild-type or mutant LDLR (G615V and C201F). Relative expression and the ability of those cells to express LDLR were assayed by immunoblotting with a specific antibody against the LDLR. For wild-type LDLR only one band was detected, corresponding to the mature form (apparent molecular weight ~160 kDa). For mutant G615V and C201F two bands were detected, though the amount of mature protein was lower compared to the wild-type receptor and it could be seen a small amount of the precursor form (apparent molecular weight ~120 kDa) of the receptor protein, more evident in variant C201F (Figure 6).

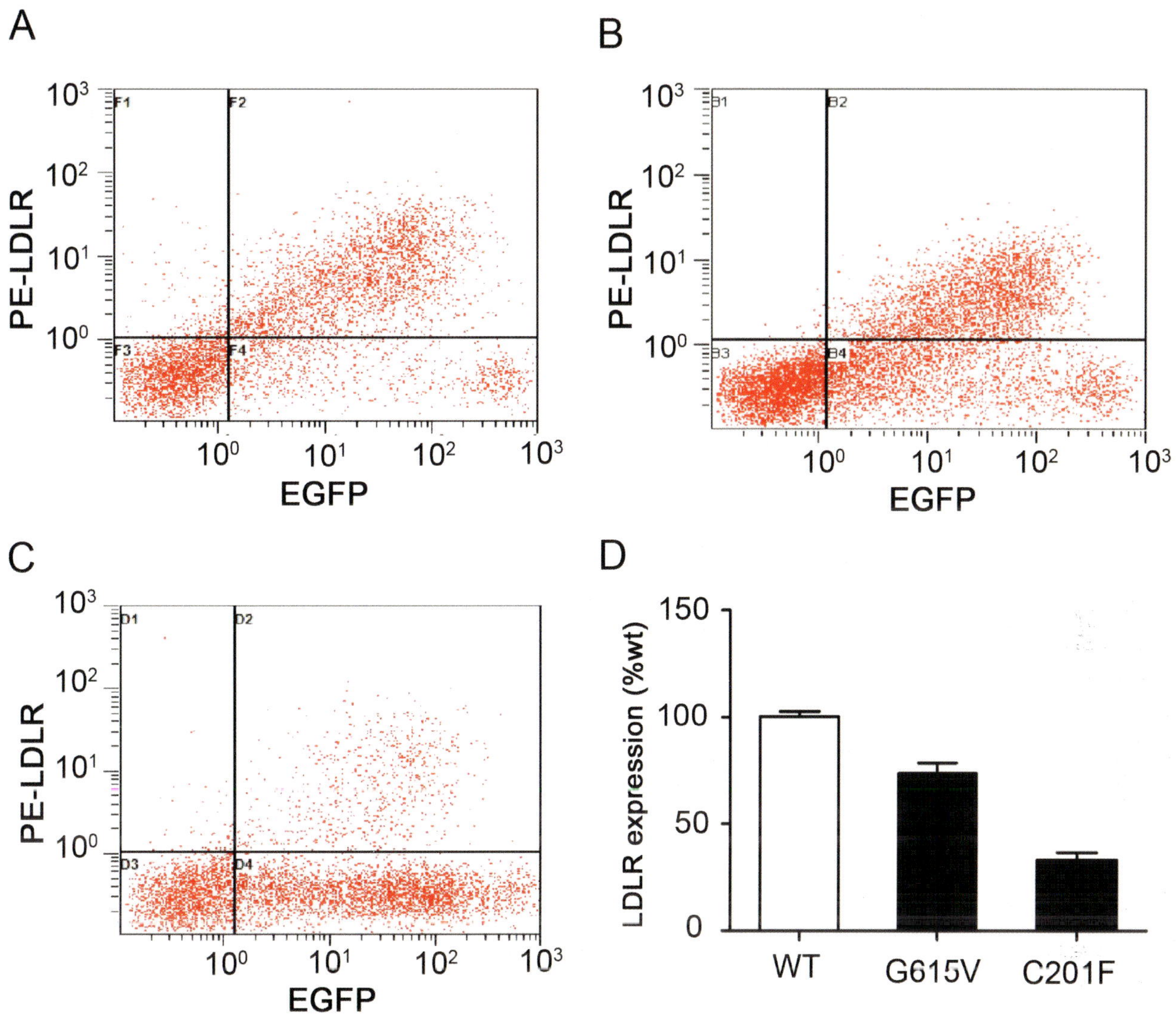

Figure 4. Flow cytometric measurements of wild-type and mutatant LDLR expression in transfected HEK-293 cells. The cells were incubated with phycoerythrin (PE)-conjugated mouse monoclonal anti-human LDLR antibody at room temperature for 30 minutes. The upper right area of the dot plots represents EGFP and LDLR double positive cells. (A) Transfected with wild-type; (B) Transfected with the G615V mutant LDLR; (C) Transfected with the C201F mutant LDLR; (D) The histogram shows the percentage of fluorescence for each of the mutations relative to wild-type. The results are representative of the means ± SD for three independent experiments.

Discussion

In the current study, two different *LDLR* gene mutations, G615V and C201F, were identified in two probands. In particular, the G615V mutation has not been reported elsewhere, while the C201F was previously found in the Netherlands [20]. However, there is no data on the *in vitro* functional consequence of the C201F mutation.

We used an *in vitro* experiment to identify the functional consequences of the *LDLR* mutations. Flow cytometry showed that the expression of cell-surface LDLR was reduced to 73.6% and 33.2% for the G615V and C201F LDLR mutations, respectively, relative to wild-type LDLR. CLSM showed that mutant proteins partially accumulated in the endoplasmic reticulum. The results of western blot showed that the amount of mature protein detected for mutants G615V and C201F was lower compared to the wild-type receptor and it could be seen a small amount of the precursor form. Therefore, both G615V and C201F mutations are classified as class 2B mutations. The incidence rate of class 2 mutations is more than 50%, which is the highest of all *LDLR* mutations that result in FH [11,21]. The endoplasmic reticulum contains many folding chaperones and enzymes that promote the folding and transport of newly synthesized proteins. These chaperones and enzymes also identify proteins unable to fold correctly and hinder them from being exported from the ER to the Golgi apparatus [19]. The accumulation of misfolded proteins in the ER can cause ER stress.

However, a portion of the mutant proteins were able to reach the cell surface and retain their function despite the G615V and C201F LDLR mutants being partially retained in the ER. Flow cytometry showed that LDL internalization was reduced to 82.6% and 33.5% for G615V and C201F LDLR mutants, respectively, relative to wild-type LDLR. Class 2 mutations are unable to remove cholesterol from the blood plasma, which eventually leads to the occurrence of atherosclerosis and coronary heart disease

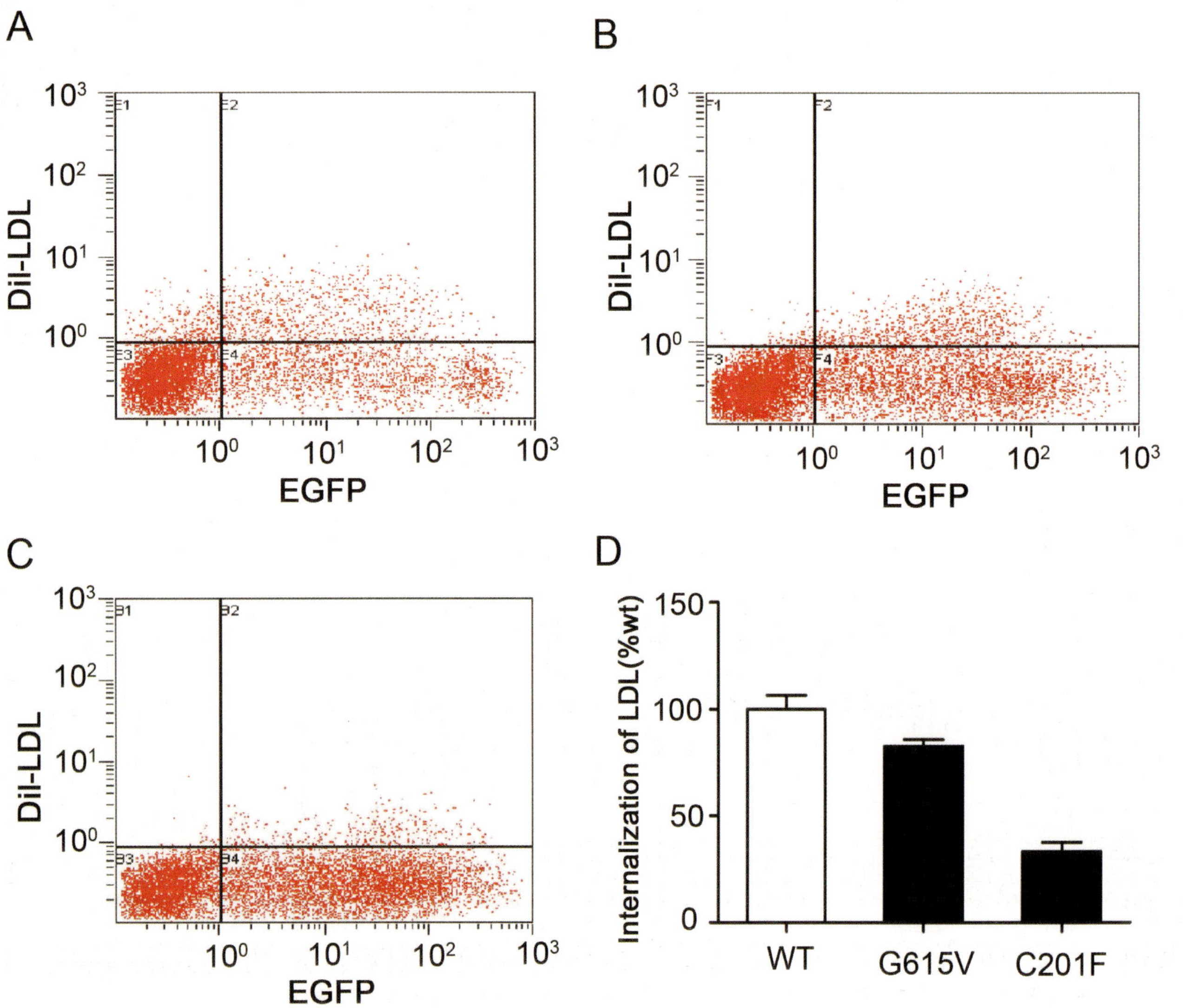

Figure 5. Flow cytometric measurements of wild-type and mutant LDLR internalization activity in transfected HEK-293 cells. The transfected cells were incubated in serum-free media containing 20 μg/ml Dil-LDL at 37°C for 4 hours. The upper-right area of the dot plots represents EGFP and LDLR double positive cells. (A) Transfected with wild-type; (B) Transfected with the G615V mutant LDLR; (C) Transfected with the C201F mutant LDLR; (D) The histogram shows the percentage of fluorescence for each of the mutations relative to wild-type LDLR. The results are representative of the means ± SD for three independent experiments.

because the LDLR is unable to reach the cell-surface. FH has therefore been classified as an ER retention disease [22].

The G615V and C201F mutations are located in different functional domains of the LDLR. G615V is located in the epidermal growth factor precursor (EGFP) homology domain, which is 35% homologous to the EGFP. This domain contains two epidermal growth factor precursor like (EGFP-like) motifs followed by a series of six YWTD (tyrosine-tryptophan-threonine-aspartate) repeats and a third EGF-like motif [10]. The YWTD repeats form a six-bladed β-propeller. Approximately 54% of all *LDLR* gene mutations that result in FH occur in the EGFP homology domain [23], which means that this domain plays an important role in the function of the LDLR. The EGFP homology domain controls lipoprotein release in low pH environments and the recycling of the receptor back to the cell surface [24]. After the receptor-ligand complexes enter the cell by endocytosis, the low pH environment of the endosome causes the LDLR to change conformation and release its ligand completing the transport process. Under neutral pH conditions at the cell surface, the LDLR extends itself in an elongated form to bind LDL due to the function of the β propeller; however, in the acidic environment of the endosomes, the LDLR folds back on itself as the β propeller and competes with LDL for binding to the ligand-binding site [25], which results in LDL being released. The G615V mutation is located in the sixth YWTD repeats of the β propeller and likely affects the function of the β propeller. Therefore, the release of LDL and the recycling of the receptor back to the cell surface are impaired, which eventually leads to FH.

The C201F mutation is located in the ligand-binding domain, which contains seven LDL receptor type A (LA) repeats that are rich in cysteine. This domain is responsible for binding lipoproteins [10]. Some studies have shown that deleting the first two LA repeats has little influence on the binding of LDL. However, deletion of any other individual LA repeat leads to more than a 50% reduction in LDL binding [26,27]. Therefore, the above results suggest that the LA repeats play a crucial role in binding

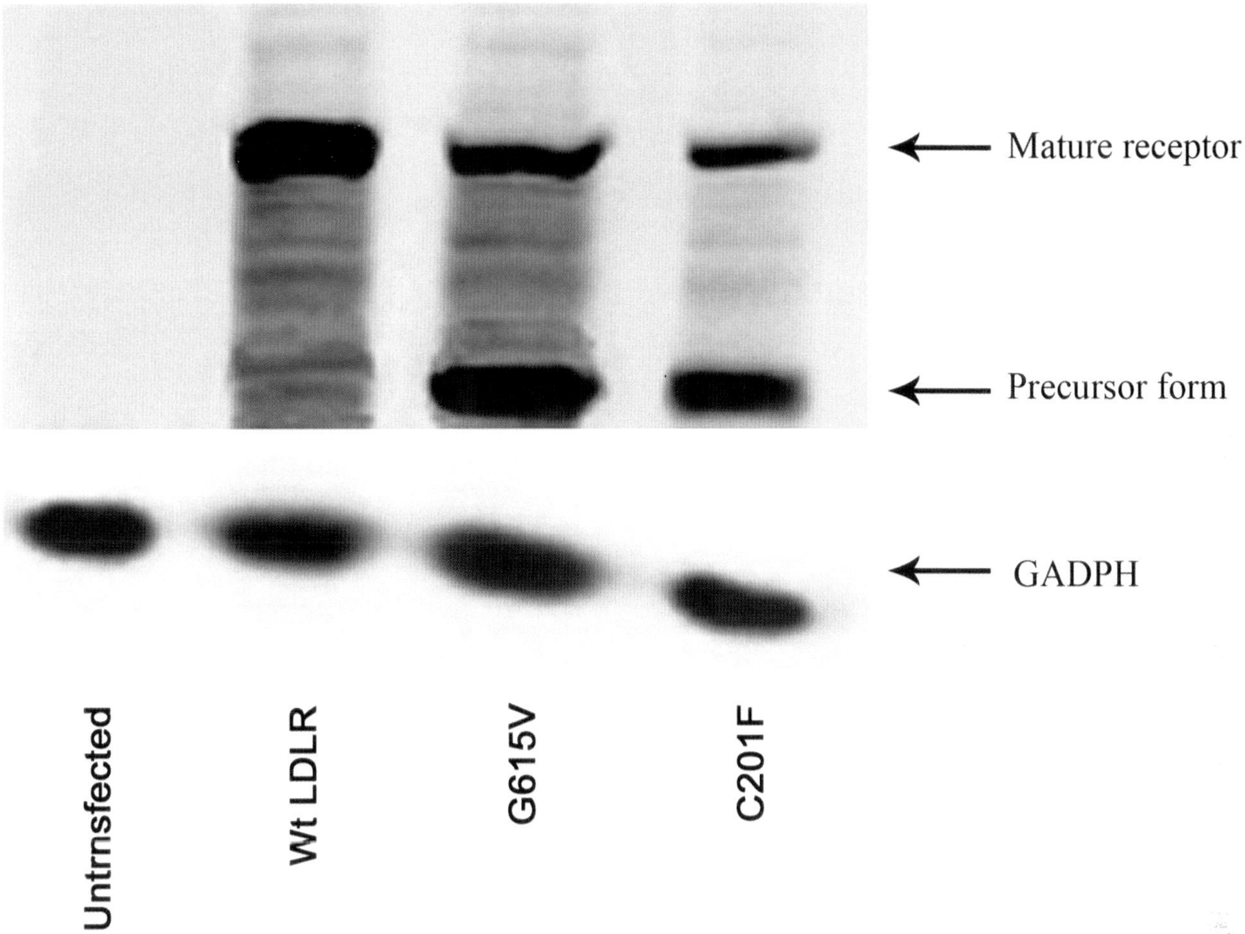

Figure 6. Western blot analysis of wild-type and mutant LDLR protein expression in transfected HEK-293 cells. Whole cell extracts (30 μg) were separated by 8% SDS-PAGE, transferred onto nitrocellulose membranes for incubation with a specific antibody against the LDLR. For wild-type LDLR only one band was detected, corresponding to the mature form. For mutant G615V and C201F two bands were detected, though the amount of mature protein was lower compared to the wild-type receptor and it could be seen a small amount of the precursor form, more evident in variant C201F.

LDL. The C201F mutation is located in the fifth LA repeat (LA5). Therefore, this mutation most likely affects LDL binding, which results in FH.

Although the LDLR activity of proband 1 was higher than that of proband 2, proband 2 had a lower level of plasma cholesterol compared to proband 1. For proband 1, the plasma TC level was 16.87 mmol/L and LDL-C was 13.93 mmol/L. For proband 2, the plasma TC level was 12.79 mmol/L and LDL-C was 10.05 mmol/L. However, in terms of the clinical phenotype of the target organ, proband 2 had a more serious phenotype than proband 1. For proband 2, the interphalangeal joints were widened and deformed, the Achilles tendons were widened. The aorta wall was thickened and the lumen was narrowed, the whole heart was enlarged, and systolic function of the heart was obviously decreased. Mild mitral regurgitation, hydropericardium, valve thickening, and left and right coronary artery diffuse stenosis were also discovered, the CFVR was reduced to 1.16. For prond 1, each cardiac chamber was within the normal range and the thickness and motion of each ventricular wall was normal, but the CFVR was reduced to 1.9.We speculate that the discrepancy between phenotype and LDLR activity in these two probands with G615V and C201F mutations may partly be influenced by other genetic and/or environment factors.

The mother of proband 1 was clinically diagnosed with heterozygous FH, but no *LDLR* gene mutation had been detected in this woman. Approximately 10%–40% of patients with a clinical diagnosis of FH do not have their *LDLR* mutation investigated [28,29]. It is possible that these patients present a polygenic basis for their LDL-C elevation without contributions from any of the classical FH genes [7]. The inconsistency between clinical phenotype and genetic testing should be further studied.

In conclusion, two *LDLR* heterozygous missense mutations, G615V and C201F, were found in this study. In particular, the G615V mutation was a novel mutation. Functional research was performed for both mutations. The results showed that the mutant LDLRs were transport defective. The level of expression of the mutant LDLR and LDL internalization were both reduced compared to wild-type LDLR. These two mutations likely result in the LDLR being retained in the ER, and thus, the LDLR was unable to successfully reach the cell surface to clear LDL leading to FH. Our research increases the mutational spectrum of FH in the Chinese population. Identifying the pathogenicity of the *LDLR* mutations is of great importance to determine the actual cause of hypercholesterolemia. Additionally, understanding the mechanisms by which these mutations result in FH could help to determine a suitable lipid-lowering therapy for each patient.

Supporting Information

Table S1 Sequences of oligonucleotide used for the amplification of *LDLR* gene.

Table S2 Sequences of oligonucleotide used for the amplification of *PCSK9* gene.

Table S3 Sequences of oligonucleotide used for the amplification of *apoB* gene.

Acknowledgments

We wish to thank Wei Cui and Sa Liu for technical assistance of flow cytometry analysis, Limin Zhao for assistance with images analysis of the confocal laser-scanning microscope.

Author Contributions

Conceived and designed the experiments: HHW LYW. Performed the experiments: HHW SYX. Analyzed the data: LYS. Contributed reagents/materials/analysis tools: XDP. Wrote the paper: HHW SWY LYW.

References

1. Leren TP, Berge KE (2011) Subjects with molecularly defined familial hypercholesterolemia or familial defective apoB-100 are not being adequately treated. PLoS One 6: e16721.
2. Goldstein JL, Hobbs HH, Brown MS (2001) Familial hypercholesterolemia. In: Scriver CR, Baudet AL, Sly WS, Valle D, eds. The metabolic basis of inherited disease. New Yrok: McGraw-Hill. 2863–2913.
3. Austin MA, Hutter CM, Zimmern RL, Humphries SE (2004) Genetic causes of monogenic heterozygous familial hypercholesterolemia: a HuGE prevalence review. Am J Epidemiol 160: 407–420.
4. Marais AD (2004) Familial hypercholesterolaemia. Clin Biochem Rev 25: 49–68.
5. Soutar AK, Naoumova RP (2007) Mechanisms of disease: genetic causes of familial hypercholesterolemia. Nat Clin Pract Cardiovasc Med 4: 214–225.
6. Benn M, Watts GF, Tybjaerg-Hansen A, Nordestgaard BG (2012) Familial hypercholesterolemia in the danish general population: prevalence, coronary artery disease, and cholesterol-lowering medication. J Clin Endocrinol Metab 97: 3956–3964.
7. Nordestgaard BG, Chapman MJ, Humphries SE, Ginsberg HN, Masana L, et al. (2013) Familial hypercholesterolaemia is underdiagnosed and undertreated in the general population: guidance for clinicians to prevent coronary heart disease: Consensus Statement of the European Atherosclerosis Society. Eur Heart J.
8. Moorjani S, Roy M, Gagne C, Davignon J, Brun D, et al. (1989) Homozygous familial hypercholesterolemia among French Canadians in Quebec Province. Arteriosclerosis 9: 211–216.
9. Rader DJ, Cohen J, Hobbs HH (2003) Monogenic hypercholesterolemia: new insights in pathogenesis and treatment. J Clin Invest 111: 1795–1803.
10. Jeon H, Blacklow SC (2005) Structure and physiologic function of the low-density lipoprotein receptor. Annu Rev Biochem 74: 535–562.
11. Hobbs HH, Brown MS, Goldstein JL (1992) Molecular genetics of the LDL receptor gene in familial hypercholesterolemia. Hum Mutat 1: 445–466.
12. Gent J, Braakman I (2004) Low-density lipoprotein receptor structure and folding. Cell Mol Life Sci 61: 2461–2470.
13. Hobbs HH, Russell DW, Brown MS, Goldstein JL (1990) The LDL receptor locus in familial hypercholesterolemia: mutational analysis of a membrane protein. Annu Rev Genet 24: 133–170.
14. Usifo E, Leigh SE, Whittall RA, Lench N, Taylor A, et al. (2012) Low-density lipoprotein receptor gene familial hypercholesterolemia variant database: update and pathological assessment. Ann Hum Genet 76: 387–401.
15. Naoumova RP, Neuwirth C, Pottinger B, Whittal R, Humphries SE, et al. (2004) Genetic diagnosis of familial hypercholesterolaemia: a mutation and a rare non-pathogenic amino acid variant in the same family. Atherosclerosis 174: 67–71.
16. Silva S, Alves AC, Patel D, Malho R, Soutar AK, et al. (2012) In vitro functional characterization of missense mutations in the LDLR gene. Atherosclerosis 225: 128–134.
17. Lin J, Wang LY, Liu S, Xia JH, Yong Q, et al. (2008) Functional analysis of low-density lipoprotein receptor in homozygous familial hypercholesterolemia patients with novel 1439 C->T mutation of low-density lipoprotein receptor gene. Chin Med J (Engl) 121: 776–781.
18. Wang L, Lin J, Liu S, Cao S, Liu J, et al. (2009) Mutations in the LDL receptor gene in four Chinese homozygous familial hypercholesterolemia phenotype patients. Nutr Metab Cardiovasc Dis 19: 391–400.
19. Sorensen S, Ranheim T, Bakken KS, Leren TP, Kulseth MA (2006) Retention of mutant low density lipoprotein receptor in endoplasmic reticulum (ER) leads to ER stress. J Biol Chem 281: 468–476.
20. Fouchier SW, Defesche JC, Umans-Eckenhausen MW, Kastelein JP (2001) The molecular basis of familial hypercholesterolemia in The Netherlands. Hum Genet 109: 602–615.
21. Leigh SE, Foster AH, Whittall RA, Hubbart CS, Humphries SE (2008) Update and analysis of the University College London low density lipoprotein receptor familial hypercholesterolemia database. Ann Hum Genet 72: 485–498.
22. Beuret N, Stettler H, Renold A, Rutishauser J, Spiess M (2004) Expression of regulated secretory proteins is sufficient to generate granule-like structures in constitutively secreting cells. J Biol Chem 279: 20242–20249.
23. Jeon H, Meng W, Takagi J, Eck MJ, Springer TA, et al. (2001) Implications for familial hypercholesterolemia from the structure of the LDL receptor YWTD-EGF domain pair. Nat Struct Biol 8: 499–504.
24. Rudenko G, Henry L, Henderson K, Ichtchenko K, Brown MS, et al. (2002) Structure of the LDL receptor extracellular domain at endosomal pH. Science 298: 2353–2358.
25. Rudenko G, Deisenhofer J (2003) The low-density lipoprotein receptor: ligands, debates and lore. Curr Opin Struct Biol 13: 683–689.
26. Russell DW, Brown MS, Goldstein JL (1989) Different combinations of cysteine-rich repeats mediate binding of low density lipoprotein receptor to two different proteins. J Biol Chem 264: 21682–21688.
27. Esser V, Limbird LE, Brown MS, Goldstein JL, Russell DW (1988) Mutational analysis of the ligand binding domain of the low density lipoprotein receptor. J Biol Chem 263: 13282–13290.
28. Civeira F, Ros E, Jarauta E, Plana N, Zambon D, et al. (2008) Comparison of genetic versus clinical diagnosis in familial hypercholesterolemia. Am J Cardiol 102: 1187–1193, 1193 e1181.
29. Palacios L, Grandoso L, Cuevas N, Olano-Martin E, Martinez A, et al. (2012) Molecular characterization of familial hypercholesterolemia in Spain. Atherosclerosis 221: 137–142.

Use of Targeted Exome Sequencing in Genetic Diagnosis of Chinese Familial Hypercholesterolemia

Wen-Feng Wu[1,2], Li-Yuan Sun[1], Xiao-Dong Pan[2], Shi-Wei Yang[1,2], Lv-Ya Wang[2]*

1 Beijing Anzhen Hospital Affiliated with Capital Medical University, Beijing, China, **2** Department of Atherosclerosis, Beijing Institute of Heart Lung and Blood Vessel Diseases, Beijing, China

Abstract

Familial hypercholesterolemia is an autosomal dominant inherited disease characterized by elevated plasma low-density lipoprotein cholesterol (LDL-C). It is mainly caused by mutations of the low-density lipoprotein receptor (*LDLR*) gene. Currently, the methods of whole genome sequencing or whole exome sequencing for screening mutations in familial hypercholesterolemia are not applicable in China due to high cost. We performed targeted exome sequencing of 167 genes implicated in the homozygous phenotype of a proband pedigree to identify candidate mutations, validated them in the family of the proband, studied the functions of the mutant protein, and followed up serum lipid levels after treatment. We discovered that exon 9 c.1268 T>C and exon 8 c.1129 T>G compound heterozygous mutations in the *LDLR* gene in the proband derived from the mother and father, respectively, in which the mutation of c.1129 T>G has not been reported previously. The mutant LDL-R protein had 57% and 52% binding and internalization functions, respectively, compared with that of the wild type. After 6 months of therapy, the LDL-C level of the proband decreased by more than 50% and the LDL-C of the other family members with heterozygous mutation also reduced to normal. Targeted exome sequencing is an effective method for screening mutation genes in familial hypercholesterolemia. The exon 8 and 9 mutations of the *LDLR* gene were pedigree mutations. The functions of the mutant LDL-R protein were decreased significantly compared with that of the wild type. Simvastatin plus ezetimibe was proven safe and effective in this preschool-age child.

Editor: Reiner Albert Veitia, Institut Jacques Monod, France

Funding: This study was supported by grants from the Natural Science Foundation of Beijing (No. 7112040) and National Natural Science Foundation of China (No. 81170810 and 81271923). The funders had no role in study design, data collection and analysis, decision to publish, or preparation of the manuscript.

Competing Interests: The authors have declared that no competing interests exist.

* E-mail: wanglvya2012@163.com

Introduction

Familial hypercholesterolemia (FH; MIM #143890) is a serious single-gene, dominant genetic disease. The main clinical manifestations are significantly elevated plasma low-density lipoprotein cholesterol (LDL-C) levels. The pathological basis of FH is LDL receptor (*LDLR*; MIM #606945) gene mutations that cause cholesterol metabolism dysfunction. Clinically, FH is divided into homozygous and heterozygous phenotypes. The latter is relatively common and leads to premature coronary heart disease; it occurs in 1:500 people in most countries. The former is rare, occurring in 1:1,000,000 births; however, its symptoms are severe [1,2]. However, as the most populous country in the world, China may bear a heavy burden of this genetic disorder. However, there is no applicable genetic screening method in clinical practice in China.

To date, 3 genes *LDLR*, apolipoprotein B (APOB), and proprotein convertase subtilisin/kexin 9 (PCSK9) have been accepted [3]. Reported mutations of FH widely spread over the coding regions of these causative genes. Genetic screening through traditional approaches, such as direct sequencing is therefore difficult. A high-throughput and cost-effective method to detect the genetic defects is needed. Whole exome sequencing has been proved to be a powerful tool to discover novel disease-related genes or genetic mutations in large genomic regions [4–6]. With the progresses on next-generation sequencing (NGS) and bioinformatics, it has been demonstrated to have higher efficiency but lower cost comparing with whole gene sequencing. However, the astronomical information amount, subsequent arduous data processing and large cost limit its widely application in practice in China. In this study, we utilized targeted exome sequencing (TES) to study genetic defects in one family, in order to establish a strategy feasible to genetic diagnosis of FH patients. We also studied the binding and internalization functions of the mutant protein and followed up the effect of lipid-lowering therapy in the pedigree.

Materials and Methods

Ethics Statement

The study was reviewed and approved by the Ethical Committee of Beijing Anzhen Hospital, and all participants signed an informed consent form. For those aged <18 years, written consent was obtained from either parent.

Study Population and Data Collection

This study was part of a large study aimed at screening FH mutations using TES in the Han Chinese population. An FH family was recruited at Beijing Anzhen Hospital in February 2013 (Figure 1). The proband (III-1) was a 5-year-old boy with distinct clinical features of skin xanthoma near the elbow, lap, and hips

(Figure 2); his parents had no apparent clinical features but had high TC and LDL-C upon physical examination. Homozygous FH was diagnosed based on the following criteria: (1) plasma or serum LDL-C>10 mmol/L; (2) presence of tendon and cutaneous xanthomas at an early age; (3) autosomal inheritance of hypercholesterolemia in relatives; (4) presence of primary hypercholesterolemia in the parents of the proband [7]. Secondary causes of hypercholesterolemia were excluded. The clinical features of members in the FH family were investigated (Table 1).

Blood Sampling and Measurements

Blood samples were obtained from participants after a 12-h fast. TC, triglycerides (TG), LDL-C, and high-density lipoprotein cholesterol (HDL-C) were measured using routine commercial kits (Beckman Coulter, Brea, CA) and a Beckman AU 4500 automated biochemical analyzer (Beckman Coulter).

Illumina Library Construction

Proband genomic DNA was extracted from whole blood using a DNA Extraction Kit (TianGen, Beijing, China) according to the manufacturer's instructions. DNA quantification was performed using a NanoDrop 2000 unit (Thermo Fisher Scientific, Wilmington, DE). DNA (minimum 3 μg) was used for the indexed Illumina libraries as per the manufacturer's protocol. A final library size of 350–400 bp, including adapter sequences, was selected.

Enrichment and Sequencing of Disease Genes

In total, 167 disease genes, including the genes relevant with blood lipids [8] and cholic acid metabolism (Table S1) were selected by a gene capture strategy using a GenCap Custom Enrichment Kit (MyGenostics, Beijing, China) according to previously described technologies [9,10]. The capture experiment was conducted according to the manufacturer's protocol. Briefly, 1 μg DNA library was mixed with Buffer BL and a GenCap hypercholesterolemia probe (MyGenostics) and heated in a polymerase chain reaction (PCR) machine at 95°C for 7 min and 65°C for 2 min. 23 μL of the 65°C pre-warmed Buffer HY (MyGenostics) was added; the mixture was held at 65°C with the PCR lid heat on for 22 h for hybridization. 50 μL MyOne beads (Life Technology, Carlsbad, CA) were washed in 500 μL 1× binding buffer thrice and re-suspended in 80 μL 1× binding buffer. 64 μL 2× binding buffer was added, the mixture

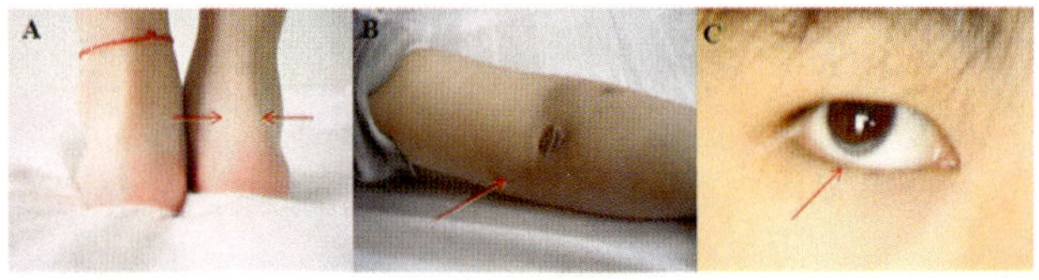

Figure 2. Clinical manifestations of the proband. (A) Achilles tendon thickening. (B) Cutaneous xanthomas on the elbow region. (C) Arcus corneae.

transferred into a tube containing 80 μL MyOne beads, and spun for 1 h on a rotator. We washed the beads once with WB1 buffer at room temperature for 15 min and WB3 buffer thrice at 65°C for 15 min. Elution buffer was used to elute the bound DNA, which was amplified as follows: 98°C for 30 s; 98°C for 25 s, 65°C for 30 s, 72°C for 30 s (15 cycles); 72°C for 5 min. We purified the PCR product using SPRI beads (Beckman Coulter) using the manufacturer's protocol. Enrichment libraries were sequenced on an Illumina HiSeq 2000 sequencer (Illumina, San Diego, CA) for 100-bp paired reads.

Bioinformatics Analysis

After sequencing, we retrieved high-quality reads from raw reads by filtering out low-quality reads and adaptor sequences using the Solexa QA package [11] and cutadapt program (http://code.google.com/p/cutadapt/), respectively. We used the SOAPaligner program [12] to align the clean read sequences to the human reference genome (hg19).

To detect exon duplication and deletions, the coverage of each position was plotted by the base positions. Higher coverage of a region denoted duplication; uncovered regions indicated deletions. After removing duplicates with Picard software [13], single-nucleotide polymorphisms (SNPs) were identified using the SOAPsnp program [12] (http://soap.genomics.org.cn/soapsnp.html). Subsequently, reads were realigned to the reference genome using the Burrows–Wheeler alignment program [14], and insertions or deletions (InDels) were identified with the Genome Analysis Toolkit [15] (http://www.broadinstitute.org/gsa/wiki/index.php/Home_Page). We annotated identified SNPs and InDels using the Exome-assistant program (http://122.228.158.106/exomeassistant). Short read alignment and candidate SNP and InDel validation was performed using MagicViewer [16]. We

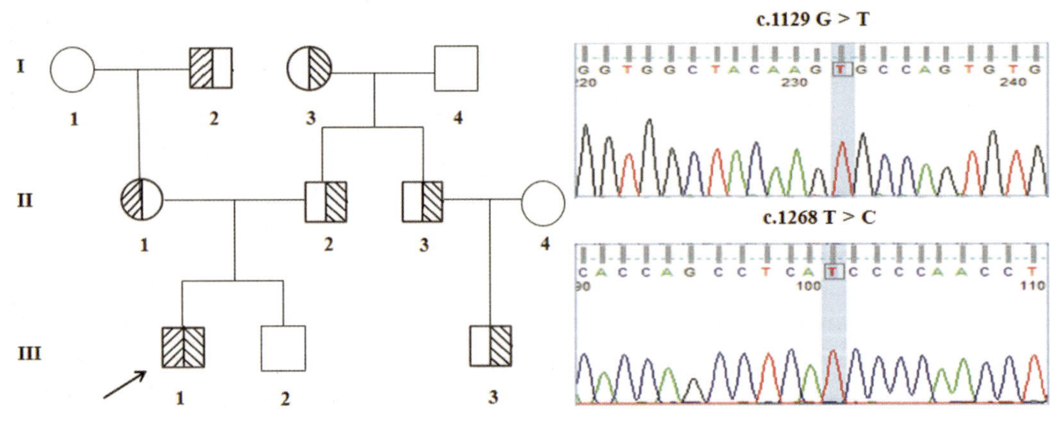

Figure 1. Pedigree and mutations of a hypercholesterolemic family. Arrow denotes the proband. Shaded and partially shaded shapes denote compound heterozygotes and heterozygotes with different mutations, respectively. The exon 8 c.1129 G>T and exon 9 c.1268 T>C mutations are depicted on the right.

Table 1. Clinical Data of the Family.

ID	Sex	Age (years)	TC (mmol/L)	TG (mmol/L)	LDL-C (mmol/L)	HDL-C (mmol/L)	Arcus corneae	Cutaneous xanthoma	Tendon xanthoma	CHD
grandmother	F	57	4.64	1.65	3.24	1.16	No	No	No	No
grandfather	M	57	6.70	0.79	5.00	1.34	Yes	No	No	No
grandmother	F	66	7.89	0.98	5.54	1.12	Yes	No	No	No
grandfather	M	68	5.12	1.09	3.11	1.92	No	No	No	No
mother	F	28	8.15	1.45	6.26	1.23	Yes	No	No	No
father	M	34	7.56	1.50	5.33	1.55	Yes	No	No	No
uncle	M	44	8.29	1.62	6.53	1.34	Yes	Yes	No	No
aunt	F	42	4.45	1.32	3.12	1.74	No	No	No	No
proband	M	2	24.65	1.35	14.80	2.86	Yes	Yes	No	No
sibling	M	0	4.51	0.51	2.60	1.54	No	No	No	No
counsin	M	23	6.56	1.14	4.60	1.48	No	No	No	No
Normal range			≤5.20	≤1.70	≤4.12	≥1.04				

Abbreviations: TC, total cholesterol; HDL-C, high-density lipoprotein cholesterol; LDL-C, low-density lipoprotein cholesterol; TG, triglyceride; M, male; F, female; CHD, Coronary heart disease.

used the PolyPhen, SIFT, PANTHER and PMUT algorithms to evaluate non-synonymous variants to determine pathogenicity [17]. Sequencing data were deposited in NIH Short Read Archive (SRR1169449).

Expanded Validation

DNA samples from all family members were obtained for Sanger sequencing. We also PCR-amplified the coding regions of the mutations identified as described for conventional direct sequencing. We used an ABI 3500 Genetic Analyzer (Applied Biosystems, Foster City, CA) to cycle-sequence purified PCR products. We analyzed the Sanger sequencing results using Mutation Surveyor (Softgenetics, State College, PA), reconfirming them using the same procedure.

Construction of Mutant

The C356G LDL-R mutant was constructed according to the protocol previously described [18].

Functional Studies of the Mutant

LDL-R binding and internalization functions were measured as previously describe [18].

Lipid-lowering Therapy, Blood Lipid Target, and Follow-up

According to whether the proband reached the target ≥50% LDL-C reduction from baseline [19], we treated him with 10 and 20 mg simvastatin daily for 2 months, and then 20 mg simvastatin plus 10 mg ezetimibe daily for the next 2 months (Figure 3). Heterozygous patients in the family received 20 mg simvastatin daily.

Blood lipids were re-examined every month until 6 months later. The subjects were followed for serious adverse reactions.

Results

General Clinical Data

The general clinical data of the family are listed in Table 1. TC and LDL-C levels in the proband (III-1) were extremely high before treatment and he exhibited typical clinical features. The maternal grandfather (I-2), paternal grandmother (I-3), mother (II-1), father (II-2), uncle (II-3), and cousin (III-3) had a clinical diagnosis of heterozygous FH and high TC and LDL-C levels when recruited; only II-3 had cutaneous xanthoma. Other family members had normal serum lipid levels. All subjects had normal HDL-C levels, no tendon xanthoma, and we confirmed that there was no evidence of coronary heart disease.

TES Identification of Candidate Mutations

We performed TES of 167 genes implicated in FH. The average sequencing depths on the targeted regions of samples that underwent TES was 640.32 (Table S2). The sample had 96.9% coverage of the targeted regions. Meanwhile, there was 92.3% and 89.3% coverage of targeted exons for 10 and 20 reads, respectively. Via SOAPsnp [13], an average 650 variants were identified in the sample. Among them were 386 non-synonymous variants, missense, nonsense, and splicing variants. This was narrowed down to 46 by excluding variants reported in HapMap 28 and the SNP release of the 1000 Genome Project with minor allele frequency>0.05. For missense variants, computational prediction by PolyPhen, SIFT, PANTHER, PMUT and consistency of genetic transmission mode further narrowed the number of candidate mutations to <8. For the 7 coding InDels initially identified in the sample using the Genome Analysis Toolkit program [15], we identified 2 compound heterozygous variants(I402T and C356G) on LDLR gene that correlated with the disease phenotype (Figure 4).

Expanded Familial Validation and Sanger Sequencing Confirmation

We validated TES results from the proband to the entire family using Sanger sequencing. Sanger sequencing of the coding region confirmed that the I402T and C356G mutations were transmitted from the paternal grandmother (I-3) and the maternal grandfather (I-2), respectively. And, the heterozygous *LDLR* mutation I402T was carried by the father (II-2), uncle (II-3), and cousin (III-3), while the heterozygous *LDLR* mutation C356G was carried by the mother (II-1). But the sibling (III-2) carried no *LDLR* mutation. So

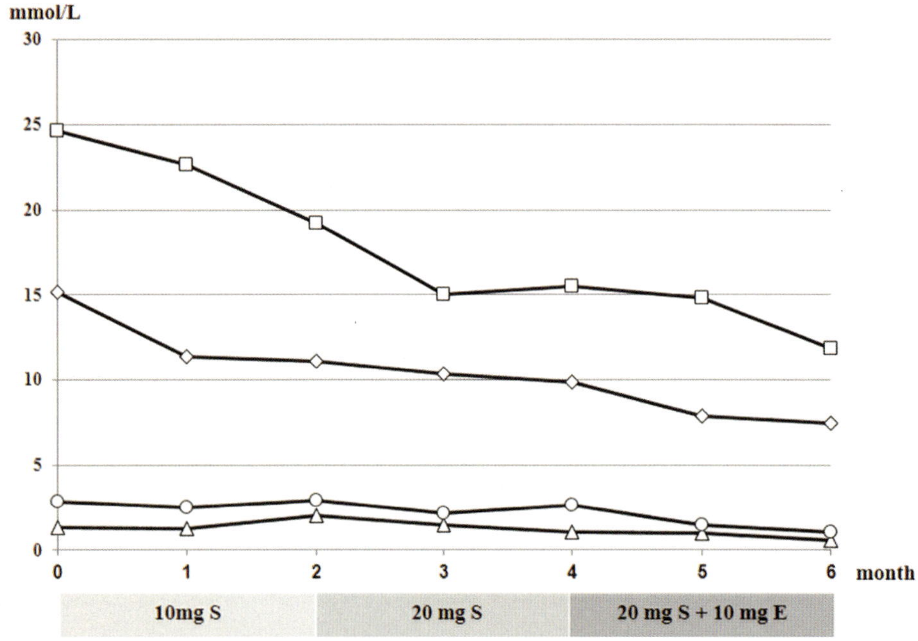

Figure 3. Serum lipid changes after lipid-lowering therapy. Plasma concentrations of TC (square), TG (triangle), LDL-C (diamond), and HDL-C (circle) in the proband. S, simvastatin; E, ezetimibe.

the proband (III-1) carried 2 compound heterozygous *LDLR* mutations (C356G and I402T) (Figure 1). Furthermore, we performed co-segregation analysis to confirm the extracted mutations in the pedigree. All mutations were confirmed to co-segregate well with the disease in the family.

Effect of C356G *LDLR* Mutation on LDL-R Function

The effects of the C356G mutation on LDL-R function was investigated by transient expression in HEK-293 cells. To measure LDL-R binding and internalization functions, HEK-293 cells were harvested 48 h after transfection and analyzed by flow cytometry. Analyses of antibody-labeled cells and measurement of activity revealed that receptors with the C356G mutation had 57%

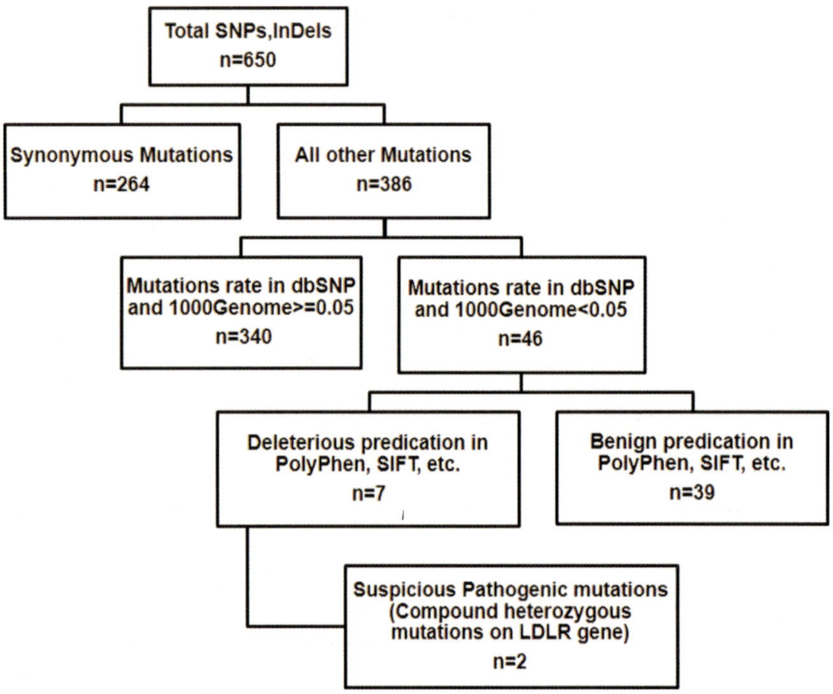

Figure 4. Flow chart of the data analysis.

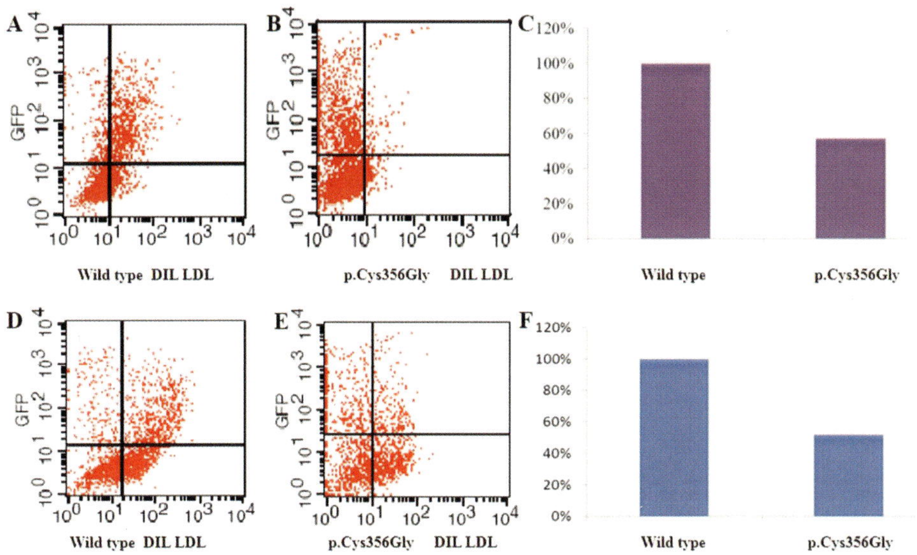

Figure 5. Characterization of C356G mutation LDL-R binding and internalization function. (A, D) Wild-type LDL-R binding and internalization function. (B, E) C356G LDL-R binding and internalization function. (C, F) Histogram of wild-type and C356G mutant LDL-R binding and internalization function.

binding and 52% internalization activity compared with that of the wild-type receptor. The majority of EGFP-positive cells could not bind and internalize LDL effectively (Figure 5, Table 2).

Family Lipid Level Follow-up

Lipid-lowering therapy was started upon the proband being diagnosed with FH. He was initially given 10 mg simvastatin daily to treat hyperlipidemia, but after 2 months, his LDL-C decreased by only 25% from baseline. We increased the dose to 20 mg daily; 2 months later, his LDL-C levels had decreased by about 35% from baseline, meaning the target level still had not been achieved. Therefore, we combined 20 mg simvastatin with 10 mg ezetimibe daily. At the end of the fifth month, his LDL-C levels had declined by 50% as compared to baseline and remained at about 7.4 mmol/L (Figure 3). After 6 months, lipid levels in heterozygous patients in the family had decreased to normal levels (Table 3). All subjects experienced no adverse reaction during treatment.

Discussion

Estimated with the prevalence of heterozygous 1/500, there should be about 2.6 million potential FH patients in China, but the definitions of patients and potential patients are inconsistent. The first reason is that both doctors and patients have poor understanding of FH, and serum lipid levels are not examined during routine physical examination of children. On the other hand, only a few laboratories in China have the capability for detecting gene(s) mutations of FH. Therefore, a significant number of FH patients are not diagnosed and treated in a timely manner. Foreign research has shown that early diagnosis and intervention can delay the occurrence of complications of atherosclerosis and coronary heart disease in FH patients [20–22]. Traditional screening for FH mutations is also infeasible because distribution of the mutation sites is scattered. Whole exome sequencing has been proved to be a powerful tool to discover novel disease-related genes or genetic mutations in large genomic regions [4–6], but clinical application in China is rarely accepted due to high cost. In the present study, we carried out TES for 167 genes implicated in FH and found that the average sequencing depth of the target genes was >640, coverage of the target region was about 97%. The data from sequencing was about 650 Mb one sample (Table S2), equal to about 10% of whole exome sequencing. Therefore, we have proved that deep exome sequencing of target 167 genes is a fast and efficient method to assist the diagnosis. The cost was saved at least 50% compared with whole exome sequencing, even less the amount of work saved. Notably, only a single sample from the proband was sufficient for identifying the causative mutation in the family; finalization could be enhanced using intra-familial mutation validation and co-segregation analysis. Therefore, there are 3 advantages of TES: 1) the genetic screening range can be reduced greatly; 2) data analysis can be performed with high

Table 2. LDL-R Function Comparisons.

Group	LDL-R function analysis (geometric mean fluorescence intensity)	
	LDL-R binding ability (%)	LDL-R internalization ability (%)
Wild-type[a]	100	100
p.Cys356Gly mutant	57±9	52±10

[a]RefSeq: NP_000518.1., NM_000527.4.
Abbreviations: LDL-R, Low-density lipoprotein receptor.

Table 3. Lipid Levels of Heterozygous Family Members after 6-month 20 mg Simvastatin Treatment.

Case No	Age (years)	Sex	TC (mmol/L)	TG (mmol/L)	HDL-C (mmol/L)	LDL-C (mmol/L)	LDL-R mutation
I-2	57	M	5.20	0.93	1.09	3.10	p.Cys356Gly (c.1129T>G)
I-3	66	F	4.75	1.21	1.13	3.87	p.Ile402Thr (c.1268T>C)
II-1	28	F	4.47	1.47	1.26	4.02	p.Cys356Gly (c.1129T>G)
II-2	34	M	5.10	0.96	1.53	3.41	p.Ile402Thr (c.1268T>C)
II-3	44	M	5.01	1.38	2.01	4.11	p.Ile402Thr (c.1268T>C)
III-3	23	M	3.87	1.19	1.67	3.17	p.Ile402Thr (c.1268T>C)
Normal range			≤5.20	≤1.70	≥1.04	≤4.12	

Abbreviations: TC, total cholesterol; HDL-C, high-density lipoprotein cholesterol; LDL-C, low-density lipoprotein cholesterol; LDL-R, LDL receptor; TG, triglyceride; M, male; F, female.

efficiency; 3) it is much less expensive than whole exome sequencing.

The latest version of the LDL-R FH database of the University College London (www.ucl.ac.uk/ldlr, accessed Jan 1, 2014) states that >1125 *LDLR* gene variants worldwide, including different point mutations, small and large fragment deletions, insertions, rearrangements, and many new mutations, were recently discovered. The I402T mutation, transmitted from the paternal grandmother in the present study, has been reported in Switzerland, France, and Malaysia [23–25], with binding and internalization functions of the mutant LDL-R protein decreasing to 59% and 54%, respectively, compared with the normal protein [26]. The C356Y mutation (nucleotide change to c.1130G>A) was first reported by Ekstrom in 1998 [27], but the C356G mutation (nucleotide change to c.1129T>G) has not been reported previously. In this study, we concentrated on the effect of the novel C356G mutation on LDL-R function. Flow cytometry revealed that receptors with the C356G mutation had 57% binding activity compared with that of the wild-type receptor. The mutant receptor also displayed 52% internalization function compared to that of the wild-type. In the LDL-R protein, the C356G mutation is located in the epidermal growth factor precursor homology domain B region, a disulfide- and cysteine-rich region. As this sequence is highly conserved, it may play an important functional role. It has been proven that the cysteine-to-glycine mutation has a marked effect on protein folding, impairing receptor function [26]. The epidermal growth factor precursor homology domain has been implicated in low-pH receptor recycling and lipoprotein release [28]; therefore, mutations in this region will disrupt the natural primary function of the uptake of cholesterol-carrying particles into cells, thus lipids remain in the blood, resulting in hyperlipidemia.

The proband was diagnosed with compound heterozygous FH and was administrated with cholesterol synthesis inhibitor, simvastatin (dose titrated from 10 to 20 mg daily), accompany with diet therapy, though evidence of simvastatin use in child is limited. Four months later, the LDL-C decreased just by less than 50%, did not reach the target. We assumed that such a reduction amount may arise from either possible statin escape [29] or the sole blocking function of cholesterol synthesis but not cholesterol absorption. We combined simvastatin with the cholesterol absorption inhibitor ezetimibe (10 mg daily); after 1 month, his LDL-C levels were reduced by 50% from baseline, consistent with the report by Catapano et al [30]. The therapy failed to lower LDL-C down to normal range. Nevertheless, the target (reduction ≥ 50%) recommended by the guideline was eventually met [19]. During treatment, the skin xanthoma partly lightened and no subject developed the adverse reactions of liver function damage and creatine phosphokinase elevation; the growth in terms of height and weight of the children was unaffected as well. This lipid-lowering therapy not only is suitable for adult patients with hyperlipidemia [31], but also is safe for this preschool-age (<6 years) compound heterozygous child.

Diagnosis of FH in China largely depends on clinical features, but patients with heterozygous mutations, such as the parents of the proband, often do not exhibit detectable clinical features. FH is detected in such patients only by measuring their cholesterol levels and by genetic diagnosis. In such patients, preventive treatment followed by early diagnosis is of great importance to avoid damage stemming from long-term elevation of cholesterol levels.

In summary, we successfully diagnosed FH genetically using next-generation sequencing methods and proved that it is a rapid, high-throughput, and efficient screening strategy. Briefly, TES of the 167 genes was sufficient and clinically useful for revealing genetic defects in patients with genetic dyslipidemia disease comprehensively.

Acknowledgments

We thank all family members for their participation in this study.

Author Contributions

Conceived and designed the experiments: LYW SWY. Performed the experiments: WFW XDP. Analyzed the data: LYS WFW. Contributed reagents/materials/analysis tools: XDP. Wrote the paper: WFW.

References

1. Kim YR, Han KH (2013) Familial hypercholesterolemia and the atherosclerotic disease. *Korean Circ J* 43: 363–367
2. Kastelein JJ, van Leuven SI, Burgess L, Evans GW, Kuivenhoven JA, et al. (2007) Effect of torcetrapib on carotid atherosclerosis in familial hypercholesterolemia. *N Engl J Med* 356: 1620–1630.

3. Chiou KR, Charng MJ (2010) Detection of mutations and large rearrangements of the low-density lipoprotein receptor gene in Taiwanese patients with familial hypercholesterolemia. *Am J Cardiol* 105: 1752–1758
4. Futema M, Plagnol V, Whittall RA, Neil HA, Simon Broome Register Group, et al. (2012) Use of targeted exome sequencing as a diagnostic tool for Familial Hypercholesterolaemia. J Med Genet 49: 644–649.
5. Vandrovcova J, Thomas ER, Atanur SS, Norsworthy PJ, Neuwirth C, et al. (2013) The use of next-generation sequencing in clinical diagnosis of familial hypercholesterolemia. Genet Med 15: 948–957.
6. Motazacker MM, Pirruccello J, Huijgen R, Do R, Gabriel S, et al. (2012) Advances in genetics show the need for extending screening strategies for autosomal dominant hypercholesterolaemia. Eur Heart J, 33: 1360–1366.
7. Bertolini S, Cassanelli S, Garuti R, Ghisellini M, Simone ML, et al. (1999) Analysis of LDL receptor gene mutations in Italian patients with homozygous familial hypercholesterolemia. Arterioscler Thromb Vasc Biol 19: 408–418.
8. Teslovich TM, Musunuru K, Smith AV, Edmondson AC, Stylianou IM, et al. (2010) Biological, clinical and population relevance of 95 loci for blood lipids. Nature 466: 707–713.
9. He J, Wu J, Jiao Y, Wagner-Johnston N, Ambinder RF, et al. (2011) IgH gene rearrangements as plasma biomarkers in Non-Hodgkin's lymphoma patients. Oncotarget 2: 178–185.
10. Wu J, Matthaei H, Maitra A, Dal Molin M, Wood LD, et al. (2011) Recurrent GNAS mutations define an unexpected pathway for pancreatic cyst development. Sci Transl Med 3: 92ra66.
11. Cox MP, Peterson DA, Biggs PJ (2010) SolexaQA: At-a-glance quality assessment of Illumina second-generation sequencing data. BMC Bioinformatics 11: 485.
12. Li R, Yu C, Li Y, Lam TW, Yiu SM, et al. (2009) SOAP2: an improved ultrafast tool for short read alignment. Bioinformatics 25: 1966–1967.
13. Li H, Handsaker B, Wysoker A, Fennell T, Ruan J, et al. (2009) The Sequence Alignment/Map format and SAMtools. Bioinformatics 25: 2078–2079.
14. Li H, Durbin R (2009) Fast and accurate short read alignment with Burrows-Wheeler transform. Bioinformatics 25: 1754–1760.
15. DePristo MA, Banks E, Poplin R, Garimella KV, Maguire JR, et al. (2011) A framework for variation discovery and genotyping using next-generation DNA sequencing data. Nat Genet 43: 491–498.
16. Hou H, Zhao F, Zhou L, Zhu E, Teng H, et al. (2010) MagicViewer: integrated solution for next-generation sequencing data visualization and genetic variation detection and annotation. Nucleic Acids Res 38(Web Server issue): W732–736.
17. Jin ZB, Mandai M, Yokota T, Higuchi K, Ohmori K, et al. (2008) Identifying pathogenic genetic background of simplex or multiplex retinitis pigmentosa patients: a large scale mutation screening study. J Med Genet 45: 465–472.
18. Wang L, Lin J, Liu S, Cao S, Liu J, et al. (2009) Mutations in the LDL receptor gene in four Chinese homozygous familial hypercholesterolemia phenotype patients. Nutr Metab Cardiovasc Dis 19: 391–400.
19. European Association for Cardiovascular Prevention & Rehabilitation, Reiner Z, Catapano AL, De Backer G, Graham I, et al. (2011) ESC/EAS Guidelines for the management of dyslipidaemias: the Task Force for the management of dyslipidaemias of the European Society of Cardiology (ESC) and the European Atherosclerosis Society (EAS). Eur Heart J 32: 1769–1818.
20. Espinheira Mdo C, Vasconcelos C, Medeiros AM, Alves AC, Bourbon M, et al. (2013) Hypercholesterolemia–a disease with expression from childhood. Rev Port Cardiol 32: 379–386.
21. Alonso R, Mata P, Zambón D, Mata N, Fuentes-Jiménez F (2013) Early diagnosis and treatment of familial hypercholesterolemia: improving patient outcomes. Expert Rev Cardiovasc Ther 11: 327–342.
22. Elis A, Zhou R, Stein EA (2013) Treatment of familial hypercholesterolaemia in children and adolescents in the last three decades. Cardiol Young 10: 1–5.
23. Ekström U, Abrahamson M, Sveger T, Lombardi P, Nilsson-Ehle P (1995) An efficient screening procedure detecting six novel mutations in the LDL receptor gene in Swedish children with hypercholesterolemia. Hum Genet 96: 147–150.
24. Khoo KL, van Acker P, Defesche JC, Tan H, van de Kerkhof L, et al. (2000) Low-density lipoprotein receptor gene mutations in a Southeast Asian population with familial hypercholesterolemia. Clin Genet 58: 98–105.
25. Amsellem S, Briffaut D, Carrié A, Rabès JP, Girardet JP, et al. (2002) Intronic mutations outside of Alu-repeat-rich domains of the LDL receptor gene are a cause of familial hypercholesterolemia. Hum Genet 111: 501–510.
26. Chang JH, Pan JP, Tai DY, Huang AC, Li PH, et al. (2003) Identification and characterization of LDL receptor gene mutations in hyperlipidemic Chinese. J Lipid Res 44: 1850–1858.
27. Ekstrom U, Abrahamson M, Wallmark A, Florén CH, Nilsson-Ehle P (1998) Mutations in the low-density lipoprotein receptor gene in Swedish familial hypercholesterolaemia patients: clinical expression and treatment response. Eur J Clin Invest 28: 740–747.
28. Jeon H, Meng W, Takagi J, Eck MJ, Springer TA, et al. (2001) Implications for familial hypercholesterolemia from the structure of the LDL receptor YWTD-EGF domain pair. Nat Struct Biol 8: 499–504.
29. Wu WF, Wang QH, Zhang T, Mi SH, Liu Y, et al. (2013) Gas chromatography analysis of serum cholesterol synthesis and absorption markers used to predict the efficacy of simvastatin in patients with coronary heart disease. Clin Biochem 46: 993–998.
30. Catapano AL, Davidson MH, Ballantyne CM, Brady WE, Gazzara RA, et al. (2006) Lipid-altering efficacy of the ezetimibe/simvastatin single tablet versus rosuvastatin in hypercholesterolemic patients. Curr Med Res Opin 22: 2041–2053.
31. Ballantyne CM, Abate N, Yuan Z, King TR, Palmisano J (2005) Dose-comparison study of the combination of ezetimibe and simvastatin (Vytorin) versus atorvastatin in patients with hypercholesterolemia: the Vytorin Versus Atorvastatin (VYVA) study. Am Heart J 149: 464–73.

A Nonsense Mutation in the Acid α-Glucosidase Gene Causes Pompe Disease in Finnish and Swedish Lapphunds

Eija H. Seppälä[1,2,3], Arnold J. J. Reuser[4], Hannes Lohi[1,2,3]*

1 Research Programs Unit, Molecular Medicine, University of Helsinki, Helsinki, Finland, **2** Department of Veterinary Biosciences and Department of Medical Genetics, University of Helsinki, Helsinki, Finland, **3** Folkhälsan Institute of Genetics, Helsinki, Finland, **4** Departments of Clinical Genetics and Paediatrics, Center for Lysosomal and Metabolic Diseases, Erasmus MC, Rotterdam, The Netherlands

Abstract

Pompe disease is a recessively inherited and often fatal disorder caused by the deficiency of acid α-glucosidase, an enzyme encoded by the *GAA* gene and needed to break down glycogen in lysosomes. This glycogen storage disease type II has been reported also in Swedish Lapphund dogs. Here we describe the genetic defect in canine Pompe disease and show that three related breeds from Scandinavia carry the same mutation. The affected dogs are homozygous for the *GAA* c.2237G>A mutation leading to a premature stop codon at amino acid position 746. The corresponding mutation has previously been reported in humans and causes infantile Pompe disease in combination with a second fully deleterious mutation. The affected dogs from both the Finnish as well as the Swedish breed mimic infantile-onset Pompe disease genetically, but also clinico-pathologically. Therefore this canine model provides a valuable tool for preclinical studies aimed at the development of gene therapy in Pompe disease.

Editor: Andrea Dardis, University Hospital S. Maria della Misericordia, Udine, Italy

Funding: This study was funded by the Academy of Finland, the Sigrid Juselius Foundation and The Jane and Aatos Erkko Foundation. The funders had no role in study design, data collection and analysis, decision to publish, or preparation of the manuscript.

Competing Interests: A DNA test for the Finnish Lapphund, Swedish Lapphund and Lapponian Herders is commercially available through Genoscoper Oy (Ltd), which is partly owned by HL. This does not alter the authors' adherence to all the PLOS ONE policies on sharing data and materials.

* E-mail: hannes.lohi@helsinki.fi

Introduction

Pompe disease, also referred to as glycogen storage disease type II, is an autosomal recessive lysosomal storage disorder caused by a deficiency of acid α-glucosidase (EC 3.2.1.20) in humans. The enzyme degrades α-1,4 and α -1,6 linkages in glycogen, maltose, and isomaltose. Deficiency of this enzyme leads to storage of glycogen inside lysosomes and eventually also to cytoplasmic glycogen storage. Ultimately, the accumulation of glycogen results in tissue destruction reflected by a spectrum of clinical phenotypes ranging from a fatal infantile form of Pompe disease to a slowly progressive late-onset form [1,2].

Canine glycogen storage disease type II was first described in a Lapland dog from Sweden by Mostafa in 1970 [3]. In the 1980s researchers from the Netherlands reported clinical and morphological data of another Swedish Lapphund family affected by the same disease [4,5]. Clinical signs and symptoms of the affected dogs included oesophageal dilation induced vomiting, progressive muscular weakness, loss of condition, clinical heart disease, and myocardial hypertrophy, the severity of which required euthanasia at about 1.5 years of age [3,4,6,7]. Pathological findings revealed accumulation of glycogen containing vacuoles in cerebral cortex, liver, and myocardial plus oesophageal smooth muscle, and ultrastructural evidence of a lysosomal glycogen storage disorder [8]. Biochemical studies demonstrated a severe deficiency of acid α-glucosidase activity in heart, skeletal muscle and liver [9]. Furthermore, it was shown that the presence of catalytically inactive acid α-glucosidase was the primary defect in canine Pompe disease and, consequently, that Swedish Lapphunds represented a homologous model of human classic infantile-Pompe disease [5,6]. However, the primary molecular genetic defect of canine Pompe disease has remained unknown for more than 40 years.

In the present study we show that a recessively inherited nonsense mutation in the acid α-glucosidase (*GAA*) gene causes Pompe disease in both Swedish and Finnish Lapphunds as it does in humans. In addition, we discovered that the same mutation occurs in Lapponian Herders although no cases in that breed have been reported as yet. Forty years after the initial cases were reported our findings have finally enabled developing a genetic test to eradicate lethal Pompe disease from the Scandinavian dog breeds. Our study has also established affected Swedish and Finnish Lapphunds as large animal models for the preclinical testing of gene therapy in Pompe disease.

Materials and Methods

Study population

Four out of seven puppies from a Finnish Lapphund litter born in 2010 were affected by slowly progressive muscle weakness and from frequent vomiting. The affected dogs show a striking mutual resemblance indicating a genetic disease and when clinical history and findings were compared to the previous literature describing inherited diseases in Lapland dogs, canine Pompe disease was strongly suspected [3,4,6]. We collected blood samples from two affected dogs. Case 1 suffered from regurgitation starting at the age of 7 months. At the age of 8 months the owner started to notice progressive muscle weakness and at the age of 12 months the dog started to vomit mucous. Constant panting, dysphonia and apathetic habitus were evident at the age of 13 months. The local veterinarian had taken radiographs of heart (age 15 months) and thorax (age 18 months) and had performed abdominal ultrasound examination (age 15 months) for case 1. Radiographs showed dilatation of the esophagus and cardiac enlargement. Ultrasound examination revealed changes in the liver. Blood chemistry showed decreased plasma alkaline phosphatase (ALP) level and increased alanine aminotransferase (GPT, ALAT), blood urea nitrogen (BUN) and glucose levels and hematology results showed increased monocyte count and increased mean platelet volume at the age of 18 months. Case 1 is currently alive at two years of age but is not expected to survive for very much longer.

The owner of case 2 reported that the dog gradually developed symptoms and loss of condition at the age of 12 months. The coat became poor quality, appetite was lost and dog was vomiting. As the symptoms progressed the local veterinarian examined the dog first time when she was 14 months old. Blood chemistry showed increased plasma ALAT and aspartate aminotransferase (GOT, ASAT) levels at the age of 15 months and they had increased further at the age of 18 months and the dog was euthanized at the age of 19 months. The common symptoms for both of these siblings were vomiting of mucous, panting, dyspnea, dysphagia, regurgitation and progressive muscle weakness. Blood was drawn also from three healthy litter mates, both parents and 18 healthy second degree relatives (Fig 1).

We also analyzed a DNA sample from a previously described Swedish Lapphund with Pompe disease born in 1979 (case four reported in [7]). This case was diagnosed at 4 months of age by measuring low acid α-glucosidase activity in peripheral blood leucocytes. The clinical symptoms started to appear at the age of 7 months and the dog was euthanized at the age of 14 months when clinical disease developed.

Mutation detection and screening

The coding exons and splice junctions of the canine *GAA* gene were amplified by PCR. The analysis included DNA from the two affected Finnish Lapphunds, their dam and an unrelated healthy 8-year-old Finnish Lapphund as control. The PCR products were purified with ExoSAP-IT kit (USB Corporation, Cleveland, Ohio) before sequencing with an ABI Prism 3730xl DNA analyzer (Applied Biosystems, Foster City, CA). Sequence data was analyzed by Sequencher® 5.0 software, (Gene Codes Corporation, Ann Arbor, MI USA). The primers are available upon request.

To determine the population frequency of the newly identified mutation we screened 95 Finnish Lapphunds, 99 Lapponian Herders and 34 Swedish Lapphunds. Most of the Finnish Lapphunds and Lapponian Herders were unrelated at the grandparental level, whereas many of the Swedish Lapphunds were related to each other. A total of 304 samples from 21 other breeds were also screened for the mutation (Table 1).

Analysis of *GAA* mRNA

Blood samples from one affected (homozygous mutant) and one unaffected (homozygous wild type) Finnish Lapphunds were collected to PAXgene Blood RNA Tubes and total RNA was purified using RNeasy Mini Kit (Qiagen AB, Scandinavia, Solna, Sweden). Then mRNA was reverse transcribed to cDNA using High Capacity RNA-to-cDNA Kit (Applied Biosystems, Foster City, CA). Part of the *GAA* cDNA was sequenced using exon-specific primers (available upon request).

Ethics statement

All samples were from privately owned pets and we obtained consent from the owners of the dogs involved in our study. We also obtained permission for blood sampling from the Animal Ethics Committee (ESLH-2009-07827/Ym-23), The State Provincial Office of Southern Finland, P.O. B150, 13101 Hämeenlinna.

Results

As part of our canine disease genomics program, we became interested in identifying the molecular basis of Pompe disease in dogs when we encountered a Finnish Lapphund litter with four affected dogs. Their symptoms and their clinical findings were consistent with those previously described in four Swedish Lapphunds with Pompe disease [3,4,7]. As a first action, we collected blood samples from two of the four affected Finnish dogs, from three of their unaffected littermates and from their parents for the purpose of DNA extraction.

Exonic sequencing of the canine *GAA* gene revealed a c.2237G>A change, compared to the reference sequence RefSeq XM_845556.2, that results in a premature stop codon p.W746* in the 15th coding exon. The nucleotide numbering reflects the cDNA numbering with +1 corresponding to the A of the ATG initiation codon; the amino acid numbering is according to XP_850649.1. The p.W746* mutation truncates the last 206 amino acids (~22% of the protein) of the canine acid α-glucosidase and its effect is very severe according to the Pompe Disease Mutation Database at www.pompecenter.nl. The two affected Finnish Lapphund littermates were both homozygous for the mutation, their parents were both heterozygous, two of their three healthy littermates were heterozygous and one was homozygous wild type (Fig. 1). In addition, ten synonymous coding variants and seven intronic variants were detected in *GAA* gene but none of them segregated with the disease.

It then became interesting to investigate if the Swedish Lapphunds that had been described back in the 1960s and 1970s, when DNA analysis was not yet possible, had the same or another Pompe disease mutation. Fortunately, a cell line established in those days from the tong tissue was successfully retrieved from storage in liquid nitrogen and could serve as a DNA source. Thereby, we were able to establish that one of the originally described Swedish Lapphunds with Pompe disease was also homozygous for the same c.2237G>A mutation.

We then aimed to screen the current Finnish and Swedish Lapphund populations, the Lapponian Herders and 22 other breeds for the occurrence of the c.2237G>A mutation. This study revealed that the mutation is present only in two Scandinavian breeds: 5% (5/95) of Finnish Lapphunds and 2% (2/99) of Lapponian Herders carry the mutation. The cohort of 34 Swedish Lapphunds did not contain any carriers.

Sequencing of the GAA mRNA from homozygous mutant Pompe case and from wild type healthy control revealed that the mutated gene is transcribed into mRNA suggesting that it does not lead to large-scale nonsense-mediated RNA decay (data not shown). This is consistent with the previous study showing that the mutated GAA protein is also present in the affected dogs, although in an inactive form [6].

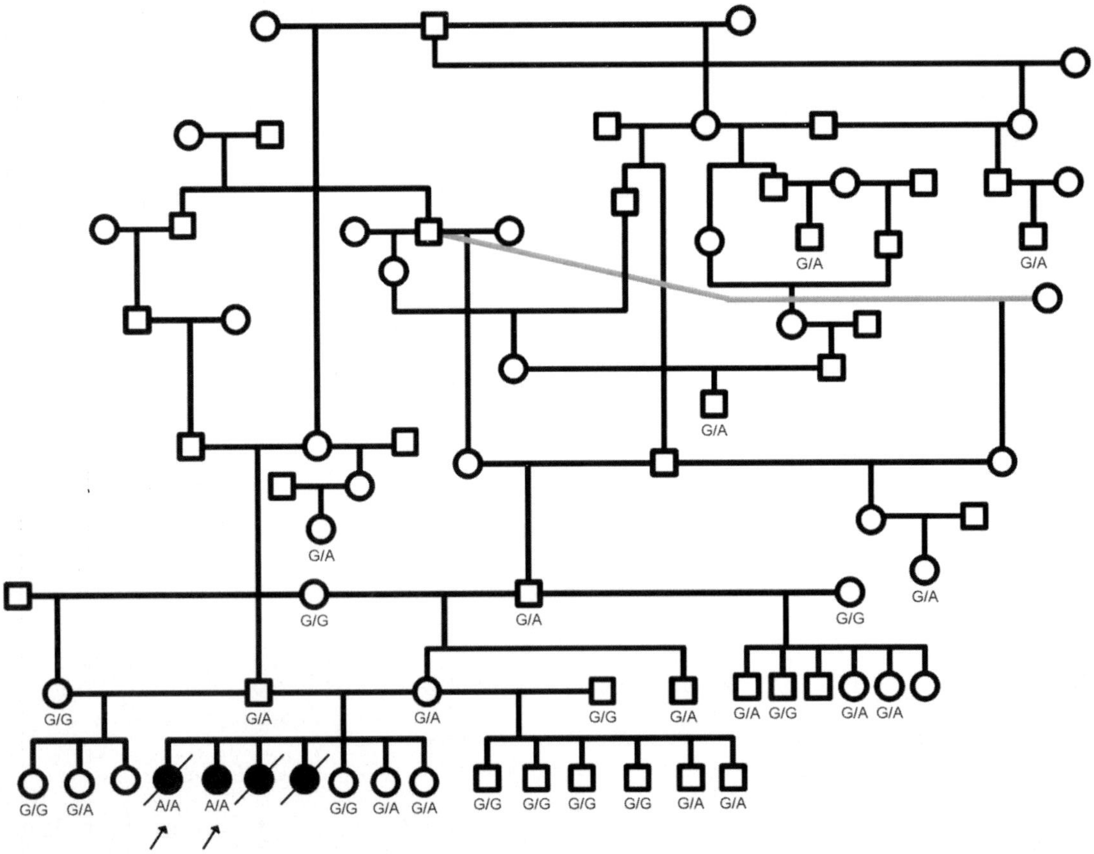

Figure 1. The pedigree of the Finnish Lapphunds affected with Pompe disease. Four puppies suffered similar symptoms and two of them (arrows) were available for genetic studies. All five mutation carriers that were identified by screening of 95 healthy Finnish Lapphunds could be traced back to the same pedigree. The *GAA* c.2237G>A genotypes of the studied dogs are shown below the gender symbol.

Discussion

Pompe disease is an autosomal recessive disorder in humans caused by mutations in the *GAA* gene (OMIM #232300, [10,11]). Acid α-glucosidase is encoded by the *GAA* gene. It is essential for the degradation of glygogen to glucose in lysosomes. Over 300 potentially pathogenic *GAA* mutations have been identified in human patients (www.pompecenter.nl). Human patients are often compound heterozygotes. A combination of two mutated alleles deleting the enzymatic function completely results in infantile-onset Pompe disease. Different combinations of other mutations in the *GAA* gene affect GAA activity and modify the onset and progression of the disease. However, at present, it is not possible to predict in all cases the clinical course based on genotype alone [12].

Besides humans, Pompe disease has also been reported in other species including cattle (OMIA 000419-9913, [13,14]), Japanese quails (OMIA 000419-93934, [15]), cats (OMIA 000419-9685, [16]), sheep (OMIA 000419-9940,[17]) and dogs (OMIA 000419-9615, [3,4]). Three breed-specific mutations in bovine *GAA* gene all causing a premature stop codon have been identified in Brahman and Beef Shorthorn cattle [18]. So far no mutations have been identified in cats, quails or sheep with Pompe disease. Until now, the genetic defect underlying canine Pompe disease has also remained unknown.

The clinical, pathological and biochemical characteristics of classic infantile Pompe disease in humans and dogs resemble each other very well [6–8]. The pathogenesis in both species implies the total absence of acid α-glucosidase activity, generalized glycogen storage leading to progressive muscular weakness, cardiac hypertrophy, cardio-respiratory failure and death. A finding unique to the disease in dogs is the megaoesophagus and its associated symptoms of regurgitation and vomiting [8]. With respect to this manifestation, the difference between humans and dogs might be related to their different posture. Swallowing difficulties are amongst the clinical manifestations of Pompe disease in humans, but are neither associated with dilatation of the oesophagus nor do they lead to vomiting.

The p.W746* nonsense mutation was first reported in combination with a second fully deleterious mutation (c.2758_2775dup) in a patient with infantile onset Pompe disease [19]. Later, four Italian infants were reported to carry this mutation in four different heteroallelic combinations with either c.525delT, c.670C>T, c.1655T>C, or c.2481+102_2646+31del [20–22]. In addition, 9/40 Italian patients with late onset forms of Pompe patients were identified as carriers of the p.W746* mutation. All of them had the most common leaky splice variant c.-32-13T>G as second mutation [23]. W746* has also been reported in heteroallelic combination with the less severe P285S variant and was in that case associated with late-onset disease [24]. The fact that W746* was rather frequently seen in humans and is now also found in dogs suggests that the chromosomal region around c.2237G is a mutation hotspot. The listing of c.2236T>G, c.2237G>C, c.2238G>C, c.2238G>A as other pathogenic mutations in human Pompe disease supports this view (www.pompecenter.nl).

Table 1. Other breeds screened for the *GAA* p.W746* mutation.

Breed	Number of samples tested
Alaskan Malamute	17
Basenji	15
Bernise Mountain Dog	16
Bichon Havanaise	16
Brasilian Terrier	14
Curly Coated Retriever	13
Dachshund, wire-haired	14
Finnish Hound	16
Finnish Spitz	21
German Shepherd	14
Irish Setter	14
Keeshond (Wolfsspitz)	15
Miniature Pincher	13
Rough Collie	11
Saluki	18
Samoyed	13
Schipperke	14
Siperian Husky	11
Spanish Water Dog	15
Staffordshire Bull Terrier	9
Whippet	15
TOTAL 21 BREEDS	304

None of the tested dogs carried the mutation.

Although the affected Swedish Lapphund born in 1979 was homozygous for the mutation and original reports indicate that there have been several cases among Swedish Lapphunds in those days [3–7], we were not able to identify any carriers from the current dogs of this breed. This might be due to too small sample size. It is also possible that the rigorous breeding program has eliminated the carriers from the modern Swedish Lapphunds. It is also worth noting that we identified carriers from Lapponian Herders although no affected cases have been reported in this breed.

The canine p.W746* mutation is shared exclusively among the three closely related breeds from Lapland reflecting a founder effect. The Finnish and Swedish Lapphunds and Lapponian Herders are all descended from the guarding and reindeer herding dogs of Sámi people from northern Scandinavia [25]. The Swedish Lapphund is one of the native Swedish breeds and the other two breeds originate from Finland. Lapphunds are very similar; the biggest difference is the coat color. In Swedish Lapphunds, only black color is accepted whereas in the Finnish Lapphunds all colors are allowed for breeding. Finnish Lapphund and Lapponian Herder were separated in the 1960s on the basis of their coat length [25]. Nowadays these two breeds differ also in overall shape.

Though Pompe disease was described already in the 1960s–1980s in Swedish Lapphunds, its existence in Finnish Lapphunds had not previously been reported by breeders. As far as we know, these Finnish Lapphund dogs are the first correctly diagnosed cases in Finland. Difficulties in diagnosing Pompe disease in Lapphunds might have caused diagnostic delay, but the moderately low mutation frequency in the Finnish Lapphund breed and the pattern of autosomal recessive inheritance appear contributing factors. Our study enables the development of a genetic test for these Scandinavian dog breeds so that this rare but fatal disease can now be eradicated.

Enzyme replacement therapy (ERT) is currently the only effective treatment for human Pompe disease. ERT has been shown to improve ventilator-free survival in patients with infantile-onset Pompe disease. Recent studies indicate that also children and adults benefit from treatment [26,27]. However, the present form of ERT does not provide a total cure. Therefore, the challenge of improving ERT or introducing alternative therapeutic interventions remains. Given the current promising achievements in the field of gene therapy this approach deserves serious investigation also for treatment of Pompe disease. Being large and well described animal models, the Finnish and Swedish Lapphunds could be instrumental in these new developments.

Acknowledgments

We would like to thank Ranja Eklund, Marianne Hoogeveen and Marjut Ritala (Genoscoper Ltd) for their excellent technical assistance. The Lapphund Club of Finland is acknowledged for their help in collection of the samples. We also like to thank all the dog owners and breeders from Finland, Sweden and Norway who participated in this study.

Author Contributions

Conceived and designed the experiments: EHS HL. Performed the experiments: EHS. Analyzed the data: EHS. Contributed reagents/materials/analysis tools: AJJR HL. Wrote the paper: EHS AJJR HL.

References

1. Hirschhorn R, Reuser AJJ (2001) Glycogen storage disease type II: Acid alpha-glucosidase (acid maltase) deficiency. In: Scriver CR, Beaudet AL, Valle D, Sly WS, editors. The Metabolic and Molecular Bases of Inherited Disease. New York: McGraw-Hill. pp. 3389–3420.
2. Kishnani PS, Beckemeyer AA, Mendelsohn NJ (2012) The new era of Pompe disease: Advances in the detection, understanding of the phenotypic spectrum, pathophysiology, and management. Am J Med Genet C Semin Med Genet 160: 1–7.10.1002/ajmg.c.31324; 10.1002/ajmg.c.31324.
3. Mostafa IE (1970) A case of glycogenic cardiomegaly in a dog. Acta Vet Scand 11: 197–208.
4. Walvoort HC, van den Ingh TS, van Nes JJ (1981) Glycogenosis type II in the dog. Berl Münch Tierärztl Wochenschr 94: 39.
5. Walvoort HC (1985) Glycogen storage disease type II in the Lapland dog. Vet Q 7: 187–190. 10.1080/01652176.1985.9693981.
6. Walvoort HC, Slee RG, Sluis KJ, Koster JF, Reuser AJ (1984) Biochemical genetics of the Lapland dog model of glycogen storage disease type II (acid alpha-glucosidase deficiency). Am J Med Genet 19: 589–598. 10.1002/ajmg.1320190323.
7. Walvoort HC, van Nes JJ, Stokhof AA, Wolvekamp WTC (1984) Canine glycogen storage disease type II (GSD II): A clinical study of four affected Lapland dogs. J Am Anim Hosp Assoc 20: 279–286.
8. Walvoort HC, Dormans JA, van den Ingh TS (1985) Comparative pathology of the canine model of glycogen storage disease type II (Pompe's disease). J Inherit Metab Dis 8: 38–46.
9. Walvoort HC, Slee RG, Koster JF (1982) Canine glycogen storage disease type II. A biochemical study of an acid alpha-glucosidase-deficient Lapland dog. Biochim Biophys Acta 715: 63–69.
10. Pompe JC (1932) Over idiopathische hypertrophie van het hart. Ned Tijdschr Geneeskd 76: 304–312.
11. Hudgson P, Gardner-Medwin D, Worsfold M, Pennington RJ, Walton JN (1968) Adult myopathy from glycogen storage disease due to acid maltase deficiency. Brain 91: 435–462.
12. Kroos M, Hoogeveen-Westerveld M, van der Ploeg A, Reuser AJ (2012) The genotype-phenotype correlation in Pompe disease. Am J Med Genet C Semin Med Genet 160: 59–68. 10.1002/ajmg.c.31318; 10.1002/ajmg.c.31318.

13. Jolly RD, Van-de-Water NS, Richards RB, Dorling PR (1977) Generalized glycogenosis in beef Shorthorn cattle - heterozygote detection. Aust J Exp Biol Med Sci 55: 14U–50.
14. O'Sullivan BM, Healy PJ, Fraser IR, Nieper RE, Whittle RJ, et al. (1981) Generalised glycogenosis in Brahman cattle. Aust Vet J 57: 227–229.
15. Matsui T, Kuroda S, Mizutani M, Kiuchi Y, Suzuki K, et al. (1983) Generalized glycogen storage disease in japanese quail (coturnix coturnix japonica). Vet Pathol 20: 312–321.
16. Sandstrom B, Westman J, Ockerman PA (1969) Glycogenosis of the central nervous system in the cat. Acta Neuropathol 14: 194–200.
17. Manktelow BW, Hartley WJ (1975) Generalized glycogen storage disease in sheep. J Comp Pathol 85: 139–145.
18. Dennis JA, Moran C, Healy PJ (2000) The bovine alpha-glucosidase gene: Coding region, genomic structure, and mutations that cause bovine generalized glycogenosis. Mamm Genome 11: 206–212.
19. Beesley CE, Child AH, Yacoub MH (1998) The identification of five novel mutations in the lysosomal acid a-(1-4) glucosidase gene from patients with glycogen storage disease type II. Hum Mutat 11: 413.
20. Pittis MG, Donnarumma M, Montalvo AL, Dominissini S, Kroos M, et al. (2008) Molecular and functional characterization of eight novel GAA mutations in Italian infants with Pompe disease. Hum Mutat 29: E27–36. 10.1002/humu.20753.
21. Nascimbeni AC, Fanin M, Tasca E, Angelini C (2008) Molecular pathology and enzyme processing in various phenotypes of acid maltase deficiency. Neurology 70: 617–626. 10.1212/01.wnl.0000299892.81127.8e.
22. Pittis MG, Montalvo AL, Miocic S, Martini C, Deganuto M, et al. (2003) Identification of four novel mutations in the alpha glucosidase gene in five italian patients with infantile onset glycogen storage disease type II. Am J Med Genet A 121A: 225–230. 10.1002/ajmg.a.20164.
23. Montalvo AL, Bembi B, Donnarumma M, Filocamo M, Parenti G, et al. (2006) Mutation profile of the GAA gene in 40 italian patients with late onset glycogen storage disease type II. Hum Mutat 27: 999–1006. 10.1002/humu.20374.
24. Bali DS, Tolun AA, Goldstein JL, Dai J, Kishnani PS (2011) Molecular analysis and protein processing in late-onset pompe disease patients with low levels of acid alpha-glucosidase activity. Muscle Nerve 43: 665–670. 10.1002/mus.21933; 10.1002/mus.21933.
25. Jackson T (2003) Finnish Lapphund comprehensive owner's guide. Allenhurst, NJ, , USA: Kennel club books, Inc.p 9–31.
26. Kishnani PS, Corzo D, Nicolino M, Byrne B, Mandel H, et al. (2007) Recombinant human acid [alpha]-glucosidase: Major clinical benefits in infantile-onset pompe disease. Neurology 68: 99–109. 10.1212/01.wnl.0000251268.41188.04.
27. van der Ploeg AT, Clemens PR, Corzo D, Escolar DM, Florence J, et al. (2010) A randomized study of alglucosidase alfa in late-onset Pompe's disease. N Engl J Med 362: 1396–1406. 10.1056/NEJMoa0909859.

Mosaicism of Podocyte Involvement Is Related to Podocyte Injury in Females with Fabry Disease

Michael Mauer[1,2], Emily Glynn[3], Einar Svarstad[4,5], Camilla Tøndel[5,6], Marie-Claire Gubler[7], Michael West[8], Alexey Sokolovskiy[3], Chester Whitley[1], Behzad Najafian[3]*

1 Department of Pediatrics, University of Minnesota, Minneapolis, United States of America, **2** Department of Medicine, University of Minnesota, Minneapolis, United States of America, **3** Department of Pathology, University of Washington, Seattle, United States of America, **4** Department of Medicine, Haukeland University Hospital, Bergen, Norway, **5** Department of Clinical Medicine, University of Bergen, Bergen, Norway, **6** Department of Pediatrics, Haukeland University Hospital, Bergen, Norway, **7** U983, Université René Descartes, Hôpital Necker-Enfants Malades AP-HP, Paris, France, **8** Division of Nephrology, Department of Medicine, Dalhousie University, Halifax, Nova Scotia, Canada

Abstract

Background: Fabry disease. an X-linked deficiency of α-galactosidase A coded by the GLA gene, leads to intracellular globotriaosylceramide (GL-3) accumulation. Although less common than in males, chronic kidney disease, occurs in ~15% of females. Recent studies highlight the importance of podocyte injury in Fabry nephropathy development and progression. We hypothesized that the greater the % of podocytes with active wild-type GLA gene (due to X-inactivation of the mutant copy) the less is the overall podocyte injury.

Methods: Kidney biopsies from 12 treatment-naive females with Fabry disease, ages 15 (8–63), median [range], years were studied by electron microscopy and compared with 4 treatment-naive male patients.

Results: In females, 51 (13–100)% of podocytes (PC) per glomerulus had no GL-3 inclusions, this consistent with a non-Fabry podocyte phenotype (NFPC). In PC with GL-3 inclusions [Fabry podocyte phenotype (FPC)], GL-3 volume density per podocyte was virtually identical in females and males, consistent with little or no cross-correction between FPC and NFPC. %NFPC per glomerulus (%NFPC/glom) correlated with age in females ($r = 0.65$, $p = 0.02$), suggesting a survival disadvantage for FPC over time. Age-adjusted %NFPC/glom was inversely related to foot process width (FPW) ($r = -0.75$, $p = 0.007$), an indicator of PC injury. GL-3 volume density in FPC in females correlated directly with FPW.

Conclusions: These findings support important relationships between podocyte mosaicism and podocyte injury in female Fabry patients. Kidney biopsy, by providing information about podocyte mosaicism, may help to stratify females with Fabry disease for kidney disease risk and to guide treatment decisions.

Editor: Stuart E. Dryer, University of Houston, United States of America

Funding: This work was supported by an NIH RDCRN U54 grant (5U54NS065768-04) and an investigator initiated grant from Genzyme, a Sanofi Company. The funder provided support in the form of research grants for authors [BN, MM, and MLW], and travel support and honoraria for authors [BN, MM, CT, and MLW] but did not have any additional role in the study design, data collection and analysis, decision to publish, or preparation of the manuscript. The specific roles of these authors are articulated in the 'author contributions' section.

Competing Interests: BN is a consultant to Genzyme and Amicus Therapeutics, receives investigator initiated research support from Genzyme and Roche, and honoraria and travel support from Genzyme. BN is also a member of the Medical Advisory Board of Amicus Therapeutics. MM is a consultant to Genzyme, and receives investigator initiated research support, honoraria, and travel support from Genzyme. MM is also a member of the Genzyme funded FDA mandated Fabry Registry Board. This interest for MM has been reviewed and managed by the University of Minnesota in accordance with its conflict of interest policies. MM is also a consultant to Amicus. CT and ES received travel support and speakers honoraria from Shire and Genzyme. MLW has received research support, honoraria, and/or travel support from Actelion, Amicus, Excelsior Pharmaceuticals, Genzyme, Glaxo SmithKline, Shire, and Sumitomo Pharma. Behzad Najafian is a PLOS ONE Editorial Board member, and commercial affiliations do not alter the authors' adherence to PLOS ONE Editorial policies and criteria.

* Email: najafian@u.washington.edu

Introduction

Fabry disease is a storage disease caused by deficiency of the α-galactosidase A (αGal A) enzyme that hydrolyzes the terminal α-galactosyl moieties from glycolipids and glycoproteins. This leads to the accumulation of its substrates, predominately globotriaosylceramide (GL-3) in various cell types and organs, causing a constellation of complications including skin lesions, strokes, cardiac arrhythmias and cardiomyopathy, neuropathies and renal failure. [1] αGal A is encoded by the GLA gene located on the X chromosome locus Xq21.3-q22. Similar to other X-linked diseases, the complications are typically less frequent and more variable in severity in females, [2,3,4] although they can be as severe as in male patients. [5,6] A significant proportion of female patients suffer from important complications, including 40% with clinical renal disease (mainly proteinuria) [7] and about 15% with serious renal events. [2] Fabry disease is associated with significant life expectancy reductions in both sexes. [8] It is of great importance to understand the factors associated with disease severity in females. Currently, there are no reliable tests to identify females at greater risk to develop kidney failure, thus justifying earlier treatment with enzyme replacement therapy (ERT). Podocytes are terminally differentiated cells with pivotal role in preserving glomerular structure and function. [9] Recent studies suggest that GL-3 accumulation in podocytes plays an important role in the pathophysiology of Fabry nephropathy. [10] These cells are also much more resistant to ERT than most other kidney cell types. [11,12] Similar to other "terminally differentiated cells" podocytes do not easily regenerate following injury [13]. Continuous podocyte loss leads to progressive reduction of these cells in the glomeruli, this eventually reaching critical levels causing irreversible glomerular scarring [14]. Despite recent evidence that higher doses of ERT during childhood may result in partial to almost complete clearance of podocytes from GL-3 inclusions, [15] there is no consensus as to when to initiate ERT, especially in females, and the relative clinical effectiveness of the different licensed ERT doses remain unsettled. [16,17,18] We hypothesized that podocytes, due to random X-inactivation, are heterogeneously involved by Fabry disease in female patients and that this heterogeneity could influence podocyte injury. Herein we describe a method to quantify the % of podocytes with the Fabry phenotype and report an inverse relationship in females between age-adjusted % podocytes with no GL-3 inclusions in glomeruli and foot process width, a sensitive indicator of podocyte injury [19], supporting a relationship between X-inactivation and podocyte injury in females with Fabry disease. We also found no evidence of cross-correction between podocytes without and with the Fabry phenotype in females with Fabry disease.

Methods

These studies were performed in accordance with principles of the Declaration of Helsinki and were reviewed and approved by the Institutional Review Board of the University of Minnesota, Comité. de Protection des Personnes "Ile-De-France II." and the Regional Ethics Committee of Western Norway. Informed consents approved by the institutional board review committees were obtained prior to these studies.

Subjects and Clinical Parameters

Kidney biopsies from 12 ERT-naive females with Fabry disease, age 15 (8–63) years were studied by electron microscopy for distribution of podocyte involvement by the Fabry phenotype. Biopsies were obtained for assessment of the severity of the lesions of Fabry nephropathy in order to aid clinical decision-making regarding ERT initiation and/or as a baseline biopsy prior to ERT initiation. Biopsies from 4 ERT-naive males with Fabry disease, age 14 (7–18), were studied for comparison; 7/16 patients presented here were included in our previous publications. [10,15] The demographic and clinical data of all patients are presented in Table 1.

9/12 female and 3/4 male patients had results of GLA mutation analysis in their medical records confirming the diagnosis of Fabry disease (Table 1). The diagnosis of Fabry disease in the other patients was based on family history or clinical findings with or without reduced leukocyte αGal A activity and confirmed by the kidney biopsy findings. Protein excretion per gram creatinine (UPCR) was based on urine samples obtained close to the date of biopsy. GFR was estimated by the plasma clearance of iohexol where available or by creatinine clearance. Except for one of the patients where we were not able to find information about the use of renin-angiotensin system blockers, none of the patients were receiving these drugs.

Biopsies from 6 healthy living kidney donors, age 37 (16–52) were used to estimate normal control values for podocyte foot process with (FPW), as described below.

Biopsy Tissue Preparation and Electron Microscopy

Electron microscopy specimens were fixed in 2.5% glutaraldehyde, and embedded in PolyBed. Random glomerular sections were prepared as previously described. [20] Thin sections were mounted on formvar coated copper slot grids. Overlapping digital low magnification (~10,000 x) images of the entire glomerular profiles were obtained using a JEOL CX100 electron microscope for the podocyte mosaicism studies. High magnification (~30,000 x) images were obtained according a systematic uniform random sampling protocol for estimation of fraction of the volume (Vv) of PC cytoplasm occupied by GL-3 inclusions [Vv(Inc/PC)], Vv of inclusions/glomerular mesangial cell [Vv(Inc/Mes)], Vv of inclusions/glomerular endothelial cell [Vv(Inc/Endo)], and podocyte average FPW as previously described [10,20].

Identification of Podocytes with and without the Fabry Phenotype

Observers were masked to any of the patient characteristics. Montages of complete glomerular profiles were prepared from the above images in Adobe Photoshop software (Adobe Photoshop CS5 Extended, version 12.0×32). Twice digital magnification was applied to the images. Podocyte nuclei were identified and glomerular profiles with less than 10 podocyte nuclei (n = 3) were excluded from these studies. The cytoplasmic profiles surrounding each podocyte nucleus were carefully examined for presence of GL-3 inclusions. Podocyte nuclear profiles with cytoplasmic GL-3 inclusions, consistent with Fabry phenotype podocytes (FPC) or without cytoplasmic GL-3 inclusions, consistent with non-Fabry phnotype podocytes (NFPC) cytoplasmic GL-3 inclusions were counted in each glomerulus and %NFPC/glom was calculated. The maximum number of immediately adjacent podocytes, including podocytes on the other side of the same capillary loop, which were NFPC was recorded as an estimate of the size of podocyte mosaic patches on the section.

Electron Microscopy Stereology

Based on the best quality of tissue preservation and images, one glomerulus per biopsy was arbitrarily selected for detailed GL-3 volume density measurement in podocytes with visible nuclei on the section. Boundaries of nuclei and cell membranes, excluding the tertiary foot processes were traced using the magnetic lasso tool in separate layers in Adobe Photoshop (Figure 1). Similarly, the most convex points of cytoplasmic GL-3 inclusions were connected using the magnetic lasso tool to draw a polygon around the GL-3 inclusion aggregates in a separate layer. The tracings were colored differentially for nuclei, cytoplasm and inclusions (Figure 1). The observed magnification was calculated from the average of 10 horizontal and 10 vertical random measurements performed on images from a SPI grating carbon replica #02902-AB (Structure Probe, Inc., West Chester, PA, USA) with horizontal and vertical lines 0.463 μm apart obtained at the same magnification as for the montage images. Subsequently, the measurement tool of the software was calibrated. The area of cell, nucleus and inclusion aggregate profiles were obtained separately for each podocyte profile with a visible nucleus from the Adobe Photoshop measurement log. The fractional volume of GL-3 inclusions per each nucleated podocyte profile with GL-3 inclusions [Vv(Inc/

Table 1. Clinical characteristics of subjects.

Case	Sex	Age (year)	UPCR (mg/g)	UACR (mg/g)	GFR (ml/min/1.73 m²)	GLA Mutation	Mutation Type	Aangiokeratoma	Corneal Opacity
1	F	8	40	NA	NA*	NA	NA	+	+
2	F	11	0.02	53	105	c.800T>G (p.M267R)	Missense	+	+
3	F	12	29	NA	109	W236X	Nonsense	−	−
4	F	13	0	NA	97	Y216D	Missense	−	+
5	F	13	60	5	100	NA	NA	+	−
6	F	14	62	11	90	c.800T>G (p.M267R)	Missense	NA	NA
7	F	16	30	12	127	NA	NA	−	−
8	F	34	150	NA	118	R301Q	Missense	+	−
9	F	34	100	5	99	R112C	Missense	−	+
10	F	39	100	NA	78	1270T	Missense	+	+
11	F	39	40	ND	99	N215S	Missense	+	−
12	F	63	1150	NA	46	C.427G>C p.Ala143Pro	Missense	+	−
13	M	7	0	NA	183	Y216D	Missense	+	+
14	M	16	92	12	112	c.1212_1214delAAG	Deletion	+	+
15	M	18	251	135	96	c.800T>G(p. M267R)	Missense	+	+
16	M	23	102	NA	111	NA	NA	NA	NA

Abbreviations: UPCR = urine protein/creatinine ratio; UACR = urine albumin/creatinine ratio; GFR = glomerular filtration rate; NA = data not available; *Serum creatinine within the normal range; F = female; M = male; ND = Not detectable.

FPC)] was estimated as follows: $V_V(Inc/FPC) = \frac{A_{inclusions} \times 100}{A_{cell} - A_{nucleus}}$.
The overall average glomerular volume fraction of GL-3 inclusions per podocytes [Vv(Inc/PC)], endothelial cells [Vv(Inc/Endo)] and mesangial cells [Vv(Inc/Mes)] were estimated using unbiased stereology methods as previously detailed. [10] For clarity, we emphasize that Vv(Inc/FPC) is an estimate of GL-3 inclusion density in nucleated podocyte profiles with GL-3 inclusions, while Vv(Inc/PC) is an estimate of the same parameter in all visible podocyte profiles regardless of GL-3 content and including the podocytes with and without visible nuclei over 3 (1–3), median (range), glomeruli per biopsy. Average foot process width (FPW) was also estimated using unbiased stereology methods as detailed elsewhere. [10,20,21] In order to compare podocyte injury in FPC *vs.* NFPC in female patients with Fabry disease, FPW was separately estimated in systematically and uniformly obtained electron micrographs with and without FPC.

Statistical Analyses

Statistica 8.0 (Statsoft, Inc.) was used for statistical analysis. Comparison between groups was made by student t-test after confirming homogeneity of variances. Relationships between variables were evaluated using Pearson correlation. Partial correlations were performed to control for confounding variables. Random effects model variance component analysis was performed to estimate % contribution of biopsies (inter-subject) and glomeruli (intra-subject) variations to total variance of %NFPC per glomerulus (%NFPC/glom). $p<0.05$ was considered statistically significant.

Results

Electron Microscopy Examination of Kidney Biopsies

Examination of electron micrographs from all biopsies allowed easy and reliable distinction between male and female patients by the identification in females of podocytes with visible nuclei without GL-3 cytoplasmic inclusions, termed non-Fabry podocytes (NFPC) (Figure 1) in contrast with podocytes containing GL-3 inclusions, termed Fabry phenotype podocytes (FPC). However, mosaicism of the Fabry phenotype was not easily identifiable in the other glomerular or extra-glomerular cells, perhaps, at least in part, due to uncertainty about cellular boundaries (*e.g.*, mesangial or endothelial cells). In 4 female patient biopsies, no GL-3 inclusions were identified in endothelial and/or mesangial cells, thus, comments about mosaicism could not be made in those cell types. In 7/12 female patient biopsies, parietal epithelial cell profiles with no GL-3 inclusions were identified while occasional parietal epithelial cells with enlarged cytoplasm had abundant GL-3 inclusions. Characteristic lamellar GL-3 inclusions were not easily identified in proximal tubular epithelial cells. Distal tubular epithelial cells showed variable GL-3 inclusions in both males and females. Thus, this variability could not be accounted for X-inactivation mosaicism in those cells.

Distribution of GL3 Inclusions among Podocytes in Males and Females

54 (27–87) podocytes per biopsy were examined for presence of GL-3 inclusions in female patients. 51 (13–100)% of podocyte profiles per biopsy with visible nuclei and no GL-3 inclusions, were classified as NFPC in these females. NFPC were distributed as

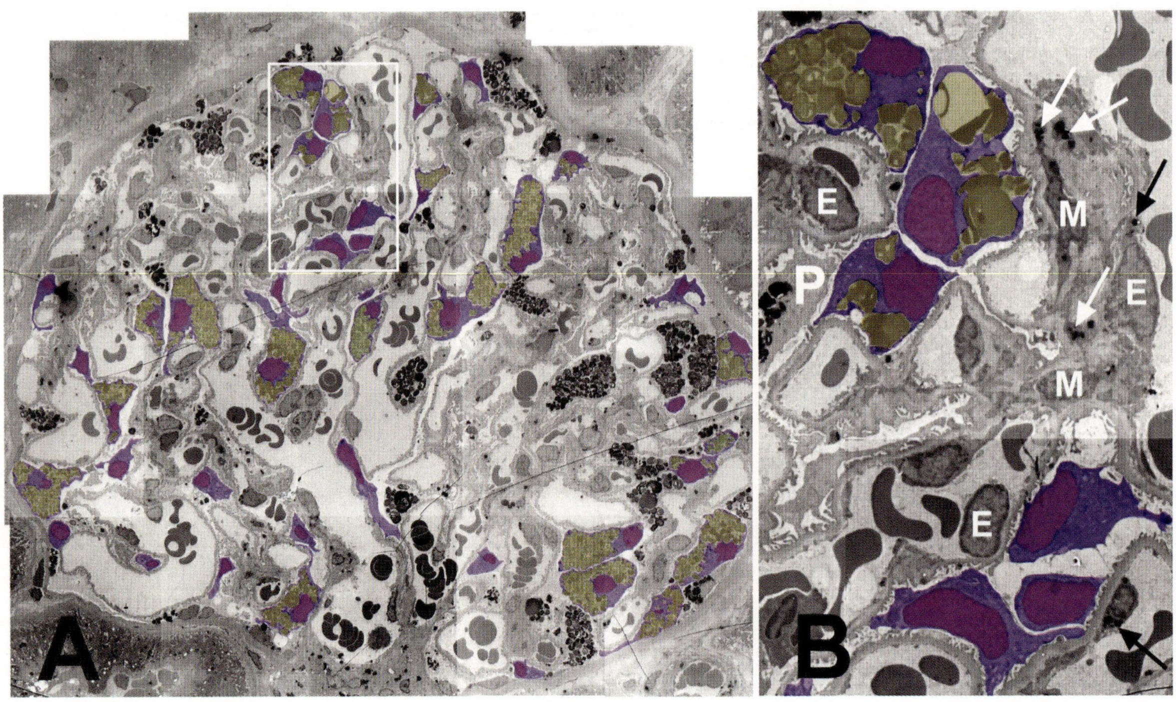

Figure 1. Mosaicism of podocyte Fabry phenotype in a glomerulus from a female patient with Fabry disease. (**A**) Montage image of a glomerulus (~3,000×). Podocyte bodies with visible nuclei are colored blue, podocyte nuclei purple, and GL-3 inclusions yellow. The white rectangle is magnified in B. (**B**) Magnified view of three podocyte profiles without (at the bottom) and three other podocyte profiles with GL-3 inclusions (on the top). Arrows show GL-3 inclusions in mesangial (M) cells (black) and endothelial (E) cells. P is a podocyte profile with no visible nucleus on this section.

single cells among FPC or in patches composed of 2–6 podocytes (Figure 1).

Two biopsies from female patients (one with 3 and another with 2 glomeruli) had no GL-3 inclusions in podocytes with visible nuclei (cases #9 and #11, Table 1). Case #9 showed rare podocyte profiles that were filled with GL-3. However, because these GL-3 containing podocytes had no visible nuclei they were not included in calculation of %NFPC per glomerulus. This case had a missense mutation (R112C) with GFR, UPCR and UACR values all within the normal range (Table 1). Clinical examination revealed corneal opacities, but no angiokeratoma. Echocardiograms showed normal left ventricular size and function with an estimated ejection fraction of 55–60% and normal right ventricular size and systolic function. Case #11 had distal tubular cells with GL-3 inclusions. This case had a cardiac variant mutation (N215S) with normal GFR and UPCR values and no detectable albumin in the urine (Table 1). The diagnosis of Fabry disease was made based on known family history. Clinical examination revealed angiokeratoma, but no corneal opacities. Clinically, she was asymptomatic. No echocardiograms were available from this case. None of these two subjects had a history of stroke. In order to determine whether random sectioning through podocytes may have obscured the observation of GL-3 inclusions in podocyte profiles 4 male patients with Fabry disease were similarly studied, 1–3 (median 2.5) glomeruli, containing 18–36 (median 22) podocyte profiles per glomerulus with visible nuclei were examined (Table 1). All podocyte profiles from these glomeruli contained abundant GL-3 inclusions, consistent with FPC, except for two very small profiles in a 7-year-old boy. The volume fraction of GL-3 inclusions per FPC [Vv(Inc/FPC)] was nearly identical in males (0.56±0.11) and females (0.53±0.13; $p = 0.54$).

Inter- and Intra-subject Variations of Podocyte Phenotype Mosaicism

Biopsies from 9 female patients with more than one glomerulus (3 (2–5), median (range)) available for electron microscopy were used to compare inter- and intra- subject variability of podocytes with the Fabry the phenotype. The %NFPC/glom in 2–4 glomeruli per biopsy in female patients is shown in Figure 2. Variance component analysis showed that only 9.6% of total variance in podocyte Fabry phenotype mosaicism originated from inter-glomerular (intra-subject) variation, while the vast majority of variance lay in differences in this parameter among the subjects.

Relationships Between % Podocytes with no GL-3 Inclusions and Female Patient Characteristics, Renal Function and Other Glomerular Structural Parameters

Values of %NFPC/glom, Vv(Inc/PC), volume fraction of GL-3 inclusions per mesangial cells [Vv(Inc/Mes)], volume fraction of inclusions per endothelial cells [Vv(Inc/Endo)], and foot process width (FPW) are provided in Table 2. The average %NFPC/glom was calculated in biopsies from female patients with more than one available glomerulus. There was a direct relationship between age and %NFPC/glom ($r = 0.65$; $p = 0.02$, Figure 3). No statistically significant relationship was found between %NFPC/glom and urine albumin/creatinine ratio (UACR) (available in 6/12 patients), urine protein creatinine ratio (UPCR) or glomerular filtration rate (GFR). As expected, %NFPC/glom was inversely related to Vv(Inc/PC) ($r = -0.70$, $p = 0.02$) for all podocytes. Simple linear regression analysis revealed no statistically significant relationships between %NFPC/glom and foot process width, Vv(Inc/Endo), Vv(Inc/Mes). However, adjusted for age, significant inverse relationships were found between %NFPC/glom and FPW ($r = -0.75$, $p = 0.007$), and Vv(Inc/Mes) ($r = 0.70$, $p = 0.02$), but not with Vv(Inc/Endo).

To better visualize the relationships between %NFPC/glom and FPW and UPCR, 10 female patients were grouped into 5 age-matched pairs, 3 pairs with identical ages and the 2 other pairs with ages no more than 2 years apart. Except for one pair, in each pair, the subject with lower %NFPC/glom had greater FPW value, suggestive of an inverse relationship between the extent of podocyte injury and the number of NFPC in age-matched Fabry females (Figure 4). Even an 8 year old female with 20% NFPC/glom (case #1) had greater FPW than an 11 year old (case #2) with 50% NFPC/glom. The one exception was a pair with greater FPW in a 14 year old girl with 22% NFPC/glom (case #6) compared to a 16 years old with 13% %NFPC/glom (case #7) (Figure 4). The relationships between %NFPC/glom and UPCR among the above pairs paralleled the relationships between %NFPC/glom and FPW, except for cases #2 and #3 with almost identical %NFPC/glom (50 and 52%, respectively) and slightly (~15%) greater UPCR for case#2 (Figure 4). However, the relationship between %NFPC and UPCR remained not statistically significant after age adjustment. Also, when adjusted for age, Vv(Inc/FPC) in females correlated with FPW ($r = 0.64$, $p = 0.03$). In females with Fabry disease, FPW in electron micrographs where glomerular basement membranes were covered by FPC (562±160 nm) was not statistically different from those where glomerular basement membranes were covered by NFPC (663±283 nm). On the other hand, FPW in either of these areas were greater than FPW in normal control biopsies (406±34 nm, $p = 0.037$ for FPC and $p = 0.048$ for NFPC).

Discussion

We recently demonstrated that the fraction of the volume of podocytes occupied by GL-3 [Vv(Inc/PC)] increases with age in children with Fabry disease and is directly correlated with FPW and to proteinuria,[9] the latter a strong predictor of renal disease risk among Fabry disease patients.[23] Increased FPW is a common concomitant of injury in podocytes and is seen in a variety of conditions known to be associated with injury in these cells. [21,22], [23] Thus careful examination of this cell in Fabry disease is important. This is the first study to provide unbiased electron microscopic morphometric measures of the heterogeneity of podocyte involvement in females with Fabry disease, almost certainly as a result of X-inactivation. Gubler *et al* first described the heterogeneous distribution of GL-3 inclusions in podocytes in 3 females with Fabry disease. [24] Valbuena *et al* also described variable podocyte GL-3 accumulation in 4 females with Fabry disease. [25] However, no quantitative assessment of podocyte GL-3 or statistical analyses was provided in these reports. Similar to these studies, [24,25] we found that a distinction between Fabry and non-Fabry phenotype, consistent with cells carrying active mutant or wild-type GLA, respectively, could be easily made in podocytes but not in other renal cells of female patients. This could be due to distinct borders of podocyte cell bodies from their neighbor cells, or because podocytes are apparently very long lived [26] and may thus retain GL-3 inclusions for years while other cell types are more frequently replaced.

Importantly, we documented, through unbiased morphometric measurements, that the average fraction of podocyte cytoplasm occupied by GL-3 was virtually identical in male and female patients, suggesting that FPC do not benefit from the enzymatic activity of the adjacent NFPC or from the generally higher residual plasma αGal A in females than on males. [27] [28,29].

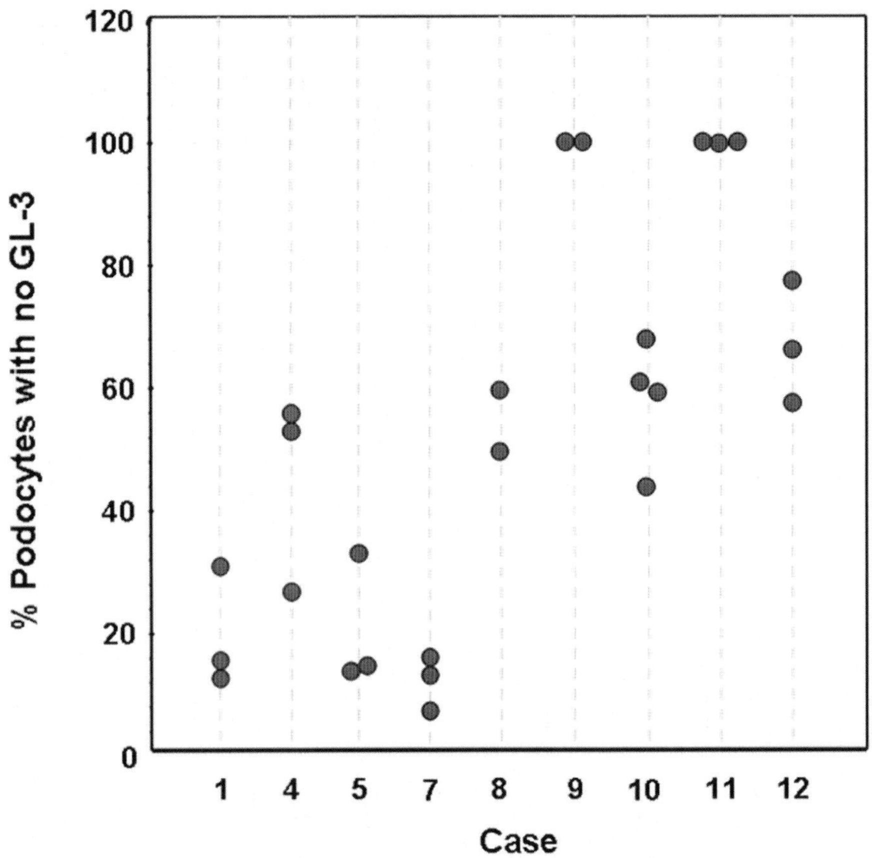

Figure 2. Intra- and inter-subject variability of podocyte mosaicism for Fabry phenotype in females. X axis shows case numbers (see Table 1). Each vertical dashed line represents a biopsy and each circle represents % podocytes with no GL-3 inclusions in one glomerulus.

Also important, we found that inter-glomerular variation in podocyte phenotype mosaicism in a given female Fabry patient's renal biopsy is much smaller than inter-patient variation. This suggests that estimation of podocyte phenotypic mosaicism even in a single glomerulus is representative of this phenomenon in the biopsy and validates the study of podocyte phenotype mosaicism in a few glomeruli. It also suggests that podocyte mosaciasm in females is established relatively early in embryogenesis. It should be noted that in these studies we used random profiles of glomeruli. Although we observed NFPC in patches of up to 5 cells in these two-dimensional glomerular cross-sections, these patches are likely larger in three dimensions. Nonetheless we posit that these patches are not very large, otherwise we might have expected greater inter-glomerular variability as a result of random sectioning through glomeruli.

This study is the first to show a quantitative relationship in females with Fabry disease between the X-inactivation phenomenon and podocyte injury manifest as increased FPW. Although X-inactivation may play a role in the clinical phenotypic expression of X-linked diseases, a direct link between skewed X-inactivation and severity of the Fabry phenotype has been controversial. Dobrovolny *et al.* reported that the trend line between the age and the Mainz severity score index (MSSI) [30] was steeper in 10 Fabry females with *vs.* 28 without unfavorably skewed X-inactivation in leukocytes, urinary and salivary cells. This suggested that random X-inactivation could influence the severity of the Fabry phenotype in female patients. [31] In contrast, Maier *et al.* found that in 46% of the 28 Fabry females studied, skewed X-inactivation did not correlate with phenotype severity. [4] Similarly, in a more recent study, while confirming random X-inactivation in leukocytes in ~82% of 77 female Fabry patients, there was no relationship between X-inactivation ratios and age, αGal A activity, MSSI scores, cardiac involvement, neuropathic pain or proteinuria. [32] We did not find a statistically significant relationship between % NFPC/glom and UPCR. However, in regression models including UPCR among the predictor variables, UPCR accounted for much less of the variance for rates of GFR decline in women than in men with Fabry disease. [33] Also, increased UPCR can reflect parameters other than podocyte injury, such as impaired tubular reabsorption reabsorption of filtered protein. However, after adjusting for age, we documented a significant inverse relationship between %NFPC/glom and FPW, a widely accepted indicator of podocyte injury. Thus, having more NFPC in glomeruli was associated with less podocyte injury. However, having a greater proportion of NFPC in older females with Fabry disease is not necessarily indicative of less podocyte injury. In fact, the observed increase in the %NFPC/glom with age in female patients in the current study is suggestive of progressive FPC loss with aging due to a survival disadvantage caused by the Fabry phenotype. Thus, glomeruli of older female patients may have fewer total podocytes than those of younger females with lesser %NFPC/glom, a hypothesis that remains to be tested in future studies. On the other hand, our side-by-side comparisons of age-matched female pairs revealed a robust inverse relationship between %NFPC/glom and FPW. However, given that Fabry disease is genetically heterogeneous, with more

Table 2. Glomerular Structural Parameters.

Case	Sex	Age (year)	%NFPC/glom	Vv(Inc/PC)	Vv(Inc/Mes)	Vv(Inc/Endo)	Vv(Inc/FPC)	FPW* (nm)
1	F	8	20	0.28	0.03	0.08	0.50	524
2	F	11	50	0.43	0.02	0	0.62	426
3	F	12	52	0.21	0	0	0.42	372
4	F	13	45	0.20	0	0.03	0.42	464
5	F	13	21	0.26	0.03	0.03	0.68	663
6	F	14	22	0.38	0.07	0.02	0.53	602
7	F	16	13	0.51	0.03	0.02	0.67	461
8	F	34	55	0.43	0.01	0.01	0.70	620
9	F	34	100	0	0	0.01	0	427
10	F	39	58	0.21	0.01	0	0.35	654
11	F	39	100	0.02	0.01	0	0	441
12	F	63	68	0.16	0.04	0.06	0.48	673
13	M	7	8**	0.21	0.01	0.09	0.58	369
14	M	16	0	0.44	0.10	0.37	0.56	551
15	M	18	0	0.50	0.16	0.21	0.61	823
16	M	23	0	0.34	0.56	0.27	0.65	714

Abbreviations: %NFPC/glom = % non-Fabry podocytes per glomerulus; Vv(Inc/PC) = volume fraction of GL3 inclusions per podocyte; Vv(Inc/Mes) = volume fraction of GL3 inclusions per mesangial cell; Vv(Inc/Endo) = volume fraction of GL3 inclusions per endothelial cell; Vv(Inc/FPC) = volume fraction of GL3 inclusions per Fabry podocytes; FPW = foot process width; F = female; M = male; *Normal values for FPW obtained from biopsies from 6 healthy living donors was 406±34 nm. **The biopsy contained two very small podocyte profiles with no GL3 inclusions, most likely due to random sectioning.

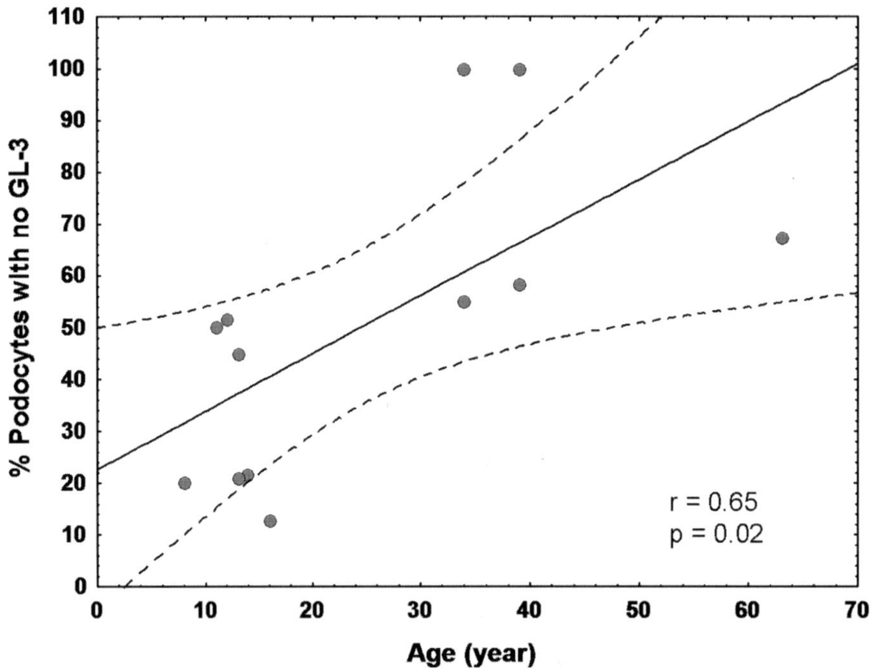

Figure 3. Relationship between age and % podocytes with no GL-3 in females. Dashed lines represent 0.95 confidence interval.

than registered 600 mutations, [34] it should be expected that attempts to explain all phenotype variation by a single parameter such as mosaicism will necessarily be overambitious. [35,36] Nevertheless, it will be interesting to examine if a relationship can be found between podocyte mosaicism status in the kidney and skewed X-inactivation in other organs or cell types, especially that of leukocytes. However, some of the cases presented in this study were from historical archived material and no simultaneous blood samples or skin biopsies had been obtained for x-inactivation studies at the time other biopsies were performed.

The relationship between podocyte mosaicism and podocyte injury in female Fabry patients suggests that the status of podocyte X-inactivation, after making adjustment for the age of the patient, could help to identify females with greater risk of progression of Fabry nephropathy. Although it would be desirable to use less invasive methods to obtain information about the proportion of cells with active mutant GLA, the status of mosaicism may be cell type and organ specific. Moreover, as outlined above, studies attempting to link X-inactivation in peripheral blood leukocytes and clinical manifestations of Fabry females have produced contradictory results. [4,31] Thus far, renal biopsy may be the only reliable way to obtain information about podocyte mosaicism in these patients.

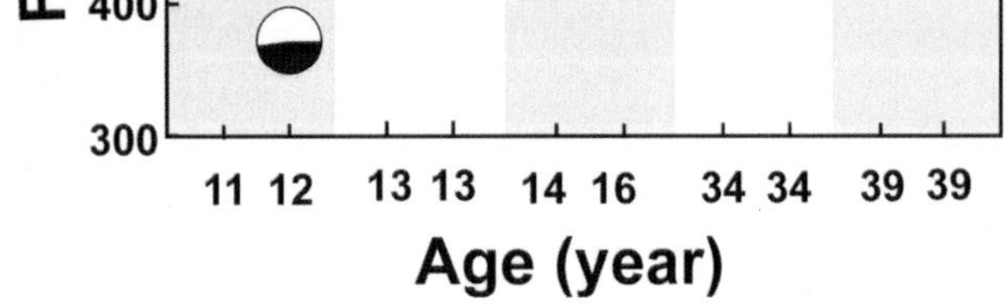

Figure 4. Relationships between podocyte mosaicism and foot process width in age-matched paired females. Each vertical grey or white band represents an age-matched pair. Each pie chart represents %NFPC/glom as white and %FPC/glom as black area. Abbreviation: FPW: foot process width.

Importantly, the present study showed that not only podocyte mosaicism for Fabry phenotype and podocyte injury are linked in female patients, but also podocyte injury in these patients is not limited to FPC and extends to NFPC, evidenced by increased FPW in GBM areas covered by NFPC compared with normal control biopsies. This is consistent with experimental studies performed by Matsusaka et al. where following administration of the immunotoxin LMB2 to the mice chimeric for hCD25 (LMB2 receptor), not only hCD25+ podocytes, but also hCD25- podocytes were injured and showed foot process widening, suggesting that specific injury to some podocytes can induce non-specific injury to other podocytes, [14] a phenomenon that if severe enough could lead to a vicious cycle of podocyte loss and glomerulosclerosis.

To our knowledge, this is the first report of the finding of rare cells with GL-3 inclusions in kidney biopsies from female Fabry patients. We encountered two females, ages 34 (case #9) and 39 years (case #11), with known Fabry disease by mutation analysis with very rare kidney cells with GL-3 inclusions. One (case #11), had a cardiac variant GLA mutation (N215S) [37] and the other (case #9) had a missense mutation (R112C). Thus, in contrast to males, the finding of even rare cells with GL3 inclusions in kidney biopsies from females should raise strong suspicion for Fabry disease. Notably, both of these subjects had very mild phenotypes, raising suspicion that the favorable skewed X-inactivation (predominantly affecting the mutant copy of GLA) observed in kidney biopsies may have also been present in other organs, especially since R112C mutation has been associated with classical Fabry disease causing ESRD [38], while case #9 in the present study had normal renal function and no history of cardiac disease or strokes. We did not have access to blood samples or other biopsies from these subjects to do correlative studies with our findings in kidney biopsies.

This study has some limitations. Although, it is the largest kidney biopsy study of females with Fabry disease, given the heterogeneity of Fabry mutations and clinical manifestations, additional studies are needed to confirm our results. We did not examine the status of X-inactivation in podocytes directly, rather we studied their apparent phenotype as to presence/absence of GL-3 inclusions in cell body profiles as a surrogate for X-inactivation. However, the easy discrimination between males and females on biopsies based on podocyte mosaicism supports validity of this surrogate. We cannot exclude the possibility of overestimation of %NFPC/glom in this study due to missing GL-3 inclusions in a single section through podocyte cell bodies. However, among 4 biopsies examined from male patients, only 2 of 98 podocyte nucleated profiles, both of very small size, had no GL-3 inclusions. Thus, we believe the extent of %NFPC/glom overestimation due to random sectioning is trivial.

In summary, this is the first study showing that mosaicism of podocytes in females with Fabry disease is related to podocyte injury. The extent of podocyte mosaicism for the Fabry phenotype is quite uniform among the glomeruli. The fraction of the cell body occupied by GL-3 in affected podocytes in females is the same as in males, indicating the absence of significant cross-correction. The relative number of podocytes without the Fabry phenotype increases with age in female patients, suggesting either a disproportionate loss of Fabry-affected podocytes over time and/ or selection bias. Information about podocyte mosaicism in kidney biopsies may be useful to identify females with Fabry disease with increased risk of developing progressive podocyte and nephron loss. The methodology we introduced is applicable to future longitudinal biopsy studies to test this hypothesis.

Acknowledgments

Special thanks to Frieda Maiers, Ann Palmer and Paul Murry for their help with electron microscopy images and histologic measurements, Cathy Bagne for clinical coordinator assistance, and Kristina Chayet for secretarial assistance.

Author Contributions

Conceived and designed the experiments: MM BN. Performed the experiments: MM EG AS BN. Analyzed the data: AS BN. Contributed reagents/materials/analysis tools: MM ES CT MG MW CW. Contributed to the writing of the manuscript: MM BN EG ES CT MG AS MW CW.

References

1. Zarate YA, Hopkin RJ (2008) Fabry's disease. Lancet 372: 1427–1435.
2. Wilcox WR, Oliveira JP, Hopkin RJ, Ortiz A, Banikazemi M, et al. (2008) Females with Fabry disease frequently have major organ involvement: lessons from the Fabry Registry. Mol Genet Metab 93: 112–128.
3. MacDermot KD, Holmes A, Miners AH (2001) Anderson-Fabry disease: clinical manifestations and impact of disease in a cohort of 60 obligate carrier females. J Med Genet 38: 769–775.
4. Maier EM, Osterrieder S, Whybra C, Ries M, Gal A, et al. (2006) Disease manifestations and X inactivation in heterozygous females with Fabry disease. Acta Paediatr Suppl 95: 30–38.
5. Wang RY, Lelis A, Mirocha J, Wilcox WR (2007) Heterozygous Fabry women are not just carriers, but have a significant burden of disease and impaired quality of life. Genet Med 9: 34–45.
6. Gibas AL, Klatt R, Johnson J, Clarke JT, Katz J (2008) Disease rarity, carrier status, and gender: a triple disadvantage for women with Fabry disease. J Genet Couns 17: 528–537.
7. Deegan PB, Baehner AF, Barba Romero MA, Hughes DA, Kampmann C, et al. (2006) Natural history of Fabry disease in females in the Fabry Outcome Survey. J Med Genet 43: 347–352.
8. Mehta A, Ricci R, Widmer U, Dehout F, Garcia de Lorenzo A, et al. (2004) Fabry disease defined: baseline clinical manifestations of 366 patients in the Fabry Outcome Survey. Eur J Clin Invest 34: 236–242.
9. Reiser J, Sever S (2013) Podocyte biology and pathogenesis of kidney disease. Annu Rev Med 64: 357–366.
10. Najafian B, Svarstad E, Bostad L, Gubler MC, Tondel C, et al. (2011) Progressive podocyte injury and globotriaosylceramide (GL-3) accumulation in young patients with Fabry disease. Kidney Int 79: 663–670.
11. Thurberg BL, Rennke H, Colvin RB, Dikman S, Gordon RE, et al. (2002) Globotriaosylceramide accumulation in the Fabry kidney is cleared from multiple cell types after enzyme replacement therapy. Kidney Int 62: 1933–1946.
12. Germain DP, Waldek S, Banikazemi M, Bushinsky DA, Charrow J, et al. (2007) Sustained, long-term renal stabilization after 54 months of agalsidase beta therapy in patients with Fabry disease. J Am Soc Nephrol 18: 1547–1557.
13. Kriz W, LeHir M (2005) Pathways to nephron loss starting from glomerular diseases-insights from animal models. Kidney Int 67: 404–419.
14. Matsusaka T, Sandgren E, Shintani A, Kon V, Pastan I, et al. (2011) Podocyte injury damages other podocytes. J Am Soc Nephrol 22: 1275–1285.
15. Tondel C, Bostad L, Larsen KK, Hirth A, Vikse BE, et al. (2013) Agalsidase benefits renal histology in young patients with Fabry disease. J Am Soc Nephrol 24: 137–148.
16. Terryn W, Cochat P, Froissart R, Ortiz A, Pirson Y, et al. (2013) Fabry nephropathy: indications for screening and guidance for diagnosis and treatment by the European Renal Best Practice. Nephrol Dial Transplant 28: 505–517.
17. Najafian B, Mauer M, Hopkin RJ, Svarstad E (2013) Renal complications of Fabry disease in children. Pediatr Nephrol 28: 679–687.
18. Warnock DG, Mauer M (2014) Fabry Disease: Dose Matters. J Am Soc Nephrol.
19. Kriz W, Shirato I, Nagata M, LeHir M, Lemley KV (2013) The podocyte's response to stress: the enigma of foot process effacement. Am J Physiol Renal Physiol 304: F333–347.
20. Najafian B, Mauer M (2011) Quantitating glomerular endothelial fenestration: an unbiased stereological approach. Am J Nephrol 33 Suppl 1: 34–39.
21. Toyoda M, Najafian B, Kim Y, Caramori ML, Mauer M (2007) Podocyte detachment and reduced glomerular capillary endothelial fenestration in human type 1 diabetic nephropathy. Diabetes 56: 2155–2160.
22. Deegens JK, Dijkman HB, Borm GF, Steenbergen EJ, van den Berg JG, et al. (2008) Podocyte foot process effacement as a diagnostic tool in focal segmental glomerulosclerosis. Kidney Int 74: 1568–1576.
23. Topham PS, Haydar SA, Kuphal R, Lightfoot JD, Salant DJ (1999) Complement-mediated injury reversibly disrupts glomerular epithelial cell actin microfilaments and focal adhesions. Kidney Int 55: 1763–1775.
24. Gubler MC, Lenoir G, Grunfeld JP, Ulmann A, Droz D, et al. (1978) Early renal changes in hemizygous and heterozygous patients with Fabry's disease. Kidney Int 13: 223–235.
25. Valbuena C, Carvalho E, Bustorff M, Ganhao M, Relvas S, et al. (2008) Kidney biopsy findings in heterozygous Fabry disease females with early nephropathy. Virchows Arch 453: 329–338.
26. Wolf G, Chen S, Ziyadeh FN (2005) From the periphery of the glomerular capillary wall toward the center of disease: podocyte injury comes of age in diabetic nephropathy. Diabetes 54: 1626–1634.
27. Pinto LL, Vieira TA, Giugliani R, Schwartz IV (2010) Expression of the disease on female carriers of X-linked lysosomal disorders: a brief review. Orphanet J Rare Dis 5: 14.
28. Migeon BR (2006) The role of X inactivation and cellular mosaicism in women's health and sex-specific diseases. JAMA 295: 1428–1433.
29. Aerts JM, Groener JE, Kuiper S, Donker-Koopman WE, Strijland A, et al. (2008) Elevated globotriaosylsphingosine is a hallmark of Fabry disease. Proc Natl Acad Sci U S A 105: 2812–2817.
30. Whybra C, Kampmann C, Krummenauer F, Ries M, Mengel E, et al. (2004) The Mainz Severity Score Index: a new instrument for quantifying the Anderson-Fabry disease phenotype, and the response of patients to enzyme replacement therapy. Clin Genet 65: 299–307.
31. Dobrovolny R, Dvorakova L, Ledvinova J, Magage S, Bultas J, et al. (2005) Relationship between X-inactivation and clinical involvement in Fabry heterozygotes. Eleven novel mutations in the alpha-galactosidase A gene in the Czech and Slovak population. J Mol Med (Berl) 83: 647–654.
32. Elstein D, Schachamorov E, Beeri R, Altarescu G (2012) X-inactivation in Fabry disease. Gene 505: 266–268.
33. Warnock DG, Ortiz A, Mauer M, Linthorst GE, Oliveira JP, et al. (2012) Renal outcomes of agalsidase beta treatment for Fabry disease: role of proteinuria and timing of treatment initiation. Nephrol Dial Transplant 27: 1042–1049.

34. (2013) The Human Gene Mutation Database at the Institute of Medical Genetics in Cardiff.
35. Ashton-Prolla P, Tong B, Shabbeer J, Astrin KH, Eng CM, et al. (2000) Fabry disease: twenty-two novel mutations in the alpha-galactosidase A gene and genotype/phenotype correlations in severely and mildly affected hemizygotes and heterozygotes. J Investig Med 48: 227–235.
36. Eng CM, Ashley GA, Burgert TS, Enriquez AL, D'Souza M, et al. (1997) Fabry disease: thirty-five mutations in the alpha-galactosidase A gene in patients with classic and variant phenotypes. Mol Med 3: 174–182.
37. Bekri S, Enica A, Ghafari T, Plaza G, Champenois I, et al. (2005) Fabry disease in patients with end-stage renal failure: the potential benefits of screening. Nephron Clin Pract 101: c33–38.
38. Wang C, Wang Y, Zhu F, Xiong J (2013) A Missense Mutation of the alpha-Galactosidase A Gene in a Chinese Family of Fabry Disease with Renal Failure. Kidney Blood Press Res 37: 221–228.

Mutation Spectrum of Six Genes in Chinese Phenylketonuria Patients Obtained through Next-Generation Sequencing

Ying Gu[1], Kangmo Lu[2], Guanghui Yang[3], Zhong Cen[3], Li Yu[4], Lin Lin[3], Jing Hao[3], Zhigang Yang[3], Jiabao Peng[3], Shujian Cui[3], Jian Huang[5,6*]

1 Prenatal Diagnosis Center, Maternal and Child Health Care Hospital, Lianyungang, Jiangsu, China, 2 Prenatal Diagnosis Center, Chengdu Women's and Children's Central Hospital, Chengdu, Sichuan, China, 3 Shanghai Find Bio-Tech Co., Ltd., Shanghai, China, 4 Life Technologies Company, Shanghai, China, 5 National Engineering Center for Biochip at Shanghai, Shanghai, China, 6 Shanghai-MOST Key Laboratory for Disease and Health Genomics, Chinese National Human Genome Center at Shanghai, Shanghai, China

Abstract

Background: The identification of gene variants plays an important role in the diagnosis of genetic diseases.

Methodology/Principal Findings: To develop a rapid method for the diagnosis of phenylketonuria (PKU) and tetrahydrobiopterin (BH4) deficiency, we designed a multiplex, PCR-based primer panel to amplify all the exons and flanking regions (50 bp average) of six PKU-associated genes (*PAH, PTS, GCH1, QDPR, PCBD1* and *GFRP*). The Ion Torrent Personal Genome Machine (PGM) System was used to detect mutations in all the exons of these six genes. We tested 93 DNA samples from blood specimens from 35 patients and their parents (32 families) and 26 healthy adults. Using strict bioinformatic criteria, this sequencing data provided, on average, 99.14% coverage of the 39 exons at more than 70-fold mean depth of coverage. We found 23 previously documented variants in the *PAH* gene and six novel mutations in the *PAH* and *PTS* genes. A detailed analysis of the mutation spectrum of these patients is described in this study.

Conclusions/Significance: These results were confirmed by Sanger sequencing. In conclusion, benchtop next-generation sequencing technology can be used to detect mutations in monogenic diseases and can detect both point mutations and indels with high sensitivity, fidelity and throughput at a lower cost than conventional methods in clinical applications.

Editor: Cees Oudejans, VU University Medical Center, Netherlands

Funding: The authors gratefully acknowledge grant support from the National High Technology Research and Development Program of China (863 Program, 2012AA02A205), the Chinese National Key Program on Basic Research (973 Program, 2010CB529206 and 2014CB965002), the National Natural Science Foundation of China (81272306) and the Program of Shanghai Subject Chief Scientist (12XD1421400, 11JC1408800, 13431902000 and 12DZ942500). Shanghai Find Bio-Tech Co Ltd., provided support in the form of salaries for authors GY, ZC, LL, JH, ZY, JP, & SC. Life Technologies Company provided support in the form of a salary for author LY. National Engineering Center for Biochip at Shanghai provided support in the form of a salary for author JH. Otherwise, these organisations had no role in study design, data collection and analysis, decision to publish, or preparation of the manuscript. The specific roles of these authors are articulated in the 'author contributions' section.

Competing Interests: GY, ZC, LL, JH, ZY, JP, & SC are employed by Shanghai Find Bio-Tech Co Ltd., whose company provided the sequencing service. LY is employed by Life Technologies Company. JH is employed by National Engineering Center for Biochip at Shanghai. There are no patents, products in development or marketed products to declare. This does not alter our adherence to all the PLOS ONE policies on sharing data and materials.

* E-mail: huangjchgc@hotmail.com

These authors contributed equally to this work.

Introduction

Phenylketonuria (PKU), or hyperphenylalaninemia (HPA), is the most common metabolic disease in China due to autosomal recessive, inborn errors of phenylalanine metabolism. The overall incidence of PKU in China is 1/11,000 [1,2], yet the prevalence varies considerably across China with much higher rates in northern China (1/3,425 - 1/7,849) than in southern China [3–7]. The worldwide regional and ethnic variation of PKU prevalence is also apparent, ranging from 1/100,000 in the African population to 1/2,600 in the Turkish population [8]. Patients with PKU usually present with HPA and severe mental retardation unless a low phenylalanine diet is introduced early in life. PKU can be classified as classic PKU, moderate PKU, mild PKU or mild HPA, depending on the enzyme defect, genotype and severity of the disease [8]. Genetic analysis has revealed that mutations in the *PAH* gene, which encodes phenylalanine hydroxylase, result in PKU. Thus far, more than 500 mutations have been deposited in the PAH mutation database and are comprised of 60.5% missense mutations, 13.5% deletions, 11% splice site mutations, 5% nonsense mutations and 1.8% insertions (http://www.pahdb.mcgill.ca/).

A deficit in tetrahydrobiopterin (BH4), the essential cofactor required for the hydroxylation of aromatic amino acids, may cause severe HPA and PKU, also known as malignant PKU, as well as rare neurological diseases with catecholamine and serotonin deficiencies with or without HPA. The estimated incidence of these deficiencies is reported to be 1–3% of all patients with HPA [9]. Unlike disease cases caused by a *PAH* mutation, patients with BH4 deficiency and HPA mainly have causal autosomal recessive mutations in the genes encoding the BH4 biosynthesis enzymes, including *PTS* (6-pyruvoyl-tetrahydropterin synthase) and *GCH1* (GTP cyclohydrolase I), or the BH4 regeneration enzymes, including *PCBD1* (pterin-4a-carbinolamine dehydratase gene) and *QDPR* (dihydropteridine gene). Mutations are distributed across all the exons in each of these four genes without any identified hotspots [10]. GTP cyclohydrolase I feedback regulatory protein (GFRP) interacts with GCH1 in the liver [11]. Thus, GFRP may also play roles in phenylalanine metabolism, although no mutations have yet been found in this gene in humans.

Since next-generation sequencing (NGS) platforms first arrived on the market in 2005, their advantages over the classic Sanger sequencing method for genetic research have been demonstrated, including the ability not only to produce massive amounts of data in parallel but also to measure each base pair to an unprecedented depth. However, several weaknesses of NGS have prevented its application in clinical molecular labs, including the high cost, long sequencing time (2–3 days), high level of infrastructure complexity and poor sample scalability. Recently, a benchtop sequencer, the Ion Torrent Personal Genome Machine (PGM), has been developed to overcome most of these disadvantages. Using semiconductors and non-optical sequencing technology in the PGM, multiple genomic loci and samples can be sequenced on one chip in just two hours of machine running time [12]. Therefore, this technology has greatly reduced the time and cost of sequencing each sample at each locus. Furthermore, this technology has already been successfully applied to sequencing several cancer-related genes [13–15]. However, because this platform is rather novel for NGS, few publications have described its application in the mutational analysis of single gene disorders [16,17].

In this study, we aimed to use this simple, fast, scalable and cost-effective PGM platform to study the mutational spectra of six genes in 35 Chinese patients with PKU. The development of methodology for data optimization and analysis and the advantages and disadvantages of this platform in monogenic mutational analysis are discussed in detail.

Methods

Patients

The cohort study consisted of 93 subjects from 32 families, including 33 patients diagnosed with PKU and two patients diagnosed with BH4 deficiency according to the diagnostic criteria published in Blau et al., 2011 [18]. Samples from 29 complete pedigrees, termed core families, and six incomplete pedigrees, termed non-core families, were available for this study. No consanguineous families were included in this study. The project and protocol for the investigation involving humans and animals were approved by the ethics committee of the Chinese National Human Genome Center at Shanghai. All patients provided their written informed consent to participate in this study according to the Declaration of Helsinki.

DNA extraction, primer design and multiplex PCR

Genomic DNA was extracted from peripheral blood leukocytes using a QIAamp DNA Mini Kit (Qiagen). To directly sequence the 39 exons of *PAH, PTS, GCH1, QDPR, PCBD1* and *GFRP* genes, including 50 bp in the intron-exon boundaries, 108 pairs of primers were designed using the freely available software Primer Premier 5.0. Known variants were not included in the primer sequences (dbSNP build 138). Multiplex PCR was performed to reduce the number of amplification reactions. Each primer (at a final concentration of 10 μM) and 100 ng of genomic DNA were mixed together with 0.2 mM dNTPs and 10× buffer to a final reaction volume of 25 μl. Between 13 and 23 primer pairs with similar annealing temperatures were combined in one reaction, and the PCR amplification conditions varied for each multiplex PCR (95°C for 5 min followed by 30 cycles of 95°C for 30 s, the annealing temperature (Set 1: 58°C, Set 2: 56°C, and Set 3: 50°C) for 30 s and 72°C for 30 s. A final elongation step of 72°C for 5 min was added in each case. The resulting amplicons were then purified using Ampure Beads, and the concentration was measured using the Qubit dsDNA HS Assay kit (Life Technologies) and the fragment size was detected using Agilent 2100 Bioanalyzer. Amplicons were then mixed in equal amounts.

Library construction and Ion Torrent sequencing

The template preparation was performed according to the Ion OneTouch System protocol (PNMAN0006957, Rev. 6.0) according to manufactory instructions. Briefly, an input concentration of one DNA template copy per Ion Sphere Particle (ISP) was added to the emulsion PCR master mix. The emulsion preparation was followed by DNA clonal amplification using the Ion OneTouch instrument (Life Technologies). The ISPs were then recovered, and the template-positive ISPs were enriched using Dynabeads MyOne Streptavidin C1 beads (Life Technologies) in the Ion OneTouch ES instrument (Life Technologies). ISP enrichment was qualified using the Ion Sphere quality control kit (Life Technologies) and a Qubit 2.0 fluorometer (Life Technologies). The complete ISP samples were loaded on either Chip 314 or Chip 316 and prepared for sequencing using the Ion PGM 200 sequencing kit protocol (PN4474246, Rev. D). The sequencing runs were performed using 520 flows for 130 cycles.

Data analysis and variant prioritization pipeline

After the PGM run was complete, the data were processed using the Ion Torrent pipeline software Torrent Suite v3.4 (Life Technologies) to generate sequence reads. Barcode primers were used to identify the reads from different samples. After sorting, the adaptor sequences were removed from the reads. The sequence of each read was trimmed by 2 bp past the expected primer-indexed sequence length to accommodate a possible (or 99.7% likely) 2 bp insertion, because the 2 bp insertion has a 99.7% chance of occurring in our study. We further removed a few unqualified sequences from the primary data using a local dynamic programming algorithm, including very short reads of less than 20 bp (1.67% of the sequences, Figure 1) and reads with a quality score less than 20 (Figure 1), to increase the specificity of the read alignment. The remaining sequences were considered clean reads and were used for further analysis.

The clean reads were aligned against the human genome (HG19) reference sequence retrieved from the NCBI database (Build 37) using the BWA (Burrows Wheeler Aligner) Multi-Vision software package. Sequence variants, including indels, splice sites and single nucleotide variations (SNV), were identified using VarScan v2.3.5 software. The previously identified SNPs were determined using the NCBI dbSNP, HapMap or 1000 Human Genome Project databases. The well-known disease causing mutations were confirmed in the PAH mutations database (http://www.pahdb.mcgill.ca/), the Human Gene Mutation Database at the Institute of Medical Genetics in Cardiff (HGMD. http://www.ghmd.cf.ac.uk/) and previous publications.

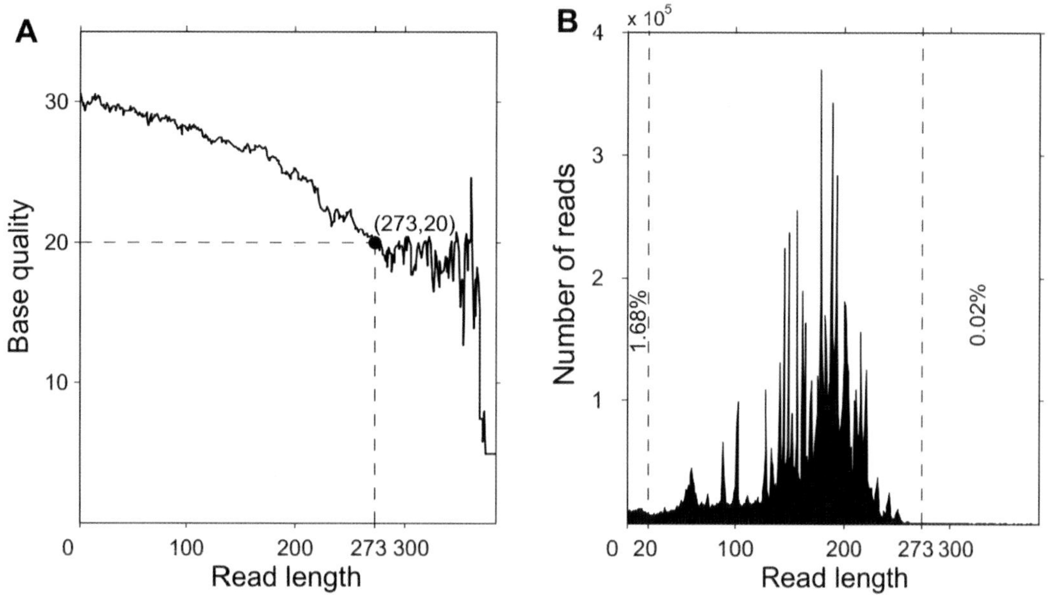

Figure 1. Selection criteria for trimmed reads. (A) The relationship between base quality and read length in the raw data. (B) The relationship between number of reads and read length in the raw data.

All the sequence data (fastq) have been deposited in the NCBI SRA database; the accession number is SRR1171639 and the file name is "PKU research PGM data."

Sanger sequencing

The sample preparation and Sanger sequencing were performed by Life Technologies. Sanger sequencing was performed using the BigDye Terminator v1.1 Cycle Sequencing kit. After ethanol purification, the samples were run on an ABI 3730 sequencer. The chromatograms of the Sanger sequencing results were analyzed using SeqMan software.

Results

Multiplex PCR, high-throughput sequencing, alignment and coverage

To quickly discover DNA variants of the causal genes involved in genetic disorders and to sequence all the bases in the exons and intron-exon boundaries of the six genes (*PAH, PTS, GCH1, QDPR, PCBD1* and *GFRP*) involved in PKU and BH4 deficiency, 108 primer pairs were designed for multiplex PCR to amplify 39 exons containing 9,967 base pairs. The amplicons ranged in size from 103 to 267 bp (Table S1). To distinguish the sequences from different samples, we added a 10-bp barcode sequence to the 5′ end of each primer. After optimizing the PCR amplification conditions, we could use eight-time PCR reactions to amplify all the exons in each sample (Figure S1). The enriched DNA was used for library construction and then sequenced at single-base resolution using the Ion Torrent system. The total length of all PCR amplification products (PCR product + barcode sequence) from the six genes was approximately 22 kb (22,887 bp). In each sequence run, we obtained approximately 1.5 M reads (average read length was 200 bp) totaling 300 Mb of sequence using the Ion 316 chip. To obtain an average of 1,000-fold coverage of the targeted regions, 15 samples can be pooled in one sequence run using one Ion 316# chip.

Using the primer panel, we amplified all the exons in 93 samples from 35 PKU or BH4 deficiency patients and their parents (32 families) and 26 samples from healthy adults as controls. The PCR products were purified using magnetic beads (Agencourt NO.A63882, Beckman, Beverly, USA), and the enriched DNA from 15 samples was pooled together with same amount of each sample. After library construction, the pooled DNA library was sequenced using the Ion 316# chip. We obtained a total of 11,507,388 raw reads. To retain the high-quality reads for further analysis, we filtered all the raw data according to strict criteria (Figure 2) that removed the following: (1) the lower quality reads that were polluted by linker or adapter sequences; (2) the barcode sequence of each read; (3) those reads shorter than 20 bp (Figure 1A) because short reads are likely to align to multiple loci in the human genome; and (4) those reads longer than 273 bp because the majority of the bases after 273 bp had quality scores less than 20 (Figure 1B). (5) A final modification was performed because the reads obtained from the Ion Torrent sequencer are uneven in length; those reads longer than the expected amplicon size were cut to a length of the expected size plus 2 bp to analyze the potential insertion of 1 to 2 bp, which occurred in the overwhelming majority of reads in our study using the Ion Torrent system (Figure S2). For example, if the expected amplicon size was 103 bp, then the read was trimmed to 105 bp. After applying these filters, we obtained 8,420-375,137 high-qualitytrimmed reads per sample (Table S2). On average, 69.7% of the clean reads mapped uniquely to the human reference genome (HG19), with 93.9% of these reads mapping to the expected amplicon regions and 94.8% mapping to exon regions. We found that the average depth of coverage of all the 39 exons was 858.6-fold (Table S2) in 93 samples. The highest average depth of coverage was 3,069-fold in sample PKUD120003, and the lowest average depth of coverage was 74-fold in sample PKUD130082 (Table S2). Thus, the coverage and read depth should be adequate to reliably detect DNA variants within the majority of the targeted regions.

To evaluate the enrichment efficiency of the multiplex PCR, we analyzed the relationship between the mean percentage of

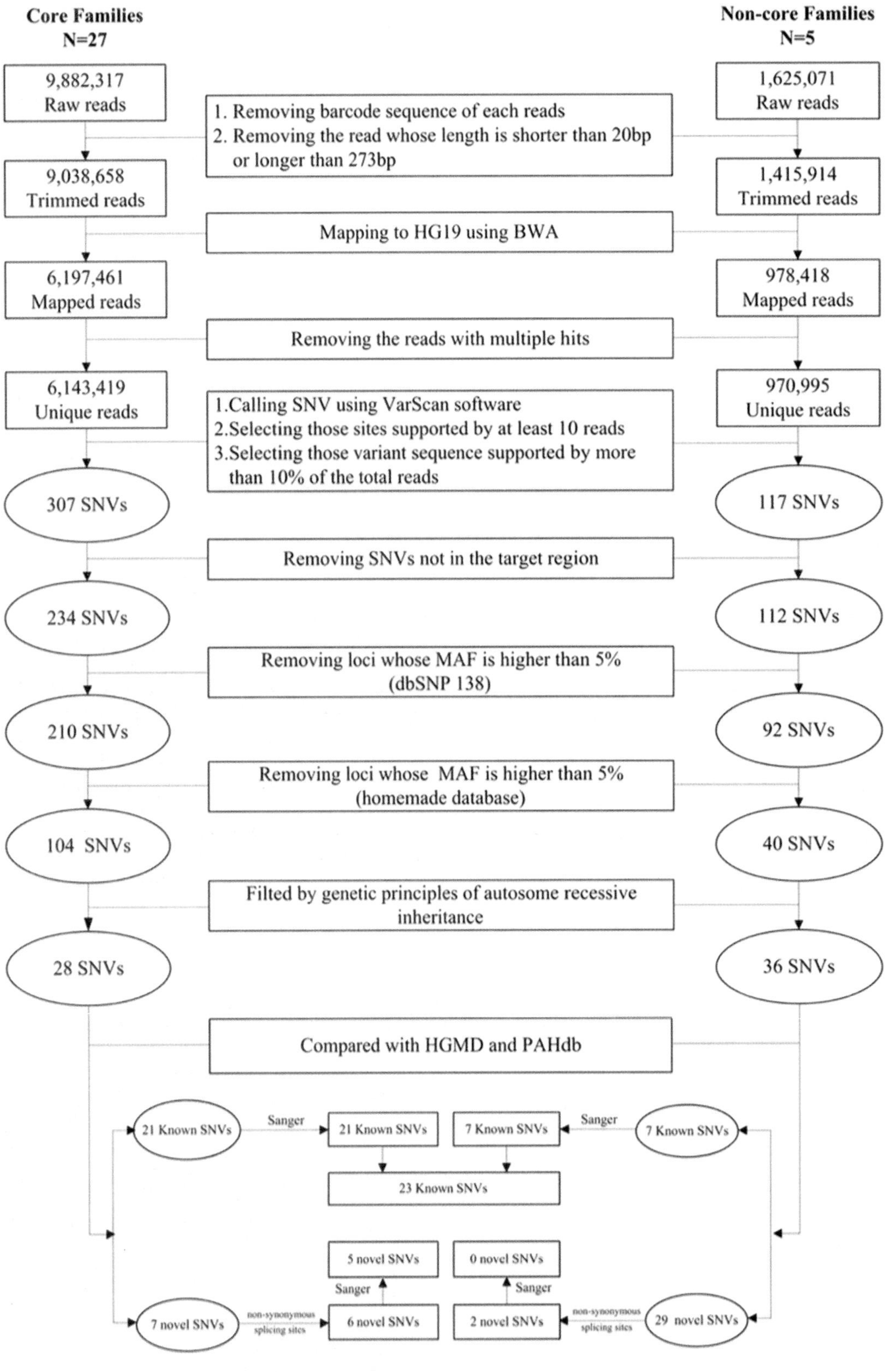

Figure 2. Flowchart for the process of screening and identifying single nucleotide variations (SNVs) in six genes by PGM sequencing.

coverage and mean depth of coverage of unique reads matched onto the six genes in all 93 samples using sequencing. Our results showed that the mean percentage of coverage and mean depth of coverage at the *PAH* gene (13 exons) in these samples was 99.3% and 1,466-fold, respectively (Figure 3A and Table S3). We also found that the mean percentage of coverage and mean depth of coverage at the other genes, including *GCH1* (6 exons) and *QDPR* (7 exons), were more than 93% and 1,200-fold, respectively (Figure 3B and 3C, Table S3), while the mean coverage and depth at the *PTS* (6 exons), *PCBD1* (4 exons) and *GFRP* (3 exons) genes were more than 90% and 200-fold, respectively (Figure 3D–3F, Table S3). However, we found that exon 4 in the *GCH1* gene and exon 1 in the *QDPR* gene had lower mean percentage of coverage (78.5% and 65.8%) and mean depth of coverage (32.7-fold and 36.9-fold), while exon 1 in the *PCBD1* gene had lower mean percentage of coverage (64.2%) and higher mean depth of coverage (340-fold) than the other exons. To explain these results, we analyzed the GC content of the 39 exons and evaluated the relationships between the GC content, mean percentage of coverage and mean depth of coverage. The findings showed that the exons with lower percentage of coverage (less than 90%) had lower (less than 40%) or higher (more than 60%) GC content, suggesting that the lower percentage of coverage was associated with excessively high or low GC content that can affect amplification and sequencing efficiency (Figure 4).

Identification of DNA variant sites

To identify the variants in the six genes in each sample, the high-quality, unique reads were mapped to HG19 using BWA software, and the variants were called using VarScan software [19] according to the following procedure (Figure 2): (1) exclusion of sites not in the target regions, (2) selection of sites supported by at least 10 reads, (3) classification of heterozygous sites as those supported by 10–90% of the total reads at that site, with all other sites classified as homozygous and (4) selection of the loci whose Minor Allele Frequency (MAF) is less than 5% according to the dbSNP database or an in-house database from the 26 normal adults sequenced using the Ion Torrent system. Following this procedure, we identified 117 single-nucleotide variants (SNVs), of which 104 were from the 27 core families, 40 were from the five non-core families, and 27 were found in both groups (Figure 2).

Identification of disease-causing substitution mutations for the diagnosis of PKU

To identify disease-causing mutations using the genetic principles of autosomal recessive inheritance (AR), we first selected those homozygous variant sites in patient samples that differed from the parental genotypes (Table S4). We then selected those heterozygous variant sites in the patient samples that represented one paternal allele and one maternal allele (Table S4). In our study, the majority of identified mutations fit into one of these two categories. After applying these selection criteria, we obtained 59 potential substitution mutations, of which 29 were from the 27 core families, 36 were from the five non-core families, and five were found in both groups (Figure 2, Table S4).

Next, these potential mutations were compared with the known disease-causing mutations deposited in disease databases, including the Human Gene Mutation Database (HGMD) [http://www.biobase-international.com/product/hgmd] and the mutation database for the human phenylalanine hydroxylase gene (PAHdb) [http://www.mcgill.ca/pahdb]. The 29 SNVs identified from the 27 core families included 21 known and 8 novel mutations, while the 36 SNVs identified from the five non-core families included seven known and 26 novel mutations (Figure 2, Table S4). From these novel potential mutations, we selected those sites with non-synonymous variants or proximity to splice sites. We finally obtained eight novel potential mutations, of which six were from the core families and two were from the non-core families (Figure 2, Table S4).

Furthermore, to validate the variants identified by NGS, we amplified all 31 candidate sites with potential mutations, including 23 known (21 from core family and 7 from non-core family) and 8 novel sites (6 from core family and 2 from non-core family), and their flanking sequences using the same primers used in NGS (Figure 2). We then sequenced the PCR products by Sanger sequencing using an ABI 3730 DNA Analyzer (Applied Biosystems). The results confirmed 23 (100%) of the 23 known mutations and five (62.5%) of the 8 novel mutations. The three SNVs that were not validated had a variant allele frequency of approximately 10%, suggesting that the Ion Torrent method used for mutation analysis provides high accuracy and a very low false-positive rate (Table S4).

In the current study, we found one homozygous mutation in exon 7 of the PAH gene in sample PKUD120001 from F1 (Table S5, Figure 5A and 5B). In addition, the majority of identified

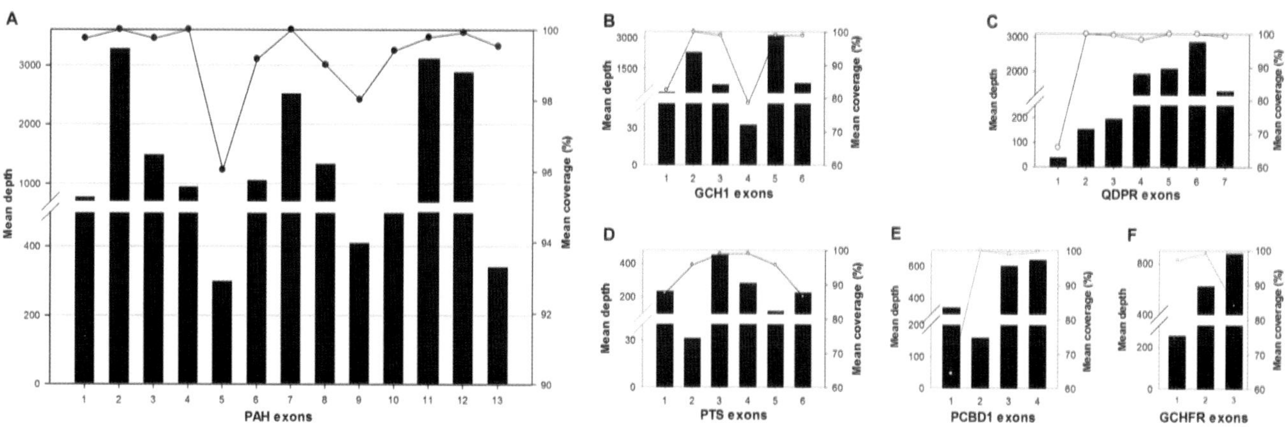

Figure 3. Mean depth of coverage and percentage of coverage of each exon of the six genes from all reads sequenced using a PGM. (A), (B), (C), (D), (E) and (F) indicate data from the *PAH, GCH1, QDPR, PTS, PCBD1* and *GCHFR* genes, respectively. The black columns indicate the mean depth of coverage, and the black circles indicate the mean percentage of coverage in each exon.

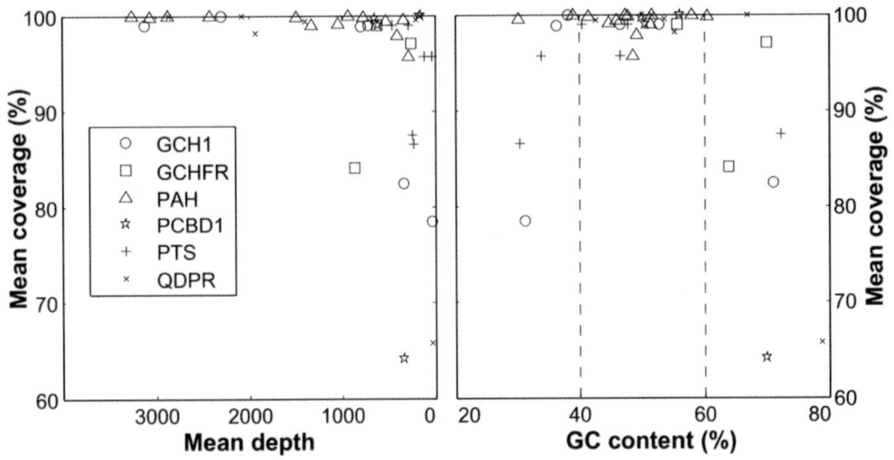

Figure 4. Comparison of GC content, read depth and coverage. The relationship between mean read depth and mean coverage (left) and the relationship between GC content and mean coverage (right) in each exon of the *PAH, GCH1, QDPR, PTS, PCBD1* and *GCHFR* genes. Exons with low coverage have relatively low read depth and excessively low (less than 40%) or high (more than 60%) GC content.

mutations were found in heterozygous variants in this study, of which one was the paternal allele while the other was the maternal allele. The representation result was displayed in Figure 5C and 5D.Four validated novel mutations present in heterozygous variants included two missense mutations (c.875C>T and c.971T>A) (Figure S3A, S3B and Table 1), one frameshift deletion (c.669delC) (Figure S3C and Table 1) and one substitution at the intron 10 splice site (IVS10-13T>G) (Figure S3D and Table 1). To predict the phenotypic effects of the mutations at the protein level, evolutionary conservation analysis was performed and revealed that the two novel missense variants (c.875C>T and c.971T>A) were highly conserved across species, especially in mammals (Figure S4). Furthermore, these two non-synonymous substitutions (c.875C>T and c.971T>A) were predicted by to be damaging mutations (SIFT score = 0) by SIFT v2.0 (http://blocks.fhcrc.org/sift/SIFT.html) according to the standard which the score of the damaging substitution of amino acid predicted by SIFT is ≤0.05. These results showed that the detected novel mutations may play a role in the progression of the disease.

Identifying disease-causing indel mutations

Given that the short insertions and deletions (indel) analysis is more difficult than variant identification; we integrated the results obtained by the two different algorithms. Firstly, all of the uniquely reads mapped to HG19 using BWA were used for calling indels using VarScan software. This analysis uncovered 498 indels, including 493 from the core families and 205 from the non-core families (Figure S5 left). In addition, the raw data were also analyzed using TMAP v3.4.1 and VariantCaller v3.4.5 software. This analysis identified 53 potential indels (Figure S5 right). We selected those loci that localized to coding sequences or splice sites and then we obtained 147 and 14 potential indels by BWA-VarScan and TMAP- VariantCaller, respectively. This selection process led to the identification of six potential indels. These six indels were validated by PCR-based Sanger sequencing, and three of them were confirmed (Figure S5 and Table S5).

Discussion

Since arriving on the market in 2011, the Ion Torrent PGM, a benchtop sequencer, has already been successfully used for the targeted resequencing of cancer genes, such as *BRCA* [15], *BRAF* [14], *POLE* and *POLD1* [13]. However, only limited research has been conducted using this semiconductor sequencing platform in monogenic disease studies [16,17]. To date, more than 7,000 single gene disorders have been identified in humans, and PKU is the most common inborn error of metabolism disease in China and is caused by mutations in the *PAH, PTS, GCH1, QDPR, PCBD1* and *GFRP* genes [20]. In this study, our aim was to construct a method for the rapid detection of all the nucleotide mutations in these six genes causing PKU disease. Together, 39 exons of these six genes were sequenced in 35 patients with either PKU or BH4 deficiency using the PGM system. After stringent read-filtering and the optimization of substitution and indel detection, 23 known substitution mutations in the *PAH* gene and five novel mutations in the *PAH* and *PTS* genes were identified. All of these mutations were confirmed by Sanger sequencing.

High-quality reads were selected in a strict manner to ensure quality results. When weak signals (quality scores less than 15) were detected during the sequencing step, the extension of that read was stopped. A weak signal could be due to problems in the emulsion PCR, such as one watery drop within the water-oil emulsion containing several Ion Sphere Particals (ISP) or bad amplification in one ISP. When the raw data were analyzed, these short reads often mapped to multiple positions. In this study, we removed those reads less than 20 bp to increase the alignment efficiency (Figure 1B). In addition, we found some reads with lower quality base pairs (scores less than 20) at positions past 273 bp (Figure 1B). These low-quality bases were also trimmed to ensure accurate results.

The sequencing coverage was lower in several exons than in the other exons. To explain this result, we analyzed the GC content and found that the regions with lower coverage (less than 80%) had excessively low (less than 40%) or high (more than 60%) GC content. The imbalanced GC content may explain why the multiplex PCR did not achieve uniform amplification of every amplicon [15]. Although the PCR conditions were optimized to amplify all the coding regions, it was difficult to avoid cross reaction because different primer pairs were mixed in one reaction. This method could have resulted in low PCR specificity when amplifying certain regions of the genes. Adjusting the maximum number of pooled samples per chip [15] and minimizing other artificial effects, such as unequal loading, would

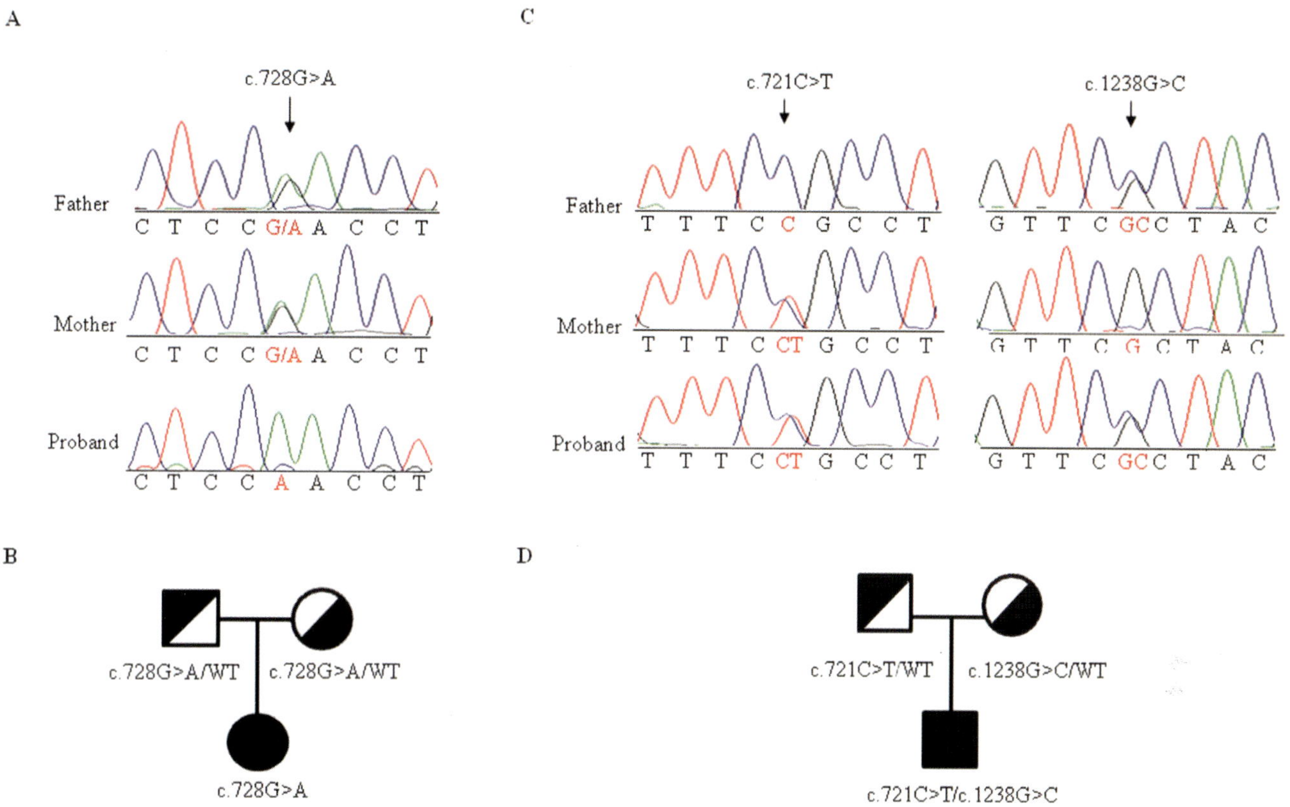

Figure 5. The representative mutation types observed based on the genetic principles of autosomal recessive inheritance. (A) A homozygous missense mutation of G to A in exon 7 of the PAH gene. The parents of this patient were confirmed to be heterozygous carriers for this mutation. (B) The family pedigree of the patient described in panel A. (C) A heterozygous missense mutation of T to A in exon 7 and a heterozygous mutation of G to A in exon 12 of the *PAH* gene. The father of this patient was a heterozygous carrier with a C allele in exon 12, while the mother was a heterozygous carrier with a T allele in exon 7. (D) The family pedigree of the patient described in panel C.

reduce non-specific amplification and false-negative variant detection.

PGMs have been reported to be biased toward the detection of indels; 92.1% of the novel indels called using the PGM in this study were of this class (Figure S2), and most of these indels could not be confirmed by Sanger sequencing. Although some of these indels fell within the context of homopolymers or tri-nucleotide repeats as observed in previous publications [16,21], others were randomly distributed throughout the sequenced genes. To accurately identify the indels, we used two different analysis software packages to call indels in this study. The overlapping results were validated by Sanger sequencing, and 50% (three indels) were confirmed (Table S5).

Another advantage of using the PGM sequencer is the cost and time efficiency of the workflow, which was consistent with previous reports [15,16]. Using the barcode system, six genes from 15 individuals can be sequenced simultaneously in two hours. Therefore, only 24 hours were required to sequence all the coding regions of these six genes from 93 individuals using a 314 or 316 chip, which greatly reduces the labor and time requirements compared to the cumbersome and lengthy Sanger sequencing method. Furthermore, with the newly developed 318 chip, more samples and regions could be sequenced in an improved 1G high-throughput setting.

In screening for actual disease-causing mutations, complete core families have an advantage over non-core families. The presence of data from both unaffected parents aids in the removal of unrelated SNVs when following the autosomal recessive inheritance principles. The removal rate was 73% (76/104) in the core families, but only 10% (4/40) in the non-core families. Therefore, when dealing with massive data produced by NGS for the study of monogenic diseases, collecting DNA from a complete pedigree would help to remove false-positive results and identify potential disease-causing changes.

In this study, in addition to the identification of 23 known mutations, we found six novel mutations, including five point mutations and one novel short deletion, that were supported by high read quality and depth and were confirmed by Sanger sequencing. Among these novel mutations, three novel missense mutations (P292L and I324N in the *PAH* gene and K91R in the *PTS* gene) and one nonsense mutation (Y414X), were located in the enzymes' catalytic domains and may affect protein function; however, further *in vitro* functional analysis is necessary to support this hypothesis. We also found one frame-shift mutation (N223fsdelC for the deletion of c.669delC) that result in the premature termination of protein translation. This terminated PAH protein would lack part of the catalytic domain and the entire tetramerization domain [1]. Thus, this mutation is highly likely to be a disease-causing mutation. Moreover, the IVS10-13T>G mutation is located in a region related to intron 10 splicing. Mutations within this region, such as IVS10-11G>A and IVS10-13T>G, have been suggested in PAHdb to be splice mutations. A functional study of the IVS10-11G>A mutation was performed *in vitro* and demonstrated that the mutant protein was functionally dead [22]. Despite these supportive observations,

Table 1. Spectrum of PAH and PTS mutations.

Gene	ID	Variants		Locations	Characters	Type	Number of	Frequency	Family
		cDNA	Protein		of mutation		alleles	(%)	
PTS	1	c.259C>T	p.P87S	Exon 5	Missense	Known	2	3.28	Core
PTS	2	c.272A>G	p.K91R*	Exon 5	Missense	Novel	1	1.64	Core
PAH	3	c.208_210delTCT	p.S70del	Exon 3	Deletion	Known	1	1.64	Core
PAH	4	c.284_286delTCA	p.I95del	Exon 3	Deletion	Known	1	1.64	Core
PAH	5	c.442-1G>A	IVS4-1G>A	Intron 4	Splicing	Known	1	1.64	Core
PAH	6	c.482T>C	p.F161S	Exon 5	Missense	Known	2	3.28	Core
PAH	7	c.498C>A	p.Y166X	Exon 5	Nonsense	Known	1	1.64	Core
PAH	8	c.611A>G	p.Y204C	Exon 6	Missense	Known	3	4.92	Core
PAH	9	c.669delC	p.N223Kfs	Exon 6	Deletion	Novel	1	1.64	Core
PAH	10	c.699C>A	p.F233L	Exon 6	Missense	Known	1	1.64	Core
PAH	11	c.716G>A	p.G239D	Exon 7	Missense	Known	1	1.64	non-core
PAH	12	c.721C>T	p.R241C	Exon 7	Missense	Known	6	9.84	Core/non-core
PAH	13	c.727C>T	p.R243X	Exon 7	Nonsense	Known	1	1.64	Core
PAH	14	c.728G>A	p.R243Q	Exon 7	Missense	Known	10	16.39	Core/non-core
PAH	15	c.740G>T	p.G247V	Exon 7	Missense	Known	1	1.64	non-core
PAH	16	c.823C>T	p.P275S	Exon 7	Missense	Known	1	1.64	Core
PAH	17	c.833C>A	p.T278N	Exon 7	Missense	Known	1	1.64	Core
PAH	18	c.842+1G>A	IVS7+1G>A	Intron 7	Splicing	Known	1	1.64	Core
PAH	19	c.875C>T	p.P292L*	Exon 8	Missense	Novel	1	1.64	Core
PAH	20	c.971T>A	p.I324N*	Exon 10	Missense	Novel	1	1.64	Core
PAH	21	c.977G>A	p.W326X	Exon 10	Nonsense	Known	1	1.64	Core
PAH	22	c.1006C>T	p.Q336X	Exon 10	Nonsense	Known	1	1.64	Core
PAH	23	c.1045T>G	p.S349A	Exon 10	Missense	Known	2	3.28	Core
PAH	24	c.1066-11G>A	IVS10-11G>A	Intron 10	Splicing	Known	1	1.64	Core
PAH	25	c.1066-13T>G	IVS10-13T>G*	Intron 10	Splicing	Novel	1	1.64	Core
PAH	26	c.1068C>A	p.Y356X	Exon 11	Nonsense	Known	5	8.20	Core/non-core
PAH	27	c.1197A>T	p.V399V	Exon 11	Splicing	Known	4	6.56	Core/non-core
PAH	28	c.1222C>T	p.R408W	Exon 12	Missense	Known	1	1.64	Core
PAH	29	c.1238G>C	p.R413P	Exon 12	Missense	Known	4	6.56	Core/non-core
PAH	30	c.1242C>A	p.Y414X*	Exon 12	Nonsense	Novel	1	1.64	Core
PAH	31	c.1301C>A	p.A434D	Exon 12	Missense	Known	2	3.28	Core
Total							61	100.00	

* indicates stop code.

further analysis, such as minigene construction, is essential to validate the functional effect of the IVS10-13T>G mutation.

In this study, we analyzed a total of 93 samples from 35 PKU and BH4 deficiency patients and their parents (32 families), of which 29 patients were from 27 core families and six patients were from five non-core families. Using this dataset, we identified 23 known variants in the *PAH* gene that included 21 mutations from the core families and seven mutations from the non-core families (Table S5). Consistent with previous PKU analyses, several of the most prevalent mutations discovered in our analysis, R243Q, R241C, Y356X, V399V and R413P (Table 1), matched the predominant type of PKU-associated mutation found in the Asian population [1,7]. These results suggest that these mutations are not only found in northern China but also in the central Chinese population. The migration of people from northern to southern China in recent years because of unbalanced economic development may account for the extended geographical distribution of these mutations. The mutation detection rate of 90.1% detected in this study is comparable to the 94.3% rate calculated in previous publications [1].

Despite sequencing the entire *PAH* coding region by NGS and Sanger sequencing, incomplete mutation profiles were identified in nine patients using strict criteria based on the genetic principles of autosomal recessive inheritance; six of these patients were from core families, and three were from non-core families (Table S5 with gray marks). In each of these cases, we only detected one disease-causing mutation in one allele. This observation may be due to the inability to detect additional mutations that are located in regions that were not sequenced in this study, for example, the 5′ or 3′ untranslated regions near promoters or non-coding RNA binding sites, intronic sequences far from intron/exon boundaries or large deletions. For the unsolved cases with BH4 deficiency, mutations may be located in the low coverage regions of the five genes. Possibly, other undiscovered, novel PKU-causing genes exist. Misdiagnosis may be rare, but it is also a possible explanation for the failure to identify additional disease-causing mutations in some individuals. Whole-exome sequencing will be applied in these cases after diagnosis is confirmed in future studies.

Conclusion

This study is the first study to investigate the feasibility of using the PGM platform to study the common metabolic diseases PKU and BH4 deficiency. A detailed analysis of the mutation spectrum that was obtained by sequencing the coding regions of six genes was described. Four novel, potential disease-causing mutations were identified in the *PAH* gene. Further improvements in the PGM analysis pipeline and chip 318 would overcome the aforementioned shortcomings. As a cost- and time-effective sequencing method, the PGM would be an easy-to-use and robust platform for clinical studies of monogenic disorders.

Supporting Information

Figure S1 Detection of PCR products from the 108 primer pairs by agarose gel electrophoresis. (Top) PCR products from the 108 primer pairs. (Bottom) Products from eight multiplex PCR reactions using the 108 primer pairs. I includes 15 primer pairs; II, III, IV and V include 14 different primer pairs; VI includes 23 primer pairs; VII includes 13 primer pairs; and VIII includes one primer pair.

Figure S2 Distribution of insertion/deletion variant (indels) sizes detected by a PGM.

Figure S3 The result of six novel mutations in the PAH gene confirmed by Sanger sequencing. (A), (B), (C), (D), (E) and (F) indicate c.272A>G/c.259C>T, c.669delC/c.823C>A, c.875C>T/c.728G>A, c.971T>A/c.1066-11G>A, c.1066-13T>G/c.728G>A and c.1242C>A/c.611A>G, respectively. Red indicates the novel allele.

Figure S4 Evolutionary conservation analysis of the six alleles with novel mutations. Representative reads aligned to the reference sequence (top) in exon 8 of the *PAH* gene. The boxes indicate the position with the substitution mutation (c.875C>T) as supported by 66 high-quality reads. (B) Representative reads aligned to the reference sequence (top) in exon 10 of the *PAH* gene. The boxes indicate the position with the substitution mutation (c.971T>A) as supported by 445 high-quality reads. (C) Evolutionary conservation analysis of the sequence fragment with a variant (p.P292L) in the *PAH* gene from seven species by ClustalW alignment. (D) Evolutionary conservation analysis of the sequence fragment with a variant (p.I324N) in the *PAH* gene from seven species by ClustalW alignment.

Figure S5 Venn diagrams of the number of indels detected by the two algorithms.

Table S1 List of primers in this study.

Table S2 Overview of PGM sequencing performance in all samples.

Table S3 The relationship between mean depth and mean coverage.

Table S4 List of potential variants in 93 samples.

Table S5 Phenotype and genotype in 32 kindred including 35 patients.

Author Contributions

Conceived and designed the experiments: J. Huang. Performed the experiments: GY LY J. Hao ZY JP SC. Analyzed the data: J. Huang ZC GY LL. Contributed reagents/materials/analysis tools: YG KL. Wrote the paper: J. Huang.

References

1. Song F, Qu YJ, Zhang T, Jin YW, Wang H, et al. (2005) Phenylketonuria mutations in Northern China. Mol Genet Metab 86 Suppl 1:S107–118.
2. Gu XF, Wang ZG (2004) Screening for phenylketonuria and congenital hypothyroidism in 5.8 million neonates in China. Zhonghua Yu Fang Yi Xue Za Zhi 38: 99–102.
3. Wang Z, Zhang Q (2006) Screening and treatment of hypothyrosis phenylketonuria in Jiangxi Province. Chinese journal of Birth Health & Heredity 14: 111–112.
4. Li ZY (2005) Study oon phenylketonuria in 138,988 neonatal patients. HeiLong Jiang Medicine Journal 29: 554–559.
5. Li L, Liu FX, Xiang HL (2009) Analyzing on screening and the effect of prevention from neonatal disorders. Chinese journal of Child Health Care 17: 464–465.
6. Chen GQ, Tian Y (2006) Clinical analysis of 48 children with phenylketonuria. Journal of Applied Clinical Pediatrics 21: 483–484.
7. Zhou YA, Ma YX, Zhang QB, Gao WH, Liu JP, et al. (2012) Mutations of the phenylalanine hydroxylase gene in patients with phenylketonuria in Shanxi, China. Genetics and molecular biology 35: 709–713.
8. Mitchell JJ, Trakadis YJ, Scriver CR (2011) Phenylalanine hydroxylase deficiency. Genetics in Medicine 13: 697–707.
9. Chiu YH, Chang YC, Chang YH, Niu DM, Yang YL, et al. (2012) Mutation spectrum of and founder effects affecting the PTS gene in East Asian populations. J Hum Genet 57:145–152.
10. Thöny B, Blau N (2006) Mutations in the BH 4 -Metabolizing Genes GTP Cyclohydrolase I, 6-Pyruvoyl-Tetrahydropterin Synthase, Sepiapterin Reductase, Carbinolamine-4a-Dehydratase, and Dihydropteridine Reductase. Hum Mutat 27:870–878.
11. Niederwieser A, Blau N, Wang M, Joller P, Atarés M, et al. (1984) GTP cyclohydrolase I deficiency, a new enzyme defect causing hyperphenylalaninemia with neopterin, biopterin, dopamine, and serotonin deficiencies and muscular hypotonia. Eur J Pediatr 141:208–214.
12. Rothberg JM, Hinz W, Rearick TM, Schultz J, Mileski W, et al. (2011) An integrated semiconductor device enabling non-optical genome sequencing. Nature 475:348–352.
13. Palles C, Cazier JB, Howarth KM, Domingo E, Jones AM, et al. (2013) Germline mutations affecting the proofreading domains of POLE and POLD1 predispose to colorectal adenomas and carcinomas. Nat Genet 45:136–144.
14. Yousem SA, Dacic S, Nikiforov YE, Nikiforova M (2013) Pulmonary Langerhans cell histiocytosis: profiling of multifocal tumors using next-generation sequencing identifies concordant occurrence of BRAF V600E mutations. Chest 143:1679–1684.
15. Costa JL, Sousa S, Justino A, Kay T, Fernandes S, et al. (2013) Nonoptical Massive Parallel DNA Sequencing of BRCA1 and BRCA2 Genes in a Diagnostic Setting. Hum Mutat 34:629–635.
16. Elliott AM, Radecki J, Moghis B, Li X, Kammesheidt A (2012) Rapid detection of the ACMG/ACOG-recommended 23 CFTR disease-causing mutations using ion torrent semiconductor sequencing. J Biomol Tech 23:24–30.
17. Treff NR, Fedick A, Tao X, Devkota B, Taylor D, et al. (2013) Evaluation of targeted next-generation sequencing-based preimplantation genetic diagnosis of monogenic disease. Fertil Steril 99:1377–1384.e6.
18. Blau N, Hennermann JB, Langenbeck U, Lichter-Konecki U (2011) Diagnosis, classification, and genetics of phenylketonuria and tetrahydrobiopterin (BH4) deficiencies. Mol Genet Metab 104 Suppl: S2–9.

19. Koboldt DC, Zhang Q, Larson DE, Shen D, McLellan MD, et al. (2012) VarScan 2: somatic mutation and copy number alteration discovery in cancer by exome sequencing. Genome Res 22:568–576.
20. Blau N, Erlandsen H (2014) The metabolic and molecular bases of tetrahydrobiopterin-responsive phenylalanine hydroxylase deficiency. Mol Genet Metab 82:101–111.
21. Boland JF, Chung CC, Roberson D, Mitchell J, Zhang X, et al. (2013) The new sequencer on the block: comparison of Life Technology's Proton sequencer to an Illumina HiSeq for whole-exome sequencing. Hum Genet 132:1153–1163.
22. Dworniczak B, Aulehla-Scholz C, Kalaydjieva L, Bartholomé K, Grudda K, et al. (1991) Aberrant splicing of phenylalanine hydroxylase mRNA: The major cause for phenylketonuria in parts of Southern Europe. Genomics 11:242–246.

Advantages and Versatility of Fluorescence-Based Methodology to Characterize the Functionality of LDLR and Class Mutation Assignment

Aitor Etxebarria[1], Asier Benito-Vicente[1], Ana C. Alves[2,3], Helena Ostolaza[1], Mafalda Bourbon[2,3], Cesar Martin[1]*

1 Unidad de Biofísica (CSIC, UPV/EHU) and Departamento de Bioquímica y Biología Molecular, Universidad del País Vasco, Apdo. 644, 48080 Bilbao, Spain, **2** Grupo de Investigação Cardiovascular, Unidade I&D, Departamento de Promoção da Saúde e Prevenção de Doenças Não Transmissíveis, Instituto Nacional de Saúde Dr. Ricardo Jorge, Lisboa 1649-040, Portugal, **3** Centre for Biodiversity, Functional and Integrative Genomics, Faculty of Sciences, University of Lisboa, 1749-016 Lisboa, Portugal

Abstract

Familial hypercholesterolemia (FH) is a common autosomal codominant disease with a frequency of 1:500 individuals in its heterozygous form. The genetic basis of FH is most commonly mutations within the *LDLR* gene. Assessing the pathogenicity of LDLR variants is particularly important to give a patient a definitive diagnosis of FH. Current studies of LDLR activity *ex vivo* are based on the analysis of ^{125}I-labeled lipoproteins (reference method) or fluorescent-labelled LDL. The main purpose of this study was to compare the effectiveness of these two methods to assess LDLR functionality in order to validate a functional assay to analyse *LDLR* mutations. LDLR activity of different variants has been studied by flow cytometry using FITC-labelled LDL and compared with studies performed previously with ^{125}I-labeled lipoproteins. Flow cytometry results are in full agreement with the data obtained by the ^{125}I methodology. Additionally confocal microscopy allowed the assignment of different class mutation to the variants assayed. Use of fluorescence yielded similar results than ^{125}I-labeled lipoproteins concerning LDLR activity determination, and also allows class mutation classification. The use of FITC-labelled LDL is easier in handling and disposal, cheaper than radioactivity and can be routinely performed by any group doing LDLR functional validations.

Editor: Maria Cristina Vinci, Centro Cardiologico Monzino, Italy

Funding: This work was supported by the Spanish Ministry of Economy and Competitiveness, Programa INNPACTO (grant N° IPT-2011-0817-010000) and from the Spanish Ministerio de Ciencia y Tecnología (Project BFU 2012-36241), and the Basque Government (Grupos Consolidados IT849-13 and ETORTEK Program). The authors would like to thank the Portuguese Science and Technology Foundation for A.C. Alves's PhD grant (SFRH/BD/27990/2006) and strategic project (PEst-OE/BIA/UI4046/2011). The funders had no role in study design, data collection and analysis, decision to publish, or preparation of the manuscript.

Competing Interests: The authors have declared that no competing interests exist.

* Email: cesar.martin@ehu.es

Introduction

Familial hypercholesterolemia (FH; MIM #143890) was the first genetic disease of lipid metabolism to be characterized and is mechanistically linked to the pathogenesis of coronary heart disease (CHD) [1]. FH is an autosomal codominant disorder characterized by increased plasma LDL cholesterol, tendon xanthomas, deposits of cholesterol in peripheral tissues and accelerated atherosclerosis, leading to premature coronary heart disease (CHD) [1]. FH has a heterozygous frequency of 1:500 and a homozygous frequency of 1:1,000,000, with a prevalence of 1:200,000 for compound heterozygous [2]. FH is mainly due to mutations in the LDL receptor (*LDLR*; MIM #606945) gene, which is responsible for the uptake of LDL particles into cells [1]. To date, more than 1,300 different mutations in the *LDLR* gene have been identified worldwide [3] but not all of them have been proved to affect receptor activity. Mutations have been assigned to different classes depending on their effect: class 1 mutations result in no detectable LDL receptor protein [4]; class 2 mutations cause either complete (class 2a) or partial (class 2b) block of transport of the LDL receptor from the ER [5]; class 3 mutations result in defective LDL binding [6]; class 4 mutations cause defective clustering in clathrin coated pits [7,8] and class 5 mutations result in recycling defective receptors [9]. In order to provide a definite and complete diagnosis of FH, *LDLR* mutations should be assessed both for activity and class type mutation.

In a recently reported study, *in silico* analysis of 443 described missense variants predicted a loss of LDLR activity in 89% of the described variants using at least one *in silico* method [10]. However, it is well recognized that *in silico* software has several limitations and has to be used with caution [11]. Functional validation of these LDLR variants must be assessed in order to identify which mutations lead to a functional loss of receptor activity. Once characterized, unequivocal genetic diagnosis of FH is possible, allowing the implementation of adequate treatment (either early initiation or intensification) to reduce the increased cardiovascular risk characteristic of these patients. The early identification and treatment of FH patients is especially important for young patients in whom the physical stigmata are not yet developed and so CHD can be prevented. Current methodologies, which determine LDLR functionality ex *vivo*, are based on the use of radioactivity or flow cytometry. LDL uptake and degradation of ^{125}I-labeled LDL is commonly determined in radioactivity-based methods, and very similarly, binding and uptake of LDL are determined by flow cytometry when using fluorescent-labelled LDL [6,12–17]. Both methods are used indistinctly, probably depending on the research laboratory facilities or because there is a traditional used methodology in the laboratory.

To compare the suitability of both techniques in the determination of LDLR activity with regard to sensitivity, reproducibility and practical considerations, we have conducted an inter-laboratory comparative study. Data obtained by ^{125}I assays in one of the laboratories [11] have been compared with data obtained by FITC-labelled LDL in another laboratory. We have also analysed whether the use of FITC-labelled LDL and flow cytometry is a reliable assay for the functional characterization of LDLR variants and whether the advantages of the fluorescence assay can be extended to the assignment of LDLR class type mutation. In both type of experiments CHO-*ldlA7* cells transfected with the plasmids encoding wild-type (wt) or *LDLR* variants p.Val429Leu (c.1285G>C), p.Trp490Arg (c.1468T>C), p.Ser648Pro (c.1942T>C), p.Pro685Ser (c.2053C>T) and p.Val859Met (c.2575G>A) have been used. Confocal laser microscopy was used to determine the cellular localization, class type mutation and biological activity of the mutant LDLR.

Materials and Methods

Variant nomenclature

For sequence analysis the reference sequence used was NM_000527.4 and cDNA numbering was considered following the Human Genome Variation Society nomenclature, with nucleotide c.1 being A of the ATG initiation codon p.1 [18,19].

In silico analysis

The predicted effects of *LDLR* alterations were assessed using the following open access software: PolyPhen-2 [20], Sorting Tolerant From Intolerant (SIFT) [21], Consensus Deleteriousness score of missense SNVs (Condel) [22], Mutation taster [23], Grantham Score [24] and PhyloP [25]. The PolyPhen-2 programs give predictions of "Probably Damaging", "Possibly Damaging" and "Benign". The programs SIFT and CONDEL predict whether an amino acid substitution would be "Deleterious" or "Neutral". The program Mutation Taster gives a prediction of "Disease Causing" or "Polymorphism". The program Grantham Score predicts, in a numerical form, whether an amino acid substitution is: conservative (0–50), moderately conservative (51–100), moderately radical (101–150), or radical (≥151). The program PhyloP (phylogenetic p-value) gives a prediction in a numerical form between −14.1 and 6.4 (the higher the value the most conserved the nucleotide is between species).

Site-directed mutagenesis

Individual point mutations leading to p.Val429Leu, p.Trp490Arg, p.Ser648Pro, p.Pro685Ser and p.Val859Met LDLR variants were generated as described before [11]. Presence of the desired nucleotide alteration was confirmed by PCR and restriction enzyme digestion of the appropriate fragments and the integrity of the remaining LDLR cDNA sequence of all constructs was verified by direct sequence analysis.

Expression of LDLR proteins *in vitro*

LDLR-deficient Chinese hamster ovary (CHO) cell line *ldlA7* (CHO-*ldlA7*) (kindly provided by Dr. Monty Krieger, Massachu-

Table 1. Results obtained by the different bioinformatics tools for each alteration under study.

				Pathogenicity prediction			
cDNA	**Protein**	**phyloP**	**Grantham score**	**SIFT**	**Polyphen-2**	**Mutation Taster**	**CONDEL**
c.1285G>C	p.Val429Leu	3.84	Conservative	Tolerated	Benign	Disease Causing	Neutral
c.1468T>C	p.Trp490Arg	4.48	Moderate radical	Deleterious	Probably damaging	Disease Causing	Deleterious
c.1942T>C	p.Ser648Pro	0.93	Moderate conservative	Deleterious	Probably damaging	Polymorphism	Neutral
c.2053C>T	p.Pro685Ser	5.72	Moderate conservative	Deleterious	Probably damaging	Disease Causing	Deleterious
c.2575G>A	p.Val859Met	−0.76	Conservative	Deleterious	Probably damaging	Polymorphism	Deleterious

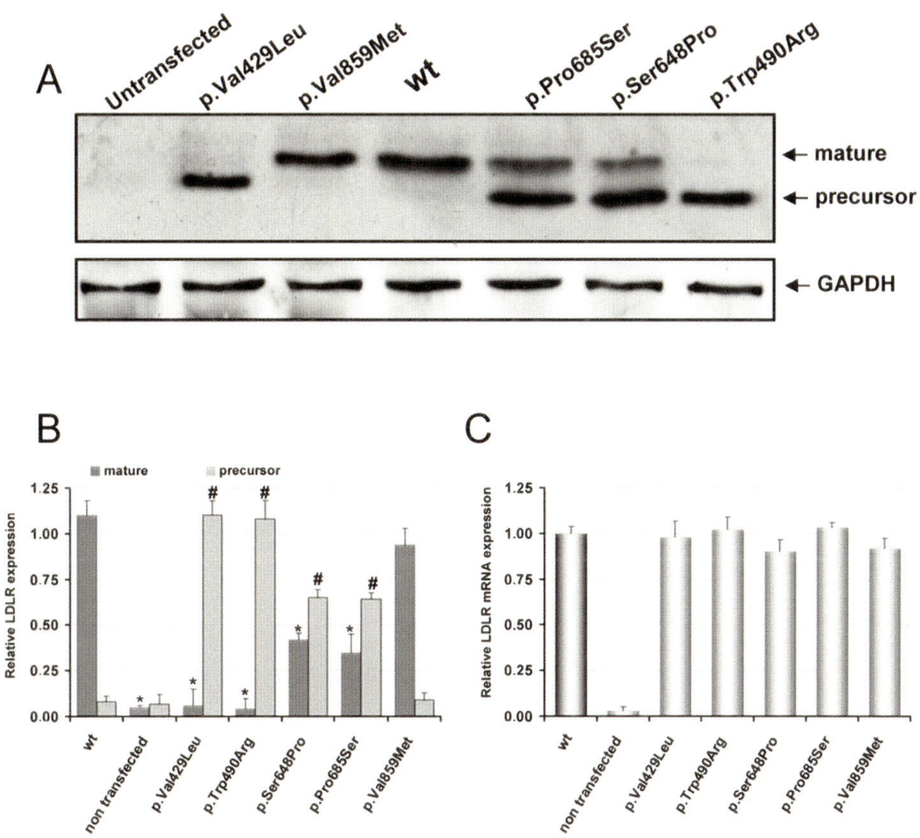

Figure 1. Protein and mRNA expression of wt LDLR and LDLR variants in CHO-*ldlA7* transfected cells. Cells were transfected with the corresponding plasmids carrying the mutations of interest, LDLR was overexpressed for 48 h and then (A) protein expression was analyzed by Western blot, (B) the relative band intensities of both mature and precursor LDLR forms were calculated as the ratio of 160 kDa or 130 kDa LDLR band intensity to that of GAPDH (C) relative LDLR mRNA expression determined by qRT-PCR (normalised to GAPDH). A representative experiment from three independently performed assays is shown in (A). The values in (B) and (C) represent the mean of triplicate determinations (n = 3) and (n = 2), respectively; error bars represent ± SD. Levels of significance were determined by a two-tailed Student's t-test, and a confidence level of greater than 95% ($p<0.05$) was used to establish statistical significance. *$p<0.001$ compared to the LDLR wt 160 kDa band and #$p<0.001$ compared to LDLR wt 130 kDa band using a Student's t-test.

setts Institute of Technology, Cambridge, MA) was cultured in Ham's F-12 medium supplemented with 5% FBS, 2 mM L-glutamine, 100 units/mL penicillin, and 100 µg/mL streptomycin. CHO-*ldlA7* cells were plated into 24 well culture plates, and transfected with plasmids carrying the *LDLR* mutations using Lipofectamine LTX and Plus Reagent (Invitrogen) according to the manufacturer's instructions. Transfected cells were maintained in culture during 48 h to achieve maximal LDLR expression.

Western blot analysis

Cell lysates were prepared, protein concentration determined, and fractionated by electrophoresis on non-reducing 8.5% SDS-PAGE for semi-quantitative immunoblotting. Membranes were immunostained with rabbit polyclonal anti-LDLR antibody (1:2000) (Cayman Chemical, Cat. No. 10007665) for 16 h at 4°C and rabbit polyclonal IgG anti-GAPDH antibody (1:1000) (Santa Cruz Biotechnology, Cat. No. SC-25778) for 1 h at room temperature and counterstained with a horseradish peroxidase-conjugated anti-rabbit antibody (Cell Signalling, Cat. No: 7074s). The signals were developed using SuperSignal West Dura Extended Substrate (Pierce Biotechnology, Rockford, IL, USA). ChemiDoc XRS (Bio-Rad, Hercules, CA, USA) was used to detect the signals, and Quantity One Basic 4.4.0 software (Bio-Rad) was used to quantify band intensities. The concentrations of the antibodies were optimized to achieve low background and a linear dose-dependent increase in signal intensity. The relative band intensities for the mature and precursor forms of LDLR protein expressed for the different constructs was calculated as the ratio between the LDLR 160 kDa or 130 kDa bands to that of GAPDH.

Real-time Quantitative PCR

CHO-*ldlA7* cells (0.5×10^6) were seeded in 6-well tissue-culture plates overnight and transfected as described before. 48 h post-transfection, RNA was harvested from cells using TRIzol Reagent (Invitrogen), and cDNA was synthesized from 1 µg of RNA using Affinity Script qRT-PCR cDNA synthesis kit (Stratagene, Agilent Technologies, USA) according to the manufacturer's instructions. The qRT-PCR was performed in triplicates using the Brilliant-III Ultra Fast SYBR Green QPCR. Primers were purchased from Integrated DNA Technologies (Cat. No. Hs.PT.58.3621384 for LDLR and, the primer sequences used to amplify hamster GAPDH gene were 5′-CATGTTCCAGTATGACTCCACTC-3′ and 5′-GGCCTCACCCCATTTGATGT-3′). Reactions were performed in the Applied Biosystems 7900HT Fast Real-Time PCR System, the real-time PCR program consisted of 40 cycles (95°C for 15 s and 60°C for 1 min) after initial 10 min incubation

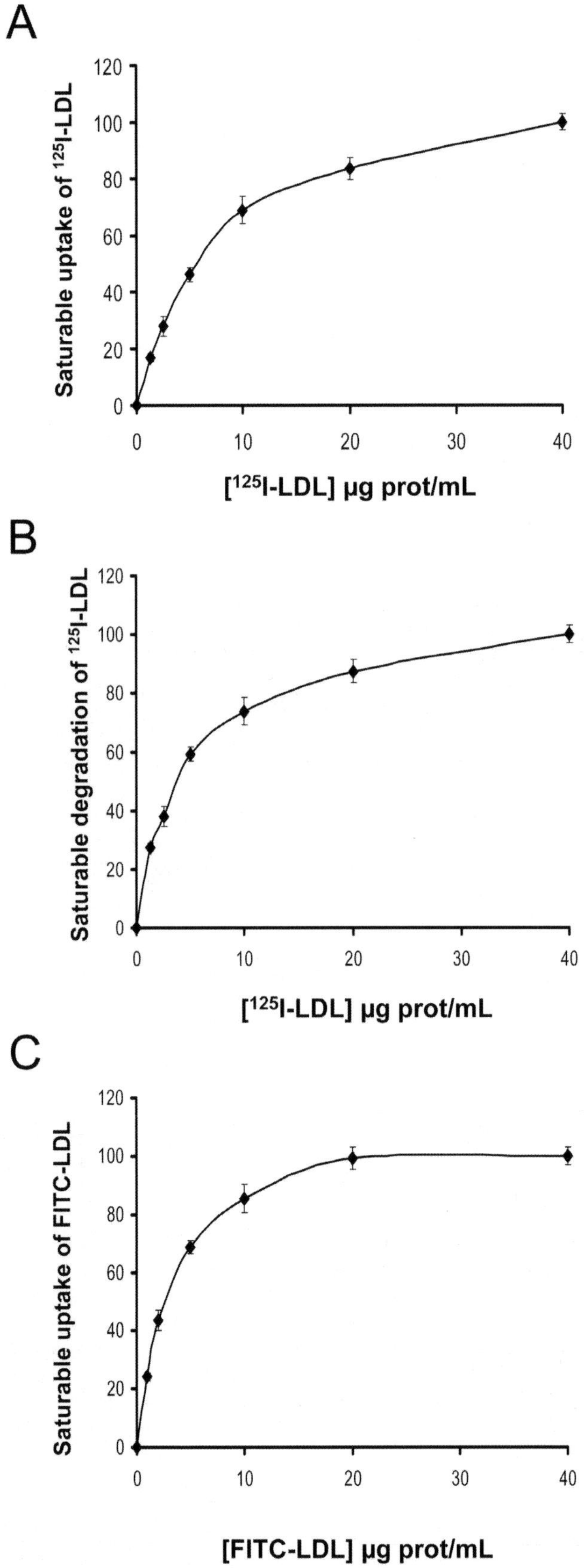

Figure 2. Saturable uptake and degradation of labeled-LDL in CHO-*ldlA7* transfected cells with wt LDLR. (A) saturable uptake of ^{125}I-LDL, (B) saturable degradation of ^{125}I-LDL and, (C) saturable uptake of FITC-LDL. For analysis of ^{125}I-LDL uptake (binding plus internalization) and degradation, CHO-*ldlA7* transfected cells expressing wt LDLR were incubated for 4 h at 37°C with increasing concentrations of ^{125}I-LDL as indicated. Subsequently, cells were assayed for cell associated radioactivity (uptake) and degradation of the protein component of LDL. Values were corrected for non-saturable association or degradation determined in the presence of an excess of unlabeled LDL (1 mg/mL). For analysis of FITC-LDL uptake, CHO-*ldlA7* transfected cells expressing wt LDLR were incubated for 4 h at 37°C with increasing concentrations of FITC-LDL as indicated. 10,000 cells were acquired in a Facscalibur and values of LDL uptake were calculated as described in Material and Methods. The values represent the mean of triplicate determinations (n = 3); error bars represent ±SD.

at 95°C. Reactions were conducted in triplicate, and expression of all transcripts relative to GAPDH was determined.

Uptake and degradation of ^{125}I-LDL

LDL catabolism in CHO-*ldlA7* cells carrying wt or LDLR variants was determined by using ^{125}I-labelled LDL as previously described [12,26]. Each LDLR variant expressing CHO-*ldlA7* cells were seeded on day 1 in 12-well plates (2×10^5 cells/dish) in triplicates to determine the ability of uptake (binding plus internalization) or degrade ^{125}I-labelled LDL. To achieve maximum LDLR expression, on day 2 cells were washed and preincubated for 12 h in growth medium containing 10% (v/v) lipoprotein-deficient serum (LPDS, Chemicon) and sterols (90 µg/mL of cholesterol and 9 µg/mL of 25(OH)-cholesterol). On day 3, cells were washed and incubated for 4 h at 37°C in medium containing 5% LPDS and different concentrations of ^{125}I-LDL. LDL uptake, determined at 37°C, accounts for both binding and internalization of LDL particles. Saturable uptake and degradation of ^{125}I-LDL were determined as the difference in cell-associated radioactivity (uptake) or the acid-soluble non-iodine radioactivity in the medium (degradation) between cells incubated with ^{125}I-LDL in the presence or absence of an excess (1 mg/mL) of unlabeled LDL, as described before [16,27]. Experiments were repeated at least twice with triplicate samples for each cell line. Data is shown as the percentage of maximum obtained for wt LDLR at 4 h.

Lipoprotein labelling with FITC

LDL was labelled with FITC as previously described [28]. Briefly, LDL (1 mg/mL) in 0.1 M $NaHCO_3$ (pH 9.0) were mixed with 10 µl/mL of FITC (2 mg/mL in dimethyl sulfoxide). The mixture was gently mixed by slow rocking at room temperature for 2 h. The unreacted dye was removed by gel filtration on a sephadex G-25 column equilibrated with PBS EDTA-free buffer. All fractions were assayed for protein content with bovine serum albumin as standard (Pierce BCA protein assay, Pierce).

Quantification of LDLR activity by flow cytometry

Transfected CHO-*ldl*A7 cells were grown in 24 well culture plates. 48 h after transfection, cells were incubated for 4 h, at 37°C or at 4°C with 20 µg/mL FITC-LDL to determine LDLR activity or LDL-LDLR binding, respectively. After incubation with FITC-LDL, CHO-*ldl*A7 cells were washed twice in PBS-1%BSA, fixed on 4% formaldehyde for 10 min and washed again twice with PBS-1%BSA. The quenching of external fluorescence, which distinguishes internalized from surface-adherent FITC-LDL particles, can be accomplished with the use of vital dyes such as Trypan blue [29], which is not able of penetrating intact cell membranes. This procedure allows to remove extracellular fluorescence by quenching and to determine the intensity of the

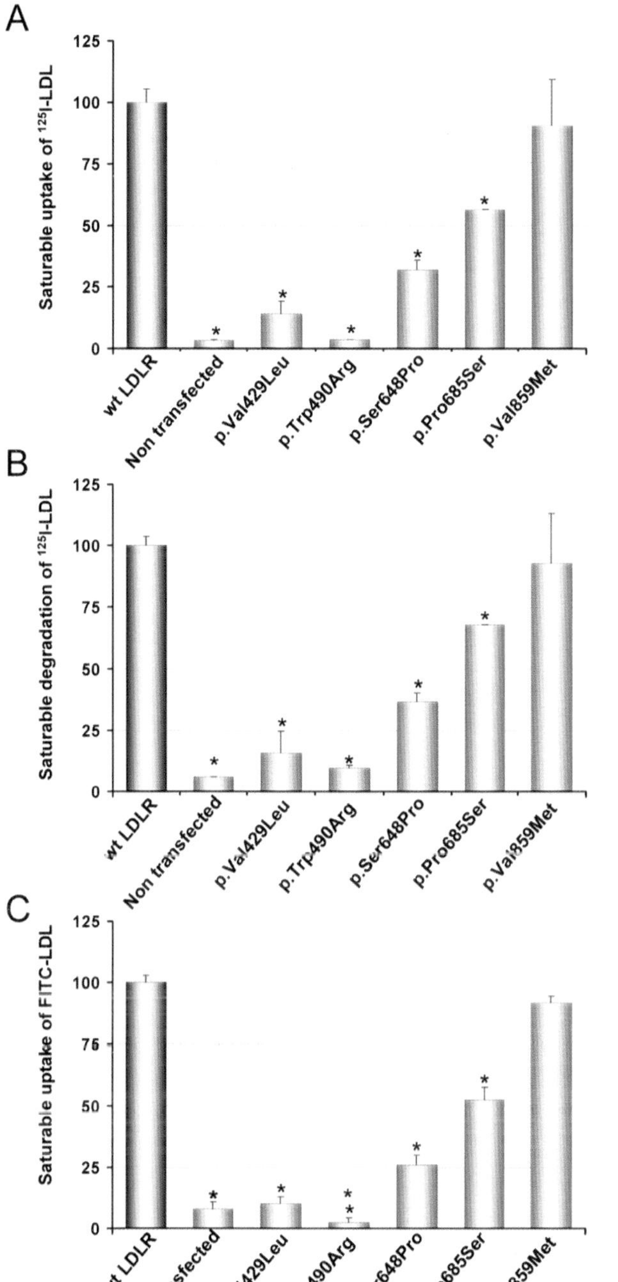

Figure 3. Uptake and degradation of labeled-LDL in CHO-*ldlA7* transfected cells with wt or different LDLR variants. (A) Uptake of ^{125}I-LDL, (B) degradation of ^{125}I-LDL and, (C) uptake of FITC-LDL. For analysis of ^{125}I-LDL uptake (binding plus internalization) and degradation, CHO-*ldlA7* transfected cells expressing wt LDLR were incubated for 4 h at 37°C with 20 µg/mL of ^{125}I-LDL as indicated. Subsequently, cells were assayed for cell associated radioactivity (uptake) and degradation of the protein component of LDL. Values were corrected for non-saturable association or degradation determined in the presence of an excess of unlabeled LDL (1 mg/mL). For analysis of FITC-LDL uptake, CHO-*ldlA7* transfected cells expressing wt LDLR were incubated for 4 h at 37°C with 20 µg/mL of FITC-LDL as indicated. 10,000 cells were acquired in a Facscalibur and values of LDL uptake were calculated as described in Material and Methods. The values represent the mean of triplicate determinations (n = 3); error bars represent ±SD. *p<0.001 compared to LDLR wt using a Student's t-test.

remaining fluorescent particles inside the cells that is not affected by the external quencher. Therefore, to determine the amount of internalized LDL, Trypan blue solution (Sigma-Aldrich, Steinheim, Germany) was added to a final concentration of 0.2% directly to the samples, eliminating the extracellular signal due to the non internalized LDLR-LDL complexes. Fluorescence intensities were measured by flow cytometry, in a Facscalibur Flow cytometer according to the manufacturer instructions as previously described [30]. For each sample, fluorescence of 10,000 events was acquired for data analysis. All measurements have been performed at least in triplicate. Uptake efficiency was corrected using the data of mature protein expression quantified by Western blot and data is shown as the percentage of maximum obtained for wt LDLR.

Quantification of LDLR expression by flow cytometry

To determine cell surface expression of LDLR by FACS, transfected CHO-*ldl*A7 cells grown during 48 h were incubated with a mouse primary antibody anti-LDLR (1:100; 5 mg/L; Progen Biotechnik GmbH, Cat. No. 61087) for 1 h, at room temperature, then, washed twice with PBS-1%BSA and incubated with a secondary antibody Alexa Fluor 488-conjugated goat anti-mouse IgG (1:100; Molecular Probes; Cat. No. A-11001). As negative controls, non transfected CHO-*ldl*A7 cells or transfected with the wt LDLR were stained with the same primary anti-LDLR antibody (Progen Biotechnik GmbH, Cat. No. 61087), which is negative for CHO-*ldl*A7 cells and, with mouse IgG2b, kappa monoclonal [MPC-11]-isotype control (abcam; Cat. No. ab18457) in identical conditions. As shown in Figure S1, isotype control antibody has no specificity for CHO-*ldl*A7 cells transfected or not with LDLR. For each sample, fluorescence of 10,000 events was acquired for data analysis. All measurements have been performed at least in triplicate. LDLR expression efficiency was corrected using the data of mature protein expression quantified by Western blot and data is shown as the percentage of maximum obtained for wt LDLR.

Confocal Laser Scanning Microscopy (CLSM)

CLSM was used to analyze expression of LDLR and colocalization of LDLR with endoplasmic reticulum (ER). Briefly, cells grown in coverslips were transfected with the *LDLR* containing plasmids and cultured for 48 h, at 37°C in 5% CO_2. Then, the medium was removed and glass slides washed twice with PBS-1%BSA. For these studies non labelled lipoproteins (20 µg/mL LDL) were added and cells were incubated at 37°C for additional 4 h. Cells were fixed with 4% paraformaldehyde during 10 min and washed three times with PBS-1%BSA and permeabilized with 1% TritonX-100 for 30 min at room temperature. Samples were then washed and blocked in PBS-10% FBS for 1 h and washed in PBS-1%BSA three times. Then, samples were incubated for 16 h at 4°C with the appropriate primary antibodies: chicken pAB anti-calreticulin (abcam; Cat. No. ab18457), and mouse mAB anti-LDLR (Progen Biotechnik GmbH, Cat. No. 61087) for calreticulin and LDLR colocalization; and, Rabbit pAB Anti-Apolipoprotein B (abcam; Cat. No. ab20737) for ApoB-100 and LDLR colocalization; followed by incubation with the appropriate fluorescent secondary antibodies: Alexa Fluor 594 Goat Anti-Chicken IgG (Molecular probes; Cat. No. sc-11042), Alexa Fluor 488 Rabbit Anti-Mouse IgG (Molecular probes; Cat. No. A-11059), Texas Red goat anti-mouse IgG (Molecular probes; Cat. No. T-862) or Alexa Fluor 488 Goat Anti-Rabbit IgG (Molecular probes; Cat. No. A-11008). Coverslips were mounted on a glass slide and samples were visualized using a confocal microscope (Olympus IX 81) with sequential excitation

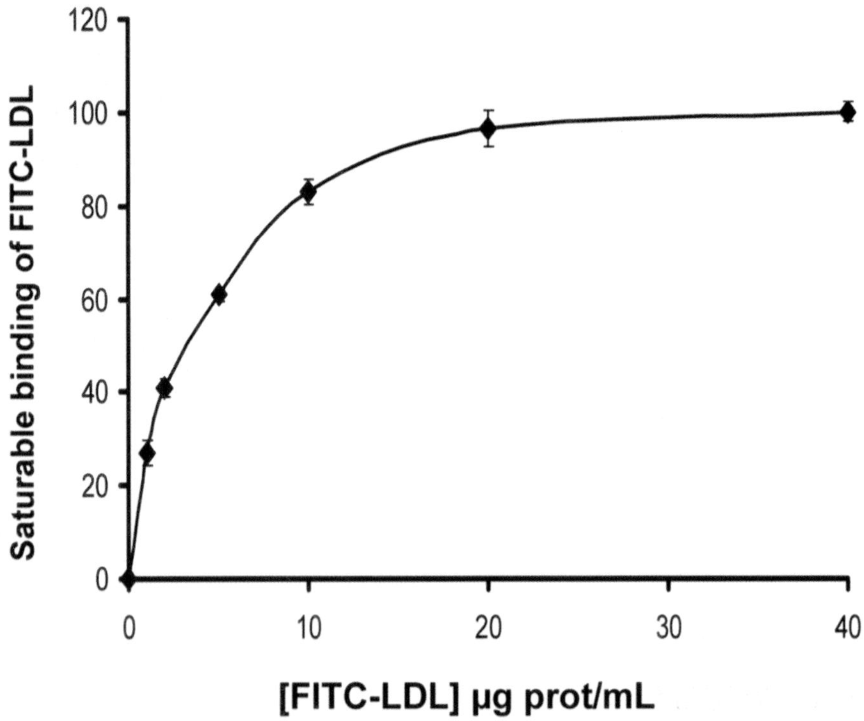

Figure 4. Saturable binding of FITC-LDL in in CHO-*ldlA7* transfected cells with wt LDLR. For analysis of FITC-LDL binding, CHO-*ldlA7* transfected cells expressing wt LDLR were incubated for 4 h at 4°C with increasing concentrations of FITC-LDL as indicated. 10,000 cells were acquired in a Facscalibur and values of LDL uptake were calculated as described in Material and Methods. The values represent the mean of triplicate determinations (n = 3); error bars represent ±SD.

and capture image acquisition with a digital camera (Axiocam NRc5, Zeiss). Images were processed with Fluoview v.50 software.

Statistical analysis

All measurements were performed at least 3 times, with n = 3 unless otherwise stated, and results are presented as mean ± standard deviation (S.D.). Levels of significance were determined by a two-tailed Student's t-test, and a confidence level of greater than 95% ($p<0.05$) was used to establish statistical significance.

Results

In silico analysis

The results obtained by different software packages are presented in Table 1.

Expression of LDLR variants in CHO-*ldl*A7 cells

Expression of LDLR in the CHO-*ldl*A7 transfected cells was assayed by immunoblotting and qRT-PCR. As shown in Figure 1A (upper panel), only the band corresponding to the LDLR mature form is detected in wt LDLR and p.Val859Met variants (Fig. 1, lanes 4 and 3, respectively); For variants p.Val429Leu and p.Trp490Arg only the band corresponding to the precursor form of the protein was detected (Fig. 1, lanes 2 and 7). In variants p.Ser648Pro and p.Pro685Ser both mature and precursor forms of LDLR were detected, being the expression of the mature protein lower compared to the wt receptor (Fig. 1, lanes 5 and 6). The extent of protein expression was determined by quantitative densitometric analysis using cytosolic GAPDH protein expression as internal control (Figure 1B). LDLR mRNA levels in the transfected cells with wt protein and LDLR variants were determined by qRT-PCR after RNA extraction as described in *Materials and Methods*. As shown in Figure 1C, the relative LDLR mRNA expression (normalised to GAPDH) of the LDLR variants resulted similar than the wt.

Uptake and degradation of ^{125}I-LDL and uptake of FITC-LDL in wt LDLR CHO-*ldlA7* transfected cells

Cell lines expressing wt LDL receptor were assayed for their ability to mediate specific, saturable uptake and degradation of ^{125}I-LDL or FITC-LDL uptake. Cells were incubated with labeled-LDL at different concentrations as indicated in *Materials and Methods*. As shown in Fig. 2, saturable activity of LDLR was reached at LDL concentrations above 10 µg/mL LDL for both ^{125}I-LDL and FITC-LDL. Statistically significant values of uptake and degradation of ^{125}I-LDL (Fig. 2A and B) or uptake of FITC-LDL (Fig. 2C) were determined at concentrations as low as 1 µg/mL. Accordingly, from these results it may be inferred that LDLR uptake activity can be determined by both methods with similar threshold of sensitivity.

Uptake and degradation of ^{125}I-LDL or FITC-LDL uptake by LDLR variants in transfected CHO-*ldlA7* cells

Cell lines expressing wt LDL receptor or the LDLR to p.Val429Leu, p.Trp490Arg, p.Ser648Pro, p.Pro685Ser and p.Val859Met variants were assayed separately by each laboratory for their LDL uptake activities [11]. For this purpose, transfected cells were incubated with 20 µg/mL of the corresponding labeled-LDL for 4 h at 37°C as indicated in *Materials and Methods*. Cells expressing variants p.Val429Leu and p.Trp490Arg showed virtually no LDL uptake or degradation of ^{125}I-LDL (Fig. 3A and B) and did not show any statistically significant uptake of

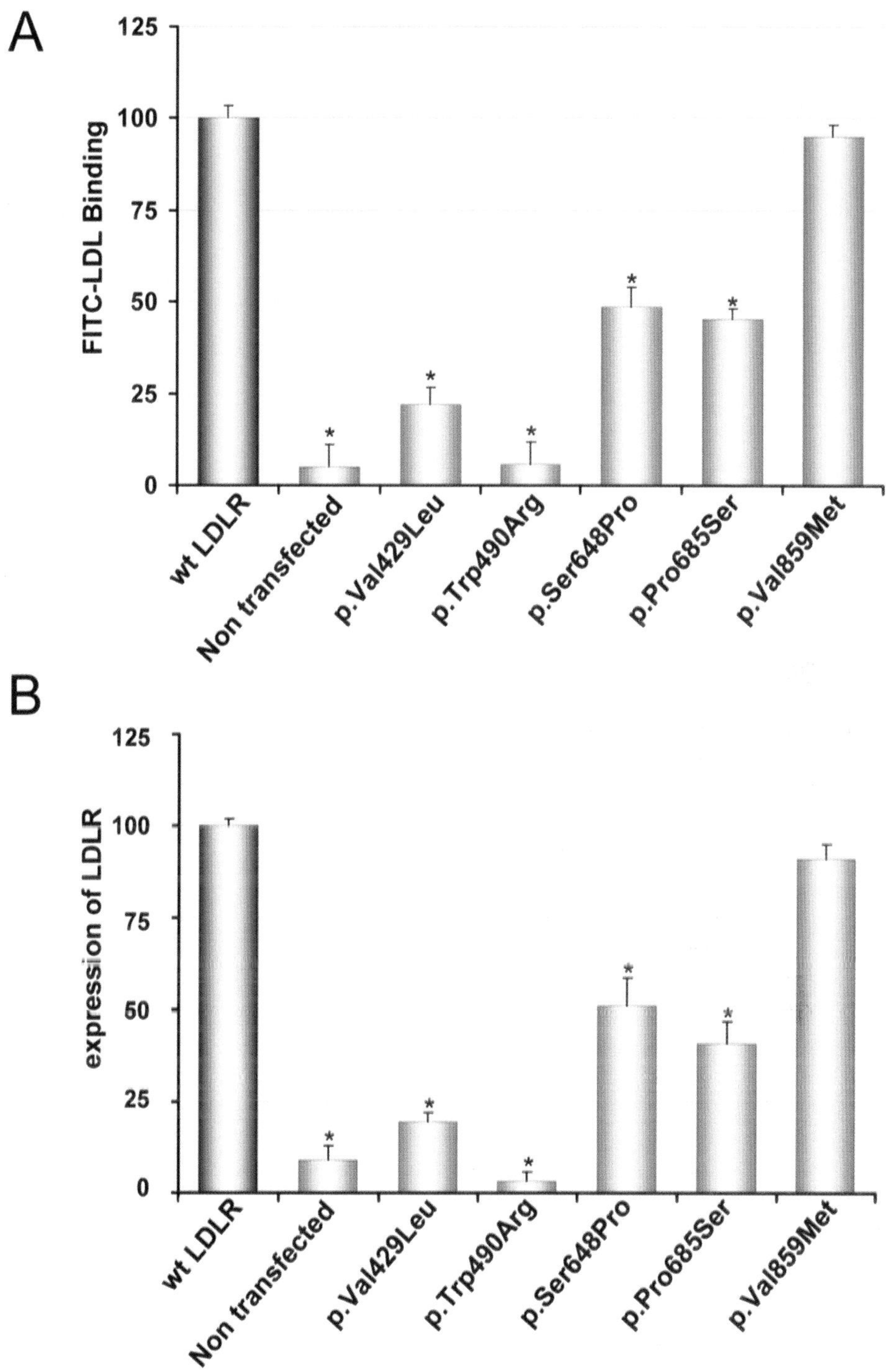

Figure 5. FITC-LDL binding and LDLR expression in CHO-*ldlA7* transfected cells with wt or different LDLR variants. (A) For analysis of FITC-LDL binding, CHO-*ldlA7* transfected cells with different LDLR variants were incubated for 4 h at 4°C with 20 µg/mL of FITC-LDL as indicated. (B) For analysis of LDLR expression, transfected cells were incubated for 48 h and then the LDLR expression at cellular membrane was determined as described in Material and Methods. 10,000 cells were acquired in a Facscalibur and values of LDL uptake were calculated as described in Material and Methods. The values represent the mean of triplicate determinations (n = 3); error bars represent ±SD. *$p<0.001$ compared to LDLR wt using a Student's t-test.

FITC-LDL when compared with non transfected CHO-*ldlA7* cells (Fig. 3C). Cells expressing variants p.Ser648Pro and p.Pro685Ser were impaired in both uptake and degradation, showing only 32% and 56%, of ^{125}I-LDL uptake capacity, respectively, and 26% and 52% uptake of FITC-LDL, respectively, when compared to cells expressing wt LDLR (Fig. 3A, and C). p.Val859Met variant presented a similar activity than the wt, both determined by uptake of ^{125}I-LDL and FITC-LDL (Fig. 3A and

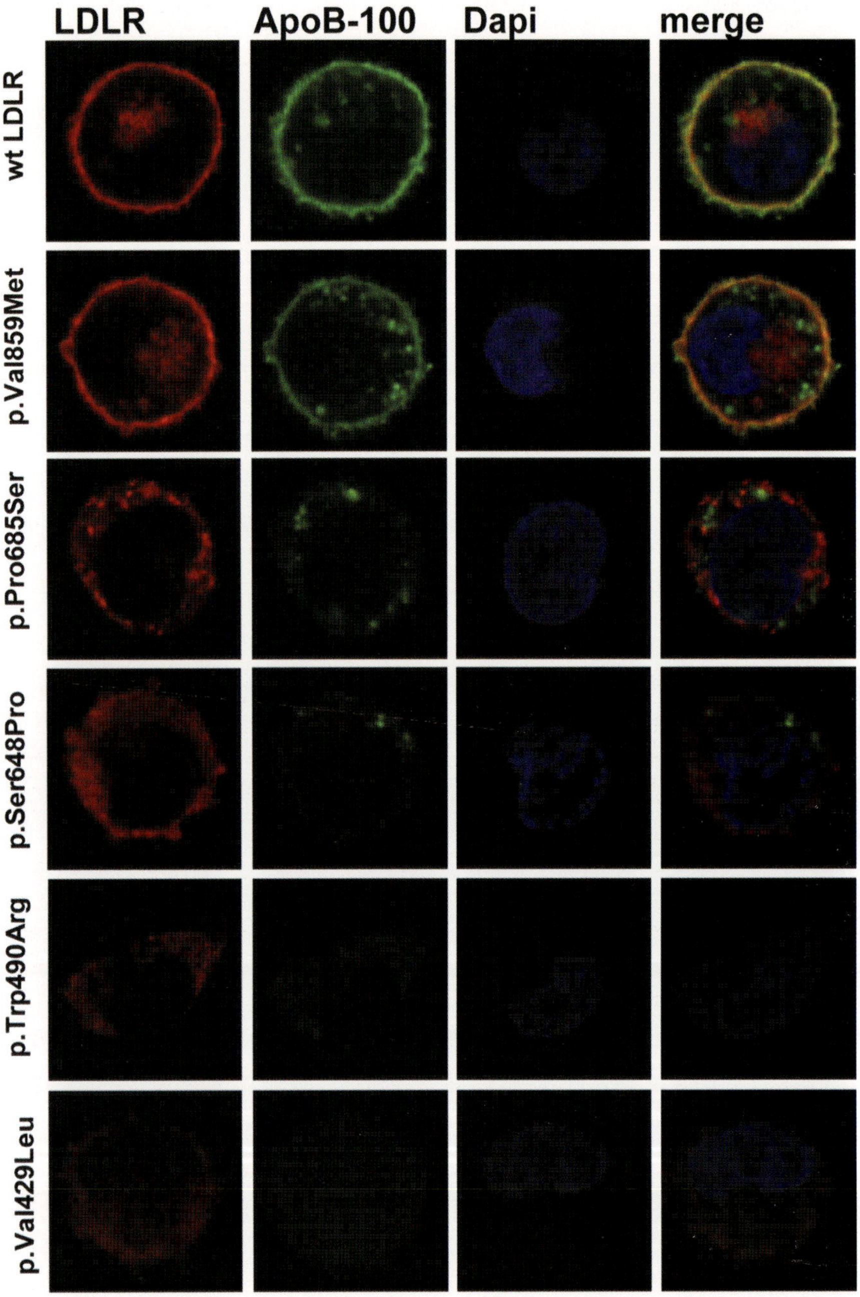

Figure 6. LDLR expression of the different variants at cell surface in CHO-*ldlA7* transfected cells. For confocal analysis of LDLR at cellular membrane and LDL uptake, CHO-*ldlA7* transfected cells were immunostained as described in Material and Methods with anti-hLDLR antibody and anti-ApoB100 antibody. Texas Red and Alexa Fluor 488 labeled secondary antibodies were used to visualize LDLR or LDL, respectively. Dapi was used to stain nuclei. The images show a representative individual cell.

C). Once again, we observed similar results when comparing data obtained by radioactivity labeling or by fluorescent labeling.

Binding of FITC-LDL to LDLR variants in CHO-*ldlA7* cells

In order to explain whether the LDL uptake differences obtained with the LDLR variants were correlated with differences in LDL binding, we used flow cytometry to determine FITC-LDL binding efficiency for each variant. Cells were incubated with 20 μg/mL FITC-LDL for 4 h at 4°C as described in *Materials and Methods*. This LDL concentration was chosen because binding saturation of FITC-LDL is achieved at [LDL] >10 μg/mL (Fig. 4). As depicted in Fig. 5A the variants p.Val429Leu, p.Trp490Arg, p.Ser648Pro and p.Pro685Ser showed a diminished binding capacity respective to wt (wt: 100±5; p.Val429Leu: 22±4, p.Trp490Arg: 5.8±5, p.Ser648Pro: 48±5 and p.Pro685Ser: 45±3) (Fig. 5A), while the binding efficiency of p.Val859Met was similar to the wt (wt: 100±5; p.Val859Met: 95±3, $p>0.26$). Therefore, the binding data were in agreement with the uptake values obtained for the different LDLR variants.

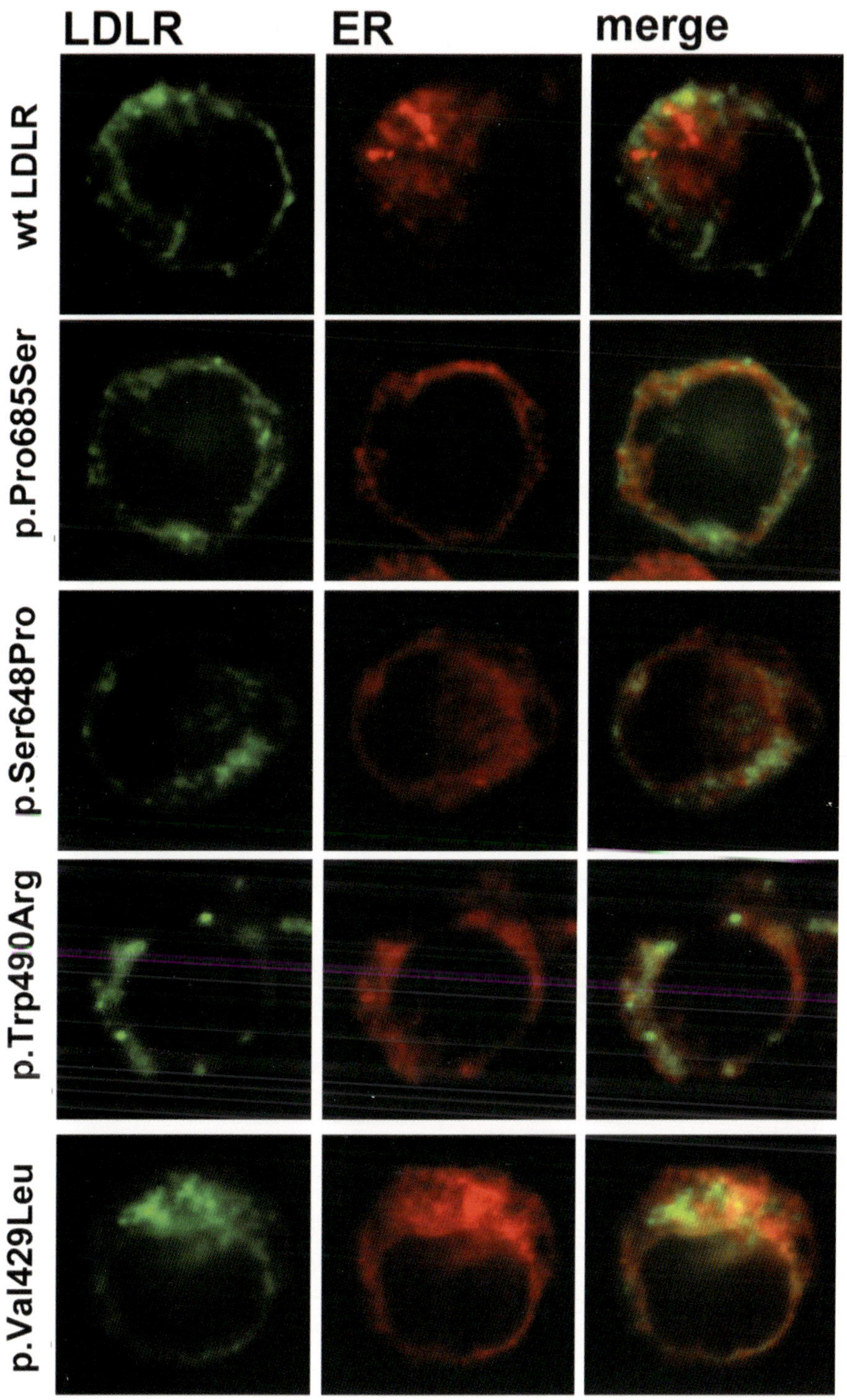

Figure 7. LDLR colocalization wit ER of the different variants in CHO-*ldlA7* transfected cells. For confocal analysis of colocalization of LDLR with ER, CHO-*ldlA7* transfected cells were immunostained as described in Material and Methods with anti-hLDLR antibody and anti-calreticulin antibody. Alexa Fluor 488 and Texas Red labeled secondary antibodies were used to visualize LDLR or calreticulin, respectively. The images show a representative individual cell.

Expression of LDLR variants in CHO-*ldlA7* cells

The surface expression of the LDLR was quantified by flow cytometry (Fig. 5B). For p.Val859Met variant the amount of LDLR detected was very similar to the wt LDLR (wt: 100±2; p.Val859Met: 91±4; $p>0.15$) (Fig. 5B). For p.Pro685Ser and p.Ser648Pro variants LDLR expression was approximately the half with respect to wt (wt: 100±2; p.Pro685Ser: 41±6 and p.Ser648Pro: 51±7). In the case of p.Val429Leu and p.Trp490Arg variants there was not significant receptor expression, which agrees with the data of LDL uptake and binding (Fig. 3 and Fig. 5A).

Intracellular localization of LDLR variants and class mutation assignment

Confocal microscopy was used to corroborate the failure of receptor expression or LDLR class mutation. Cells expressing wt or LDLR variants were incubated with LDL for 4 h and then immunostained with the appropriate antibodies to determine LDLR and LDL localization within the cell. Texas Red or FITC-conjugated secondary antibodies were used to visualize LDLR and LDL, respectively. As shown in Fig. 6, p.Ser648Pro and p.Pro685Ser variants showed a diminished receptor expression and, p.Trp490Arg and p.Val429Leu variants did not express significant amount of receptor. In agreement with the LDLR expression results obtained by cytometry, confocal images of p.Val859Met variant showed a pattern of LDLR expression similar to the wt. Additionally, we analyzed the intracellular localization of these variants to figure out their class defect, thus colocalization of these variants with calreticulin, a specific marker of the endoplasmic reticulum (ER) was assayed (Fig. 7) According to the results, colocalization of p.Trp490Arg and p.Val429Leu with ER indicates that these LDLR variants are class 2a mutant receptors with a completely defective transport from the ER to the Golgi apparatus. Regarding p.Pro685Ser and p.Ser648Pro variants, confocal images showed a partial retention of LDLR in the ER, thus the transport to the membrane is partially blocked indicating that these variants belong to class 2b mutant receptors.

A detailed analysis of p.Trp490Arg (Figure S2) shows that Trp490 residing in the YWTD repeat maintains apolar interactions with the surrounding amino acids which can not be maintained when substituted by Arginine in p.Trp490Arg mutant. Regarding p.Val429Leu, as shown in Figure S3, it is possible that the replacement of Val by a bigger amino acid as leucine does not allow the correct folding of two β-sheets. These effects may be responsible of retention of the two mutants in the ER, thus causing class 2a defects. The partial retention of LDLR in the ER occurring in class 2b mutants p.Ser648Pro and p.Pro685Ser may be related to structural modifications introduced by the amino acid replacement (Figures S4 and S5). Regarding p.Ser648Pro mutant, in wt LDLR, S648 is located in the first β-sheet of the sixth YWTD blade, adjacent to a proline that facilitates a turn to form the central barrel of the β-propeller. The replacement of Ser648 by Pro, leading two consecutive prolines, could disturb in someway the structure of the β-propeller (Figure S4). Pro685, located in the EGF-C domain of the LDL-receptor, has been identified as one of the necessary residues involved in the packing of this domain [31]. It has been described that Pro685 establishes hydrophobic interactions into a groove of the β-propeller with Val529 and Tyr532. As shown in Figure S5, the replacement of Pro685 by a serine could interfere in these interactions due to its polarity.

Discussion

CHD is the most common type of heart disease and the leading cause of global morbidity and mortality in adults contributing to at least one in every three deaths each year [32–34]. FH patients, if untreated, have an increased risk of developing premature CHD but this can be prevented by early identification and consequent implementation of lipid lowering medication. There are a number of criteria for diagnosing FH phenotypically in adults, but clinical identification is not sufficient to identify a FH patient [35]. Increasing emphasis on genetic testing has become a clear example of how new genome technologies can contribute to the benefit of patients, but only the identification of a functional FH-causing mutation in an individual provides a definitive diagnosis. To date, more than 1300 genetic variants in the *LDLR* have been described so far, and approximately 80–90% have been designated as potentially pathogenic [3,10,36] although the great majority do not have functional studies [3]. The early and definitive identification of FH is important to improve patient prognosis by the implementation of adequate treatment to prevent premature CHD, especially effective in younger individuals. [37] and, would also save large amounts of money to health services [38].

Nowadays, studies of LDLR functionality *ex vivo* are carried out mainly by radioactivity assays based on measurement of binding, uptake and degradation of ^{125}I-labeled LDL or by fluorescence-based procedures. For many years the reference method to estimate LDLR activity has been the radioactive assay [39]. However approaches using fluorescently-labelled LDL have also been described and allow determination of LDL binding and uptake by flow cytometry [11,14,30]. Radioactive assay has the advantage of being very sensitive, but it also has serious drawbacks such as the risk of exposure to radioisotopes for experimenters and colleagues, or the difficulties and ethical considerations of nuclear waste elimination procedures. In contrast, the use of fluorimetric assays based on covalent labelling of LDL with fluorophores such as FITC overcomes many of the aforementioned problems associated with radiolabeling. Labeling of LDL with FITC is an inexpensive procedure, approximately 40 times cheaper than ^{125}I-labeling, and stable fluorophore-protein complex can be obtained, quickly and simply and radioactivity-handling drawbacks are avoided.

In this work we have validated the fluorimetric assay by comparing LDLR activities of previously validated variants by the reference method [39] with the activities of the same variants determined by FACS. In LDLR activity characterization (binding and uptake) by ^{125}I-labeling and FITC-LDL, the results were very similar, both in sensitivity as in accuracy (Fig. 2 and 4). In addition, flow cytometry allowed the quantification of LDLR expression at the cell surface (Fig. 4 and 5), providing a better characterization of the defect associated to each mutation. In fact, by complementation of flow cytometry assays with confocal microscopy, which allows detection of the subcellular localization of the LDLR synthesized, it is possible to assign the class type of each variant studied.

To conclude, the data presented here show that flow cytometry using FITC-labeled LDL is a reliable and accurate methodology to determine LDLR activity. This method combined with the use of confocal microscopy offers the possibility of class type assignment for LDLR mutants, thus contributing to improve the diagnosis of FH. In sum, fluorescence-based methodology is a highly recommendable option to be used for the functional analysis of LDLR variants before reporting any variant for genetic testing.

Furthermore, the increasing genotyping results obtained by the next generation sequencing technique is providing a higher number of variants that will need functional validation. Thus, the validated methodology will be of great importance to validate functionally the described and novel alterations in order to provide an accurate diagnosis of FH.

Supporting Information

Figure S1 Specificity of LDLR antibody in in wt LDLR transfected and non transfected CHO-*ldl*A7 cells. Cells grown during 48 h were incubated with a mouse primary antibody anti-LDLR or with mouse IgG2b, kappa monoclonal [MPC-11]-isotype control as described in *Materials and Methods*. 10,000 cells were acquired in a Facscalibur and values of LDL uptake were calculated as described in Material and Methods. The values represent the mean of triplicate determinations (n = 3); error bars represent ±SD. *p<0.001 compared to LDLR wt using a Student's t-test.

Figure S2 Structure of the blades maintained by the Trp located in the YWTD repeats of the β-propeller. (A) Hydrophobic contacts of the Trp with the surrounding residues, and the water mediated hydrogen bound between the indol group of tryptophan and one carboxylate group of an adjacent Asp maintain the blade-structures. (B) Replacement of Trp490 by an Asn impairs hydrophobic interactions. This figure was prepared with PyMOL (DeLano scientifics) (PDB:1N7D).

Figure S3 Structure of the Val429 and surrounding amino acids (A). Val429 allows the correct packing of the structure maintaining hydrophobic contacts. Leu429 introduces very little change in size, but maybe sufficient to impair a correct folding of the protein (B). This figure was prepared with PyMOL (DeLano scientifics) (PDB:1IJQ).

Figure S4 Structure of the β-propeller central barrel (A). The prolines located at the beginning of each β-sheet allow a better turn to form the barrel. Two consecutive prolines could disturb the structure (B). This figure was prepared with PyMOL (DeLano scientifics) (PDB:1N7D) (PDB:3S06).

Figure S5 Structure of the interface of β-propeller in green and EGF-C in blue (A). Pro685 establishes hydrophobic contacts with β-propeller. Ser685, due to its polarity could disturb this contact (B). This figure was prepared with PyMOL (DeLano scientifics) (PDB:1N7D) (PDB:3S06).

Acknowledgments

Technical and human support provided by SGIker (Analytical and High-Resolution Microscopy in Biomedicine Service of the UPV/EHU) and Rocío Alonso for excellent technical assistance are gratefully acknowledged. We thank Prof. A. Gómez-Muñoz for flow cytometry facilities, and Dr. Monty Krieger for kindly providing *CHO-ldlA7* cells.

Author Contributions

Conceived and designed the experiments: MB CM. Performed the experiments: AE AB-V ACA. Analyzed the data: MB HO CM. Contributed to the writing of the manuscript: CM MB.

References

1. Goldstein JL HH, Brown MS (2001) Familial hypercholesterolemia; C.R. Scriver ALB, W.S. Sly and D. Valle, Editors, editor. New York McGraw-Hill.
2. Ned RM, Sijbrands EJ (2011) Cascade Screening for Familial Hypercholesterolemia (FH). PLoS Curr 3: RRN1238.
3. Usifo E, Leigh SE, Whittall RA, Lench N, Taylor A, et al. (2012) Low-density lipoprotein receptor gene familial hypercholesterolemia variant database: update and pathological assessment. Ann Hum Genet 76: 387–401.
4. Hobbs HH, Leitersdorf E, Goldstein JL, Brown MS, Russell DW (1988) Multiple crm- mutations in familial hypercholesterolemia. Evidence for 13 alleles, including four deletions. J Clin Invest 81: 909–917.
5. Goldstein JL, Brown MS, Anderson RG, Russell DW, Schneider WJ (1985) Receptor-mediated endocytosis: concepts emerging from the LDL receptor system. Annu Rev Cell Biol 1: 1–39.
6. Hobbs HH, Brown MS, Goldstein JL (1992) Molecular genetics of the LDL receptor gene in familial hypercholesterolemia. Hum Mutat 1: 445–466.
7. Davis CG, Lehrman MA, Russell DW, Anderson RG, Brown MS, et al. (1986) The J.D. mutation in familial hypercholesterolemia: amino acid substitution in cytoplasmic domain impedes internalization of LDL receptors. Cell 45: 15–24.
8. Lehrman MA, Goldstein JL, Brown MS, Russell DW, Schneider WJ (1985) Internalization-defective LDL receptors produced by genes with nonsense and frameshift mutations that truncate the cytoplasmic domain. Cell 41: 735–743.
9. Beglova N, Jeon H, Fisher C, Blacklow SC (2004) Cooperation between fixed and low pH-inducible interfaces controls lipoprotein release by the LDL receptor. Mol Cell 16: 281–292.
10. Leigh SE, Foster AH, Whittall RA, Hubbart CS, Humphries SE (2008) Update and analysis of the University College London low density lipoprotein receptor familial hypercholesterolemia database. Ann Hum Genet 72: 485–498.
11. Silva S, Alves AC, Patel D, Malho R, Soutar AK, et al. (2012) In vitro functional characterization of missense mutations in the LDLR gene. Atherosclerosis 225: 128–134.
12. Knight BL, Soutar AK (1982) Changes in the metabolism of modified and unmodified low-density lipoproteins during the maturation of cultured blood monocyte-macrophages from normal and homozygous familial hypercholesterolaemic subjects. Eur J Biochem 125: 407–413.
13. Leren TP, Tonstad S, Gundersen KE, Bakken KS, Rodningen OK, et al. (1997) Molecular genetics of familial hypercholesterolaemia in Norway. J Intern Med 241: 185–194.
14. Ranheim T, Kulseth MA, Berge KE, Leren TP (2006) Model system for phenotypic characterization of sequence variations in the LDL receptor gene. Clin Chem 52: 1469–1479.
15. Romano M, Di Taranto MD, Mirabelli P, D'Agostino MN, Iannuzzi A, et al. (2011) An improved method on stimulated T-lymphocytes to functionally characterize novel and known LDLR mutations. J Lipid Res 52: 2095–2100.
16. Sun XM, Patel DD, Knight BL, Soutar AK (1997) Comparison of the genetic defect with LDL-receptor activity in cultured cells from patients with a clinical diagnosis of heterozygous familial hypercholesterolemia. The Familial Hypercholesterolaemia Regression Study Group. Arterioscler Thromb Vasc Biol 17: 3092–3101.
17. Tada H, Kawashiri MA, Noguchi T, Mori M, Tsuchida M, et al. (2009) A novel method for determining functional LDL receptor activity in familial hypercholesterolemia: application of the CD3/CD28 assay in lymphocytes. Clin Chim Acta 400: 42–47.
18. den Dunnen JT, Antonarakis SE (2000) Mutation nomenclature extensions and suggestions to describe complex mutations: a discussion. Hum Mutat 15: 7–12.
19. Taschner PE, den Dunnen JT (2011) Describing structural changes by extending HGVS sequence variation nomenclature. Hum Mutat 32: 507–511.
20. Adzhubei IA, Schmidt S, Peshkin L, Ramensky VE, Gerasimova A, et al. (2010) A method and server for predicting damaging missense mutations. Nat Methods 7: 248–249.
21. Ng PC, Henikoff S (2003) SIFT: Predicting amino acid changes that affect protein function. Nucleic Acids Res 31: 3812–3814.
22. Gonzalez-Perez A, Lopez-Bigas N (2011) Improving the assessment of the outcome of nonsynonymous SNVs with a consensus deleteriousness score, Condel. Am J Hum Genet 88: 440–449.
23. Schwarz JM, Rodelsperger C, Schuelke M, Seelow D (2010) MutationTaster evaluates disease-causing potential of sequence alterations. Nat Methods 7: 575–576.
24. Grantham R (1974) Amino acid difference formula to help explain protein evolution. Science 185: 862–864.
25. Pollard KS, Hubisz MJ, Rosenbloom KR, Siepel A (2010) Detection of nonneutral substitution rates on mammalian phylogenies. Genome Res 20: 110–121.
26. Goldstein JL, Brown MS (1974) Binding and degradation of low density lipoproteins by cultured human fibroblasts. Comparison of cells from a normal subject and from a patient with homozygous familial hypercholesterolemia. J Biol Chem 249: 5153–5162.
27. Soutar AK, Knight BL, Patel DD (1989) Identification of a point mutation in growth factor repeat C of the low density lipoprotein-receptor gene in a patient with homozygous familial hypercholesterolemia that affects ligand binding and intracellular movement of receptors. Proc Natl Acad Sci U S A 86: 4166–4170.
28. Dardik R, Varon D, Tamarin I, Zivelin A, Salomon O, et al. (2000) Homocysteine and oxidized low density lipoprotein enhanced platelet adhesion to endothelial cells under flow conditions: distinct mechanisms of thrombogenic modulation. Thromb Haemost 83: 338–344.
29. Hed J, Hallden G, Johansson SG, Larsson P (1987) The use of fluorescence quenching in flow cytofluorometry to measure the attachment and ingestion phases in phagocytosis in peripheral blood without prior cell separation. J Immunol Methods 101: 119–125.
30. Etxebarria A, Palacios L, Stef M, Tejedor D, Uribe KB, et al. (2012) Functional characterization of splicing and ligand-binding domain variants in the LDL receptor. Hum Mutat 33: 232–243.
31. Jeon H, Meng W, Takagi J, Eck MJ, Springer TA, et al. (2001) Implications for familial hypercholesterolemia from the structure of the LDL receptor YWTD-EGF domain pair. Nat Struct Biol 8: 499–504.
32. Minino AM, Xu J, Kochanek KD, Tejada-Vera B (2009) Death in the United States, 2007. NCHS Data Brief: 1–8.
33. Terzic A, Waldman S (2011) Chronic diseases: the emerging pandemic. Clin Transl Sci 4: 225–226.
34. Waldman SA, Terzic A (2011) Cardiovascular health: the global challenge. Clin Pharmacol Ther 90: 483–485.

35. Alves AC, Medeiros AM, Francisco V, Gaspar IM, Rato Q, et al. (2010) Molecular diagnosis of familial hypercholesterolemia: an important tool for cardiovascular risk stratification. Rev Port Cardiol 29: 907–921.
36. Haase A, Goldberg AC (2012) Identification of people with heterozygous familial hypercholesterolemia. Curr Opin Lipidol 23: 282–289.
37. Nordestgaard BG, Chapman MJ, Humphries SE, Ginsberg HN, Masana L, et al. (2013) Familial hypercholesterolaemia is underdiagnosed and undertreated in the general population: guidance for clinicians to prevent coronary heart disease: consensus statement of the European Atherosclerosis Society. Eur Heart J 34: 3478–3490a.
38. Brice P, Burton H, Edwards CW, Humphries SE, Aitman TJ (2013) Familial hypercholesterolaemia: a pressing issue for European health care. Atherosclerosis 231: 223–226.
39. Brown MS, Goldstein JL (1975) Regulation of the activity of the low density lipoprotein receptor in human fibroblasts. Cell 6: 307–316.

The Effect of Recombinant Human Iduronate-2-Sulfatase (Idursulfase) on Growth in Young Patients with Mucopolysaccharidosis Type II

Zbigniew Żuber[1], Agnieszka Różdżyńska-Świątkowska[2], Agnieszka Jurecka[3,4]*, Anna Tylki-Szymańska[5]

1 Department of Pediatrics, S. Louis Regional Children's Hospital, Cracow, Poland, **2** Anthropology Laboratory, The Children's Memorial Health Institute, Warsaw, Poland, **3** Department of Molecular Biology, University of Gdańsk, Gdańsk, Poland, **4** Department of Medical Genetics, The Children's Memorial Health Institute, Warsaw, Poland, **5** Department of Pediatrics, Nutrition and Metabolic Diseases, The Children's Memorial Health Institute, Warsaw, Poland

Abstract

Mucopolysaccharidosis type II (MPS II; Hunter syndrome) is an X-linked, recessive, lysosomal storage disorder caused by deficiency of iduronate-2-sulfatase. Early bone involvement leads to decreased growth velocity and short stature in nearly all patients. Our analysis aimed to investigate the effects of enzyme replacement therapy (ERT) with idursulfase (Elaprase) on growth in young patients with mucopolysaccharidosis type II. Analysis of longitudinal anthropometric data of MPS II patients (group 1, n = 13) who started ERT before 6 years of age (range from 3 months to 6 years, mean 3.6 years, median 4 years) was performed and then compared with retrospective analysis of data for MPS II patients naïve to ERT (group 2, n = 50). Patients in group 1 received intravenous idursulfase at a standard dose of 0.58 mg/kg weekly for 52–288 weeks. The course of average growth curve for group 1 was very similar to growth pattern in group 2. The average value of body height in subsequent years in group 1 was a little greater than in group 2, however, the difference was not statistically significant. In studied patients with MPS II, idursulfase did not appear to alter the growth patterns.

Editor: Raphael Schiffmann, Baylor Research Institute, United States of America

Funding: The authors have no support or funding to report.

Competing Interests: The authors have declared that no competing interests exist.

* E-mail: ajurecka@gmail.com

Introduction

Mucopolysaccharidosis type II (MPS II, Hunter syndrome, OMIM# 309900) is caused by the deficiency of the enzyme iduronate-2-sulfatase (I2S; EC 3.1.6.13) that is responsible for breaking down heparan and dermatan sulfate (HS and DS) within the cells [1]. It is a rare and life-limiting X-linked recessive disorder that affects approximately 1 in 77,000 newborn boys [2,3]. Girls are affected rarely [4].

MPS II leads to profound disruption in the normal mechanism of growth and development and a major feature of this disorder is abnormal bone and cartilage development [1]. These abnormalities arise from a lack of skeletal remodeling, disordered endochondral and intramembranous ossification, disruption of normal elastogenesis and the infiltration by GAGs [5]. It has been shown that inflammation secondary to GAG accumulation is a critical aspect of MPS disorder and contributes to the bone disease [6].

Infants with MPS II appear normal at birth, and early developmental milestones may also be within normal range; in the first years of life height of most patients with MPS II is above 50th percentile and in some cases is over the 97th percentile. However, growth velocity decreases with age: by the age of 8 years, height is below the 3rd percentile and nearly all patients exhibit growth retardation before puberty [7,8].

Currently, both hematopoietic stem cell transplantation (HSCT) and enzyme replacement therapy (ERT) using idursulfase (recombinant human 2IS, Elaprase, Shire Human Genetic Therapies, Inc., Lexington, MA, USA) are available for MPS II. ERT has been shown to be effective in ameliorating some of the clinical manifestation of MPS disease. Long-term effect of ERT on the natural history of growth patterns is less clear and detailed data on the impact of ERT on growth are very limited [9–11].

The aim of this study was to analyze the effect of ERT with idursulfase on growth in 13 young MPS II patients who began ERT before the age of 6 years.

Materials and Methods

Study design

The study objective was to evaluate the effectiveness of idursulfase on body height in young patients with MPS II by comparing a natural growth pattern in children with MPS II naïve to ERT with growth of MPS II patients who started ERT before 6 years of age.

All patients were enrolled at The Children's Memorial Health Institute (CMHI) in Poland. The clinical decisions for the patients were made by the clinicians/researchers (ATS, ZZ).

Patients

All patients enrolled in the study had to have a diagnosis of MPS II confirmed by the biochemical determination of iduronate-2-sulfatase deficiency in leukocytes and by molecular analysis. The patients were divided in two following groups:

Group 1. The first group consisted of 13 patients who had a diagnosis of MPS type II confirmed by biochemical and molecular analysis and started ERT before the age of 6 years. The demographic characteristics of these thirteen MPS II patients are listed in Table 1.

Group 2. The second group consisted of 50 patients who were naïve to ERT.

Since 1989 till 2009, a longitudinal growth study was performed at The Children's Memorial Health Institute (CMHI), Warsaw, Poland. The study population contained patients with MPS II (n = 50) aged from 0.5 to 21 years (mean 8.2 years, median 8.5 years). All patients had the severe (neurological) form of disease. All patients were born at term, and presented with the typical clinical features of MPS and had a diagnosis of MPS type II confirmed by biochemical and molecular analysis (median age of diagnosis 3 years).

All patients were naïve to ERT during the time of the study. These patients can be divided into two groups: 1) patients who have never been treated with idursulfase as they died before the introduction of ERT in Poland and 2) patients who received ERT later in life, but had anthropometric measurements performed before the introduction of ERT. In general, patients in group 1 were more recently diagnosed than patients in group 2, but there was no selection bias.

Ethical consideration

The protocol was approved by the human-subjects institutional review board at The Children's Memorial Health Institute. Written informed consent had to be provided by the parents or legal guardians.

Elaprase treatment

All patients received weekly intravenous infusions idursulfase (Elaprase, Shire Human Genetic Therapies, Lexington, MA) at a standard dose of 0.58 mg/kg. The treatment was done according to the standard care and was administered by the clinicians/ researchers (ATS, ZZ).

Evaluation of efficacy

The primary efficacy endpoint variable was body height. This efficacy measure was taken once periodically during treatment (at weeks 24, 48, 72, 96 weeks and annually after the 96th week). Until the age of 3 years length was measured in the supine position using a liberometer (accuracy to 1 mm). The same measurements of the older children were performed as standing height using a stadiometer (accuracy to 1 mm). Weight was measured using an electronic scale accurate within 0.05 kg. A non-stretchable tape was used to assess head and chest circumference (accuracy to 5 mm). The same anthropologist performed all assessments.

Statistical analysis

The data for group 1 and 2 was divided into 24 calendar age classes. Children between 6 and 36 months of life were then categorized into age groups of 3 months, while patients between 3 and 21 years of life into groups of 1 year. The degree and direction of deviations of studied features in children with MPS II were analyzed using the data standardization method and the calculated values were presented as z-scores.

All measurements were standardized for age and gender using the Polish body growth reference charts [12]. The resulting z-scores were used in all calculations. Descriptive statistics, including means and z-scores were calculated using Statistica 7 PL (Statsoft, Poland). Two-tailed t-tests were used to compare mean standardized values for body height between groups 1 and 2.

Table 1. Patient characteristics (demographic, molecular characteristics and clinical phenotypes).

Patient No.	Age (y.) Diagnosis	Age (y.) Baseline	Age (y.) Current	Total idursulfase exposure (week)	Mutations	Phenotype
1	2	5.75	11	198	deletion of IDS gene	neurological
2	4	5.5	11	159	c.1001 A>C	neurological
3	4	4.5	7.5	156	intragenic inversion	neurological
4	3	4	8	164	c.998C>T p.Ser333Leu	neurological
5	2	4	8	188	c.950_95delCT	neurological
6	3	3.5	8	188	c.998C>T	neurological
7	3	3	7	188	intragenic inversion	neurological
8	3	4	8	188	c.1135_1136insGTAA p.Pro379Argfsx8	neurological
9	3	4	8	164	Ivs2+29G→C	neurological
10	1	2	deceased	52	deletion xq28	neurological
11	2	3	5	92	c.1007G>A p.Gly336Glu	neurological
12	1/12	3/12	6	288	c.1568A>G	attenuated
13	3	3	6.5	164	c.998C>T p.Ser333Leu	neurological

The study has been reported according to STROBE guidelines.

Results

Patients

Thirteen patients (patients 1–13, Table 1) were born at term and received a diagnosis of MPS II at a mean age of 2.5 years (ranging from 1 month to 4 years, median 3 years). They began ERT with idursulfase at a mean age of 3.6 years (range from 3 months to 6 years, median 4 years). All were Caucasian. Twelve patients were classified as neurological (92.3%) and one as attenuated (7.7%).

Of the 13 enrolled patients, all completed the study. All patients received weekly intravenous infusions of idursulfase for 52 to 288 weeks. All 13 patients completed at least 52 weeks of treatment, 1 patient (7.7%) completed 288 weeks, 1 patient (7.7%) 198 weeks, 4 patients (30.8%) 188 weeks, 3 patients (23.1%) 164 weeks, and 4 patients 159, 156, 92, and 52 weeks, respectively. All patients were compliant with idursulfase treatment and the compliance with weekly infusions was 100%. All infusions were administered in hospital settings.

Clinical studies (measures of skeletal growth)

Figure 1 presents individual growth curves for patients from group 1 and 2 on the reference growth charts. Individual data for this study was standardized in order to show the actual degree and direction of deviations compared with the Polish reference charts. Figure 2 presents the mean standardized values for the body height in the calendar age groups. The results show the existence of characteristic downward trend in degree and direction of deviations in MPS II boys who started enzyme replacement therapy before 6 years of age. This course of average growth curve for MPS II ERT group was similar to growth pattern in MPS naïve group. Although the average z-score value of body height in subsequent years in MPS II ERT group was a bit greater than in MPS II naïve group this difference was not statistically significant.

Discussion

There is a scarcity of literature reporting detailed anthropometric data of both untreated children with MPS disorders as well as children receiving ERT [8–10,13] with only two studies dealing exclusively with impact of ERT on growth (Table 2) [9,10].

Schulze et al compared annual growth rates before and during ERT in 18 patients. Group 1 included nine patients who started ERT before 10 years of age; group 2 contained nine patients aged more than 10 years at the start of ERT [9]. All patients had received weekly or biweekly ERT or placebo for 1 year, followed by ERT for more than 3 years. For patients in group 1, the mean (±SD) height increase was 14.6±5.5 cm during 3 years of ERT. Patients in group 2 had a mean height increase of 8.1±1.7 cm after 3 years of ERT compared with an increase of 1 cm in the year before ERT [9]. The authors concluded that ERT seemed to have a positive influence on growth in patients with MPS II with most benefit in patients beginning ERT before the age of 10 years.

In a recent study, Jones et al, performed an analysis to investigate the effects of ERT on growth in patients enrolled in HOS – the Hunter Outcome Survey. This study showed that the slope after treatment (slope = –0.005) was significantly improved compared with before treatment (slope = –0.043) (difference = 0.038, p = 0.004) [10]. Analysis of covariates (age at treatment start, cognitive involvement, presence of puberty at the start of ERT, mutation type, functional classification), showed a significant influence on growth of mutation type (height deficit in terms of z-scores most pronounced in patients with deletions/large rearrangements/nonsense mutations, p<0.0001) and age (most pronounced in 12–15-year group, p<0.0001) [10]. The authors concluded that idursulfase treatment improves growth rate in patients with Hunter syndrome.

The results of the above-mentioned studies do not seem consistent with our results.

In our study of 13 patients with MPS II all measurements were performed by the same anthropology specialist using appropriate equipment and based on appropriate general population standards. The majority of our patients (85%) received ERT for at least 156 weeks. One of the key observations from comparing treated and naïve patients is that there was no statistically significant difference in the mean increase in body height between these two groups.

Although, some authors suggested improvement in growth rates in patients treated with ERT, our data does not support this notion. The reason for this difference may be a less detailed assessment and shorter observation time in other studies (Table 2). In large international studies, height is measured in different hospitals, by different people, which may have an impact on the quality of measurements. What's more, study groups are very heterogenous, for example in a study by Jones et al study group consisted of 892 males form 116 different countries around the world. These patients have not been divided into different groups depending on their IQ. Another often occurring problem is z-score, which is calculated in comparison to the CDC growth charts. The most recent publications, which focus on the problem of using international standards, show that global growth charts are inadequate in comparison to the regional charts [14–18]. Z-score should be calculated based on reference standards valid for the country of origin of the patient.

Body height, defined as a measurement of total body length in an upright position, describes the complicated structure of ontogeny. Process of growth is non- linear with both periodic and chaotic elements, which are specific for growth pattern in human species. Velocity and rate of growth change during ontogeny and growth rate differs in particular age classes. Generally, growth can be characterized as a period of accelerated growth divided by periods of slow growth. Individuals grow according to genetically determined pattern. The growth pattern contains the following stages: infancy with rapid postnatal spurt immediately after birth; childhood followed by a small mid-growth spurt at the age of 6–7 years; juvenile and adolescence with its marked pubertal growth spurt. Patients with MPS II, despite the disease, show the same general growth pattern, characteristic for the human species. In connection with the above-mentioned facts, it is a misapprehension to analyze growth of chronically ill patients assuming that: the rate of growth is constant (study by Schulze-Frenking) or the slope of z-score values is constant in subsequent years (HOS study) [9,10]. It is also inappropriate to analyze the process of growth for all individuals with different age in one age group like in HOS study (8–15 years). Between 12 to 15 years there is a marked acceleration of growth in human growth pattern and ignoring this fact makes the above-mentioned studies unconvincing. Growth process in MPS II patients is undoubtedly different from the growth pattern in healthy population and therefore the most appropriate method of analyze the effects of treatment is to compare the growth of ERT treated patients with patients naïve to ERT.

It is important to remember that ERT is a treatment with partial effects in specific body compartments [19]. Although it can be a life-lengthening therapeutic measure, it does not seem to alter

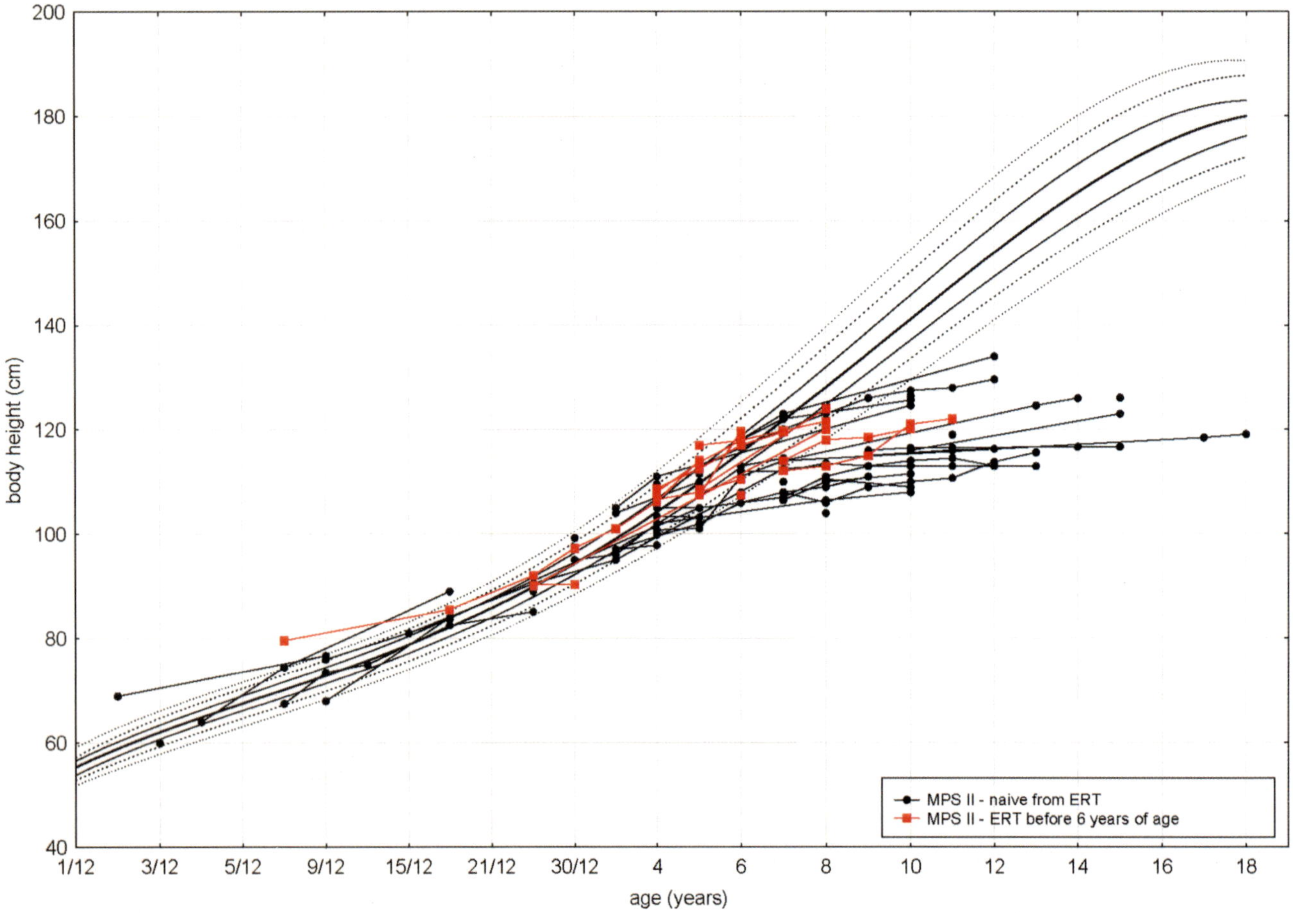

Figure 1. Growth curves for patients with MPS II who started ERT before 6 years of age (red marks) and patients naïve to ERT (black marks) on references growth charts for healthy population.

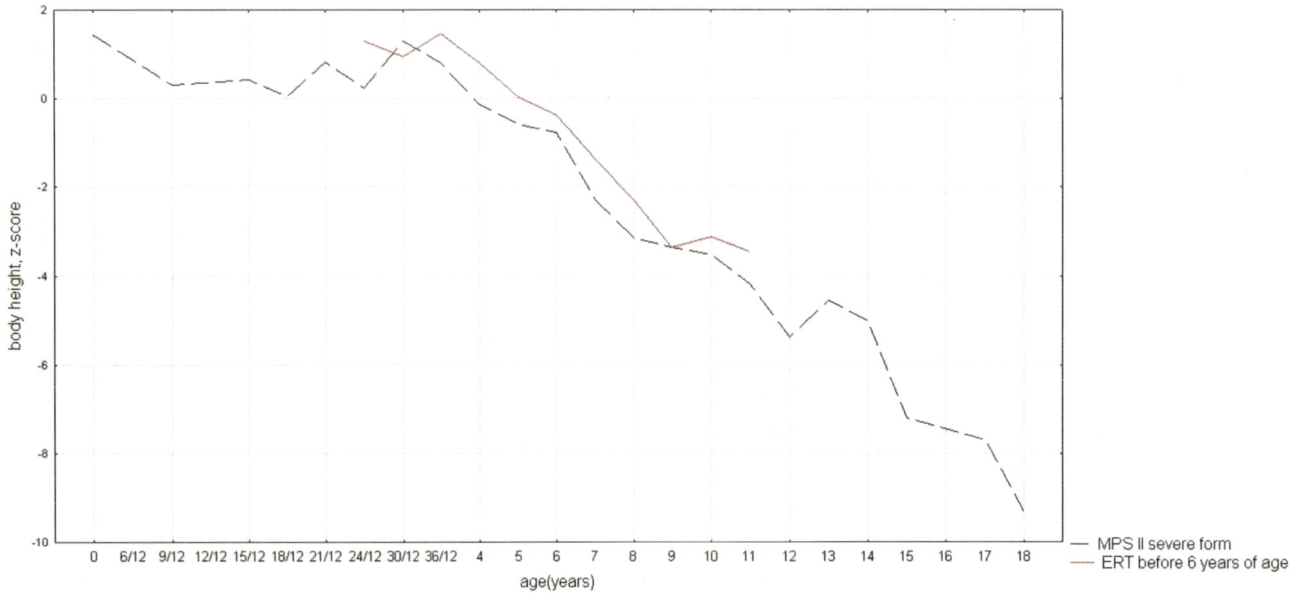

Figure 2. Comparison of growth patterns of patients with mucopolysaccharidosis type II who started enzyme replacement therapy before 6 years of age and patients who were naïve to ERT.

Table 2. Comparison of studies addressing effect of ERT on growth in patients with mucopolysaccharidosis type II.

	Schulze et al, 2011	Jones et al, 2013	Current study
Study group	18	133	13
	Germany & UK	different countries around the world	Poland
Age at ERT	2 groups	variable	< 6 y
introduction	< 10 y, > 10 y		
Severity of the disease	attenuated	?	neurological (88%) attenuated (7.7%)
Method	no detailed description	no detailed description	one anthropology specialist, precise measurements
z-score	calculated in comparison to the CDC growth charts	calculated in comparison to the CDC growth charts	calculated in comparison to the regional reference charts
Age classes	yes	no	yes
Data analysis			
Conclusions	ERT seemed to have a positive influence on growth in patients with MPS II with most benefit in patients beginning ERT before the age of 10 years.	Idursulfase treatment improves growth rate in patients with Hunter syndrome.	Idursulfase did not appear to alter the growth patterns.

the natural history of the skeletal disorder in MPS II and children will still endure the skeletal changes of the disease.

Conclusion

No apparent difference was observed between the growth rates in treated patients and the untreated disease. New approaches for the management and treatment of MPS disorders are necessary to influence skeletal abnormalities.

Acknowledgments

The authors acknowledge the contribution of the study patients and their families who gave their time and participated in this study. We also thank all study personnel.

Author Contributions

Conceived and designed the experiments: ZÅ AR-Åš AJ ATS. Performed the experiments: ZÅ AR-Åš AJ ATS. Analyzed the data: ZÅ AR-Åš AJ ATS. Contributed reagents/materials/analysis tools: ZÅ AR-Åš AJ ATS. Wrote the paper: ZÅ AR-Åš AJ ATS.

References

1. Neufeld EF, Muenzer J (2001) The mucopolysaccharidoses. In: Scriver CR, Beaudet AL, Sly WS, editors. The metabolic and molecular basis of inherited disease. New York: McGraw-Hill. pp. 3421–3452.
2. Baehner F, Schmiedeskamp C, Krummenauer F, Miebach E, Bajbouj M, et al. (2005) Cumulative incidence rates of the mucopolysaccharidoses in Germany. Journal of Inherited Metabolic Disease 28: 1011–1017.
3. Poorthuis BJ, Wevers RA, Kleijer WJ, Groener JE, de Jong JG, et al. (1999) The frequency of lysosomal storage diseases in The Netherlands. Human Genetics 105: 151–156.
4. Scarpa M, Almassy Z, Beck M, Bodamer O, Bruce IA, et al. (2011) Mucopolysaccharidosis type II: European recommendations for the diagnosis and multidisciplinary management of a rare disease. Orphanet journal of rare diseases 6: 72.
5. Hinek A, Wilson SE (2000) Impaired elastogenesis in Hurler disease: dermatan sulfate accumulation linked to deficiency in elastin-binding protein and elastic fiber assembly. The American journal of pathology 156: 925–938.
6. Simonaro CM, D'Angelo M, He X, Eliyahu E, Shtraizent N, et al. (2008) Mechanism of glycosaminoglycan-mediated bone and joint disease: implications for the mucopolysaccharidoses and other connective tissue diseases. The American journal of pathology 172: 112–122.
7. Schwartz IV, Ribeiro MG, Mota JG, Toralles MB, Correia P, et al. (2007) A clinical study of 77 patients with mucopolysaccharidosis type II. Acta Paediatrica 96: 63–70.
8. Rozdzynska A, Tylki-Szymanska A, Jurecka A, Cieslik J (2011) Growth pattern and growth prediction of body height in children with mucopolysaccharidosis type II. Acta Paediatr 100: 456–460.
9. Schulze-Frenking G, Jones SA, Roberts J, Beck M, Wraith JE (2011) Effects of enzyme replacement therapy on growth in patients with mucopolysaccharidosis type II. Journal of Inherited Metabolic Disease 34: 203–208.
10. Jones SA, Parini R, Harmatz P, Giugliani R, Fang J, et al. (2013) The effect of idursulfase on growth in patients with Hunter syndrome: data from the Hunter Outcome Survey (HOS). Molecular Genetics and Metabolism 109: 41–48.
11. Muenzer J, Beck M, Eng CM, Giugliani R, Harmatz P, et al. (2011) Long term, open-labeled extension study of idursulfase in the treatment of Hunter syndrome. Genet Med 13: 95–101.
12. Cieslik J, Kaczmarek M, Kaliszewska-Drozdowska MD (1994) [Dziecko Poznanskie' 90. Wzrastanie, dojrzewanie, normy i metody rozwoju.]. Poznan: Wydawnictwo Naukowe Bogucki.
13. Muenzer J, Beck M, Giugliani R, Suzuki Y, Tylki-Szymanska A, et al. (2011) Idursulfase treatment of Hunter syndrome in children younger than 6 years: results from the Hunter Outcome Survey. Genet Med 13: 102–109.
14. Bonthuis M, van Stralen KJ, Verrina E, Edefonti A, Molchanova EA, et al. (2012) Use of national and international growth charts for studying height in European children: development of up-to-date European height-for-age charts. PloS one 7: e42506.
15. Saari A, Sankilampi U, Hannila ML, Kiviniemi V, Kesseli K, et al. (2011) New Finnish growth references for children and adolescents aged 0 to 20 years: Length/height-for-age, weight-for-length/height, and body mass index-for-age. Annals of Medicine 43: 235–248.
16. Rosario AS, Schienkiewitz A, Neuhauser H (2011) German height references for children aged 0 to under 18 years compared to WHO and CDC growth charts. Annals of Human Biology 38: 121–130.
17. Juliusson PB, Roelants M, Hoppenbrouwers K, Hauspie R, Bjerknes R (2011) Growth of Belgian and Norwegian children compared to the WHO growth standards: prevalence below -2 and above +2 SD and the effect of breastfeeding. Archives of Disease in Childhood 96: 916–921.
18. Kulaga Z, Grajda A, Gurzkowska B, Gozdz M, Wojtylo M, et al. (2013) Polish 2012 growth references for preschool children. European Journal of Pediatrics 172: 753–761.
19. Burrow TA, Hopkin RJ, Leslie ND, Tinkle BT, Grabowski GA (2007) Enzyme reconstitution/replacement therapy for lysosomal storage diseases. Current Opinion in Pediatrics 19: 628–635.

27

From Mind to Mouth: Event Related Potentials of Sentence Production in Classic Galactosemia

Inge Timmers[1,2], Bernadette M. Jansma[2,3], M. Estela Rubio-Gozalbo[1,4]*

1 Department of Pediatrics, Maastricht University Medical Center, Maastricht, The Netherlands, **2** Department of Cognitive Neuroscience, Maastricht University, Maastricht, The Netherlands, **3** Maastricht Brain Imaging Center, Maastricht University, Maastricht, The Netherlands, **4** Laboratory of Genetic Metabolic Diseases, Maastricht University Medical Centre, Maastricht, The Netherlands

Abstract

Patients with classic galactosemia, an inborn error of metabolism, have speech and language production impairments. Past research primarily focused on speech (motor) problems, but these cannot solely explain the language impairments. Which specific deficits contribute to the impairments in language production is not yet known. Deficits in semantic and syntactic planning are plausible and require further investigation. In the present study, we examined syntactic encoding while patients and matched controls overtly described scenes of moving objects using either separate words (minimal syntactic planning) or sentences (sentence-level syntactic planning). The design of the paradigm also allowed tapping into local noun phrase- and more global sentence-level syntactic planning. Simultaneously, we recorded event-related potentials (ERPs). The patients needed more time to prepare and finish the utterances and made more errors. The patient ERPs had a very similar morphology to that of healthy controls, indicating overall comparable neural processing. Most importantly, the ERPs diverged from those of controls in several functionally informative time windows, ranging from very early (90–150 ms post scene onset) to relatively late (1820–2020 ms post scene onset). These time windows can be associated with different linguistic encoding stages. The ERP results form the first neuroscientific evidence for language production impairments in patients with galactosemia in lexical and syntactic planning stages, i.e., prior to the linguistic output phase. These findings hence shed new light on the language impairments in this disease.

Editor: Kevin Paterson, University of Leicester, United Kingdom

Funding: This work was supported by a Maastricht University Incentive to B. M. Jansma in the context of supporting "Woman in higher positions in science" and a Galactosemia Research Fund grant to M. E. Rubio-Gozalbo. The funders had no role in study design, data collection and analysis, decision to publish, or preparation of the manuscript.

Competing Interests: The authors have declared that no competing interests exist.

* E-mail: estela.rubio@mumc.nl

Introduction

Patients with classic galactosemia, an inborn error of galactose metabolism, have speech and language production impairments, whereas comprehension is relatively preserved [1,2]. Such impairments can be burdensome to patients as they might hamper communication and hence social interactions. Nevertheless, underlying language processing components and neural correlates of these impairments are poorly understood.

In classic galactosemia, there is a deficiency of the enzyme activity that converts galactose-1-phosphate (Gal-1-P) into UDP-galactose (i.e., the galactose-1-phophate uridyl transferase [GALT] enzyme). This is due to mutations in the GALT gene, located on the short arm of chromosome 9. A galactose-restricted diet resolves the neonatal toxic symptoms, but cannot prevent the emergence of cognitive difficulties such as lowered intelligence, memory problems, slower general information processing and impaired speech and language production [1,3–10], while receptive language or comprehension is relatively preserved [1]. Voice and motor speech disorders (e.g., childhood apraxia of speech or dysarthria) have been reported [9,11–14] as well as problems with word retrieval, grammar and vocabulary (the latter impairments are related to the planning of a message and not with the verbal output of a message) [2,5,6]. Although patients can experience a broad spectrum of cognitive impairments, the speech and language impairments cannot be solely explained by lower cognitive abilities in general [1,2,6] (e.g., some patients with low intelligence have no language impairments, while others with average intelligence have language impairments [1]). Hitherto, the main focus of research, diagnosis and treatment has been on speech (output) difficulties (e.g., on voice disorders or childhood apraxia of speech [9,11–13]). However, speech (output) impairments cannot solely explain the language impairments. Language production is a complex process comprising multiple processing stages prior to the output stage [15–17]. In galactosemia, nonetheless, it has never been studied how language production is affected. In this study, we took a cognitive point of view, examining language production using psycholinguistic models. In the remainder of this manuscript we will refer to 'language production' as specified in the field of linguistics and cognitive neuroscience, namely describing the cognitive phases that are involved in planning a message prior to the articulation.

Psycholinguistic models of language production suggest cognitive stages in which relevant language information is planned over time. First, an intended message has to be transferred into a conceptual/semantic representation. Appropriate lexical entries are selected and retrieved as well as the corresponding grammatical and syntactic information. Structural syntactic frames are constructed and assembled or filled in producing a well-formed utterance. Finally, the message is encoded and articulated [15,18]. The language production process has been investigated in many picture naming experiments using reaction times (see [19] for a review) and event related potentials (ERPs, derivatives of the electroencephalogram [20]). This way, sensitive time windows have been suggested for the language production stages. It has been shown that conceptual information is activated around 120 ms after stimulus onset [21], followed by semantic processing. This is followed by syntactic encoding approximately 90 ms later, serving as input to phonological encoding after another 40 ms. The processes are not fully serial but might overlap in time, suggesting cascading information flow over time [16,22–24]. Each of the planning steps can be linked to specific brain areas within a cortical network [16,25,26]. Ignoring other potentially relevant factors for a moment, any type of impairment might therefore be directly related to dysfunction within this network. Lesions within specific areas may affect production and comprehension separately [27,28], whereas disruptions of connectivity between areas may delay or disturb language processing [29]. Few imaging studies have been conducted in galactosemia, observing anatomical brain abnormalities, such as white matter abnormalities, cerebral and cerebellar atrophy [30,31], but it remains uncertain whether specific areas or networks might be particularly affected.

A screening of our patient cohort's medical files suggested a syntactic deficit in the galactosemia patients as their utterances were described as short, simple and frequently as syntactically incorrect. Necessary steps in syntactic encoding are identification and activation of grammatical information associated with the concepts (e.g., whether it is a noun or adjective; lexical selection), the assignment of syntactic relations or grammatical functions to each word (e.g., subject versus object; function assignment), inflection of words (e.g., *-s* for plural, *-ed* for past tense) and assembly of words into so called syntactic structural frames, i.e., syntactic plans (constituent assembly) [15,18]. It deduces that in syntactic planning more local phrasal-level planning (first steps described) can be distinguished from more global sentence-level planning (assembly into a frame and utterance). Especially in multi-word utterances, it is believed that the scope of planning is incremental such that the utterance can be initiated as soon as certain elements are available [15,17,32,33]. The amount of advance planning is suggested to be in terms of functional phrases [33], but is also dependent on the cognitive load of the utterance and the cognitive capacity of the speaker [15,34,35]. In healthy controls, syntactic processing has been studied in the context of syntactic anomalies or syntactic complexity during comprehension (P600 and left anterior negativity [LAN] ERP components) [36,37]. In terms of brain areas, syntactic encoding and sentence processing have been related to the left inferior frontal gyrus (LIFG, encompassing Broca's area) [25,38–40]. In comprehension research, studies assume that the LIFG is retrieving and integrating lexical information from long term memory, most likely from left temporal areas [36,41–43]. A similar process can be assumed for speech planning in which concepts have to be integrated into proper syntactic and phonological frames (see [39], for first empirical indications using intracranial electrophysiology).

In the present study, we aimed to investigate whether patients with galactosemia have impairments in sentence production by recording high temporal resolution ERPs during a language task. This method allowed us to track the neural activity related to the entire language planning process from the intention to speak onwards, across sensitive time windows. Comparing the patients' ERP (i.e., morphology of the wave, amplitude and latency of components) with that of healthy controls gives us an indication on whether syntactic encoding is intact, delayed, or malfunctioning at a millisecond time resolution. An experimental paradigm was used that elicits overt utterances in response to an animated scene in a relatively natural manner. Through different instructions, the reports of the scene varied in syntactic complexity [38,40], allowing us to study syntactic effects within the ERP. The content of the scenes differed from trial to trial (i.e., the geometrical figure, colour of the figures and verb) and not all information was available from the scene onset (i.e., the verb; the actor could either '*bump into*' or '*fly towards*' the other figure; both scene variations start visually identical, and diverge at a certain point). The participants therefore could not anticipate the action of the figure, ensuring active generation of the utterances (instead of only automated processes). Further, it allowed us to tap into both early local phrasal-level planning of noun phrases (starting immediately after scene onset, associated with initiation of planning the first elements of the utterance that are already available: the first nouns and corresponding adjectives) and on later global sentence-level planning (when all relevant information is at hand, including the verb; adding the construction of the utterance). Time windows of any deviations, relative to the visual stimulation, give information on whether differences are related to early conceptual, early local syntactic, or rather late global syntactic or articulatory processing. Specifically, variation with syntactic complexity would reflect time windows relevant for syntactic encoding during sentence production. Moreover, relevant cognitive functions (i.e., visual memory, attention, working memory) were studied independently using standardized tests and related to the ERP data in order to exclude possible confounding of these more basic functions.

Materials and Methods

Ethics statement

The Medical Ethical Committee of Maastricht University Hospital/Maastricht University (azM/UM) gave ethical clearance for this study. All participants, and for minors also both parents/caregivers, gave written informed consent.

Participants

Twenty-four adolescent patients with galactosemia and twenty-one healthy controls participated in this study. Classic galactosemia was diagnosed by GALT enzyme activity assay and/or GALT-gene mutation analysis. Two participants (both patients) were excluded because of difficulties executing the ERP task. Patient characteristics can be found in Table 1. Of the remaining 22 patients, 15 were female and 7 male, mean age 14.9 years (SD 2.2 y, range 10.8–19.1 y). The control group consisted of 14 females and 7 males mean age 14.2 years (SD 1.8 y, range 11.4–17.0 y). Neither gender nor age differed significantly between the groups [$F(1,41) = .01$, $p = .92$ and $F(1,41) = 1.07$, $p = .31$, respectively]. Participants had no other relevant health conditions, all had normal or corrected to normal vision, and were native Dutch speakers.

Neuropsychological tests

The Rey Osterreith Complex Figure was used to assess visuomotor skills (Copy subtest), short term visual memory (Immediate Recall) and long term visual memory (Delayed Recall and Recognition) [44]. The Bourdon-Vos test was used to measure sustained attention skills (mean reaction time [RT]) [45]. The Digit Span (Forward and Backward) addressed verbal working memory skills [46].

Table 1. Galactosemia patient characteristics.

	N	Mean	SD	Range of values
Age at diagnosis (in days)	22	12.4	14.3	0–60
Age at introduction of diet (in days)	22	12.2	14.4	0–60
GALT activity (in % of mean reference value)[1,2]	20	0.60	0.57	ND[3] - 1.83
Urine galactose level (in μmol/mmol creatinine)[4]	22	12.0	21.1	ND[3] – 96
Urine galactitol level (in μmol/mmol creatinine)[4]	22	132.0	22.8	94 – 187
Special education[5]	22	68.2%		
Speech therapy[5]	22	86.4%		
Motor therapy[5]	22	50.0%		
GALT gene mutation	10	50%	Q188R/Q188R	
	5	25%	Q188R/other[6]	
	5	25%	other[7]	

GALT enzyme activities indicate that all patients have the classic galactosemia type. Urine galactose and galactitol levels indicate adequate dietary compliance.
[1]GALT activity was measured at diagnosis;
[2]In case the GALT activity is not reported, it was confirmed by the treating physician to be severely decreased;
[3]ND = not detected;
[4]Urine levels were measured within three months of testing;
[5]At some point in life;
[6]Q188R/L195P (n = 4) or Q188R/S135W (n = 1);
[7]L195P/K229N (n = 3) or 400Tdel/unknown (n = 2).

Language paradigm during EEG recording

Visually animated scenes were presented to the participants. Each scene consisted of three geometrical shapes (square, triangle, or circle) having one of three different colours (red, blue or green). In each trial, one of the three geometrical figures performed an action upon another figure (one figure moves towards or bumps into another figure; described by either 'to fly towards' or 'to bump into'). Participants were asked to either passively watch the scene (control task, 'C') or to describe the animated scene overtly using one of two possible responses that varied in syntactic complexity: using separate words, 'W' (e.g., *"triangle", "red", "square", "green", "to bump into"*; minimal syntactic planning) or using sentences, 'S' (e.g., *"The red triangle bumps into the green square."*; sentence-level syntactic planning) [38,40]. Participants were asked to keep the naming format of the phrases constant over trials. In the word 'W' naming format, lexical access of words is required, but virtually no syntactic encoding. In the sentence 'S' naming format, in contrast, syntactic encoding is required on local noun phrase level (e.g., inflection of adjectives) and on sentence level (e.g., inflection of the verb, determination of the word order, constructing and filling in of the syntactic frame). The control ('C') condition was added in this study to receive relevant information for the required non-linguistic resources (e.g., visual processes, attention).

Procedure

The study was conducted in two sessions. In the first session, the neuropsychological tests were conducted in all participants after explanation and written informed consents were given (by the participant and both parents/caregiver). In the second session, the language paradigm and EEG recordings took place. After a brief explanation, participants were prepared and seated in an electrically-shielded, sound-attenuated room in front of a computer monitor. The session started with the control task 'C', followed by instructions and a practice version of the language task (consisting of 18 practice trials per condition) and the main language experiment.

The main language task consisted of three runs in a blocked design. Each run comprised two blocks which were randomized within the run and counter-balanced between participants to exclude order effects. Each block started with a brief instruction reflecting the expected naming format (i.e., either 'SENTENCE' or 'WORD') followed by 32 trials of different scene displays, of which the content (figures, colours, action and arrangement) was randomized. Per condition and participant, a total of 96 trials were recorded. The control task consisted of three consecutive runs, having a total of 108 trials. Figure 1 gives a schematic overview of the sequences of events within a trial. The duration of animation in the scene differed (955 or 1885 ms) depending on the action format ('to fly towards' or 'to bump into', respectively). The difference in animation durations is caused by a different amount of action frames (10 versus 18 frames, where the actual 'bump' event occurred at frame 14, at 1520 ms after scene onset). Note that the movements in the scenes are visually identical until they diverge at the moment the 'to fly towards' trials freeze while 'to bump into' trials continue. Participants were instructed to start the description as fast and accurate as possible. The next trials started via a self-paced button push (USB-keyboard key), except for the control trials which had a fixed 2000 ms interval between trials. Control trials had approximately the same duration as the linguistic trials.

Electroencephalography (EEG) recording

The EEG recording was done using an elastic cap in which 32 tin electrodes were mounted (Electro-Cap International (ECI), Inc.), positioned according to the international 10–20 system [47]. Twenty electrodes - F3, Fz, F4, FC3, FCz, FC4, C3, Cz, C4, CP3, CPz, CP4, P3, Pz, P4, O1, Oz, O2, T3 and T4 - were measured as active leads, AFz was used as the ground electrode. The left mastoid (A1) was used as online reference. Offline the signal was re-referenced to the average signal of both mastoids. Vertical eye movements and blinks were monitored by two electrodes placed at the left upper and lower orbital ridge. Horizontal eye movements were recorded with electrodes placed on the left and right cantus.

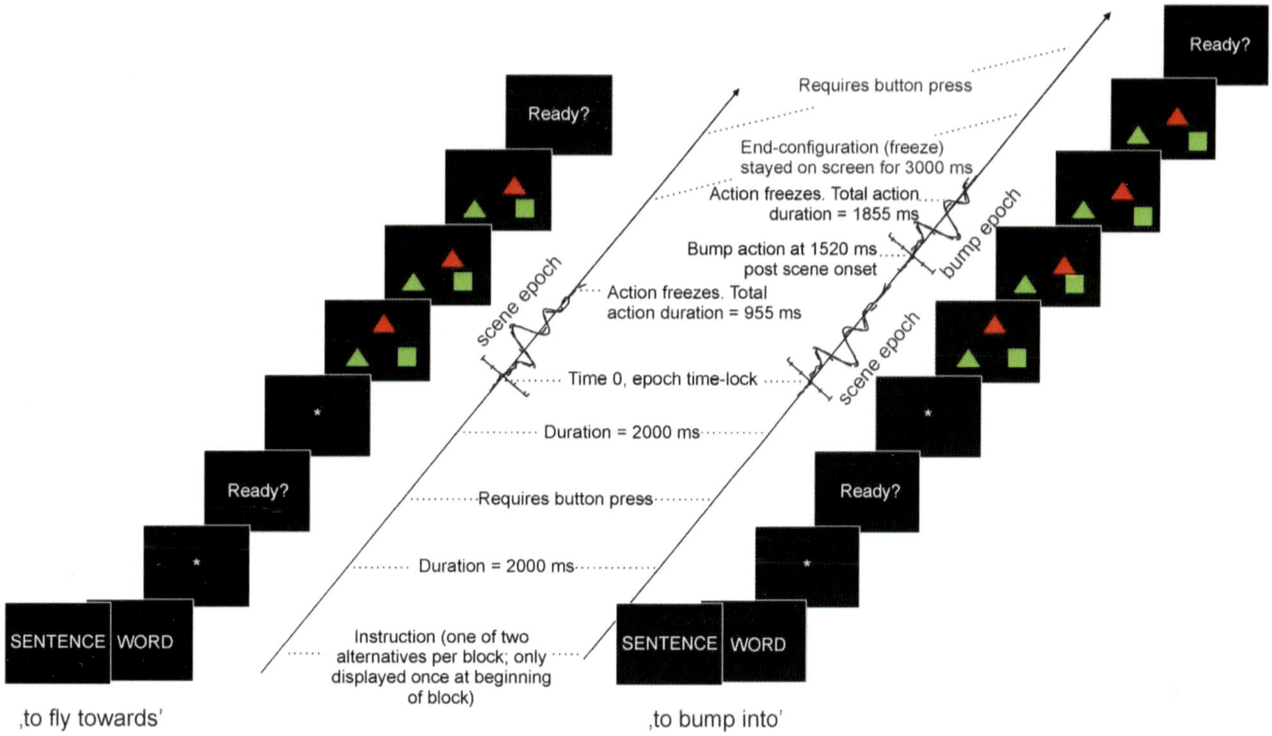

Figure 1. Overview of the sequences of events within trials. Timing of events within an experimental trial, separated for the two action formats ('to fly towards' and 'to bump into'). Time is displayed upwards. The block started with the instruction cue ('WORD' or 'SENTENCE'), a fixation cross, a ready sign, and a randomized sequence of trials. For each trial type screenshots are displayed to illustrate the actual moving time period of the objects along with the moments of expected response of the participant, and the corresponding ERP epochs of interest (time-locked to scene onset and the bump event, respectively).

The impedance of all electrodes was kept below 5 kΩ. Data acquisition was done using Brain Vision Recorder software (Brain Vision, MedCaT B.V.) and the signal was amplified using a 0.05–50 Hz band pass and sampled at a 500 Hz interval. The scene onset as well as the voice onset triggered a TTL pulse directly into the EEG recordings. The voice onset pulse was initiated whenever the sound pressure level reached a certain threshold (individually adjusted to each subject) and was transferred via a microphone.

Analyses

The number of errors and self-corrections were computed using the recorded audio data and manual (online) scores. Errors were defined as any deviation from the expected utterance (i.e., incorrect figure, colour, action, naming format or ordering). Self-corrections were defined as any overt corrective effort during the response utterance. The voice onset time (VOT) was determined as the time between the scene onset and the onset of the voice response; the total speech time (TST) was cautiously estimated as the time between the onset of the voice response and the button push indicating when participants were ready to continue. VOTs<0.5 seconds and >4.5 seconds and TSTs<2 seconds and >10 seconds were considered outliers and discarded from analysis. The neuropsychological data were standardized using norm data and classified according to the guidelines of Lezak [48]. A repeated measures General Linear Model was used to analyze the behavioural data (VOT, TST, errors and self-corrections) having Condition ('W' versus 'S') as the within-subject factor and Group (patients, controls) as between-subject factor. The standardized neuropsychological data were analyzed using frequency tables (for the classified data) and univariate GLM to examine group differences.

With respect to the EEG data, trials in which the participant's response was absent were excluded from analysis. The EEG data were epoched from −200 to 2500 ms post scene onset (to include the entire interval from onset of visual scene to the end of the display/onset of articulation), band-pass filtered from 0.3–30 Hz (zero phase, 24 dB) and baseline corrected (from −200 to 0 ms). Large visual artefacts were removed. In addition, data were decomposed using the infomax Independent Component Analysis (ICA) in EEGlab [49]. This method disentangles brain- and artefact-related processes by searching for maximally independent components [50]. Stereotype artefact-related components reflecting eye movements, noise and muscle activity were subsequently removed. On average, 84.5% of all trials (SD 5.2%) were kept for analysis [no difference between groups, $F(1, 41) = .000$, $p = .988$]: mean 96 trials in 'C', 79 in 'W' and 78 in 'S'. The remaining components (the cleaned data) were back-projected into the ERP. In the back-projected ERPs, epochs were divided in two time ranges: one interval related to the scene onset (−200 to 1000 ms after scene onset), and one related to the bump event (−200 to 800 ms after the bump event, or 1320 to 2320 ms post scene onset) (see also Figure 1). Note that in the bump epoch, only 'to bump into' trials were included (and no 'to fly towards' trials), corresponding to on average 49 trials in 'C', 39 in 'W' and 40 in 'S'. The bump epochs were baseline corrected (−200 to 0 ms after the bump event). Based on visual inspection of the grand averages, target peak ERP components and corresponding time windows were specified on which we conducted mean amplitude analyses.

ERP statistics were performed on the mean amplitude data per time window, condition, and participant using repeated measures GLM with Condition as within-subjects factor ('C', 'W', 'S'), and two within-subject topographical factors Laterality (left, central, right) and Anterior-Posterior (F, FC, C, CP, P, O). Based on visual inspection, additional analyses were performed on subsets of electrodes. Group was added as the between-subjects factor (patients, controls). Pearson's correlations were used to examine the relationship between the ERP data and behaviour (on-line measures of reaction times and accuracy) and other cognitive functions (off-line neuropsychological tests); and with patient characteristics (e.g., mutation, rest activity of the enzyme). Where necessary, corrections were made for multiple testing (Bonferroni) and for sphericity violations (Greenhouse Geisser). Age and gender were added as covariates in all analyses but the ones performed on standardized data. An alpha of 0.05 was used as significance level.

Results

Neuropsychological test results

The patients scored significantly lower compared to controls on the following subtests: Rey Complex Figure Copy, Immediate and Delayed Recall and Recognition; Bourdon-Vos total RT and number of errors; and Digit span $[.000<p<.027]$. However, when the Rey Complex Figure Copy score was subtracted from the Immediate Recall score (not standardized, to control for visuo-motor differences), the groups did not differ $[p=.75]$. Examining the slope of the three Bourdon-Vos RTs (not standardized, to examine the sustainability of attention), the groups did not differ either $[p=.25]$. The groups did not differ on the number of omissions and corrections on the Bourdon-Vos $[p=.91$ and $p=.33$, respectively]. Table 2 gives an overview of the neuropsychological data of the patient group (control data is not presented for clarity reasons).

Behavioural data language paradigm

Accuracy. The number of errors differed between groups, $[F(1,39)=12.24, p=.001]$: the patients made more errors than the controls. There was no difference in the number of errors between the word 'W' versus the sentence 'S' condition $[F(1,39)=2.143, p=.151]$. The number of self-corrections showed no group difference $[F(1,39)=0.063, p=.801]$, but a condition effect. More self-corrections were made in 'S' compared to 'W' $[F(1,39)=27.78, p<.001]$ (Figure 2).

Reaction times. The patients had longer VOTs and longer TSTs compared to controls $[F(1,37)=5.28, p=.027$ and $F(1,37)=13.154, p=.001$, respectively]. The TST was longer in 'S' $[F(1,37)=26.406, p=<.001]$. No condition effect for the VOT was observed in either group $[F(1,37)=.061, p=.807]$.

Correlations behavioural data and neuropsychological data. In both groups, lower scores on the Rey Complex Figure (Immediate and Delayed Recall) were related to more errors [patients: $-.543<r<-.490$, $.009<p<.021$; controls: $-.550<r<-.478$, $.010<p<.028$]. In patients, lower performance on the Rey Immediate recall task was associated with longer TSTs $[r=-.651, p=.001]$.

ERP data

The ERP waveforms depict the planning phase of the utterance from scene onset onwards. Figure 3 shows the grand average waveforms of the patients with galactosemia versus the matched controls for the entire epoch interval of −200 to 2500 ms after scene onset (averaged across conditions). Separate lines are shown for the two action formats 'to fly towards' and 'to bump into'. The figure illustrates that the scenes (and the corresponding ERPs) were identical until approximately 1000 ms post scene onset and start to diverge relatively late. Visual inspection of the grand averages showed a clear ERP morphology during the first thousand milliseconds post scene onset, followed by a relatively steady period (in which no event related activity is visible). Another subset of ERP components was observable at a relatively late time

Table 2. Classified neuropsychological data of the patients with galactosemia.

	Very low	Low	Below average	Average	Above average	High	Very high
Expected distribution	2.3%	7.4%	17.7%	45.2%	17.7%	7.4%	2.3%
Rey Complex Figure							
Copy	68.2%	13.6%	18.2%[1]				
Time to copy	-	8.3%	91.7%[1]				
Immediate Recall	59.1%	22.7%	9.1%	4.5%	4.5%	-	-
Delayed Recall	54.5%	27.3%	9.1%	9.1%	-	-	-
Recognition	27.3%	18.2%	18.2%	31.8%	4.5%	-	-
Bourdon-Vos							
Total RT	-	59.1%	27.3%	13.6%	-	-	-
Number of omissions			59.1%	36.4%	4.5%		
Number of corrections			4.5%	45.5%	50.0%		
Number of errors			36.4%	63.3%	-		
Digit Span							
	42.9%	23.8%	14.3%	19.0%	-	-	-

Presented are the percentages of patients scoring within the particular classifications as described in Lezak [48]: $z<-2$ very low; $-2<z<-1.3$ low; $-1.3<z<-0.6$ below average; $-0.6<z<0.6$ average; $0.6<z<1.3$ above average; $1.3<z<2$ high; $z>2$ very high. Note that the expected distribution reflects percentages based on the normal distribution.

[1]Below average or higher.

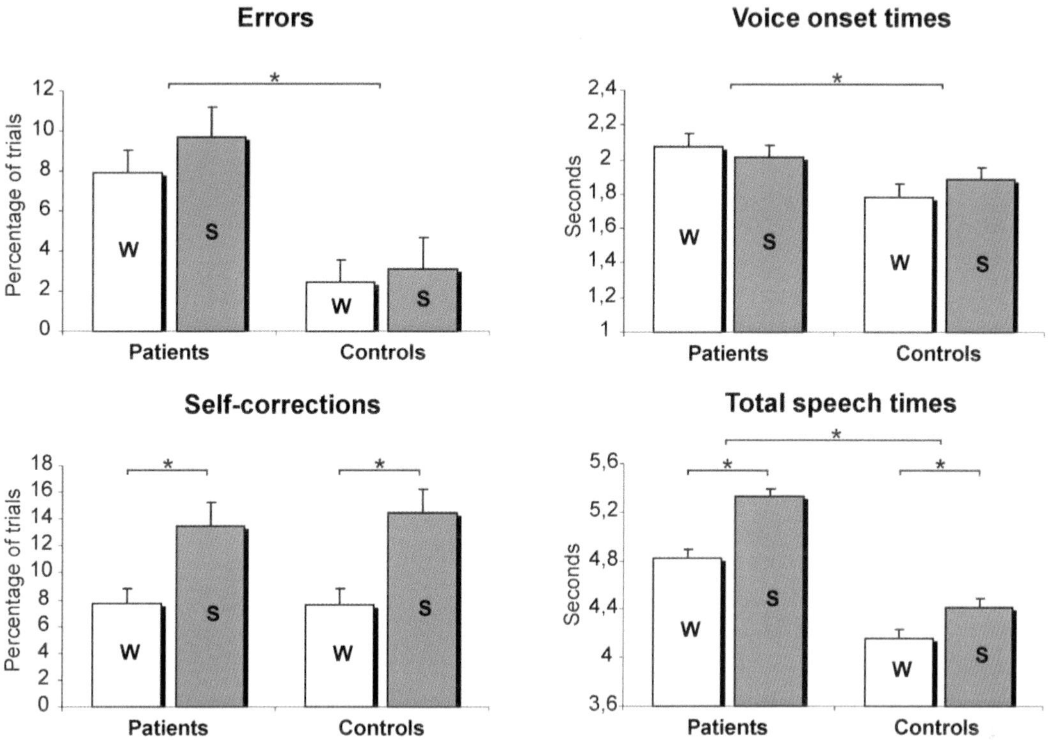

Figure 2. Behavioural data. Behavioural data per group and per condition. 'W' = Word condition; 'S' = Sentence condition. Presented are estimated marginal means with standard error (SE) bars. Asterisks indicate significant effects ($P < .05$).

interval (from approximately 1500 ms after scene onset onwards), restricted to the bump trials. Analyses were directed towards these two epochs of interest: −200 to 1000 ms after the scene onset (before the action format and thus the verb is available; local syntactic planning) and −200 to 800 ms after the bump event (when the verb is available, corresponding to 1320 to 2320 ms after scene onset, limited to the bump trials; global sentence-level syntactic planning). As the arrows in Figure 3 depict, there are several time points at several electrodes where groups and/or conditions differ, starting early in time. The overall morphology, however, was quite similar (see also topographies in Figure 3). Statistical analyses were carried out across several time windows with labels 'scene' referring to components following scene onset, and label 'bump' referring to components following the 'bump' event: 90–150 ms (referred to as *P1 scene*), 100–160 ms (*N1 scene*), 180–240 ms (*P2 scene*) and 350–650 ms (*P3 scene*) post scene onset; 70–170 ms (*N1 bump*), 180–280 ms (*P2 bump*) and 300–500 ms (*P3 bump*) post bump event. Note that the labels P1, N1, P2 and P3 are used for descriptive purposes.

Time windows of interest post scene onset

Time window 90–150 ms – P1 scene. A positive component was observed with a maximum around 120 ms post scene onset and an occipital scalp distribution. Analyses were restricted to the occipital plane (O). A Group effect [$F(1, 39) = 6.00$, $p = .019$] was visible and significant in all three conditions ('C': $p = .032$, 'W': $p = .021$, 'S': $p = .021$), with the patients' ERP being more positive. The patients but not the controls showed a trend in the Condition effect [$F(1.59, 30.23) = 2.91$, $p = .081$]. Simple contrasts in the patients data revealed that 'C' differed from both 'W' and 'S' [$p = .004$ en $p = .024$, respectively] (see Figure 4A).

Time window 100–160 ms – N1 scene. At anterior sites, a negative component was observed at 100–160 ms after scene onset, with a maximum at 130 ms. Analyses were restricted to F3, Fz, F4. No clear condition effect was revealed. The Group effect was not significant either [$F(1,39) = 3.47$, $p = .070$].

Time window 180–240 ms – P2 scene. A positive component was observed peaking around 210 ms after scene onset. Analyses showed that this component was largest over midline fronto-central and parietal sites. Because of interactions between Condition and the topographical factors, the analysis was further conducted on sub-regions.

At the right side of the scalp (F4, FC4, C4, CP4, P4) there was a Condition effect [$F(1.95,76.03) = 7.93$, $p = .001$]. Follow-up analyses showed that 'C' differed from both 'W' and 'S' [$p = .001$ and $p = .007$, respectively]. There was no difference between 'W' and 'S'. Recordings at right posterior electrodes (CP4, P4) revealed a Group effect [$F(1,39) = 4.62$, $p = .038$]. Follow-up analyses showed that the patients' ERP signal in the linguistic conditions (but not in passive watching) was more positive compared to controls ['W': $F(1,39) = 4.31$, $p = .044$; 'S': $F(1,39) = 4.97$, $p = .032$] (see Figure 4B).

Only in controls, better sustainability of attention (lower slope of the Bourdon Vos reaction times) was associated with a larger linguistic condition effect (i.e., difference in mean amplitudes between 'C' and both 'W' and 'S' at FC4) ['C'-'W': $r = -.444$, $p = .044$; 'C'-'S': $r = -.754$, $p < .001$].

Time window 350–650 ms – P3 scene. During this time window, a large long-lasting positive activity was observed, with a maximum at posterior sites. Analyses indicated interactions between the Condition effect and the electrode locations. Therefore, further analyses were performed on sub-regions.

In central and parietal regions (FC, C, CP, P), a Condition effect was observed [$F(1.98,77.34) = 21.19$, $p < .001$]. Pair wise compar-

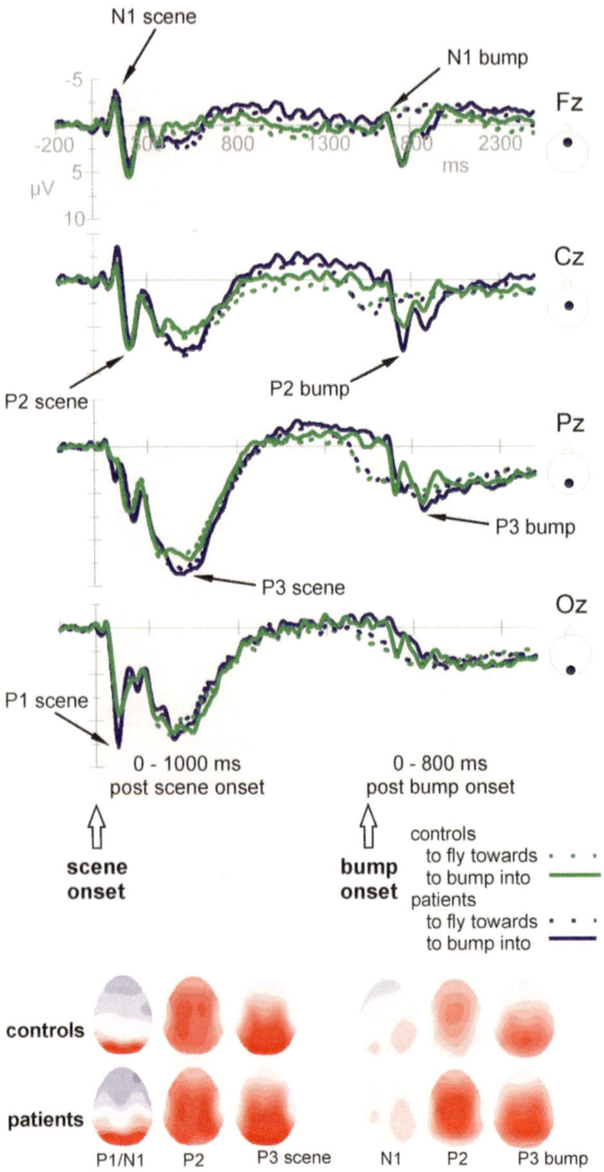

Figure 3. Overview of ERPs and topographies. Top: Grand average ERPs of the patients with galactosemia (blue) and the healthy controls (green) across the midline of the scalp (F = Frontal, C = Central, P = Parietal, O = Occipital). The lines are averaged across conditions, but separate for the two action formats: solid lines represent the 'to bump into' format; dashed lines the 'to fly towards' format. The two epochs of interest are highlighted: the post scene onset epoch (where scenes of both action formats, and their corresponding ERPs, are still identical) and the post bump event epoch (where the analyses were limited to the 'to bump into' trials, as the 'to fly towards' trials do not show an ERP morphology during this time window). Negative voltage is plotted up in this and all subsequent figures. Bottom: Overview of the topographical distributions over the scalp of the components of interest, for each group seperately. Both the ERPs and the corresponding topographies illustrate an overall similar morphology for the patients and controls.

isons showed that 'C' differed from 'W' and 'S' [both $p<.001$]. The groups did not differ significantly and the Condition effect was the same for both groups. At frontal regions (F), a difference was observed between 'S' and 'W' [$F(1,39)=4.838$, $p=.034$]. However, this effect was only present in the controls [$F(1,18)=7.589$, $p=.013$] and not in the patients [$F(1,19)=.022$, $p=.884$] (see Figure 4C). At the frontal site, there is a trend towards a difference in amplitudes between groups [$F(1,39)=2.625$, $p=.113$].

In controls, larger syntactic complexity effects (i.e., mean amplitude difference between 'S' and 'W' at Fz) were associated with shorter TSTs (in 'S') [$r=-.462$, $p=.035$]. In patients, longer VOTs (in 'S') were associated with smaller syntactic complexity effects [$r=-.474$, $p=.030$].

Time windows of interest post bump event

Time window 70–170 ms – N1 bump. At anterior sites, a negative component was visible at 70–170 ms after the bump event, on average peaking at 130 ms. Analyses were restricted to frontal and fronto-central electrodes (F FC). There was no significant Condition effect [$F(1.83,71.36)=1.96$, $p=.151$], nor any interaction effects. The groups did not differ either [$F(1,39)=0.65$, $p=.43$].

Time window 180–280 ms – P2 bump. Around 230 ms post bump event, a large positive component was observed. The topographic distribution was fronto-central. Analyses therefore were restricted to these electrodes (F FC C). In addition to Condition and Group effects, interaction effects were found between the factor Anterior-Posterior and both Group and Condition.

Sub-analyses revealed only a marginal Condition effect in the FC plane [$F(2.0,77.91)=2.94$, $p=.059$], while the Group effect was significant ($F(1,39)=9.42$, $p=.004$]. In the central plane (C), there was a clear Condition effect [$F(1.99,77.71)=9.24$, $p<.001$], where 'C' differed from both 'W' and 'S' [$p=.000$ and $p=.006$, respectively]. The two linguistic conditions did not differ [$p=.214$]. The Group effect was significant [$F(1,39)=12.88$, $p=.001$], reflected in more positive amplitudes in the patients' ERP compared to controls (see Figure 5A).

Only in controls, larger linguistic condition effects (i.e., difference between non-linguistic and linguistic conditions at Cz) were associated with shorter VOTs ['C'-'W' effect: $r=-.497$, $p=.033$; 'C'-'S' effect: $r=-.633$, $p=.002$] and with fewer errors ['C'-'W' effect: $r=-.517$, $p=.016$; 'C'-'S' effect: $r=-.602$, $p=.004$]. Only in patients, better visual memory performance (Rey Complex Figure Immediate and Delayed Recall) was related to larger linguistic condition effects ('C'-'W') [$r=.570$, $p=.006$; $r=.611$, $p=.003$, respectively].

Time window 300–500 ms – P3 bump. Between 300 and 500 ms post bump event, a large positive component was observed. The component was broadly distributed, with a maximum over posterior sites (CP P). Analyses were performed on F FC C CP P electrode lines. In addition to a significant Condition effect, there were interactions between the Anterior-Posterior topographical factor and the Condition factor. The groups differed across the entire scalp [$F(1,39)=11.21$, $p=.002$; in all conditions, 'C': $p=.046$, 'W': $p=.010$, 'S' $p=.001$].

Sub-analyses revealed a Condition effect that was present in all planes (except for F), but was largest at posterior sites [P: Condition $F(1.95,76.03)=9.08$, $p<.001$]. Follow up analyses showed that 'C' differed from both 'W' and 'S' [$p<.001$ and $p=.002$, respectively]. Posterior, the linguistic conditions did not deviate. Anterior, however, 'W' and 'S' differed significantly [FC: $p=.025$], with 'S' being more positive than 'W'. There was no interaction between Group and Condition (see Figure 5B).

Only in controls, better sustainability of attention was associated with larger syntactic complexity effects (i.e., difference in mean amplitude between 'S' and 'W' at FCz) [$r=.498$, $p=.022$].

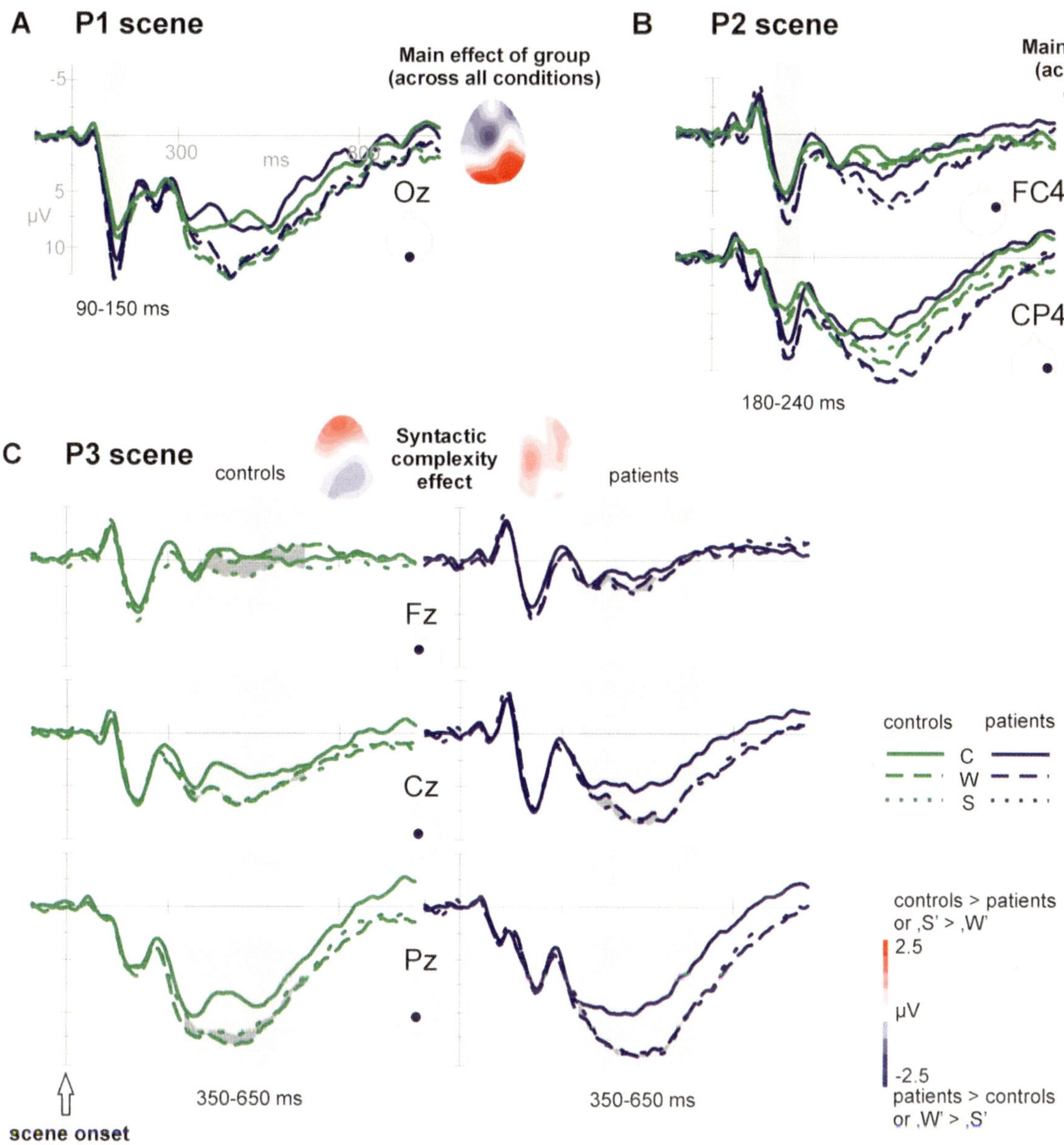

Figure 4. Overview of the ERP effects in the post scene onset epoch. A) Grand average waveforms of the occipital midline electrode (Oz) displaying the P1 Group effect (patients>controls) within the time window 90–150 ms post scene onset. This group effect (difference between groups) is also displayed in the topography. B) Grand average waveforms of two right-hemispheric electrodes (i.e., FC4, CP4) displaying the P2 Group effect (patients>controls; also displayed in the topography) and the lexical access effect ('W'='S'>'C') within the time window 180–240 ms post stimulus. C) Grand averages of the anterior P3 syntactic complexity effect ('S'>'W'; highlighted in dark grey), significant in controls but not in patients, within the time window 350–650 ms post scene onset. The corresponding topographies of the syntactic complexity effect also show the effect in the controls, while no clear effect is observable in the patients.

Associations between outcome data and patient characteristics

There were no significant correlations between the patient characteristics (i.e., age at introduction diet, GALT enzyme activity, urine galactose and galactitol values) and the ERP data. Inspection of correlations with behavioural data revealed that older age at introduction of diet was related to longer TSTs [$r=.689$, $p=.001$]. Further, higher urine galactitol values were correlated with the shorter VOTs [$r=-.514$, $p=.017$]. Better verbal working memory scores (Digit Span) were related to lower galactitol values in urine [$r=-.471$, $p=0.031$].

Differential effects for patients with different genotypes were explored (homozygous for Q188R versus other mutations). The GALT enzyme activity and urine galactose and galactitol values did not differ across groups. The Q188R homozygous group had longer VOTs [only in the 'W' condition, $F(1,18)=5.213$, $p=.036$]. No differences in neuropsychological scores were found, but the groups differed with respect to the ERP effects: the syntactic complexity effect (i.e., difference between the linguistic conditions in the P3 bump time window) was greater in the 'other mutation' group compared to the homozygous group [$F(1,19)=13.362$, $p=.002$].

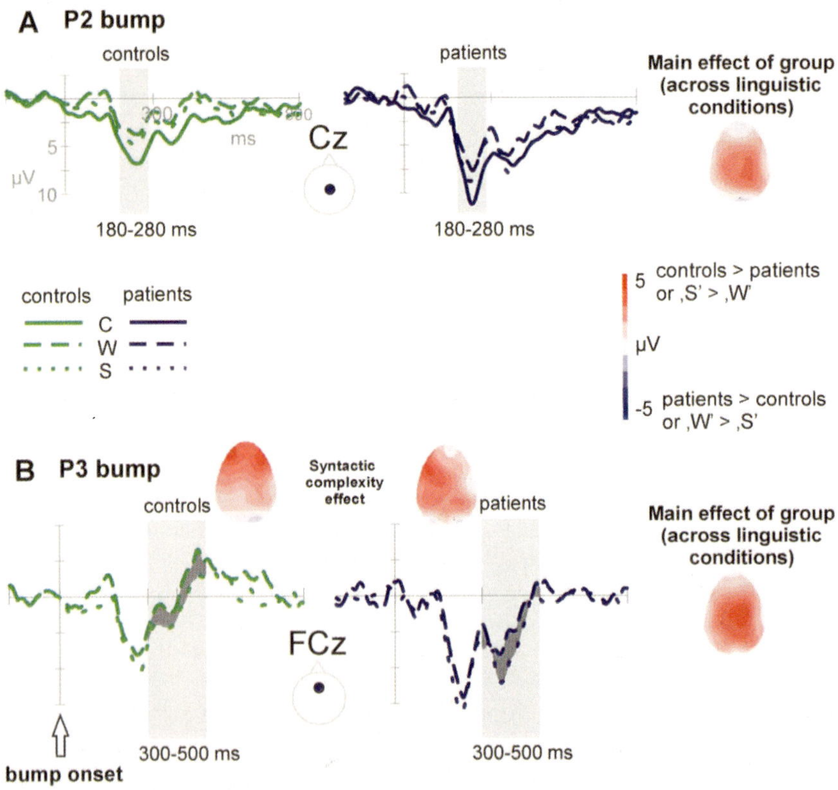

Figure 5. Overview of the ERP effects in the post bump event epoch. A) Grand average waveforms of the central midline electrode (Cz) displaying the P2 bump group effect (patients>controls; also reflected in the topography) and the P2 bump linguistic condition or lexical access effect ('W' = 'S'<'C') within the time window 180–280 ms post bump event. B) Grand averages of the fronto-central midline electrode (FCz) reflecting the P3 bump syntactic complexity effect ('S'>'W'; reflected in the dark grey fill in the ERPs and in the corresponding topographies) and the P3 group effect (patients>controls; see also topography) within time window 300–500 ms post bump event.

Discussion

This study is the first to apply theories, methods, and experimental paradigms from cognitive neuroscience to study language production impairments in classic galactosemia. This approach reveals impairments in several language production stages prior to articulation in these patients.

Behavioural data

The adolescent participants described animated scenes using different syntactic complexity formats: either separate words ('W') or complete sentences ('S'). Both groups required more self-corrections and speaking time in the sentence condition as compared to the word condition, suggesting that the intended complexity variation of syntactic planning was successful. Several outcome measures are found to deviate in patients compared to matched controls. The patients made more errors than controls (8.8% versus 2.8% of all trials). They needed more time to prepare (VOT 2.0 versus 1.8 seconds) and to finish the utterance (TST averaged across conditions: 5.1 versus 4.3 seconds), indicating that the patients were both slower and less accurate. Interestingly, in both groups, the error rates and voice onset times did not differ across the sentence and the word condition. The finding that the speaking time is modulated by syntactic complexity, but the voice onset time is not, suggests that most of the syntactic planning occurs after the initiation of the utterance.

ERP components of healthy controls

The ERPs reflect the entire information processing sequence, including visual processing of the figures and their movements, and the language planning process. We will first discuss the effects of the condition modulations in the control group only, in order to make inferences on their functional relevance. Several time windows showed a condition modulation, before and after the action format (the verb) became clear, reflecting the early initiation of the utterance and the incremental nature of the language planning.

The ***P1 scene*** is, with respect to distribution and latency, most likely an instance of the occipital P100, traditionally associated with visual and attention processes [51,52]. The P1 has also been linked to motion processing of visual stimuli (i.e., influenced by on- and offset, linked to V1) [53] and to conceptual processes [21,54]. There was no modulation with condition, indicating similar requirements for motion processing, attention and conceptualisation across the conditions in this study. The ***P2 scene*** component is most likely a P200, traditionally observed over anterior sites [52] and linked to lexical access of words during picture naming [55,56] or word reading [57]. Along this line, the observed effect likely reflects lexical access, as the linguistic conditions ('W' and 'S') do not differ in lexical requirements or P2 modulation, but differ from passive viewing (not requiring lexical access). Although the scene just started at this point, it is already clear which figure is the actor and which object is involved in the action, while the action format - verb - is still ambiguous. Therefore, lexical access is most likely restricted to access of the first noun phrase (actor). The idea that planning starts with the onset of the visual stimuli is consistent with the idea that language production is (at least partly) driven by visual input or visual attention [58–60]. The long lasting and widely distributed ***P3 scene*** resembles a P300. Anterior, the P3 showed variation with syntactic complexity. The timing and direction of the effect is in line with previous reports of the P300 reflecting integration of working memory and attention, both necessary for updating incoming information over time [61]. The observed ERP variation with syntactic complexity at the frontal midline (where 'S' is more positive than 'W') can be explained by the need for more attention- and memory-related resources in case of higher syntactic complexity, or could be a direct indication for more complex syntactic processing. At this time point, the action format (verb) is still ambiguous as differentiation between the two potential verbs can only happen after appropriate visual input (the bump, at 1520 ms after scene onset). Based on this, we conclude that syntactic planning reflected by the P3 must be restricted to local syntactic processing (i.e., retrieval of syntactic information about the actor/noun, inflection of the adjective). As there was no syntactic complexity effect in the VOT, we can assume that the utterance is initiated prior to syntactic planning once the first element of lexical access is in (noun or noun phrase) [32,33]. Larger P3 syntactic complexity effects were associated with shorter TSTs, indicating that more advanced local syntactic planning decreases the speaking time or increases the efficiency of the language process. In the following time window, the ERP shows activity around baseline (approximately 900 to 1400 ms post scene onset), presumably reflecting neural activity without clearly measurable events (eventually due to high variation in cognitive processing within and between groups). Then, divergence across action formats (verbs) occurs both scene-wise and ERP-wise. Time-locked to the moment of the bump, another set of ERP components arise (in the 'to bump into' trials only, presumably because the lack of a clear temporal event in the 'to fly towards' trials). During the fronto-central ***P2 bump*** component, we observed a condition pattern identical to that of the *P2 scene* component: the two linguistic conditions differed from passive watching, but not from each other. Now, all information is available (including the verb), making lexical access of the verb possible in an unambiguous way. Larger linguistic condition effects (i.e., difference between non-linguistic and linguistic conditions) were related to shorter VOTs and less errors, indicating that larger linguistic condition effects are associated with more accurate and faster performance. Finally, the large and widely distributed ***P3 bump*** component probably reflects a P300. Again, this post-bump P3 showed a similar pattern as the post-scene P3: variation with syntactic complexity. At this point, not only local but also global syntactic planning is required in the sentence condition (i.e., combination and integration of all noun phrases and the verb into a well-formed sentence), reflected in the larger P3 amplitudes. To sum, the functional interpretation of the ERPs in healthy controls is such that it starts with a set of components related to processing of moving visual information/conceptualisation (*P1 scene*), lexical access of the noun phrases (*P2 scene*) and local syntactic planning of the noun phrases (*P3 scene*). When all information, including the verb, is available, the ERP continues with similar components related to lexical access of the verb (*P2 bump*) and to syntactic planning on a more global sentence-level (*P3 bump*).

Relatively few studies have examined overt naming during ERPs recording, especially not using multi-word utterances [22,55,62,63]. Marek et al. [62] elicited multi-word utterances and sentences and found a posterior P3-like component (350–500 ms post stimulus) reflecting syntactic complexity (in addition to increasing conceptual complexity, as the used paradigm did not disentangle the two). In the present study, conceptual complexity was kept constant, suggesting that the observed P3 modulations speak to syntactic complexity proper. The production P3's that are found in the current study and the described previous studies, might therefore be analogous to the P600/SPS in syntactic comprehension [37,64,65], albeit with a more anterior distribution of the syntactic effect. The finding that both instances of the P3 in this study (post scene and post bump event) display the syntactic complexity effect provides additional support for a role for syntactic encoding in this component.

Psycholinguistic models of speech processing assume incremental planning of an utterance [15,17,35]. In our study, the utterance seems to be initiated after lexical access of the first noun, but prior to syntactic planning of this noun phrase (as the VOT did not vary with syntactic complexity). Our results therefore support the idea that an utterance can be initiated before the visual stimulation is finished (and before all necessary information is available). In addition, by means of ERP variations, we could look into the linguistic planning phase. Well before voice onset and before the visual input of the scene is complete, we observed activation related to local syntactic planning. When all information was available, there was continuation of syntactic encoding (on a more global, sentence-level). Although this paradigm was originally implemented using PET [38,40], this study demonstrates its suitability for high temporal resolution methods, since it allows us to disentangle this early local and later more global planning.

ERP components of patients with galactosemia

The patient ERPs showed a similar morphology compared to that of the matched controls, suggesting a generally intact neural network of cognition and language processing. The patient ERP differed from those of controls in several time windows. In the ***P1 scene*** component, related to attention, visual integration of moving objects and conceptualisation processes, the patients showed higher amplitudes in all three conditions (classically interpreted as more effortful processing) compared to controls. The fact that the patients differ in all conditions from controls, including passive watching, suggests early visual or attention processing deficits or an increased effort to integrate moving objects over time. Moreover, the patients showed a difference between linguistic and non-linguistic conditions ('W'/'S' versus 'C') that was not present in controls, suggesting linguistic effects in this early time window, likely reflecting impaired conceptualization. This is the first evidence that the patients diverge at an early stage in cognitive information processing from healthy controls during the preparation of language. In the ***P2 scene***, associated with lexical access, the patients showed the same pattern of condition effects as the controls (difference between control condition and both language conditions). Posterior, the patients showed greater amplitudes in both language-related conditions compared to controls, suggesting difficulties with lexical access. During the ***P3 scene***, the patients did not show the syntactic effect. The finding that the controls showed this syntactic variation but the patients did not can be interpreted as a ceiling effect for the patients: the sentence condition does not diverge from the word condition, as the ceiling level of memory/attention resources is already reached in the word condition (descriptively corroborated by the grand averages showing that in the patient ERP both the 'W' and 'S' condition are in the same range as the 'S' condition in controls). It could be that the patients perform less efficient advance syntactic planning. In controls, larger syntactic complexity effects (i.e., more advance syntactic planning) were associated with shorter TSTs. The patients needed more speaking time compared to controls, also indicative of less (efficient) advance syntactic planning. Different from the controls, smaller syntactic complexity effects were related to longer VOTs, suggesting that for the patients, less advance syntactic planning is related to slower or later initiation of the utterance. The patient' ERP further deviates from controls in the ***P2 bump*** component, providing additional support for impaired lexical access in the patients. Finally, the groups differed from each other during the ***P3 bump*** component, with the patients having larger mean amplitudes compared to controls. The syntactic variation was also present in the patients (opposite to the *P3 scene* component, where only the controls showed this variation). Two explanations are: they require more resources when engaging sentence-level syntactic planning (explaining the higher amplitudes) or, they compensate for earlier impairments in local syntactic planning by engaging in both local and sentence-level syntactic planning at a later (post bump) planning phase causing the higher amplitudes. We cannot disentangle between these alternatives at the moment.

The finding that there were no significant (or minor) differences in the ERP morphology between the groups in passive watching confirms an overall comparable cognitive system, suggesting that behavioural language impairments of the patients are not part of a severe general impairment. This assumption receives empirical support by the observed difference in ERPs between groups for the linguistic task. These differences cannot be explained merely by differences in the visual processing between conditions, but must be related to higher language function – as this was the task manipulation. Besides language planning the effects could be explained by variation in attentional or memory resources. Such variation across different naming formats cannot be excluded.

We investigated whether the observed impairments were purely linguistic in nature or whether they can be explained by other cognitive difficulties by looking into their neuropsychological test profile and by comparing the ERP with test results of specific cognitive functions. As reported in the result section and consistent with previous reports [5–8], the patients scored lower on several neuropsychological tests. The patients were slower (Bourdon-Vos reaction times [45]) and had difficulties with the visuo-motor task (Rey Complex Figure Copy subtest [44], among other things requiring the integration of a multitude of components into a unifying whole). Important as well is that visual working memory, when corrected for the visuo-motor differences, was not significantly worse in the patients. Therefore, visual working memory (keeping the visual scene online and actively in mind) cannot explain the behavioural and ERP-related differences between the groups. Verbal working memory performance [46], however, was lower in the patients, potentially adding to the language impairments. Importantly, verbal working memory scores were not correlated to the behavioural and ERP effects during the language task. The lack of correlation suggested that verbal working memory did not directly contribute to the observed ERP effects. Interestingly, several domains that are affected in the patients with classic galactosemia (i.e., visuo-motor skills, motion processing) require some form of integration of information over time. Such an integration deficit may also lead to the difficulties in constructing syntactic frames as well as difficulties to access and fill in the right words into these frames [18].

Correlations with patient variables (i.e., GALT enzyme activity, age at introduction diet, urine galactose and galactitol values) were far from robust, consistent with previous studies failing to find predictive value for these variables [6,31,66]. We observed that patients homozygous for the Q188R mutation performed worse on certain aspects compared to patients with other mutations, which is in line with other, but not all, studies [66]. Patients with the Q188R/Q188R mutation had longer VOTs and showed smaller syntactic complexity effects in the P3 bump ERP component.

Previous studies in classic galactosemia have reported general cognitive slowing and diffuse white matter abnormalities [4,30,67], theoretically linked to deficient galactosylation of cerebrosides (an important component of myelin) [68]. In line with these findings, our study showed longer reaction times for the patients (both the time needed to prepare and to finish the utterance). In the ERP data, we did not find any delays in the overall evolution of the ERP components. The morphology of the signal was similar for patients and controls. We observed amplitude differences, suggesting an alteration in the neural activity related to a certain cognitive processing phase, which indicates that brain abnormalities might be more clustered than previously suggested. Within the *P3 scene* time window we see a comparable onset of the component, but the P3 seems to be extended in time for patients compared to matched controls. As depicted in Figure 4C, for controls the ERP signal for the 'W' and 'S' conditions catches up sooner with the signal of the 'C' condition, especially more posterior. This overall ERP pattern of the patients suggests that the local neural circuits work within time windows that are comparable to those of healthy controls. However, the larger amplitudes in the patient ERPs indicate aberrant neural activation patterns. Accumulating metabolites or resulting deficiencies that alter neuronal signalling might be involved herein (e.g., myo-inositol [69]). In contrast, the overall integration problem might result from problems of long distance neural communication possibly associated with myelin abnormalities compromising information transfer [30,67]. However, whether abnormal cell signalling and/or brain connectivity is affected and in which specific regions requires further investigation.

To summarize, patients with classic galactosemia show difficulties in this language production task, both behaviourally (less accurate and slower) and in their ERPs, compared to healthy controls. The ERP deviations start already around the time that attention is directed towards the relevant moving objects and conceptual knowledge of these objects becomes available, suggesting that these processes are affected by the disease. The ERP differences continue throughout the consecutive linguistic preparation phases, indicating affected lexical access and impaired syntactic planning (both local and sentence-level syntactic planning). We conclude that, although anecdotal reports have appeared on weak word retrieval and sentence construction, this study is the first to provide neuro-cognitive evidence for language impairments in patients with classic galactosemia. These impairments affect the planning of language, which occurs prior to the output stage. Based on the ERP data, we suggest that these impairments are related to problems in lexical access and syntactic planning of an utterance. These findings are relevant for speech and language therapies within this patient group, deserving further investigation.

Acknowledgments

We kindly acknowledge the Dutch Galactosemia Patient Organization for their cooperation and assistance during the preparation of this study, and the participants and their parents for their time, effort and cooperation. We thank Francesco Gentile for the preparation of the experimental stimuli and support with the analyses, and the anonymous reviewers for providing useful comments and suggestions.

Author Contributions

Conceived and designed the experiments: IT BMJ MER. Performed the experiments: IT. Analyzed the data: IT. Contributed reagents/materials/ analysis tools: IT BMJ MER. Wrote the paper: IT. Added to the discussion on interpretations of results: IT BMJ MER. Critical revisions of manuscript: BMJ MER. Final approval of initial manuscript: IT BMJ MER. Consideration and discussing of reviewers' comments and suggestions: IT BMJ MER. Revision of manuscript and writing rebuttal letter: IT. Final approval of revisions and rebuttal letter: IT BMJ MER.

References

1. Potter NL, Lazarus JAC, Johnson JM, Steiner RD, Shriberg LD (2008) Correlates of language impairment in children with galactosaemia. Journal of Inherited Metabolic Disease 31: 524–532.
2. Waisbren SE, Norman TR, Schnell RR, Levy HL (1983) Speech and language deficits in early-treated children with galactosemia. Journal of Pediatrics 102: 75–77.
3. Schadewaldt P, Hoffman B, Hammen H, Kamp G, Schweitzer-Krantz S, et al. (2010) Longitudinal Assessment of Intellectual Achievement in Patients with Classical Galactosemia. Pediatrics 125: e374–e381.
4. Widhalm K, Miranda-da-Cruz BD, de Sonneville LMJ (2002) Information processing characteristics and uridine treatment in children with classical galactosemia. Nutrition Research 22: 257–270.
5. Schweitzer S, Shin Y, Jakobs C, Brodehl J (1993) Long-term outcome in 134 patients with galactosemia. European Journal of Pediatrics 152: 36–43.
6. Waggoner DD, Buist NRM, Donnell GN (1990) Long-Term Prognosis in Galactosemia: Results of a Survey of 350 Cases. Journal of Inherited Metabolic Disease: 802–818.
7. Antshel KM, Epstein IO, Waisbren SE (2004) Cognitive strengths and weaknesses in children and adolescents homozygous for the galactosemia Q188R mutation: a descriptive study. Neuropsychology 18: 658–664.
8. Doyle CM, Channon S, Orlowska D, Lee PJ (2010) The neuropsychological profile of galactosaemia. Journal of Inherited Metabolic Disease 33: 603–609.
9. Potter NL (2011) Voice disorders in children with classic galactosemia. Journal of Inherited Metabolic Disease 34: 377–385.
10. Waisbren SE, Potter NL, Gordon CM, Green RC, Greenstein P, et al. (2012) The adult galactosemic phenotype. Journal of Inherited Metabolic Disease 35: 279–286.
11. Shriberg LD, Potter NL, Strand EA (2010) Prevalence and Phenotype of Childhood Apraxia of Speech In Youth with Galactosemia. Journal of Speech, Language, and Hearing Research.
12. Robertson A, Singh RH, Guerrero NV, Hundley M, Elsas LJ (2000) Outcomes analysis of verbal dyspraxia in classic galactosemia. Genetics in Medicine 2: 142–148.
13. Nelson CD, Waggoner DD, Donnell GN, Tuereck JM, Buist NRM (1991) Verbal Dyspraxia in Treated Galactosemia. Pediatrics 88: 349–350.
14. Webb AL, Singh RH, Kennedy MJ, Elsas LJ (2003) Verbal dyspraxia and galactosemia. Pediatric Research 53: 396–402.
15. Bock K (1995) Sentence Production: From Mind to Mouth. In: Miller JL, Eimas PD, editors. Speech, Language, and Communication Handbook of perception and cognition. San Diego, CA, , US: Academic Press. pp. 181–216.
16. Indefrey P (2011) The spatial and temporal signatures of word production components: a critical update. Frontiers in Psychology 2: doi: 10.3389/fpsyg.2011.00255.
17. Levelt WJM (1989) Speaking: From Intention to Articulation. Cambridge, MA: The MIT Press.
18. Bock K, Levelt W (1994) Language Production: Grammatical Encoding. In: Gernsbacher MA, editor. Handbook of Psycholinguists. San Diego: Academic Press. pp. 945–984.
19. Levelt WJM, Roelofs AS, Meyer A (1999) A theory of lexical access in speech production. Behavioral and Brain Sciences 22: 1–75.
20. Kutas M, Schmitt BM (2003) Language in Microvolts. In: Banich MT, Mack M, editors. Mind, brain, and language: Multidisciplinary perspectives. NJ: Lawrence Erlbaum Associates. pp. 171–209.
21. Rahman RA, Sommer W (2008) Seeing what we know and understand: How knowledge shapes perception. Psychonomic Bulletin & Review 15: 1055–1063.
22. Jansma BM, Rodriguez-Fornells A, Möller J, Münte TF (2004) Electrophysiological studies of speech production. In: Pechman T, Habel C, editors. Multidisciplinary approaches to language production. Berlin: Mouton de Gruyter. pp. 361–395.
23. Schmitt BM, Schiltz K, Zaake W, Münte TF, Kutas M (2000) The time course of conceptual and syntactic encoding during language production estimated by event related potentials. Journal of Cognitive Neuroscience: 29B.
24. van Turennout M, Hagoort P, Brown CM (1997) Electrophysiological evidence on the time course of semantic and phonological processes in speech production. Journal of Experimental Psychology: Learning, Memory, and Cognition 23: 787–806.
25. Hickok G (2009) The functional neuroanatomy of language. Physics of Life Reviews 6: 121–143.
26. Price CJ (2010) The anatomy of language: a review of 100 fMRI studies published in 2009. Cognitive Neuroscience 1191: 62–88.
27. Rogalski E, Cobia D, Harrison TM, Wieneke C, Thompson CK, et al. (2011) Anatomy of Language Impairments in Primary Progressive Aphasia. The Journal of Neuroscience 31: 3344–3350.
28. Friederici AD (2006) The Neural Basis of Language Development and Its Impairment. Neuron 52: 941–952.
29. Glasser MF, Rilling JK (2008) DTI tractography of the human brain's language pathways. Cerebral cortex 18: 2471–2482.
30. Nelson MD, Wolff JA, Cross CA, Donnell GN, Kaufman FR (1992) Galactosemia: Evaluation with MR Imaging. Radiology 184: 255–261.
31. Kaufman FR, McBride Chang C, Manis FR, Wolff JA, Nelson MD (1995) Cognitive functioning, neurologic status and brain imaging in classical galactosemia. European Journal of Pediatrics 154: S2–5.
32. Allum PH, Wheeldon LR (2007) Planning scope in spoken sentence production: the role of grammatical units. Journal of experimental psychology Learning, memory, and cognition 33: 791–810.
33. Allum PH, Wheeldon L (2009) Scope of Lexical Access in Spoken Sentence Production: Implications for the Conceptual-Syntactic Interface. Journal of Experimental Psychology-Learning Memory and Cognition 35: 1240–1255.
34. Wagner V, Jescheniak JD, Schriefers H (2010) On the flexibility of grammatical advance planning during sentence production: Effects of cognitive load on multiple lexical access. Journal of experimental psychology Learning, memory, and cognition 36: 423–440.
35. Meyer AS (1996) Lexical access in phrase and sentence production. Journal of Memory and Language 35: 477–496.
36. Hagoort P (2003) How the brain solves the binding problem for language: a neurocomputational model of syntactic processing. Neuroimage 20: S18–S29.
37. Kaan E, Harris A, Gibson E, Holcomb P (2000) The P600 as an index of syntactic integration difficulty. Language and Cognitive Processes 15: 159–201.
38. Indefrey P, Brown CM, Hellwig F, Amunts K, Herzog H, et al. (2001) A neural correlate of syntactic encoding during speech production. Proceedings of the National Academy of Sciences of the United States of America 98: 5933–5936.
39. Sahin NT, Pinker S, Cash SS, Schomer D, Halgren E (2009) Sequential Processing of Lexical, Grammatical, and Phonological Information Within Broca's Area. Science 326: 445–449.
40. Indefrey P, Hellwig F, Herzog H, Seitz RJ, Hagoort P (2004) Neural responses to the production and comprehension of syntax in identical utterances. Brain and Language 89: 312–319.
41. Vosse T, Kempen G (2000) Syntactic structure assembly in human parsing: a computational model based on competitive inhibition and a lexicalist grammar. Cognition 75: 105–143.
42. Snijders TM, Vosse T, Kempen G, Van Berkum J, Petersson KM, et al. (2009) Retrieval and unification of syntactic structure in sentence comprehension: an FMRI study using word-category ambiguity. Cerebral cortex 19: 1493–1503.
43. Hagoort P (2005) On Broca, brain, and binding: a new framework. Trends in Cognitive Sciences 9: 416–423.
44. Meyers JE, Meyers KR (1995) Rey Complex Figure Test and Recognition Trial: Professional Manual. Odessa: Psychological Assessment Resources, Inc.
45. Vos PG (1988) Bourdon-Vos-Test [Bourdon Vos Test]. Lisse: Swets & Zeitlinger.
46. van Haasen PP, de Bruyn EEJ, Pijl YL, Poortinga YH, Spelberg HC, et al. (1986) WISC-R, Wechsler Intelligence Scale for Children - Revised, Nederlandstalige uitgave. Deel I. Testinstructie; Deel II. Scoring en Normen; Deel III. Verantwoording. Lisse: Swets & Zeitlinger.
47. Jasper HH (1958) The ten-twenty electrode system of the International Federation. Electroencephalogr Clin Neurophysiol 10: 370–375.
48. Lezak MD (1995) Neuropsychological Assessment, 4th edition. New York, NY: Oxford University Press.
49. Delorme A, Makeig S (2004) EEGLAB: an open source toolbox for analysis of single-trial EEG dynamics. Journal of Neuroscience Methods 134: 9–21.
50. Makeig S, Onton J (2009) ERP features and EEG dynamics: an ICA perspective. In: Luck SJ, Kappenman E, editors. Oxford Handbook of Event-Related Potential Components. New York: Oxford University Press.
51. Coles MGH, Rugg MD (1995) Event-related brain potentials: an introduction. In: Rugg M, Coles M, editors. Electrophysiology of Mind: Event-Related Brain Potentials and Cognition. New York, US: Oxford University Press. pp. 1–26.
52. Luck SJ (2005) An Introduction to the Event-Related Potential Technique: MIT Press.
53. Mercier M, Schwartz S, Michel CM, Blanke O (2009) Motion direction tuning in human visual cortex. European Journal of Neuroscience 29: 424–434.
54. Rabovsky M, Sommer W, Rahman RA (2011) Depth of Conceptual Knowledge Modulates Visual Processes during Word Reading. Journal of Cognitive Neuroscience [Epub ahead of print].
55. Strijkers K, Costa A, Thierry G (2009) Tracking Lexical Access in Speech Production: Electrophysiological Correlates of Word Frequency and Cognate Effects. Cerebral Cortex 20: 912–928.
56. Costa A, Strijkers K, Martin C, Thierry G (2009) The time course of word retrieval revealed by event-related brain potentials during overt speech. Proceedings of the National Academy of Sciences of the United States of America 106: 21442–21446.
57. Bles M, Alinka A, Jansma B (2007) Neural aspects of cohort-size reduction during visual gating. Brain Research 1150: 143–154.
58. Meyer AS, Lethaus F (2004) The use of eye tracking in studies of sentence generation. In: Henderson JM, Ferreira F, editors. The interface of language, vision, and action: What we can learn from free-viewing eye tracking. New York: Psychology Press. pp. 191–211.

59. Bock K (1982) Toward a cognitive psychology of syntax: Information processing contributions to sentence formulation. Psychological Review 89: 1–47.
60. Mortensen L, Meyer AS, Humphreys GW (2008) Speech planning during multiple-object naming: Effects of ageing. The Quarterly Journal of Experimental Psychology 61: 1217–1238.
61. Kok A (2001) On the utility of P3 amplitude as a measure of processing capacity. Psychophysiology 38: 557–577.
62. Marek A, Habets B, Jansma BM, Nager W, Münte TF (2007) Neural correlates of conceptualisation difficulty during the preparation of complex utterances. Aphasiology 21: 1147–1156.
63. Koester D, Schiller NO (2008) Morphological priming in overt language production: Electrophysiological evidence from Dutch. Neuroimage 42: 1622–1630.
64. Hagoort P, Brown C, Groothusen J (1993) The syntactic positive shift (SPS) as an ERP measure of syntactic processing. Language and Cognitive Processes 8: 439–483.
65. Osterhout L, Holcomb PJ (1992) Event-Related Brain Potentials Elicited by Syntactic Anomaly. Journal of Memory and Language 31: 785–806.
66. Shield JP, Wadsworth EJ, MacDonald A, Stephenson A, Tyfield L, et al. (2000) The relationship of genotype to cognitive outcome in galactosaemia. Archives of Disease in Childhood 83: 248–250.
67. Dubroff JG, Ficicioglu C, Segal S, Wintering NA, Alavi A, et al. (2008) FDG-PET findings in patients with galactosaemia. Journal of Inherited Metabolic Disease 31: 533–539.
68. Lebea PJ, Pretorius PJ (2005) The molecular relationship between deficient UDP-galactose uridyl transferase (GALT) and ceramide galactosyltransferase (CGT) enzyme function: a possible cause for poor long-term prognosis in classic galactosemia. Medical Hypotheses 65: 1051–1057.
69. Berry GT (2011) Is prenatal myo-inositol deficiency a mechanism of CNS injury in galactosemia? Journal of Inherited Metabolic Disease 34: 345–355.

Permissions

All chapters in this book were first published in PLOS ONE, by The Public Library of Science; hereby published with permission under the Creative Commons Attribution License or equivalent. Every chapter published in this book has been scrutinized by our experts. Their significance has been extensively debated. The topics covered herein carry significant findings which will fuel the growth of the discipline. They may even be implemented as practical applications or may be referred to as a beginning point for another development.

The contributors of this book come from diverse backgrounds, making this book a truly international effort. This book will bring forth new frontiers with its revolutionizing research information and detailed analysis of the nascent developments around the world.

We would like to thank all the contributing authors for lending their expertise to make the book truly unique. They have played a crucial role in the development of this book. Without their invaluable contributions this book wouldn't have been possible. They have made vital efforts to compile up to date information on the varied aspects of this subject to make this book a valuable addition to the collection of many professionals and students.

This book was conceptualized with the vision of imparting up-to-date information and advanced data in this field. To ensure the same, a matchless editorial board was set up. Every individual on the board went through rigorous rounds of assessment to prove their worth. After which they invested a large part of their time researching and compiling the most relevant data for our readers.

The editorial board has been involved in producing this book since its inception. They have spent rigorous hours researching and exploring the diverse topics which have resulted in the successful publishing of this book. They have passed on their knowledge of decades through this book. To expedite this challenging task, the publisher supported the team at every step. A small team of assistant editors was also appointed to further simplify the editing procedure and attain best results for the readers.

Apart from the editorial board, the designing team has also invested a significant amount of their time in understanding the subject and creating the most relevant covers. They scrutinized every image to scout for the most suitable representation of the subject and create an appropriate cover for the book.

The publishing team has been an ardent support to the editorial, designing and production team. Their endless efforts to recruit the best for this project, has resulted in the accomplishment of this book. They are a veteran in the field of academics and their pool of knowledge is as vast as their experience in printing. Their expertise and guidance has proved useful at every step. Their uncompromising quality standards have made this book an exceptional effort. Their encouragement from time to time has been an inspiration for everyone.

The publisher and the editorial board hope that this book will prove to be a valuable piece of knowledge for researchers, students, practitioners and scholars across the globe.

List of Contributors

Michela Zanetti, Rocco Barazzoni and Annamaria Semolic
Clinica Medica, Department of Medical, Surgical and Health Sciences, University of Trieste, Trieste

Mariagrazia Zenti, Federica Zardi and Enzo Bonora
Endocrinology, Diabetes and Metabolism, University and Azienda Ospedaliera Universitaria Integrata of Verona, Verona, Italy

Michele Giuseppe Messa
Nephrology, University and Azienda Ospedaliera Universitaria Integrata of Verona, Verona, Italy

Maurizio Fonda and Luigi Cattin
Diabetes and Metabolic Diseases Unit, Department of Medical, Surgical and Health Sciences, University of Trieste, Trieste, Italy

Gianpaolo Russi and Luca Scarano
Immunohematology and Transfusion Unit, Ospedale Santa Maria Nuova, Reggio Emilia, Italy

Aurelie Nguyen Dinh Cat, Brigitte Escoubet, Vincent Agrapart, Violaine Griol-Charhbili and Frederic Jaisser
Inserm U872 Team 1, Paris, France

Aurelie Nguyen Dinh Cat, Vincent Agrapart, Violaine Griol-Charhbili and Frederic Jaisser
University Pierre et Marie Curie, Paris, France

Brigitte Escoubet
AP-HP Hôpital Bichat, Paris, France
Centre d'Explorations Fonctionnelles-Imagerie, Bichat Federative Research Institute 02, University Denis Diderot, Paris, France

Trenton Schoeb, Wenguang Feng, Edgar Jaimes and David G. Warnock
University of Alabama at Birmingham, Birmingham, Alabama, United States of America

Masahiro Sugawara, Hidemi Ohye, Chisato Tomoda and Takahiko Kogai
Endocrinology and Diabetes Division, Department of Medicine, Veterans Affairs Greater Los Angeles Health Care System, David Geffen School of Medicine at University of California Los Angeles, Los Angeles, California, United States of America

Masahiro Sugawara
Primary Care Service, Department of Medicine, Veterans Affairs Greater Los Angeles Health Care System, David Geffen School of Medicine, University of California Los Angeles, Los Angeles, California, United States of America

Yoshimasa Kamata
Department of Pathology, Hirosaki University School of Medicine, Hirosaki, Japan

Gholam H. Pezeshkpour and Farhad Moatamed
Department of Pathology, Veterans Affairs Greater Los Angeles Health Care System, David Geffen School of Medicine, University of California Los Angeles, Los Angeles, California, United States of America

Jenny Shin, Katrina Epperson and Kasturi Haldar
Center for Rare and Neglected Diseases, University of Notre Dame, Notre Dame, Indiana, United States of America

Nicole M. Yanjanin and Forbes D. Porter
Program in Developmental Endocrinology and Genetics, NICHD, National Institutes of Health, DHHS, Bethesda, Maryland, United States of America

Jennifer Albus, Laura Borgenheimer, Natalie Bott, Erin Brennan, Daniel Castellanos, Melissa Cheng, Michael Clark, Margaret Devany, Courtney Ensslin, Nina Farivari, Shanik Fernando, Lauren Gabriel, Rani Gallardo, Moriah Castleman, Olimpia Gutierrez, Allison Herschel, Sarah Hodge, Anne Horst, Mary Howard, Evan James, Lindsey Jones, Mary Kearns, Mary Kelly, Christine Kim, Kinzie Kiser, Gregory Klazura, Chris Knoedler, Emily Kolbus, Lauren Lange, Joan Lee, Eileena Li, Wei Lu, Andrew Luttrell, Emily Ly, Katherine McKeough, Brianna McSorley, Catherine Miller, Sean Mitchell, Abbey Moon, Kevin Moser, Shane O'Brien, Paula Olivieri, Aaron Patzwahl, Marie Pereira, Craig Pymento, Erin Ramelb, Bryce Ramos, Teresa Raya, Stephen Riney, Geoff Roberts, Mark Robertshaw, Frannie Rudolf, Samuel Rund, Stephanie Sansone, Lindsay Schwartz, Ryan Shay, Edwin Siu, Timothy Spear, Catherine Tan, Marisa Truong, Mairaj Uddin, Jennifer VanTrieste, Omar Veloz and Elizabeth White
NPC Consortium for Community-Based Assessment of Patient Records, Cape Town, South Africa

Thaneas Prabakaran, Rikke Nielsen and Erik I. Christensen
Section of Cell Biology, Department of Anatomy, Aarhus University, Aarhus, Denmark

Jakob V. Larsen and Claus M. Petersen
Department of Medical Biochemistry, Aarhus University, Aarhus, Denmark

Søren S. Sørensen
Department P, Rigshospitalet, Copenhagen, Denmark

Ulla Feldt-Rasmussen
Department of Medical Endocrinology, Rigshospitalet, Copenhagen, Denmark

Moin A. Saleem
Children's Renal Unit and Academic Renal Unit, University of Bristol, Southmead Hospital, Bristol, United Kingdom

Pierre J. Verroust
UMRS 592, Institut de la Vision, Paris, France

Roeland Huijgen, Sjoerd B. J. Verhoeven, Maud N. Vissers and John J. P.Kastelein
Department of Vascular Medicine, Academic Medical Center (AMC), Amsterdam, The Netherlands

Iris Kindt
Foundation for the Identification of Persons with Inherited Hypercholesterolemia, Amsterdam, The Netherlands

Eric J. G. Sijbrands
Department of Cardiovascular Genetics and Department of Pharmacology, Vascular and etabolic Diseases, Erasmus Medical Center, Rotterdam, The Netherlands

Barbara A. Hutten
Department of Clinical Epidemiology, Biostatistics and Bioinformatics, Academic Medical Center (AMC), Amsterdam, The Netherlands

Ulrike Mütze, Skadi Beblo, Carmen Rohde and Wieland Kiess
Department of Women and Child Health, Hospital for Children and Adolescents, University Hospital, University of Leipzig, Leipzig, Germany

Linda Kortz, Joachim Thiery and Uta Ceglarek
Clinical Chemistry and Molecular Diagnostics, Institute of Laboratory Medicine, University Hospital, University of Leipzig, Leipzig, Germany

Linda Kortz and Uta Ceglarek
LIFE - Leipzig Research Center for Civilization Diseases, University Leipzig, Leipzig, Germany

Claudia Matthies and Berthold Koletzko
Division Metabolic Diseases and Nutritional Medicine, Dr. von Hauner Children's Hospital, Ludwig-Maximilians-University of Munich, Munich, Germany

Mathias Bruegel
Institute of Laboratory Medicine, Ludwig-Maximilians-University of Munich, Munich, Germany

Xu Wang, Liyuan Sun, Jie Lin and Lu-Ya Wang
The Key Laboratory of Remodeling-related Cardiovascular Diseases, Capital Medical University, Ministry of Education, and Beijing Institute of Heart Lung and Blood Vessel Diseases, Beijing Anzhen Hospital of the Capital University of Medical Sciences, Beijing, People's Republic of China

Xin Li, Yong-Biao Zhang, Feng Zhang and Duen-Mei Wang
CAS Key Laboratory of Genome Sciences and Information, Beijing Institute of Genomics, Chinese Academy of Sciences, Beijing, People's Republic of China

Patrick Solverson, Sangita G. Murali and Denise M. Ney
Department of Nutritional Sciences, University of Wisconsin, Madison, Wisconsin, United States of America

Suzanne J. Litscher and Robert D. Blank
Geriatrics Research, Education, and Clinical Center, William S. Middleton Veterans Hospital, Madison, Wisconsin, United States of America
Division of Endocrinology, Diabetes and Metabolism, Department of Medicine, University of Wisconsin, School of Medicine and Public Health, Madison, Wisconsin, United States of America

Trond P. Leren and Knut Erik Berge
Medical Genetics Laboratory, Department of Medical Genetics, Oslo University Hospital Rikshospitalet, Oslo, Norway

Mireia Mora, Felicia A. Hanzu, Gloria B. Aranda and Irene Halperin
Department of Endocrinology and Nutrition, Hospital Clinic, Barcelona, Spain
Laboratory of Endocrine Disorders, Institut d'Investigacions Biomèdiques August Pi ISunyer (IDIBAPS), Barcelona, Spain

Mireia Mora, Felicia A. Hanzu, Marta Pradas-Juni and Gloria B. Aranda and Eduardo Fernández-Rebollo
Spanish Biomedical Research Centre in Diabetes and Associated Metabolic Disorders (CIBERDEM), Barcelona, Spain

Marta Pradas-Juni and Eduardo Fernández-Rebollo
Diabetes and Obesity Research Laboratory - Institut d'Investigacions Biomèdiques August Pi i Sunyer (IDIBAPS), Barcelona, Spain

Manuel Puig-Domingo
Department of Endocrinology and Nutrition, Hospital Germans Trias i Pujol Research Institut and Hospital, Universitat Autònoma de Barcelona, Badalona, Spain
Sira Aguiló
Department of Internal Medicine, Hospital Clínic, Barcelona, Spain

Saskia M. Rombach, Carla E. M. Hollak and Gabor E. Linthorst
Department of Endocrinology and Metabolism, Division of Internal Medicine, Academic Medical Center, Amsterdam, The Netherlands

Johannes M. F. G. Aerts, Ben J. H. M. Poorthuis, Johanna E. M. Groener, Wilma Donker-Koopman, Erik Hendriks, Mina Mirzaian, Sijmen Kuiper and Frits A. Wijburg
Department of Medical Biochemistry, Academic Medical Center, Amsterdam, The Netherlands

Andreas D. Kistler, Rudolf P. Wüthrich and Andreas L. Serra
Division of Nephrology, University Hospital, Zürich, Switzerland

Andreas D. Kistler
Division of Nephrology and Hypertension, University of Miami Miller School of Medicine, Miami, Florida, United States of America

Justyna Siwy and Harald Mischak
Mosaiques Diagnostics and Therapeutics AG, Hannover, Germany

Frank Breunig and Christoph Wanner
Division of Nephrology, University Hospital, Würzburg, Germany

Praveen Jeevaratnam and Derralynn A. Hughes
Department of Haematology, Hampstead Campus, University College Medical School, London, United Kingdom

Alexander Scher
Proteomics Core Facility, Faculty of Medicine, University of Geneva, Geneva, Switzerland

William Mullen
School of Life Sciences, College of Medical, Veterinary and Life Sciences, University of Glasgow, Glasgow, United Kingdom

David G. Warnock
Department of Medicine, University of Alabama at Birmingham, Birmingham, Alabama, United States of America

Harald Mischak
BHF Glasgow Cardiovascular Research Centre, University of Glasgow, Glasgow, United Kingdom

Sadik H. Kassim, Luk H. Vandenberghe, Christian Hinderer, Peter Bell, Hongwei Yu and James M. Wilson
Gene Therapy Program, Department of Pathology and Laboratory Medicine, University of Pennsylvania, Philadelphia, Pennsylvania, United States of America

Hui Li, Dawn Marchadier, Aisha Wilson, Debra Cromley, Valeska Redon and Daniel J. Rader
Institute for Translational Medicine and Therapeutics, University of Pennsylvania, Philadelphia, Pennsylvania, United States of America

Alex Langford-Smith, Kia J. Langford-Smith, Fiona L.Wilkinson and Brian W. Bigger
Stem Cell and Neurotherapies, School of Biomedicine, Faculty of Medical and Human Sciences, University of Manchester, Manchester, United Kingdom

Simon A. Jones and J. E. Wraith
Genetic Medicine, St. Mary's Hospital, Manchester, United Kingdom

Robert F. Wynn
Blood and Marrow Transplant Unit, Royal Manchester Children's Hospital, Manchester, United Kingdom

John Marshall, Karen M. Ashe, Dinesh Bangari, KerryAnne McEachern, Wei-Lien Chuang, Joshua Pacheco, Diane P. Copeland, Ronald K. Scheule and Seng H.Cheng
Applied Discovery Research, Genzyme Corporation, Framingham, Massachusetts, United States of America

Robert J. Desnick
Genetics and Genomic Sciences, Mount Sinai School of Medicine, New York, New York, United States of America

James A. Shayman
Internal Medicine - Nephrology, Genzyme Corporation, University of Michigan, Ann Arbor, Michigan, United States of America

Karen Broekhuizen, Mireille N. M. van Poppel and Willem van Mechelen
Department of Public and Occupational Health, EMGO+ Institute for Health and Care Research, VU University Medical Centre, Amsterdam, The Netherlands

Lando L. Koppes
Division of Work and Employment, TNO, Hoofddorp, The Netherlands

Iris Kindt
Foundation for the Identification of Persons with Inherited Hypercholesterolemia, msterdam, The Netherlands

Johannes Brug
EMGO+ Institute for Health and Care Research, VU University Medical Centre, Amsterdam, The Netherlands

Katja Heinicke and Ronald G. Haller
Neuromuscular Center, Institute for Exercise and Environmental Medicine, Texas Health Presbyterian Hospital, Dallas, Texas, United States of America
Department of Neurology and Neurotherapeutics, University of Texas Southwestern Medical Center, Dallas, Texas, United States of America

Ivan E. Dimitrov, Sergey Cheshkov, Jimin Ren and Craig R. Malloy
Advanced Imaging Research Center, University of Texas Southwestern Medical Center, Dallas, Texas, United States of America

Ivan E. Dimitrov
Philips Medical Systems, Cleveland, Ohio, United States of America

Ronald G. Haller
Department of Neurology, North Texas VA Medical Center, Dallas, Texas, United States of America

Say-Hean Lye, Jagdish Kaur Chahil, Pramod Bagali and Livy Alex
INFOVALLEYI I Group of Companies, Jalan Tasik, MINES Resort City, Selangor, Malaysia

Jamunarani Vadivelu, Wan Azman Wan Ahmad, Siew-Pheng Chan, Meow-Keong Thong and Rosmawati Mohamed
Faculty of Medicine, University of Malaya, Kuala Lumpur, Malaysia

Shamsul Mohd Zain
The Pharmacogenomics Laboratory, Department of Pharmacology, Faculty of Medicine, University of Malaya, Kuala Lumpur, Malaysia

Haihong Wang, Shengyuan Xu, Liyuan Sun, Xiaodong Pan, Shiwei Yang and Luya Wang
Department of Atherosclerosis, Beijing Institute of Heart Lung and Blood Vessel Disease, Beijing Anzhen Hospital Affiliated with Capital Medical University, Beijing, China

Wen-Feng Wu, Li-Yuan Sun and Shi-Wei Yang
Beijing Anzhen Hospital Affiliated with Capital Medical University, Beijing, China

Wen-Feng Wu, Xiao-Dong Pan, Shi-Wei Yang and Lv-Ya Wang
Department of Atherosclerosis, Beijing Institute of Heart Lung and Blood Vessel Diseases, Beijing, China

Eija H. Seppälä and Hannes Lohi
Research Programs Unit, Molecular Medicine, University of Helsinki, Helsinki, Finland
Department of Veterinary Biosciences and Department of Medical Genetics, University of Helsinki, Helsinki, Finland
Folkhälsan Institute of Genetics, Helsinki, Finland

Arnold J. J. Reuser
Departments of Clinical Genetics and Paediatrics, Center for Lysosomal and Metabolic Diseases, Erasmus MC, Rotterdam, The Netherlands

Michael Mauer
Department of Pediatrics, University of Minnesota, Minneapolis, United States of America,
Department of Medicine, University of Minnesota, Minneapolis, United States of America

Emily Glynn, Alexey Sokolovskiy and Behzad Najafian
Department of Pathology, University of Washington, Seattle, United States of America

Einar Svarstad
Department of Medicine, Haukeland University Hospital, Bergen, Norway

Einar Svarstad and Camilla Tøndel
Department of Clinical Medicine, University of Bergen, Bergen, Norway

Camilla Tøndel
Department of Pediatrics, Haukeland University Hospital, Bergen, Norway

Marie-Claire Gubler
Division of Nephrology, Department of Medicine, Dalhousie University, Halifax, Nova Scotia, Canada

Ying Gu
Prenatal Diagnosis Center, Maternal and Child Health Care Hospital, Lianyungang, Jiangsu, China

Kangmo Lu
Prenatal Diagnosis Center, Chengdu Women's and Children's Central Hospital, Chengdu, Sichuan, China

Guanghui Yang., Zhong Cen, Jing Hao, Zhigang Yang, Jiabao Peng and Shujian Cui
Shanghai Find Bio-Tech Co., Ltd., Shanghai, China

Li Yu
Life Technologies Company, Shanghai, China

Jian Huang
National Engineering Center for Biochip at Shanghai, Shanghai, China
Shanghai-MOST Key Laboratory for Disease and Health Genomics, Chinese National Human Genome Center at Shanghai, Shanghai, China

Aitor Etxebarria, Asier Benito-Vicente, Helena Ostolaza and Cesar Martin
Unidad de Biofísica (CSIC, UPV/EHU) and Departamento de Bioquímicay Biología Molecular, Universidad del País Vasco, Apdo. 644, 48080 Bilbao, Spain

Ana C. Alves and Mafalda Bourbon
Grupo de Investigação Cardiovascular, Unidade I&D, Departamento de Promoção da Saúdee Prevenção de Doenças Não Transmissíveis, Instituto Nacional de Saúde Dr. Ricardo Jorge, Lisboa 1649-040, Portugal
Centre for Biodiversity, Functional and Integrative Genomics, Faculty of Sciences, University of Lisboa, 1749-016 Lisboa, Portugal

Zbigniew żuber
Department of Pediatrics, S. Louis Regional Children's Hospital, Cracow, Poland

Agnieszka Różdżyńska-Świątkowska
Anthropology Laboratory, The Children's Memorial Health Institute, Warsaw, Poland

Agnieszka Jurecka
Department of Molecular Biology, University of Gdańsk, Gdańsk, Poland
Department of Medical Genetics, The Children's Memorial Health Institute, Warsaw, Poland

Anna Tylki-Szymańska
Department of Pediatrics, Nutrition and Metabolic Diseases, The Children's Memorial Health Institute, Warsaw, Poland

Inge Timmers
Department of Pediatrics, Maastricht University Medical Center, Maastricht, The Netherlands

Inge Timmers and Bernadette M. Jansma
Department of Cognitive Neuroscience, Maastricht University, Maastricht, The Netherlands

Bernadette M. Jansma
Maastricht Brain Imaging Center, Maastricht University, Maastricht, The Netherlands

M. Estela Rubio-Gozalbo
Laboratory of Genetic Metabolic Diseases, Maastricht University Medical Centre, Maastricht, The Netherlands

Index